**EVIDENCE-BASED
ON-CALL**

# ACUTE
# MEDICINE

*This book is dedicated to Kilgore Trout,*
*Barry & Mavis and all of Bob's little babies.*

*For Churchill Livingstone:*
*Commissioning Editor:* Michael Parkinson
*Project Development Manager:* Jim Killgore
*Project Manager:* Nancy Arnott
*Designer:* Erik Bigland, Charles Simpson

# EVIDENCE-BASED ON-CALL

# ACUTE MEDICINE

Edited by

## Christopher M. Ball MA (Cantab) BM BCh MRCP

Junior Research Fellow, Centre for Evidence-based Medicine, University of Oxford and Senior House Officer, Medical Rotation, Hammersmith Hospital, UK

## Robert S. Phillips MA (Cantab) BM BCh MRCPH

Junior Research Fellow, Centre for Evidence-based Medicine, University of Oxford and Specialist Registrar in Paediatrics, Yorkshire Deanery, UK

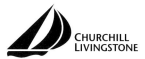

CHURCHILL
LIVINGSTONE

EDINBURGH LONDON NEW YORK PHILADELPHIA ST LOUIS SYDNEY TORONTO 2001

CHURCHILL LIVINGSTONE
An imprint of Harcourt Publishers Limited

© Oxford Medical Knowledge 2001

◢ is a registered trademark of Harcourt Publishers
Limited

First published 2001

ISBN 0443-06412-1

**British Library Cataloguing in Publication Data**
A catalogue record for this book is available from the
British Library

**Library of Congress Cataloging in Publication Data**
A catalog record for this book is available from the
Library of Congress

**Note**
Medical knowledge is constantly changing. As new
information becomes available, changes in treatment,
procedures, equipment and the use of drugs become
necessary. The editors and the publishers have taken
care to ensure that the information given in this text is
accurate and up to date. However, readers are strongly
advised to confirm that the information, especially with
regard to drug usage, complies with the latest legislation
and standards of practice.

The
publisher's
policy is to use
**paper manufactured
from sustainable forests**

Printed in Spain

# Preface

We wrote this book because we needed it — partly to find out what we *really* know about medicine, partly to improve our decision-making and patient-care, and partly to see how easy and fun it would be to put EBM into real-time practice.

This book **does not**:

- Tell you how to manage your patient. We have indicated the best management for most patients, but reckon only you (using your clinical expertise) and your patient (inputting their ideas and values) can decide what the best path to take might be.
- Give all the answers. We have given an outline on how to manage each condition, but we have not covered the nuances of management; rather we view this book as an aide-memoire, and decision support tool.
- Do pathophysiology. We have specifically looked only for outcomes that mean something to patients, in the hope that these will remain relatively constant, unlike scientific theory.
- Make arbitrary recommendations. If we cannot find any evidence, we say so; and only make a recommendation if clinical expedience demands that something be done.
- Guarantee drug doses — we have tried extremely hard to give accurate information for a typical adult patient, but encourage you to check your local formulary for more information.

It **does** give:

- Some useful facts and figures that can help you manage your patients more effectively.
- Some idea about the quality of the evidence for common clinical interventions. We have graded all our recommendations from A to D. Our grading refects *only* the weight of evidence, not the clinical importance of the recommendation*.

The ideas behind EBOC sprang from our personal struggles with understanding clinical medicine and not knowing how to find the best answers. For Chris Ball, you might call him plain distrustful. He went through medical school asking difficult questions, and got labelled as 'boorish and vitriolic'. Fortunately, Dave Sackett arrived from Canada, and showed him that evidence-based medicine offered a way of finding

---

* For example; there is Grade A evidence that EMLA cream reduces the pain of cannulation, but only Grade D evidence that intravenous fluid improves outcome in hypercalcaemia. If I were the patient – forgo the EMLA and get the saline into me.

out the answers without getting lynched. On qualifying, Chris soon realised that the biggest problem with being a clinician was that there were too many questions and too little time to find the answers. Inspired and encouraged by Dave and some other great teachers, he teamed up with smartest (and most gullible) doc he knew, Bob Phillips, and started working on ways of finding the best evidence available and getting it into clinical practice.

Bob practised 'evidence-based' medicine because he was sure there was no other way. After a year of carrying round a hundred critically appraised topics (CATs) on his Psion palmtop computer, and constantly be nagged by other clinicians for the information, *Evidence-based On-Call* was a natural progression. With a care to focus on the patient, he is sure the application of the best available evidence has saved pain, distress and possibly lives.

Evidence-based On-call is work in progress - we are sure we've missed some stuff, put emphasis on the wrong information or made some of it incomprehensible. EBOC is always on the look-out for help, comments and suggestions on how to make it better and more practical.

If you are interested in helping us create or update new material, please contact us at EBOC (info@eboc.u-net.com).

| | |
|---|---|
| Oxford | C.M.B |
| 2001 | R.S.P. |

# Acknowledgements

We give particular thanks to:

- our families for their constant love and support
- Dave Sackett for kicking us into action, and letting us run wild
- Muir Gray
- Sharon Straus, Scott Richardson, William Rosenberg and Brian Haynes
- Martin Dawes, Olive Goddard, Douglas Badenoch at the Centre for Evidence-based Medicine at the University of Oxford
- *team eboc*: Lee Bailey, Musab Hayatli, Mary Hodgkinson, Clare Wotton
- Nick Shenker
- the staff at the Cairns Library
- the Bupa Foundation, UK NHS Research and Development
- Fiona Moore and Hugh Millington; Jonathon Sheldon and the physicians at Burton Hospital for helping Chris to take an unusual career path, and letting him try out stuff on them
- Huw Edwards, John Coyle, and John Fletcher for teaching fluffy clinicians about the hard world of business
- Mike Parkinson and Jim Killgore at Churchill Livingstone for guiding this book to fruition
- Interati for creating great software.

and the many other clinicians and students who have offered advice and support as this project has developed.

# Contents

This book is designed for clinicians who want to integrate the best available evidence with their own personal skills and expertise to improve the care of their patients. It can be used by any clinician, at any stage of their training, to inform debate, assist with decisions or prop up uneven table legs.

Evidence-based medicine is the conscientious, explicit and judicious use of current best evidence in making decisions about the care of individual patients. In keeping with this, each topic covered in *Evidence-based On Call* provides not a cookbook of what to do, but a series of recommendations about issues to consider when caring for your patients.

## THE LAYOUT

Topics are arranged alphabetically, and indexed by disease area. Each topic is divided into sections based on clinical decisions: prevalence, clinical features, investigations, differential diagnosis, therapy, prevention and prognosis.

Each section is arranged in a similar way: a recommendation (with information on the level of evidence supporting it[1]), followed by a brief written summary of the evidence which supports it, and often accompanied by a table containing data derived from the original studies.

## A section layout

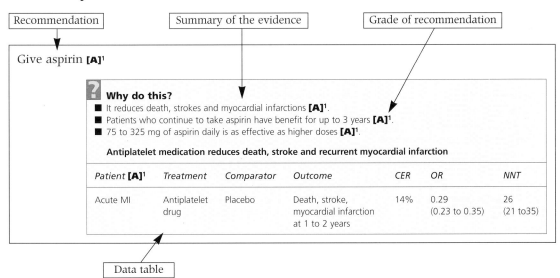

| Recommendation | Summary of the evidence | Grade of recommendation |

Give aspirin **[A]**[1]

### ? Why do this?
■ It reduces death, strokes and myocardial infarctions **[A]**[1].
■ Patients who continue to take aspirin have benefit for up to 3 years **[A]**[1].
■ 75 to 325 mg of aspirin daily is as effective as higher doses **[A]**[1].

**Antiplatelet medication reduces death, stroke and recurrent myocardial infarction**

| Patient **[A]**[1] | Treatment | Comparator | Outcome | CER | OR | NNT |
|---|---|---|---|---|---|---|
| Acute MI | Antiplatelet drug | Placebo | Death, stroke, myocardial infarction at 1 to 2 years | 14% | 0.29 (0.23 to 0.35) | 26 (21 to 35) |

Data table

[1] Our grading reflects only the weight of evidence, *not* the clinical importance of the recommendation. See **Appendix 1: Levels of Evidence** (p. 641) for further information and summary on the cover flap.

In order to get the best out of this book, the reader should be familiar with a few 'EBM' terms. There are five major concepts: number needed to treat or harm (NNT/NNH), likelihood ratios (LR+/LR–), odds ratios and relative risks (OR/RR), the number needed to follow (NNF and NNF+) and event rates. Don't worry if these are unfamiliar – a glossary is to be found at the end of the book (see **Appendix 2: Glossary**, p. 645) and more information can be gleaned from the website (www.eboncall.co.uk).

## THE PROBLEMS

There are two major deficits in this book. First, you have to trust the summary of the evidence we provide; there isn't physical space to give more supporting data! Second, it's out of date already as this was written in early 2000. To tackle the first problem, you can be reassured by the process we use to write the book, and assess the evidence we have found by looking at the critically appraised topics (CATs) – short summaries of the studies – available on the website. To address the second issue, we've put 'expiry dates' on all our material, and made up-to-date information available on the website (probably containing stuff which isn't published at the time we write).

## THE SOLUTIONS

The *Evidence-Based On Call* process takes important topics in clinical practice, turns them into a series of clinical questions, and answers them with the best evidence available. This is accomplished by the use of two independent researchers performing searches first on the 'Best Evidence' CD-ROM, then in the Cochrane Library and finally the PubMed (www.ncbi.nlm.nih.gov/entrez/query.fcgi) database. The researchers strategy looks for high quality evidence in each database in order, only progressing to the next if no quality answer to their question is found. (The search terms they have used can be found appended to the foot of each CAT.) The papers found are then appraised (using previously published criteria[2]) and summarised as CATs. Each CAT is checked by an independent researcher for accuracy, and reviewed by an experienced clinican for validity and relevance, before being made available on the website. The CATs in turn are collated by a clinician and used to produce a topic guideline, which is in turn assessed by an experienced clinician and academic expert before publication. Each article and each guide is then labelled with an expiry date.

---

[2] Sackett DS et al *Clinical epidemiology - a basic science for clinical medicine.* Philadelphia: Lippincott Williams and Wilkins; 1991 (ISBN 0-316-76599-6), the 'Users' guide to medical literature' section in JAMA running from 1992-97 available at http//:hiru.mcmaster.ca/ebm, and the policy and procedures from the journals 'Evidence-based Medicine' and 'ACP Journal Club'

The 'expiry dates' reflect the inexorable advance of clinical medicine, and the realisation that half of what we do now will be laughed at in 50 years time (but we're never sure which half...). The material in this book is slowly decaying, and it will stink in 3 years time (sooner in some cases). When the information hits its 'best before' date, the whole process of search, appraise and review rolls over again to ensure the website contains the freshest evidence we can find.

In the between time though, the literature is constantly scanned by the review editor and the team of clinicians who support the *Evidence-Based On Call* process. If an important article is found, there is no waiting for an expiry date; the process of appraisal and review moves on and the updated information is introduced.

## PREVALENCE

- A quarter of elderly patients have anaemia **[B]**[1].
- Investigations are worthwhile in all patients **[C]**[2].

 **Note**
- In anaemic patients with symptoms suggestive of GI blood loss or change in bowel habit, a cause can be found in a fifth **[A]**[3].
- This rises to two-thirds of elderly patients. Management is altered in 40% of cases **[C]**[2].

- Iron-deficiency anaemia is reasonably common in menstruating women, but rare in men until $\geq 70$ years of age **[B]**[4].

**Note**
**Iron-deficiency anaemia is common in menstruating women and the elderly**

| Age **[B]**[4] (years) | Women | Men |
| --- | --- | --- |
| 12–15 | 2% | <1% |
| 16–19 | 3% | <1% |
| 20–49 | 5% | <1% |
| 50–69 | 2% | 1% |
| ≥ 70 | 2% | 2% |

## CAUSES

Common causes of anaemia in the elderly include **[A]**[5]**[B]**[1]:

- anaemia of chronic disease
- iron-deficiency anaemia
- recent bleeding
- vitamin $B_{12}$/folate deficiency
- myelodysplastic syndrome and acute leukaemia
- chronic leukaemia, lymphoma-related disorders
- other haematological disorders (myelofibrosis, aplastic anaemia, haemolytic anaemia)
- multiple myeloma.

> **Note**
> Chronic disease, iron-deficiency and bleeding are the commonest causes of anaemia in the elderly
>
> | | Elderly inpatients [A]⁵ [B]¹ |
> |---|---|
> | Anaemia of chronic disease | 34%–44% |
> | Iron-deficiency anaemia | 15%–36% |
> | Recent bleeding | 7.3% |
> | Vitamin B$_{12}$/folate deficiency | 5.6%–8.1% |
> | Myelodysplastic syndrome and acute leukaemia | 5.6% |
> | Chronic leukaemia, lymphoma-related disorders | 5.1% |
> | Other haematological disorders (myelofibrosis, aplastic anaemia, haemolytic anaemia) | 2.8% |
> | Multiple myeloma | 1.5% |
> | No cause found | 17% |

## Iron-deficiency anaemia

Two-thirds of cases are due to upper gastrointestinal disease [B]⁶.
Common causes in the elderly include [B]⁶:

- peptic ulcer disease or erosions
- colorectal neoplasia
- gastric surgery
- hiatus hernia (> 10 cm)
- upper GI malignancy
- angiodysplasia
- oesophageal varices.

> **Note**
> Peptic ulcer disease and colorectal neoplasia are common causes of iron-deficiency anaemia in the elderly
>
> | Causes of iron-deficiency anaemia [B]⁶ | % (95% CI) |
> |---|---|
> | Upper GI disease | 60% (50% to 70%) |
> | Lower GI disease | 30% (21% to 40%) |
> | Ulcerative upper GI lesions | 36% (27% to 45%) |
> | Colorectal neoplasia | 20% (12% to 28%) |
> | Gastric surgery | 10% (4.1% to 16%) |
> | Hiatus hernia (> 10 cm) | 7.0% (2.0% to 12%) |
> | Upper GI malignancy | 6.0% (1.3% to 11%) |
> | Angiodysplasia | 5.0% (0.7% to 9.3%) |
> | Oesophageal varices | 3.0% (0.0% to 6.3%) |
> | Miscellaneous | 2.0% (0.0% to 4.7%) |
> | No cause found | 14% (7.2 %to 21%) |

## Vitamin B$_{12}$ deficiency
Common causes include [C][7]:

- pernicious anaemia
- tropical sprue
- bowel resection
- jejunal diverticula
- cobalamin malabsorption
- vegetarianism.

> **Note**
> - 12–17% of elderly people in the community have cobalamin deficiency [C][8] [C][9], but only 2% develop pernicious anaemia [B][10].
>
> **Pernicious anaemia, tropical sprue and bowel resection are the commonest causes of cobalamin deficiency**
>
> | Cause of cobalamin deficiency [C][7] | % (95% CI) |
> | --- | --- |
> | Pernicious anaemia | 76% (72% to 81%) |
> | Tropical sprue | 9.6% (6.7% to 13%) |
> | Bowel resection | 6.7% (4.2% to 9.1%) |
> | Jejunal diverticula | 1.5% (0.3% to 2.7%) |
> | Food cobalamin malabsorption | 0.7% (0.0% to 1.6%) |
> | Vegetarianism | 0.5% (0.0% to 1.2%) |
> | Unknown | 4.7% (2.6% to 6.7%) |

## Folate deficiency
Common causes include [C][7]:

- alcoholism
- malnutrition.

> **Note**
> **Alcoholism is the commonest cause of folate deficiency**
>
> | Cause of folate deficiency [C][7] | % (95% CI) |
> | --- | --- |
> | Alcoholism | 87% (80% to 93%) |
> | Malnutrition | 9.2% (4.0% to 14%) |
> | Other (including malabsorption and haemolytic anaemias) | 4.2% (0.6% to 7.8%) |

## CLINICAL FEATURES

Ask about:

- recent bleeds [A][5] [B][1]
- recent onset pallor [C][11]
- menstrual loss [B][4]
- diet and alcohol use [B][6] [C][7]
- weight loss (> 7 kg in 6 months) [C][11]

**? Why?**
**Recent pallor and weight loss make anaemia slightly more likely**

| Patient [C][11] | Target disorder (reference standard) | Diagnostic test | LR + (95% CI) | Post-test probability | LR– (95% CI) | Post-test probability |
|---|---|---|---|---|---|---|
| Suspected anaemia (pre-test probability 19%) | Anaemia (haemoglobin < 8.0 g/dl) | Recent pallor [C][11] | 2.3 (1.7 to 3.1) | 35% | 0.21 (0.11 to 0.42) | 5% |
| | | Weight loss (> 7 kg in 6 months) [C][11] | 1.5 (1.0 to 2.2) | 26% | 0.71 (0.52 to 0.99) | 14% |

- family history of anaemia [D]
- history of gastrectomy (for $B_{12}$ deficiency) [B][12] or other bowel resection [C][7]

**? Why?**
**A history of gastrectomy makes cobalamin deficiency slightly more likely**

| Patient | Target disorder (reference standard) | Diagnostic test | LR + (95% CI) | Post-test probability | LR– (95% CI) | Post-test probability |
|---|---|---|---|---|---|---|
| Undergoing cobalamin assay (pre-test probability 1.2%) | Cobalamin deficiency (Schilling test) | History of gastrectomy [B][12] | 7.4 (3.2 to 17) | 7% | 0.54 (0.33 to 0.88) | 1% |

- upper gastrointestinal symptoms (dysphagia, heartburn, nausea, vomiting) [C][13]
- lower gastrointestinal symptoms (altered bowel habit, rectal bleeding, pain relieved by defecation) [C][13].

> **? Why?**
> **Absence of upper or lower GI symptoms does not rule out disease, but makes it more likely if present**
>
> | Patient [C][13] | Target disorder (reference standard) | Diagnostic test | LR + (95% CI) | Post-test probability | LR– (95% CI) | Post-test probability |
> |---|---|---|---|---|---|---|
> | Iron deficiency anaemia (pre-test probability 60%) | Upper GI disease (gastroscopy) | Upper GI symptoms | 4.1 (1.8 to 9.6) | 86% | 0.49 (0.35 to 0.69) | 43% |
> | Iron deficiency anaemia (pre-test probability 30%) | Lower GI disease (colonoscopy) | Lower GI symptoms | 2.1 (1.1 to 4.2) | 48% | 0.73 (0.52 to 1.0) | 24% |

Do not bother asking about the following – they are of little help in diagnosing or excluding anaemia: [C][11]

- fatigue
- dizziness or palpitations
- angina
- a painful tongue
- diarrhoea or recent constipation.

Look for:

- conjunctival pallor [A][14]

> **? Why?**
> **Conjunctival pallor makes anaemia more likely, but a normal colour cannot rule it out**
>
> | Patient [A][14] | Target disorder (reference standard) | Diagnostic test | LR+ (95% CI) | Post-test probability |
> |---|---|---|---|---|
> | Inpatient (pre-test probability 18%) | Severe anaemia (haemoglobin <9 g/dl) | Pale conjunctivae | 4.5 (1.8 to 11) | 50% |
> | | | Borderline conjunctivae | 1.8 (1.2 to 2.7) | 29% |
> | | | Normal conjunctivae | 0.61 (0.45 to 0.82) | 12% |
>
> ■ Pale: little or no evidence of red colour on anterior rim which matched the fleshy part of the posterior aspect of the palpebral conjunctiva.
> ■ Borderline: neither clearly red nor clearly pale or those with one conjunctiva red and the other pale.
> ■ Normal: full or nearly full redness of the anterior rim.

- facial pallor [B][15]
- palmar pallor [B][15]
  – the more that are present, the greater the chance of anaemia [B][15].

| ? Why? | | | | | | |
|---|---|---|---|---|---|---|
| **Conjunctival pallor, facial or palmar pallor make anaemia more likely** | | | | | | |
| Patient **[B]**[15] | Target disorder (reference standard) | Diagnostic test | LR+ (95% CI) | Post-test probability | LR– (95% CI) | Post-test probability |
| Suspected anaemia (pre-test probability 19%) | Anaemia (haematocrit <0.41 men or <0.31 women) | Conjunctival pallor | 3.1 (1.4 to 6.8) | 42% | 0.65 (0.50 to 0.84) | 13% |
| | | Facial pallor | 3.6 (1.3 to 9.8) | 46% | 0.72 (0.59 to 0.89) | 14% |
| | | Palmar pallor | 2.2 (1.2 to 4.0) | 34% | 0.62 (0.46 to 0.85) | 13% |
| | | Any present | 2.3 (1.4 to 3.8) | 35% | 0.48 (0.32 to 0.72) | 10% |
| | | Two present | 3.0 (1.4 to 6.6) | 41% | 0.67 (0.52 to 0.86) | 14% |
| | | All present | 5.5 (1.3 to 23) | 56% | 0.77 (0.66 to 0.91) | 15% |

- dyspnoea **[C]**[11]

| ? Why? | | | | | | |
|---|---|---|---|---|---|---|
| **Dyspnoea makes anaemia slightly more likely** | | | | | | |
| Patient **[C]**[11] | Target disorder (reference standard) | Diagnostic test | LR+ (95% CI) | Post-test probability | LR– (95% CI) | Post-test probability |
| Suspected anaemia (pre-test probability 19%) | Anaemia (haemoglobin <8.0 g/dl) | Dyspnoea | 1.4 (1.0 to 1.8) | 25% | 0.67 (0.44 to 1.0) | 14% |

- evidence of acute bleeding **[B]**[16]
    - supine tachycardia (pulse > 100 beats/min)
    - supine hypotension (systolic blood pressure < 95 mmHg)
    - postural pulse increase of ≥ 30 beats/min or severe dizziness on sitting upright, then on standing

**Why?**
**Severe dizziness and a pulse increase > 30 beats/min on standing make a significant acute bleed more likely**

| Patient [B][16] | Target disorder (reference standard) | Diagnostic test | LR+ | Post-test probability | LR− | Post-test probability |
|---|---|---|---|---|---|---|
| Suspected acute blood loss (pre-test probability 7.3%) | Acute severe blood loss (venesection of 630–1150 ml) | Postural pulse increase > 30 beats/min, or severe postural dizziness on sitting from supine | 39 | 75% | 0.22 | 1.7% |
| | Acute severe blood loss (venesection of 630–1150 ml) | Postural pulse increase > 30 beats/min, or severe postural, dizziness on standing from supine | 49 | 79% | 0.030 | 0.24% |
| | Acute moderate blood loss (venesection of 350–600 ml) | Postural pulse increase > 30 beats/min, or severe postural dizziness on standing from supine | 44 | 78% | 0.80 | 5.9% |
| | Acute severe blood loss (venesection of 630–1150 ml) | Supine tachycardia | 4.0 | 24% | 0.92 | 6.8% |
| | Acute severe blood loss (venesection of 630–1150 ml) | Supine hypotension | 11 | 46% | 0.68 | 5.1% |
| | Acute moderate blood loss (vensection of 350–600 ml) | Supine hypotension | 4.3 | 24% | 0.90 | 6.8% |

**Note**
- Postural hypotension (fall in systolic > 20 mmHg on standing) does not usefully diagnose acute blood loss [B][16].
- Absence of supine tachycardia does not exclude moderate acute blood loss [B][16].

- koilonychia [C][11]

**Why?**
**Koilonychia makes anaemia more likely**

| Patient [C][11] | Target disorder (reference standard) | Diagnostic test | LR+ (95% CI) | Post-test probability | LR− (95% CI) | Post-test probability |
|---|---|---|---|---|---|---|
| Iron-deficiency anaemia (pre-test probability 47%) | Anaemia (haemoglobin <8.0 g/dl) | Koilonychia | 5.6 (0.67 to 46) | 83% | 0.93 (0.86 to 1.0) | 46% |

- evidence of heart failure **[D]**
- jaundice (suggesting haemolytic or megaloblastic anaemia) **[D]**
- evidence of infection or spontaneous bruising (suggesting marrow failure) **[D]**
- abdominal or rectal masses **[D]**.

Do not bother looking for the following – they are of little help at diagnosing or excluding anaemia:
- nailbed pallor **[B]**[15]
- palmar crease pallor **[B]**[15].

> **Note**
> ■ No clinician agreed with another when identifying palmar crease pallor **[B]**[15].

Perform a rectal examination **[D]** and a faecal occult blood test **[A]**[3].

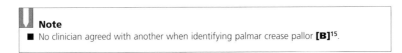

**Why?**
A positive fecal occult blood test makes a GI bleed more likely

| Patient **[A]**[3] | Target disorder (reference standard) | Diagnostic test | LR+ (95% CI) | Post-test probability | LR– (95% CI) | Post-test probability |
|---|---|---|---|---|---|---|
| Iron-deficiency anaemia (pre-test probability 19%) | Probable GI bleed (gastroscopy, colonoscopy) | Guaiac occult blood test | 2.6 (1.8 to 3.6) | 37% | 0.39 (0.22 to 0.69) | 8% |

## INVESTIGATIONS

- Blood count:
  - haemoglobin **[A]**
  - mean cell volume **[A]**[17]
  - red cell distribution width.
- Blood film.

**Why?**

**A low MCV makes iron-deficiency more likely**

| Patient [A][17] | Target disorder (reference standard) | Diagnostic test | LR+ (95% CI) | Post-test probability |
|---|---|---|---|---|
| Anaemia (pre-test probability 36%) | Iron-deficiency anaemia (bone marrow aspiration) | MCV ≤70 fl | 12 (6.1 to 19) | 87% |
| | | 70–75 fl | 3.3 (2.0 to 4.7) | 65% |
| | | 75–80 fl | 1.0 (0.69 to 1.3) | 36% |
| | | 80–85 fl | 0.91 (0.71 to 1.1) | 34% |
| | | 85–90 fl | 0.76 (0.56 to 0.96) | 30% |
| | | ≥90 fl | 0.29 (0.21 to 0.37) | 14% |

■ Patients with significant cobalamin deficiency may have neither significant anaemia nor macrocytosis [C][18].

**Macrocytosis and hypersegmented neutrophils make cobalamin deficiency more likely**

| Patient [C][18] | Target disorder (reference standard) | Diagnostic test | LR+ (95% CI) | Post-test probability | LR− (95% CI) | Post-test probability |
|---|---|---|---|---|---|---|
| Low serum cobalamin (pre-test probability 58%) | Cobalamin deficiency (response to cobalamin) | Macrocytosis (MCV > 100 fl) | 5.4 (2.6 to 11) | 89% | 0.41 (0.30 to 0.55) | 37% |
| | | Normal white cell count | 13 (4.9 to 33) | 95% | 0.15 (0.088 to 0.25) | 18% |
| | | Abnormal blood smear (macrocytosis and hypersegmented neutrophils) | 25 (3.6 to 180) | 98% | 0.34 (0.24 to 0.49) | 36% |

Combining the MCV and RDW results can help define potential causes of the anaemia (Box 1) [B][19].

| Box 1 MCV and RDW in defining potential causes of anaemia | | |
|---|---|---|
| MCV | RDW | Potential causes [B][18] |
| Low | Normal | Chronic disease |
| | | Heterogenous thalassaemia |
| Low | High | Iron deficiency |
| | | RBC fragmentation (artificial valve) |
| | | HbH |
| | | S beta-thalassaemia |
| Normal | Normal | Any chronic disease (including chronic liver disease) |
| | | Haemorrhage |
| | | Haemolysis |
| | | Transfusion |
| | | Hb AS, Hb AC |
| | | Chronic lymphocytic leukaemia with <150 × 10³ WBC |
| | | Hereditary spherocytosis |
| Normal | High | Early iron or folate (or both) deficiency |
| | | Hb SS, Hb SC |
| | | Myelofibrosis |
| | | Sideroblastic anaemia |
| High | Normal | Aplastic anaemia |
| | | Preleukaemia |
| High | High | Folate or B$_{12}$ deficiency |
| | | Immune haemolytic anaemia |
| | | Cold agglutinins with >150 × 10³ WBC |

- Urea and electrolytes [D].
- Liver function tests [D].
- Group and save serum [D].

Take the following tests before giving a blood transfusion [A].

### Microcytic anaemia
- Ferritin [A][17]

| ? Why? | | | | |
|---|---|---|---|---|
| A low ferritin makes iron-deficiency anaemia more likely, but a normal level cannot exclude it | | | | |
| Patient [A][17] | Target disorder (reference standard) | Diagnostic test | LR+ (95% CI) | Post-test probability |
| Anaemia (pre-test probability 36%) | Iron-deficiency anaemia (bone marrow aspiration) | Serum ferritin ≤ 15 µg/l | 52 (42 to 62) | 97% |
| | | 15–25 µg/l | 8.8 (7.2 to 10) | 83% |
| | | 25–35 µg/l | 2.5 (2.1 to 3.0) | 58% |
| | | 35–45 µg/l | 1.8 (1.5 to 2.2) | 50% |
| | | 45–100 µg/l | 0.54 (0.48 to 0.60) | 23% |
| | | ≥ 100 µg/l | 0.08 (0.07 to 0.09) | 4% |

**Ferritin remains useful in patients with liver cirrhosis**

| Patient [A][20] | Target disorder (reference standard) | Diagnostic test | LR+ (95% CI) | Post-test probability | LR– (95% CI) | Post-test probability |
|---|---|---|---|---|---|---|
| Liver cirrhosis and anaemia (pre-test probability 19%) | Iron-deficiency anaemia (bone marrow aspiration) | Serum ferritin < 200 µg/L | 4.3 (2.3 to 8.2) | 74% | 0.22 (0.10 to 0.49) | 13% |

**Note**
- Other investigations such as red cell protoporphyrin and transferrin saturation are less helpful at diagnosing iron-deficiency anaemia [A][5].

## Macrocytic anaemia
- Serum folate [D].
- Serum $B_{12}$ (cobalamin) [B][12].
- Urine methylmalonic acid (MMA) [B][12] or serum MMA [B][21].

**Why?**

**A normal serum cobalamin makes cobalamin deficiency unlikely**

| Patient [B][12] | Target disorder (reference standard) | Diagnostic test | LR + (95% CI) | Post-test probability | LR– (95% CI) | Post-test probability |
|---|---|---|---|---|---|---|
| Anaemia, macrocytosis, dementia or neuropathy (pre-test probability 1.2%) | Cobalamin deficiency (Schilling test) | Serum $B_{12}$ (cobalamin) < 133 pmol/l | 2.2 (1.8 to 2.6) | 2% | 0.00 (0.0 to 0.33) | 0% |

**A raised urinary or serum MMA makes cobalamin deficiency likely**

| Patient | Target disorder (reference standard) | Diagnostic test | LR + (95% CI) | Post-test probability | LR– (95% CI) | Post-test probability |
|---|---|---|---|---|---|---|
| Anaemia, macrocytosis, dementia or neuropathy (pre-test probability 1.2%) | Cobalamin deficiency (Schilling test) | Urinary MMA > 5 µg/mg creatinine [B][12] | 47 (12 to 190) | 32% | 0.19 (0.070 to 0.53) | 0.2% |
| Suspected cobalamin deficiency (pre-test probability 74%) | Cobalamin deficiency (Schilling test, bone marrow) | Serum MMA >0.34 µmol/l [B][21] | 11 (1.6 to 69) | 97% | 0.036 (0.0051 to 0.25) | 9% |

## Further investigations

### Iron-deficiency anaemia
- Gastroscopy and colonoscopy or barium enema/sigmoidoscopy [C][6].

**Why?**
- Failure to investigate upper and lower bowel misses important lesions: 16% of elderly patients with benign upper GI lesions had colonic carcinoma or adenomas in one series.
- Colonoscopy is a better test than sigmoidoscopy followed by barium enema in patients with suspected large bowel disease — there are more complete examinations and few additional investigations but no clear difference in the number of diagnoses made nor patient satisfaction. [A][6].

**Colonoscopy leads to a more complete examination and few further investigations**

| Patient [A][6] | Treatment | Comparator | Outcome | CER | RRR | NNT |
|---|---|---|---|---|---|---|
| Suspected large bowel disease | Colonoscopy | Sigmoidoscopy and barium enema | Complete examination | 36% | 87% (36% to 100%) | 3 (2 to 6) |
| | | | Further investigation required | 27% | 72% (35% to 88%) | 5 (3 to 12) |

### Cobalamin deficiency
- Intrinsic factor antibodies [C][18] [C][22].
- Schilling test [C][18].

**Why?**
**Intrinsic factor antibodies and an abnormal Schilling test make cobalamin deficiency more likely**

| Patient [C][18] | Target disorder (reference standard) | Diagnostic test | LR+ (95% CI) | Post-test probability (%) | LR– (95% CI) | Post-test probability (%) |
|---|---|---|---|---|---|---|
| Low serum cobalamin (pre-test probability 58%) | Cobalamin deficiency (response to cobalamin) | Anti-intrinsic factor antibodies | 2.6 (1.5 to 4.7) | 79 | 0.63 (0.49 to 0.80) | 48 |
| | | Abnormal Schilling test | 2.5 (1.6 to 3.8) | 70 | 0.21 (0.089 to 0.48) | 16 |

### Folate deficiency
- Dietary assessment [D].

## THERAPY

- Treat acute GI bleeding.
- Treat congestive heart failure.
- In general, chronic anaemias do not require transfusion, unless the patient is symptomatic (when it should be given slowly) [D].

> **Note**
> ■ There is little good evidence to indicate best blood transfusion practice **[B]**[23].

## Iron-deficiency anaemia

● Give iron supplements **[B]**[24] **[B]**[2], e.g. oral ferrous sulphate 200 mg three times a day **[D]**. Side-effects are common.

>  **Why do this?**
> ■ Iron supplementation increases haemoglobin levels (on average 70 g/l within 70 days) and improves exercise capacity **[B]**[24] **[B]**[25].
> ■ Watch for constipation **[B]**[24].
>
> | Patient **[B]**[25] | Treatment | Comparator | Outcome | CER | RRR | NNT |
> |---|---|---|---|---|---|---|
> | Iron-deficiency anaemia | Ferrous succinate | Placebo | Constipation | 14% | −150% (−470% to −4%) | −5 (−39 to −3) |

## Macrocytic anaemia

● Give hydroxycobalamin **[A]** 1 mg im on alternate days for 6 days **[D]**. Cobalamin can be given orally **[C]**[26] but in very high doses and with variable success **[D]**.

> **Why do this?**
> ■ Patients with pernicious anaemia or malabsorption can be successfully treated with very high dose oral cobalamin **[C]**[26].

● Give folate 5 mg orally once a day **[A]**.

Continue both until the results of vitamin assays are available, then treat as required **[D]**.

## Other haematological disorders

● Discuss with a haematologist **[D]**.

**Guideline writers**: Michael Bennett, Robert Phillips
**CAT writers**: Christopher Ball, Michael Bennett

## REFERENCES

| No | Level | Citation |
|---|---|---|
| 1 | 2c | Joosten E et al. Prevalence and causes of anaemia in a geriatric hospitalised population. Gerontology 1992; 38: 111–17 |
| 2 | 4 | Ward MC, Gundroo D, Bailey RJ et al. Effect of investigation on the management of elderly patients with iron deficiency anaemia. Age and Ageing 1990; 19: 204–6 |
| 3 | 1b | Moran A et al. Diagnostic value of a guaiac occult blood test and faecal alpha 1-antitrypsin. Gut 1995; 36: 87–9 |
| 4 | 2c | Looker AC et al. Prevalence of iron deficiency in the United States. JAMA 1997; 277: 973–6 |

| No | Level | Citation |
|----|-------|----------|
| 5 | 1b | Guyatt GH et al. Diagnosis of iron-deficiency anaemia in the elderly. Am J Med 1990; 88: 205–9 |
| 6 | 2c | Cook IJ, Pavli P, Riley JW et al. Gastrointestinal investigation of iron-deficiency anaemia. BMJ 1986; 292: 1380–2 |
| 7 | 4 | Savage DG et al. Sensitivity of serum methylmalonic acid and total homocysteine determinations for diagnosing cobalamin and folate deficiencies. Am J Med 1994; 96: 239–46 |
| 8 | 4 | Pennypacker LC et al. High prevalence of cobalamin deficiency in elderly patients. J Am Geriatr Soc 1992; 40: 1197–204 |
| 9 | 4 | Lindenbaum J et al. Prevalence of cobalamin deficiency in the Framingham elderly population. Am J Clin Nutr 1994; 60: 2–11 |
| 10 | 2b | Carmel R. Prevalence of undiagnosed pernicious anaemia in the elderly. Arch Intern Med 1996; 156: 1097–100 |
| 11 | 4 | Dawson AA et al. Evaluation of diagnostic significance of certain symptoms and physical signs in anaemic patients. BMJ 1969 3: 436–9 |
| 12 | 2b | Matchar DB et al. Performance of the serum cobalamin assay for diagnosis of cobalamin deficiency. Am J Med Sci 1994; 308: 276–83 |
| 13 | 4 | Cook IJ, Pavli P, Riley JW, et al. Gastrointestinal investigation of iron-deficiency anaemia. British Medical Journal 1986; 292: 1380–1382 |
| 14 | 1b | Sheth TN et al. The relation of conjunctival pallor to the presence of anaemia. J Gen Intern Med 1997; 12: 102–6 |
| 15 | 2b | Nardone DA et al. Usefulness of physical examination in detecting the presence or absence of anaemia. Arch Intern Med 1990; 150: 201–4 |
| 16 | 4 | McGee S et al. Is this patient hypovolemic? JAMA 1999; 281: 1022–9 |
| 17 | 1a | Guyatt GH et al. Laboratory diagnosis of iron-deficiency anaemia: an overview. J Gen Intern Med 1992; 7: 145–53 |
| 18 | 4 | Stabler SP et al. Clinical spectrum and diagnosis of cobalamin deficiency. Blood 1990; 76: 871–81 |
| 19 | 2b | Bessman JD et al. Improved classification of anaemias by MCV and RDW. Am J Clin Pathol 1983; 80: 322–6 |
| 20 | 1b | Intragumtornchai T et al. The role of serum ferritin in the diagnosis of iron deficiency anaemia in patients with liver cirrhosis. J Intern Med 1998; 243: 233–41 |
| 21 | 2b | Moelby L et al. The relationship between clinically confirmed cobalamin deficiency and serum methylmalonic acid. J Intern Med 1990; 228: 373–8 |
| 22 | 4 | Rothenberg SP et al. Autoantibodies to intrinsic factor: their definition and clinical usefulness. J Lab Clin Med 1971; 77: 476–84 |
| 23 | 2a | Hebert PC et al. Review of the clinical practice literature on allogeneic red blood cell transfusion. Can Med Assoc J 1997; 156: 11 (suppl): S9–S25 |
| 24 | 2b | Rybo E et al. Effect of iron supplementation to women with iron deficiency. Scand J Haematol 1986; 35: 103–13 |
| 25 | 2b | Gardner GW et al. Cardiorespiratory, hematological and physical performance responses of anemic subjects to iron treatment. Am J Clin Nutr 1975; 28: 982–8 |
| 26 | 4 | Berlin H et al. Oral treatment of pernicious anaemia with high dose vitamin $B_{12}$ without intrinsic factor. Acta Med Scand 1968; 184: 247–58 |

## PREVALENCE

Severe anaphylaxis is rare (~0.02% of hospital admissions) **[C]**.
Anaphylaxis may be fatal in ~1% of cases **[C]**.
Anaphylaxis is more common in certain situations **[C]**:

- general anaesthetic
- contrast radiology.

---

**Note**
- Severe anaphylaxis occurred in 0.018% of a cohort of patients from Europe and India **[C]**[1], and 0.016% of patients attending a UK emergency department **[C]**[2].
- Fatalities are rare: 0.3% (95% CI:0.0 to 0.7%) **[C]**[3] in outpatient attendees, to 7.4% (95% CI:0.0 to 17%) **[C]**[4] 'ambulance' service.
- Reactions occurred in 0.17% of contrast radiology examinations **[C]**[5]; 5% of anaphylaxis was secondary to muscle relaxants **[C]**[3].

---

Causes of anaphylaxis include **[C]**:

- foods (nuts)
- stings or bites
- drugs.

---

**Note**
**Food and insects are common causes of anaphylaxis**

| Causes **[C]**[3] **[C]**[4] | Proportion (Ranges or 95% CI) |
|---|---|
| Wasp or bee sting, or snake bite | 16.5% to 52% |
| Drugs or vaccines | 9% to 30% |
| Nuts | 7.4% to 39% |
| Unclear cause | 19% (13% to 25%) |
| Other food | 15% (9.3% to 20%) |
| Latex | 3.5% (0.7% to 6.2%) |

---

**Note**
**Certain drugs have a higher risk of anaphylaxis**

| Risk factor for possible or probable anaphylaxis **[C]**[6] | Adjusted OR (95% CI) | NNH (95% CI) |
|---|---|---|
| Glafenine | 53.8 (25.5 to 113) | 87 (42 to 190) |
| Amoxicillin | 12.3 (5.94 to 25.3) | 410 (190 to 920) |
| Diclofenac | 8.21 (3.73 to 18.1) | 630 (270 to 1700) |
| Penicillins | 7.28 (3.78 to 14.0) | 730 (350 to 1600) |
| NSAIDs | 4.19 (2.06 to 8.51) | 1400 (600 to 4300) |
| Analgesics | 3.78 (1.91 to 7.46) | 1600 (700 to 5000) |

## CLINICAL FEATURES

Symptoms of anaphylaxis are variable.
Common symptoms include [C]:

- respiratory symptoms (wheeze, breathlessness)
- cardiovascular symptoms (hypotension, arrhythmia)
- swelling or angio-oedema
- pruritus
- gut symptoms (diarrhoea, vomiting).

**Note**
Angio-oedema is common in patients with anaphylaxis [C][3]

| Symptom | Proportion (95% CI) |
|---|---|
| Angio-oedema | 87% (82% to 92%) |
| Bronchospasm | 58% (50% to 65%) |
| Hypotension | 52% (44% to 59%) |
| Pruritus | 47% (39% to 54%) |
| Vomiting | 31% (25% to 38%) |
| Conjunctivitis | 19% (13% to 24%) |
| Diarrhoea | 5.8% (2.3% to 9.3%) |

A biphasic response – symptoms 12–24 hours later – may occur [C].

**Note**
6.4% (95% CI:1.4 to 11%) of patients suffer a biphasic response [C][7].

Past history of asthma is common, and may increase risk of contrast radiography anaphylaxis [C].

**Why?**
Asthma or beta-blocker use increases the risk of anaphylaxis

| Patient | Prognostic factor | Outcome | Control rate | OR (95% CI) | NNF (95% CI) |
|---|---|---|---|---|---|
| Immunology clinic for anaphylaxis [C][3] | History of atopy/asthma | Anaphylaxis | 59% (52% to 67%) | | |
| Anaphylactoid reaction to contrast media [C][5] | Beta-blocker use or asthma | Anaphylactoid reaction | 0.16% (0.12% to 0.21%) | 3.43 (1.5 to 8.2) | 250 (84 to 1300) |

## DIFFERENTIAL DIAGNOSIS

Think about other causes of collapse.

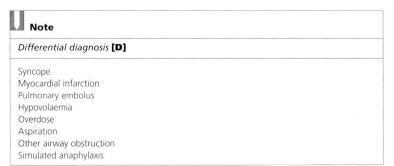

**Note**

*Differential diagnosis* **[D]**

Syncope
Myocardial infarction
Pulmonary embolus
Hypovolaemia
Overdose
Aspiration
Other airway obstruction
Simulated anaphylaxis

Many patients will have had previous episodes **[C]**.

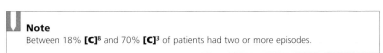

**Note**

Between 18% **[C]**[8] and 70% **[C]**[3] of patients had two or more episodes.

## INVESTIGATIONS

Don't delay treatment to investigate.
Investigations are to confirm diagnosis and identify stimuli **[C]**.

- Mast cell tryptase (within 6 h of episode) may be high.

Further investigations may be carried out in specialist outpatient
departments **[C]**.

- Skin prick testing may confirm episodes.
- IgE levels are often abnormal.
- Intradermal testing may be useful in drug-induced episodes.

**Why?**
Mast cell tryptase can rule out anaphylaxis; intradermal testing can rule it in

| Patient | Target disorder (reference standard) | Diagnostic test | LR+ (95% CI) | Post-test probability | LR− (95% CI) | Post-test probability |
|---|---|---|---|---|---|---|
| Suspected anaphylaxis (pre-test probability 64%) **[D]**[9] | Sole agent, positive passive transfer or subsequent anaesthesia | Intradermal testing | 22 (3.2 to 150) | 98% | 0.24 (0.17 to 0.35) | 30% |
| Suspected anaphylaxis (pre-test probability 39%) **[D]**[10] | Problematic subsequent general anaesthesia | Skin-prick or intradermal testing | 1.2 (1.1 to 1.4) | 44% | 0.18 (0.04 to 0.76) | 11% |
| Suspected anaphylaxis (pre-test probability 44%)**[D]** | Radioimmunoassay or intradermal testing | Mast cell tryptase >3 mg/l | 4.9 (3.6 to 6.6) | 79% | 0.066 (0.032 to 0.14) | 5% |

**Note**
**Outpatients usually have positive skin prick tests**

| Patient | Outcome | Proportion (95% CI) |
|---|---|---|
| Outpatients with anaphylaxis | Abnormal skin test or allergen-specific IgE | 69% (62% to 76%) |

## THERAPY

Assess airway, breathing and circulation.
Give im adrenaline (sc if necessary) **[A]**.

**Why?**
96% (95% CI:93 to 100%) of patients with circulatory collapse responded to adrenaline **[A]**[11].
Intravenous adrenaline has been associated with arrhythmias **[D]**.

**Note**
**Subcutaneous adrenaline is probably less reliable than intramuscular adrenaline**

| Patients | Outcome | Treatment | Control group (SD) | Experimental group (SD) | Mean difference (95% CI) |
|---|---|---|---|---|---|
| Children with history of anaphylaxis **[D]**[12] | Minutes to peak adrenaline levels | im (experimental) vs sc (control) adrenaline | 34 (40) | 8 (6) | 26 (−3 to 55) |

Strongly consider [D]:

- steroids
- antihistamines.

Strongly consider intravenous fluid [D].
Monitor cardiac and respiratory function [C].

| Why? | |
| --- | --- |
| Outcome [A]¹¹[D]³[D]⁴ | Proportion (95% CI) |
| Cardiovascular collapse | 52% to 90% |
| Respiratory symptoms | 58% to 67% |

Scrape or pinch off bee stings – don't leave them in [D].

**Why?**
Scraping or pinching off bee stings is equally good at reducing wheal and both are better than leaving them in

| Patients | Outcome | Treatment | Control group (SD) | Experimental group (SD) | Mean difference (95% CI) |
| --- | --- | --- | --- | --- | --- |
| Adults voluntarily bee stung [D]¹³ | Wheal size (mm³) | Scrape (control) vs pinch (experimental) | 80 (26) | 74 (23) | 6 (–10 to 22) |

## PREVENTION

Educate and avoid known precipitants [D].
Carry medical alert bracelet/card/letter [D].
Carry autoinjectors of adrenaline after severe cases [D].
Use prophylactic treatments prior to contrast radiography [A].

**Why?**
**Pre-treatment with hydroxazine reduces adverse effects**

| Patients | Outcome | Treatment | CER(%) | RRR(%) (95% CI) | NNT (95% CI) |
| --- | --- | --- | --- | --- | --- |
| Adults without history of anaphylaxis undergoing contrast radiography [A]¹⁴ | Adverse reaction | Hydroxyzine 100 mg orally prior to examination | 15.5 | 92 (67 to 98) | 9 (6 to 15) |

In cases of severe idiopathic anaphylaxis, preventative combination therapy may be useful [C].

**Why?**
**Few patients relapsed on prophylactic prednisolone**

| Patients | Outcome | Treatment | % (95% CI) |
|---|---|---|---|
| Adults with idiopathic anaphylaxis **[C]**[7] | Readmission to hospital | Prednisolone (if 'frequent' attacks) 60–100 mg/day | 4.9% (0% to 10%) |
| Adults with idiopathic anaphylaxis **[C]**[15] | Readmission to hospital | Prednisolone (if 'frequent' attacks) | 1.6% (0% to 3.9%) |

## PROGNOSIS

Appropriate treatment leads to survival in the vast majority of patients **[C]**.

**Note**
Fatalities are rare: 0.3% (95% CI: 0.0 to 0.7%) **[C]**[3] in outpatient attendees to 7.4% (95% CI: 0.0 to 17%) **[C]**[4] patients requiring an 'ambulance' service.

**Guideline writers**: Michael Bennett, Robert Phillips
**CAT writers**: Chris Ball, Michael Bennett

## REFERENCE

| No | Level | Citation |
|---|---|---|
| 1 | 4 | The International Collaborative Study of Severe Anaphylaxis. An epidemiologic study of severe anaphylactic and anaphylactoid reactions among hospital patients: methods and overall risks. Epidemiology 1998; 9: 141–6 |
| 2 | 4 | Stewart AG, Ewan PW. The incidence, aetiology and management of anaphylaxis presenting to an accident and emergency department. Q J Med 1996; 89: 859–64 |
| 3 | 4 | Pumphrey RS, Stanworth SJ. The clinical spectrum of anaphylaxis in north-west England. Clin Exp Allergy 1996; 26: 1364–70 |
| 4 | 4 | Soreide E, Buxrud T, Harboe S. Severe anaphylactic reactions outside hospital: etiology, symptoms and treatment. Acta Anaesthesiol Scand 1988; 32: 339–42 |
| 5 | 3b | Beta-blockers and asthma increased the risk for anaphylaxis during contrast media studies. ACP J Club 1991; 115: 92. Summary of: Lang DM et al. Increased risk for anaphylactoid reactions from contrast media in patients on beta-adrenergic blockers or with asthma. Ann Intern Med 1991; 115: 270–6 |
| 6 | 4 | van der Klauw MM, Stricker BH, Herings RM et al. A population based case-cohort study of drug-induced anaphylaxis. Br J Clin Pharmacol 1993; 35: 400–8 |
| 7 | 4 | Douglas DM, Sukenick E, Andrade WP et al. Biphasic systemic anaphylaxis: an inpatient and outpatient study. J Allergy Clin Immunol 1994; 93: 977–85 |

| No | Level | Citation |
|----|-------|----------|
| 8 | 4 | Yocum MW, Khan DA. Assessment of patients who have experienced anaphylaxis: a 3-year survey. Mayo Clin Proc 1994; 69: 16–23 |
| 9 | 4 | Fisher MM et al. The diagnosis of acute anaphylactoid reactions to anaesthetic drugs. Anaesth Intensive Care 1981; 9: 235–41 |
| 10 | 4 | Fisher MM, Bowey CJ. Intradermal compared with prick testing in the diagnosis of anaesthetic allergy. Br J Anaesth 1997; 79: 59–63 |
| 11 | 1c | Fisher MM et al. Clinical observations on the pathophysiology and treatment of anaphylactic cardiovascular collapse. Anaesth Intensive Care 1986; 14: 17–21 |
| 12 | 5 | Simons FE, Roberts JR, Gu X et al. Epinephrine absorption in children with a history of anaphylaxis. J Allergy Clin Immunol 1998; 101: 33–7 |
| 13 | 5 | Visscher PK, Vetter RS, Camazine S. Removing bee stings. Lancet 1996; 348: 301–2 |
| 14 | 1b | Bertrand PR, Soyer PM, Rouleau PJ et al. Comparative randomized double-blind study of hydroxyzine versus placebo as premedication before injection of iodinated contrast media. Radiology 1992; 184: 383–4 |
| 15 | 4 | Wiggins CA, Dykewicz MS, Patterson R. Idiopathic anaphylaxis: classification, evaluation and treatment of 123 patients. J Allergy Clin Immunol 1988; 82: 849–55 |

## PREVALENCE

Unstable angina is a common cause of chest pain [A][1].

**Note**

■ One in four patients with chest pain have unstable angina (24%; 95% CI: 21% to 27%) [A][2]; the risk is higher in elderly patients (44%: 95% CI: 42% to 45%) [A][1].

It is defined as [D] any of:
- angina for < 1 month with increasing severity, frequency or duration
- a sudden worsening of previously stable angina without change in medical therapy
- prolonged pain >10 min or recurrent angina at rest

with evidence of ischaemic heart disease, any of:
- previous myocardial infarction (MI) or angina
- transient ECG changes (ST depression or T wave inversion ≥ two leads, ST elevation, hyperacute T waves or both)
- positive exercise test or angiography.

## CLINICAL FEATURES

Ask about:
- the pain, specifically:
  - its position [B][3]

**Why?**

■ Retrosternal chest pain makes angina more likely [B][3].

  - its nature [A][2]

**Why?**

Pressure makes coronary artery disease more likely, but sharp or stabbing pain makes it less likely

| Patient [A][2] | Target disorder (reference standard) | Diagnostic test | LR + (95% CI) | Post-test probability | LR – (95% CI) | Post-test probability |
|---|---|---|---|---|---|---|
| Central or left-sided chest pain (pre-test probability 41%) | MI or unstable angina (ECG, cardiac enzymes, stress tests) | Pressure | 1.7 (1.4 to 2.0) | 54% | 0.67 (0.57 to 0.78) | 32% |
| | | Sharp or stabbing pain | 0.41 (0.29 to **0.63)** | 22% | 1.3 (1.2 to 1.5) | 48% |

**Why?**

**A pleuritic chest pain makes unstable angina or an MI unlikely**

| Patient [A][2] | Target disorder (reference standard) | Diagnostic test | LR+ (95% CI) | Post-test probability |
|---|---|---|---|---|
| Central or left-sided chest pain (pre-test probability 41%) | MI or unstable angina (ECG, cardiac enzymes, stress tests) | Pleuritic pain | 0.0 (0.0 to 0.12) | 0% |
| | | Partly pleuritic pain | 0.22 (0.13 to 0.39) | 14% |
| | | Pain not pleuritic | 1.4 (1.3 to 1.6) | 50% |

**Positional chest pain makes unstable angina or an MI less likely**

| Patient [A][2] | Target disorder (reference standard) | Diagnostic test | LR+ (95% CI) | Post-test probability |
|---|---|---|---|---|
| Central or left-sided chest pain (pre-test probability 41%) | MI or unstable angina (ECG, cardiac enzymes, stress tests) | Positional pain | 0.13 (0.030 to 0.54) | 8% |
| | | Pain partly positional | 0.31 (0.20 to 0.48) | 18% |
| | | Pain not positional | 1.4 (1.3 to 1.5) | 49% |

**Note**
- Aching or burning pain is not helpful at diagnosing or excluding MI or unstable angina [A][2].

- any exacerbating or relieving factors [B][3].

 **Why?**
- Pain brought on by exertion, or relieved by nitrates or rest make significant coronary artery disease more likely [B][3].

- a history of angina or MI [A][4] [B][5] [B][6].

 **Why?**

**Previous unstable angina or an MI makes a further episode more likely**

| Patient [A][2] | Target disorder (reference standard) | Diagnostic test | LR + (95% CI) | Post-test probability | LR – (95% CI) | Post-test probability |
|---|---|---|---|---|---|---|
| Central or left-sided chest pain (pre-test probability 41%) | MI or unstable angina (ECG, cardiac enzymes, stress tests) | Previous history of MI or angina | 2.3 (1.9 to 2.7) | 62% | 0.37 (0.30 to 0.47) | 21% |

Look for:

- chest pain that is reproduced on palpation **[A]**[2] **[B]**[4] **[B]**[5] **[B]**[6] .

| ? **Why?** Pain reproduced on palpation makes unstable angina or an MI less likely | | | | |
|---|---|---|---|---|
| Patient **[A]**[2] | Target disorder (reference standard) | Diagnostic test | LR + (95% CI) | Post-test probability |
| Central or left-sided chest pain (pre-test probability 41%) | MI or unstable angina (ECG, cardiac enzymes, stress tests) | Pain reproduced by chest-wall palpation | 0.11 (0.057 to 0.21) | 7% |
| | | Pain partially reproduced by chest wall palpation | 0.43 (0.20 to 0.94) | 24% |
| | | Pain not reproduced by chest wall palpation | 1.6 (1.4 to 1.7) | 53% |

Estimate your patient's risk of significant coronary artery disease
($\geq 50\%$ coronary artery stenosis in at least one major artery) using age
**[A]**[2] and the following symptoms (Tables 1 and 2) **[B]**[3]:

- retrosternal chest pain
- pain brought on by exertion
- pain relieved in < 10 min by rest or nitroglycerin

**Table 1   Men: probability (%) of $\geq 50\%$ coronary artery stenosis in at least one major artery**

| Symptoms | Age (years) **[B]**[3] | | | |
|---|---|---|---|---|
| | 30–39 | 40–49 | 50–59 | 60–69 |
| Asymptomatic (0 symptoms) | 2% | 6% | 10% | 12% |
| Non-anginal chest pain (1 symptom) | 5% | 14% | 22% | 28% |
| Atypical angina (2 symptoms) | 22% | 46% | 59% | 67% |
| Typical angina (all 3 symptoms) | 70% | 87% | 92% | 94% |

**Table 2   Women: probability (%) of $\geq 50\%$ coronary artery stenosis in at least one major artery**

| Symptoms | Age (years) **[B]**[3] | | | |
|---|---|---|---|---|
| | 30–39 | 40–49 | 50–59 | 60–69 |
| Asymptomatic (0 symptoms) | 0.3% | 1% | 3% | 8% |
| Non-anginal chest pain (1 symptom) | 1% | 3% | 8% | 19% |
| Atypical angina (2 symptoms) | 4% | 13% | 32% | 54% |
| Typical angina (all 3 symptoms) | 26% | 55% | 79% | 91% |

**Why?**

Increasing age increases the risk of having unstable angina or an MI

| Patient [A][2] | Target disorder (reference standard) | Diagnostic test | LR + (95% CI) | Post-test probability |
|---|---|---|---|---|
| Central or left-sided chest pain (pre-test probability: 41%) | MI or unstable angina (ECG, cardiac enzymes, stress tests) | Aged > 80 years | 3.5 (1.9 to 6.4) | 71% |
| | | Aged 70–79 years | 2.2 (1.4 to 3.4) | 61% |
| | | Aged 60–69 years | 1.8 (1.3 to 2.4) | 56% |
| | | Aged 50–59 years | 1.1 (0.83 to 1.5) | 44% |
| | | Aged 40–49 years | 0.50 (0.34 to 0.72) | 26% |
| | | Aged 30–39 years | 0.12 (0.047 to 0.28) | 8% |
| | | Aged 25–29 years | 0.10 (0.024 to 0.42) | 7% |

**Men who have chest pain are more likely to have an MI or unstable angina**

| Patient [A][2] | Target disorder (reference standard) | Diagnostic test | LR + (95% CI) | Post-test probability | LR – (95% CI) | Post-test probability |
|---|---|---|---|---|---|---|
| Central or left-sided chest pain (pre-test probability: 41%) | MI or unstable angina (ECG, cardiac enzymes, stress tests) | Male | 1.3 (1.1 to 1.5) | 48% | 0.77 (0.65 to 0.91) | 35% |

- cardiovascular risk factors [D].

Patients at low risk for an MI can be assessed in a rapid evaluation unit [B][7] by:
- CK-MB at 0, 4, 8, 12 h
- serial 12-lead ECGs
- clinical assessment at 0, 6, 12 h
- exercise ECG: if all the above negative.

**Why?**

Patients at low risk for an MI who have no CK-MB rise or further pain within 12 h are unlikely to have one

| Patient [A][8] | Target disorder (reference standard) | Diagnostic test | LR + (95% CI) | Post-test probability | LR – (95% CI) | Post-test probability |
|---|---|---|---|---|---|---|
| Low risk for MI (pre-test probability 7%) | MI (typical change in cardiac enzymes or cardiac arrest) | Cardiac enzyme rise or recurrent chest pain within 12 h | 6.8 (5.7 to 8.1) | 34% | 0.069 (0.027 to 0.18) | 0.5% |

- Patients admitted to a rapid assessment unit are not clearly less likely to be diagnosed with an MI or unstable angina [D][9], but spend on average 40 h less in hospital [D][9].
- Half the patients are still admitted to hospital (45%; 95% CI: 34% to 56%) [A][10].

Use the following clinical prediction rule (Table 3) to help determine admission to coronary care units **[A]**[11]. Look for the following risk factors:

- pain worse than prior angina or the same as the pain associated with a prior myocardial infarction
- systolic blood pressure <110 mmHg
- crackles above the bases bilaterally
- ST elevation or Q waves, not known to be old, in two or more leads
- ST segment or T wave changes, not known to be old, indicative of myocardial ischaemia.

| Table 3   Risk of major complications | |
| --- | --- |
| Group **[A]**[11] | Risk of major complication at 4 days |
| Suspected MI on ECG or suspected ischaemia on ECG and ≥2 risk factors | High |
| Suspected ischaemia on ECG and ≤1 risk factor | Moderate |
| One risk factor with no MI or ischaemia on ECG | Low |
| No risk factors | Very low |

**? Why do this?**

A clinical prediction rule can help identify patients at risk of having major complications

| Group **[A]**[11] | Risk of major complication at 4 days | % (95% CI) | NNF (95% CI) |
| --- | --- | --- | --- |
| Suspected MI on ECG or suspected ischaemia on ECG and ≥2 risk factors | High | 16% (12% to 20%) | 6 (5 to 8) |
| Suspected ischaemia on ECG and ≤1 risk factor | Moderate | 7.8% (6.0% to 9.6%) | 13 (11 to 17) |
| One risk factor with no MI or ischaemia | Low | 3.9% (2.7% to 5.2%) | 26 (19 to 37) |
| No risk factors | Very low | 0.58% (0.29% to 0.87%) | 170 (110 to 340) |

## DIFFERENTIAL DIAGNOSIS

Other common causes of chest pain include **[C]**[12]:

- MI
- pulmonary embolism
- chest infection
- musculoskeletal pain
- pericarditis.

Rarer causes include [D]:
- aortic dissection
- oesophageal spasm.

> **Note**
> MI, angina and pulmonary embolism are common causes of chest pain

| Chest pain in emergency department [A]2 [A]13 [C]12 | % |
|---|---|
| MI | 14% to 20% |
| Unstable angina | 24% (21% to 27%) |
| Stable angina | 9.0% (5.6% to 12%) |
| Pulmonary embolism | 5.8% (3.0% to 8.5%) |
| Other pulmonary disease | 5.8% (3.0% to 8.5%) |
| Chest wall pain | 5.4% (2.7% to 8.1%) |
| Pericarditis | 5.0% (2.5% to 7.6%) |
| Psychogenic | 2.9% (0.9% to 4.8%) |
| Other heart disease | 1.1% (0.0% to 2.3%) |
| Other disease | 1.1% (0.0% to 2.3%) |
| Unknown | 11% (7.5% to 15%) |

## INVESTIGATIONS

- Blood count [B]14.

> **Why?**
> A high leucocyte count or low relative lymphocyte percentage make an MI more likely

| Patient [B]14 | Target disorder (reference standard) | Diagnostic test | LR + (95% CI) | Post-test probability | LR − (95% CI) | Post-test probability |
|---|---|---|---|---|---|---|
| Central or left-sided chest pain (pre-test probability 18%) | MI (CK-MB at 24 hours) | Elevated leucocyte count | 6.8 (4.3 to 11) | 60% | 0.56 (0.45 to 0.70) | 11% |
| | | Decreased relative lymphocyte percentage | 6.3 (4.2 to 9.4) | 58% | 0.46 (0.35 to 0.61) | 9% |

- Urea, electrolytes and creatinine [D].
- Glucose [D].

- Serial cardiac enzymes, ideally CK-MB **[C]**[15] **[C]**[16]

| **Why?** Early CK-MB rise diagnoses an MI and normal levels at 20 h rule it out | | | | | | |
|---|---|---|---|---|---|---|
| Patient **[C]**[15] | Target disorder (reference standard) | Diagnostic test | LR + (95% CI) | Post-test probability | LR – (95% CI) | Post-test probability |
| Suspected myocardial infarction (pre-test probability 18%) | MI (history, ECG, CK-MB$_{act}$) | Elevated CK-MB$_{mass}$ at 3 h after symptom onset | Infinity (16 to infinity) | 100% | 0.68 (0.61 to 0.75) | 13% |
| | | At 4 h | 28 (19 to 42) | 86% | 0.45 (0.39 to 0.52) | 9% |
| | | At 6 h | 29 (19 to 44) | 86% | 0.13 (0.11 to 0.16) | 3% |
| | | At 8 h | 19 (13 to 27) | 81% | 0.063 (0.053 to 0.076) | 1% |
| | | At 12 h | 14 (11 to 18) | 75% | 0.032 (0.027 to 0.039) | 0.7% |
| | | At 20 h | 11 (8 to 16) | 71% | 0.00 (0.0 to 0.020) | 0% |

Less helpful alternatives include:
- troponin T **[A]**[17] **[B]**[18] **[C]**[15] **[C]**[16] to troponin I **[C]**[16]

| **Why?** A normal troponin T at 20 h makes an MI unlikely | | | | | | |
|---|---|---|---|---|---|---|
| Patient **[C]**[15] | Target disorder (reference standard) | Diagnostic test | LR + (95% CI) | Post-test probability | LR – (95% CI) | Post-test probability |
| Suspected myocardial infarction (pre-test probability 18%) | MI (history, ECG, CK-MB$_{act}$) | Elevated troponin T at 3 h after symptom onset | 6 (4 to 9) | 57% | 0.67 (0.59 to 0.76) | 13 |
| | | At 4 h | 11 (7 to 16) | 71% | 0.59 (0.52 to 0.67) | 9% |
| | | At 6 h | 7 (4 to 10) | 61% | 0.37 (0.31 to 0.43) | 8% |
| | | At 8 h | 9 (6 to 13) | 66% | 0.23 (0.19 to 0.27) | 5% |
| | | At 12 h | 9 (7 to 12) | 66% | 0.078 (0.064 to 0.94) | 2% |
| | | At 20 h | 9 (6 to 13) | 66% | 0.022 (0.019 to 0.027) | 0.5% |

**Why?**

**Normal CK-MB and troponin I can help rule out MI**

| Patient [C][16] | Target disorder (reference standard) | Diagnostic test | LR + (95% CI) | Post-test probability | LR – (95% CI) | Post-test probability |
|---|---|---|---|---|---|---|
| Chest pain lasting for at least 15 min within previous 24 h [C][16] (pre-test probability 37%) | MI (CK-MB$_{mass}$ at 24 h) | Troponin I at 6 h | 10 (7.3 to 14) | 59% | 0.45 (0.37 to 0.56) | 6% |
| | | Troponin I at 18 h | 15 (11 to 19) | 67% | 0.045 (0.019 to 0.11) | 1% |

- myoglobin [C][15]

**Why?**

**An elevated myoglobin diagnoses an MI, but normal levels cannot safely rule it out**

| Patient [C][15] | Target disorder (reference standard) | Diagnostic test | LR + (95% CI) | Post-test probability | LR – (95% CI) | Post-test probability |
|---|---|---|---|---|---|---|
| Suspected MI (pre-test probability 18%) | MI (history, ECG, CK-MB$_{act}$) | Elevated myoglobin at 3 h after symptom onset | 34 (23 to 49) | 88% | 0.33 (0.28 to 0.38) | 7% |
| | | At 4 h | 26 (17 to 38) | 85% | 0.24 (0.20 to 0.28) | 5% |
| | | At 6 h | 26 (17 to 39) | 85% | 0.23 (0.19 to 0.27) | 5% |
| | | At 8 h | 25 (17 to 36) | 85% | 0.26 (0.22 to 0.30) | 5% |
| | | At 12 h | 23 (16 to 31) | 83% | 0.33 (0.28 to 0.39) | 7% |
| | | At 20 h | 13 (8 to 20) | 74% | 0.63 (0.56 to 0.71) | 12% |

- Serial creatine kinase (CK) [B][14] [C][19], aspartate transaminase (AST) [A][2], lactate dehydrogenase (LDH) [A][2] taken over 24 h [A][20]

**Why?**

- 96% of MIs can be diagnosed at 24 h using CK-MB, LDH, CK and ECG changes (95 to 98%) [A][20].

**Elevated creatine kinase levels diagnose MI**

| Patient [C][19] | Target disorder (reference standard) | Diagnostic test | LR + (95% CI) | Post-test probability |
|---|---|---|---|---|
| Suspected myocardial infarction (pre-test probability 64%) | MI (ECG changes) | Highest CK ≥280 iu/l | 54 (7.7 to 380) | 99% |
| | | CK 80–279 iu/l | 4.5 (2.7 to 7.3) | 89% |
| | | CK 40–79 iu/l | 0.30 (0.16 to 0.56) | 35% |
| | | CK < 40 iu/l | 0.013 (0.0032 to 0.051) | 2.0% |

**?** **Elevated AST levels taken 12 h or more after symptom onset help diagnose MI**

| Patient [A][2] | Target disorder (reference standard) | Diagnostic test | LR + (95% CI) | Post-test probability |
|---|---|---|---|---|
| Central or left-sided chest pain (pre-test probability 41%) | MI (ECG, cardiac enzymes, stress tests) | AST taken more than 12 h after chest pain onset: ≥ 100 iu/l | 30 | 89% |
| | | 80 iu/l | 2.3 | 39% |
| | | 60 iu/l | 5.6 | 60% |
| | | 50 iu/l | 0.40 | 10% |
| | | 40 iu/l | 0.59 | 14v |
| | | 30 iu/l | 0.32 | 8% |
| | | <30 iu/l | 0.078 | 2% |

■ CK [A][2] [B][14], AST [A][2] or LDH [A][2] taken within 12 hours of symptom onset cannot safely exclude an MI.

**Cardiac enzymes taken in the emergency department cannot diagnose or exclude an MI**

| Patient [A][12] | Target disorder (reference standard) | Diagnostic test | LR + (95% CI) | Post-test probability | LR − (95% CI) | Post-test probability |
|---|---|---|---|---|---|---|
| Central or left-sided chest pain (pre-test probability 17%) | MI (ECG, cardiac enzymes) | CK > 180 | 1.8 (1.3 to 2.5) | 27% | 0.77 (0.65 to 0.91) | 14% |
| | | AST > 60 | 6.1 (3.5 to 10) | 56% | 0.43 (0.29 to 0.64) | 8% |
| | | AST > 47 | 3.4 (2.3 to 5.1) | 41% | 0.44 (0.29 to 0.68) | 8% |
| | | LDH > 200 | 2.0 | 29% | 0.59 | 11% |
| | | CK or AST abnormal | 1.7 (1.3 to 2.2) | 26% | 0.65 (0.51 to 0.82) | 12% |

**CK levels alone taken at 24 h cannot safely diagnose or exclude an MI**

| Patient [B][14] | Target disorder (reference standard) | Diagnostic test | LR + (95% CI) | Post-test probability | LR − (95% CI) | Post-test probability |
|---|---|---|---|---|---|---|
| Central or left-sided chest pain (pre-test probability 18%) | MI (CK-MB at 24 hours) | Elevated CK | 6.0 (3.7 to 9.8) | 57% | 0.62 (0.50 to 0.76) | 12% |

- A 12-lead ECG **[A]**[4] **[B]**[5] **[B]**[6] **[B]**[14] – read it carefully! **[A]**[21]

---

**Why?**
**ECG features suggestive of an MI make an MI or unstable angina more likely**

| Patient **[A]**[2] | Target disorder (reference standard) | Diagnostic test | LR + (95% CI) | Post-test probability |
|---|---|---|---|---|
| Central or left-sided chest pain (pre-test probability 41%) | MI or unstable angina (ECG, cardiac enzymes, stress tests) | Probable MI | 13 (8.5 to 20) | 73% |
| | | Ischaemia or strain not known to be old | 1.6 (1.1 to 2.3) | 25% |
| | | Ischaemia or strain or infarction but changes known to be old | 0.34 (0.13 to 0.91) | 7% |
| | | Abnormal but not diagnostic of ischaemia | 0.21 (0.066 to 0.64) | 4% |
| | | Non-specific ST or T wave changes | 0.13 (0.049 to 0.34) | 3% |
| | | Normal | 0.042 (0.0059 to 0.30) | 1% |

■ Emergency physicians can misread ECGs for patients with cardiac chest pain – missing 12% of ST elevation and 12% of T wave inversion. **[A]**[21]

---

Look for features suggestive of cardiac ischaemia:
- any ST elevation, particularly if in two or more leads or not known to be old **[A]**[4] **[B]**[5] **[B]**[6] **[B]**[14]
- any ST depression, particularly if not known to be old **[B]**[5] **[B]**[6]
- any Q waves, particularly if in two leads or more or not known to be old **[A]**[4] **[B]**[5] **[B]**[6]
- any T wave inversion, particularly if not known to be old **[B]**[5] **[B]**[6]
- any conduction defect, particularly if not known to be old **[B]**[5] **[B]**[6]

**?** **Why?**

**ST elevation or depression, Q waves and T wave inversion help diagnose MI**

| Patient | Target disorder (reference standard) | Diagnostic test | LR + (95% CI) | Post-test probability | LR − (95% CI) | Post-test probability |
|---|---|---|---|---|---|---|
| Central or left-sided chest pain [B][14] (pre-test probability 18%) | MI (CK-MB at 24 hours) | ST elevation in 2 contiguous leads | 62 (15 to 250) | 93% | 0.61 (0.51 to 0.74) | 12% |
| Attending emergency department with chest pain [B][5] (pre-test probability 20%) | MI (ECG and cardiac enzyme changes) | New ST segment elevation ≥ 1 mm | 5.7 to 54 | 59% to 93% | | |
| Anterior chest pain [B][6] (pre-test probability 12%) | | Any ST segment elevation | 11 (7.1 to 18) | 61% | 0.45 (0.34 to 0.60) | 6% |
| Attending emergency department with chest pain [B][5] (pre-test probability 20%) | | New ST depression | 3.0 to 5.2 | 43% | | |
| Anterior chest pain [B][6] (pre-test probability 12%) | | Any ST segment depression | 3.2 (2.5 to 4.1) | 31% | 0.38 (0.26 to 0.56) | 5% |
| Attending emergency department with chest pain [B][5] (pre-test probability 20%) | | New Q wave | 5.3 to 25 | 57% to 86% | | |
| Anterior chest pain [B][6] (pre-test probability 12%) | | Any Q wave | 3.9 (2.7 to 5.7) | 36% | 0.60 (0.47 to 0.76) | 8% |
| | | T wave peaking and/or inversion ≥ 1 mm | 3.1 | 44% | | |
| | | New T wave inversion | 2.4 to 2.8 | 38% to 41% | | |
| Attending emergency department with chest pain [B][5] (pre-test probability 20%) | | New conduction defect | 6.3 (2.5 to 16) | 61% | | |
| Anterior chest pain [B][6] (pre-test probability 12%) | | Any conduction defect | 2.7 (1.4 to 5.4) | 28% | 0.89 (0.79 to 1.00) | 11% |
| | | Normal ECG | 0.1 to 0.3 | 2% to 7% | | |

followed by serial ECGs [A][22] looking for:

- acute injury: ST elevation ≥ 1 mm in two contiguous limb leads, or ≥ 2 mm in two contiguous precordial leads
- acute ischaemia: ST depression ≥ 1 mm in two contiguous leads or symmetrical T wave inversion of ≥ 3 mm in two contiguous leads
- in patients with bundle-branch block: ST depression or elevation ≥ 1 mm towards deflection of main QRS deflection in two contiguous

leads, or $\geq 7$ mm away from QRS deflection and $> 50\%$ amplitude of T wave in two contiguous leads.

> **Why?**
> Abnormalities on serial ECGs help diagnose an MI or unstable angina
>
> | Patient [A][22] [B][22] | Target disorder (reference standard) | Diagnostic test | LR + (95%CI) | Post-test probability | LR – (95% CI) | Post-test probability |
> |---|---|---|---|---|---|---|
> | Chest pain (pre-test probability 52%) | MI or unstable angina (ECG at 24 hours, cardiac enzymes) | Initial ECG Serial ECG | 9.5 (5.6 to 16) 55 (18 to 170) | 91% 98% | 0.75 (0.70 to 0.79) 0.66 (0.62 to 0.70) | 44% 41% |

> **Note**
> ■ Few patients with a normal ECG go on to have life-threatening complications (1.3%; 95% CI: 0.0% to 3.0%) **[C]**[23].

- Chest X-ray **[D]**.

Arrange stress testing on discharge or as an outpatient using any of:
- exercise ECG **[A]**[24], looking for: **[A]**[24]
  - horizontal or down-sloping ST slope and 1 mm or more of depression **[B]**[3] in any lead
  - angina during test

> **Why?**
> Abnormalities on exercise ECG makes coronary artery disease more likely
>
> | Patient | Target disorder (reference standard) | Diagnostic test | LR + (95%CI) | Post-test probability | LR – (95% CI) | Post-test probability |
> |---|---|---|---|---|---|---|
> | Probable or definite stable angina (pre-test probability 51%) **[A]**[24] | Coronary artery stenosis (coronary angiography) | Exercise ECG | 3.0 (2.3 to 3.9) | 76% | 0.65 (0.59 to 0.71) | 40% |
>
> Exercise ECG: deepening ST segment depression makes coronary artery disease more likely
>
> | Patient **[B]**[3] | Target disorder (reference standard) | Diagnostic test | LR+ (95% CI) | Post-test probability |
> |---|---|---|---|---|
> | Suspected coronary artery disease (pre-test probability 51%) | Coronary artery stenosis (coronary angiography) | Non-sloping ST segment depression exercise ECG: | | |
> | | | $\geq 2.50$ mm | 39 | 98% |
> | | | 2.0 – 2.49 mm | 11 | 92% |
> | | | 1.5 – 1.99 mm | 4.2 | 81% |
> | | | 1.0 – 1.49 mm | 2.1 | 69% |
> | | | 0.5 – 0.99 mm | 0.92 | 49% |
> | | | <0.5 mm | 0.23 | 19% |

- exercise echocardiography [A][25] [A][26]

| ? Why? |
|---|
| **An abnormal exercise echocardiogram makes coronary artery disease more likely** |

| Patient | Target disorder (reference standard) | Diagnostic test | LR + (95% CI) | Post-test probability | LR – (95% CI) | Post-test probability |
|---|---|---|---|---|---|---|
| Suspected coronary artery disease (pre-test probability 64%) [A][25] | Coronary artery disease (coronary angiography) | Exercise echocardiography | 3.3 (2.9 to 3.6) | 85% | 0.16 (0.14 to 0.19) | 23% |

- scintigraphy [A][26] [B][3] – look for a reversible perfusion defect [B][3]

| ? Why? |
|---|
| **Scintigraphy makes multivessel coronary artery disease more likely** |

| Patient | Target disorder (reference standard) | Diagnostic test | LR + (95% CI) | Post-test probability | LR – (95% CI) | Post-test probability |
|---|---|---|---|---|---|---|
| Chest pain referred for further investigation (pre-test probability) 52%) [A][26] | Multi-vessel coronary artery disease (coronary angiography) | Scintigraphy | 2.5 (1.5 to 4.2) | 76% | 0.44 (0.29 to 0.67) | 36% |

| **Scintigraphy: a reversible perfusion defect makes coronary artery disease more likely** | | | | |
|---|---|---|---|---|
| Patient [B][3] | Target disorder (reference standard) | Diagnostic test | LR+ (95% CI) | Post-test probability |
| Suspected coronary artery disease (pre-test probability 51%) | Coronary artery stenosis (coronary angiography) | Scintigraphy: reversible perfusion defect fixed perfusion defect no perfusion defect | 12 1.4 0.18 | 93% 59% 16% |

- exercise SPECT (single-photon emission computed tomography) [A][25].

| ? Why? |
|---|
| **An abnormal exercise SPECT makes coronary artery disease more likely** |

| Patient | Target disorder (reference standard) | Diagnostic test | LR + (95% CI) | Post-test probability | LR – (95% CI) | Post-test probability |
|---|---|---|---|---|---|---|
| Suspected coronary artery disease (pre-test probability 76%) [A][25] | Coronary artery disease (coronary angiography) | Exercise SPECT | 2.2 (2.0 to 2.4) | 87% | 0.18 (0.16 to 0.20) | 36% |

**Note**
■ There is little difference in the cost-effectiveness of angiography, PET (positron emission tomography), SPECT, echocardiography or thallium scanning **[A]**[27].

Refer for angiography with a view to revascularisation if **[D]**[28]:
● prolonged angina with an ischaemic ECG **[D]**[28]
● abnormal stress testing
● moderate-to-severe angina after hospital discharge despite maximal anti-ischaemic therapy.

Perform angiography followed by revascularisation as soon as possible **[B]**[29].

**Why?**
Patients who live in countries that offer angiography and revascularisation within 7 days of admission compared with delayed investigation are less likely to have refractory angina, but more likely to have a stroke or major bleeding. There is no clear effect on mortality or MI **[B]**[29].

**Early angiography and revascularisation reduces refractory angina and hospital admissions**

| Patient | Treatment | Comparator | Outcome | CER | OR | NNT |
|---|---|---|---|---|---|---|
| Unstable angina **[B]**[29] | Early angiography and revascularisation | Delayed angiography and revascularisation | Refractory angina or readmission for unstable angina at 6 months | 20% | 0.64 (0.56 to 0.73) | 16 (13 to 22) |
| | | | Stroke at 6 months | 1.2% | 1.6 (1.1 to 2.4) | −140 (−840 to −61) |
| | | | Major bleeding at 6 months | 1.1% | 1.8 (1.2 to 2.7) | 120 (−460 to −55) |

**Note**
■ The shape of lesions or presence of thrombus on angiography does not clearly predict death, MI or need for revascularisation **[C]**[30].

## THERAPY

Consider admitting your patient to a chest pain observation unit **[D]**[31].

**Why do this?**
■ Patients are not clearly less likely to die or have a cardiovascular event in the next 6 months than those who have routine hospital admission **[D]**[31].

Treat symptoms rather than ECG changes **[D]**[32].

> **Why do this?**
> ■ Treating silent ischaemic compared with symptomatic disease does not clearly reduce deaths, MI, revascularisation or subsequent hospital admission **[D]**[32].

Give:
● oxygen **[D]**
● aspirin 75 to 325 mg long-term **[A]**[33] **[A]**[34].

> **Why do this?**
> ■ It reduces death, strokes and myocardial infarctions **[A]**[33].
> ■ Patients who continue to take aspirin have benefit for up to 3 years **[A]**[33].
> ■ 75–325 mg of aspirin daily is as effective as higher doses **[A]**[33].
>
> **Aspirin reduces death, strokes and MI in unstable angina**
>
> | Patient | Treatment | Comparator | Outcome | CER | ARR | NNT |
> |---------|-----------|------------|---------|-----|-----|-----|
> | Unstable angina | Aspirin | Control | Death, strokes or MI at 6–12 months | 14% | 4.92% (2.95% to 6.89%) | 20 (15 to 34) |

Alternatives include:
● ticlopidine **[A]**[35]

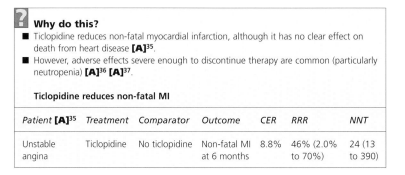

> **Why do this?**
> ■ Ticlopidine reduces non-fatal myocardial infarction, although it has no clear effect on death from heart disease **[A]**[35].
> ■ However, adverse effects severe enough to discontinue therapy are common (particularly neutropenia) **[A]**[36] **[A]**[37].
>
> **Ticlopidine reduces non-fatal MI**
>
> | Patient **[A]**[35] | Treatment | Comparator | Outcome | CER | RRR | NNT |
> |---------|-----------|------------|---------|-----|-----|-----|
> | Unstable angina | Ticlopidine | No ticlopidine | Non-fatal MI at 6 months | 8.8% | 46% (2.0% to 70%) | 24 (13 to 390) |

with **[A]**[38]
● a low-molecular weight heparin (LMWH) **[A]**[39] **[A]**[40] **[A]**[41] for as long as possible **[A]**[42] (e.g. enoxaparin 1 mg/kg daily).

### Why do this?
- LMWH reduces death and myocardial infarction [A][39] [A][42].
- LMWH is more effective than unfractionated heparin at reducing death, recurrent angina, MI or need for revascularisation, but causes more minor bleeds [A][40] [A][41]. It is also more cost-effective [A][43].

**LMWH reduces death, MI and recurrent angina, but causes more minor bleeds than heparin**

| Patient | Treatment | Comparator | Outcome | CER | RRR | NNT |
|---|---|---|---|---|---|---|
| Unstable angina [A][42] | Dalteparin | Placebo | Death, MI or revascularisation at 40 days | 24% | 24% (7% to 38%) | 18 (10 to 63) |
| Unstable angina [A][43] | Enoxaparin | Unfractionated heparin | Death, MI or recurrent angina at 30 days | 23% | 15% (3% to 26%) | 29 (16 to 160) |
| | | | Revascularisation at 30 days | 32% | 16% (7% to 25%) | 19 (12 to 49) |
| | | | Minor bleed at 30 days | 7.0% | −66% (−110% to −33%) | −21 (−38 to −15) |

- Continuing LMWH for up to 6 weeks reduces death, MI and need for revascularisation [A][42].

**Long-term LMWH reduces MI**

| Patient | Treatment | Comparator | Outcome | CER | RRR | NNT |
|---|---|---|---|---|---|---|
| Unstable angina [A][42] | LMWH for 6 weeks | Placebo | Death, MI or revascularisation at 6 weeks | 24% | 24% (7% to 38%) | 18 (10 to 63) |
| | | | MI at 6 weeks | 9.5% | 30% (1% to 51%) | 35 (18 to 680) |

- Patients who stop heparin and are not on aspirin are at increased risk of recurrent angina and urgent revascularisation over the next 4 days [A][44].

**Stopping heparin without aspirin increases recurrent unstable angina and urgent revascularisation**

| Patient | Treatment | Comparator | Outcome | CER | RRR | NNT |
|---|---|---|---|---|---|---|
| Unstable angina [A][44] | Completed 6 days of heparin, and continuing on aspirin | Completed 6 days of heparin | Recurrent unstable angina at 4 days | 13% | 65% (5% to 87%) | 12 (6 to 110) |
| | | | Urgent revascularisation at 4 days | 11% | 100% | 10 (6 to 22) |

## Less effective alternatives include:

- hirudin [A][45] [A][46]

 **Why do this?**

■ Patients who are given hirudin compared with heparin are less likely to die, have refractory angina or an MI [A][45] [A][46].

■ The risk of major bleeding is increased [A][45].

**Hirudin reduces MI, but causes more bleeding than heparin**

| Patient | Treatment | Comparator | Outcome | CER | RRR | NNT |
|---|---|---|---|---|---|---|
| Unstable angina or non-Q wave MI [A][45] | Hirudin | Heparin | Cardiovascular death, new MI or refractory angina at 7 days | 6.7% | 87% (27% to 100%) | 88 (48 to 500) |
| | | | Major bleeding at 7 days | 0.67% | −73% (−160% to −13%) | −210 (−850 to −120) |
| Unstable angina or non-Q wave MI [A][46] | Hirudin for | Heparin for 3–5 days | MI at 30 days | 6.3% | 14% (1% to 26%) | 110 (58 to 2000) |

- heparin [D][47]

**Why?**

■ Heparin is more effective than aspirin at reducing MI [A][38], but less effective than LMWH [A][40] [A][41].

■ Adding heparin to aspirin probably reduces subsequent MI or recurrent angina, but has no clear effect on bleeding or need for revascularisation [D][47].

**Heparin prevents more MI than aspirin**

| Patient | Treatment | Comparator | Outcome | CER | RRR | NNT |
|---|---|---|---|---|---|---|
| Unstable angina or non-Q wave MI [A][38] | Heparin | Aspirin | MI at 6 days | 3.8% | 77% (−3% to 95%) | 35 (18 to 440) |

with a platelet glycoprotein IIb/IIIa inhibitor for severe cases **[A]**[48] **[A]**[49].

---

**? Why do this?**

■ Patients with severe unstable angina (ECG changes or cardiac enzyme elevation) who receive eptifibatide are less likely to die or have non-fatal MI, but more likely to have severe bleeding **[A]**[48].

■ Patients with severe unstable angina (ECG changes or cardiac enzyme elevation) who receive tirofiban and heparin compared with heparin alone are less likely to have a MI or refractory ischaemia at 7 days, but not at 6 months. There is no clear increase in risk of major bleeding **[A]**[49].

**Adding glycoprotein IIb/IIIa inhibitors to standard therapy reduces mortality and further ischaemia**

| Patient | Treatment | Comparator | Outcome | CER | RRR | NNT |
|---------|-----------|------------|---------|-----|-----|-----|
| Severe unstable angina or non-Q wave MI **[A]**[48] | Eptifibatide plus standard therapy | Standard therapy | Death or non-fatal MI at 30 days | 16% | 9.0% (0.0% to 18%) | 67 (34 to 1900) |
| | | | Severe bleeding at 30 days | 0.89% | −67% (−150% to −14%) | −170 (−620 to −96) |
| Severe unstable angina or non-Q wave MI **[A]**[49] | Tirofiban and heparin | Heparin | Refractory ischaemia at 7 days | 9.3% | 27% (2% to 44%) | 30 (15 to 380) |
| | | | MI at 7 days | 3.9% | 45 (15% to 64%) | 32 (18 to 110) |

---

There is no clear benefit from using:
● a platelet glycoprotein IIb/IIIa inhibitor alone **[A]**[50].

---

**? Why?**

■ Although patients given tirofiban are less likely to die, have an MI or refractory ischaemia at 48 hours, there is no clear benefit at 1 week or 1 month **[A]**[50].

■ The risk of thrombocytopenia is increased **[A]**[50].

**Tirofiban increases the risk of thrombocytopenia**

| Patient [A][50] | Treatment | Comparator | Outcome | CER | RRR | NNT |
|---------|-----------|------------|---------|-----|-----|-----|
| Unstable angina | Tirofiban | Heparin | Thrombocytopenia at 1 month | 0.37% | −200% (−650% to −19%) | 140 (75 to 660) |

Consider starting anticoagulation (adjusted so INR 2.2 to 2.5) **[A]**[51].

> **?** **Why do this?**
> - Anticoagulation reduces rehospitalisation with unstable angina, but has no clear effect on MI or revascularisation **[A]**[51].
>
> **Dose-adjusted warfarin reduces readmissions with unstable angina**
>
> | Patient [A][51] | Treatment | Comparator | Outcome | CER | RRR | NNT |
> |---|---|---|---|---|---|---|
> | Unstable angina | Dose-adjusted warfarin aspirin | Fixed low-dose warfarin and aspirin | Rehospitalisation with unstable angina at 3 months | 17% | 58% (4.0% to 82%) | 10 (5 to 98) |

Give intravenous **[A]**[52] or buccal **[A]**[53] nitroglycerin for chest pain. (If intravenous, give 1 mg/ml; titrated from 1.5 ml/h to 12 ml/h. If 20% reduction in blood pressure or 10% decrease in heart rate, or headache, stop titration at that level.)

> **?** **Why do this?**
> - Intravenous nitroglycerin reduces ongoing ischaemia and use of sublingual nitroglycerin, but intolerable headaches and hypotension are common. There is no clear effect on mortality **[A]**[52] or myocardial infarction **[A]**[54].
> - Buccal nitroglycerin causes fewer side-effects than intravenous nitroglycerin. There is no clear difference in either the frequency of painful episodes or the need for emergency revascularisation **[A]**[53].
>
> **Intravenous nitroglycerin reduces ongoing ischaemia, but can cause intolerable side-effects**
>
> | Patient | Treatment | Comparator | Outcome | CER | RRR | NNT |
> |---|---|---|---|---|---|---|
> | Unstable angina [A][52] | Intravenous nitroglycerin | Placebo | Ongoing ischaemia at 48 h | 36% | 50% (11% to 72%) | 6 (3 to 27) |
> | | | | Use of >2 tablets of sublingual nitroglycerin at 48 h | 31% | 48% (3% to 72%) | 7 (3 to 84) |
> | | | | Intolerable side-effects at 48 h | 0.0% | | −10 (−35 to −6) |
>
> **Buccal nitroglycerin causes fewer side effects than intravenous nitroglycerin**
>
> | Patient [A][53] | Treatment | Comparator | Outcome | CER | RRR | NNT |
> |---|---|---|---|---|---|---|
> | Unstable angina | Buccal nitroglycerin | Intravenous nitroglycerin | Side-effects at 7 days | 75% | 49% (−8% to 76%) | 3 (1 to 38) |

Start a beta-blocker **[A]**[55] or a calcium-channel blocker (e.g. diltiazem **[A]**[56] **[A]**[57] or verapamil **[A]**[58]).

---

**Why do this?**

- Metoprolol reduces recurrent ischaemia, without clearly reducing MI **[A]**[55].
- Diltiazem reduces chest pain (roughly one fewer episode every 2 days) **[D]**[59], and is more effective than nitroglycerin **[A]**[60]. Fewer patients have serious headaches, but more develop AV conduction abnormalities **[A]**[60].
- Verapamil or diltiazem reduces MI, but there is no clear effect on mortality **[A]**[56] **[A]**[57] **[A]**[58].

**Metoprolol reduces recurrent ischaemia**

| Patient [A]55 | Treatment | Comparator | Outcome | CER | RRR | NNT |
|---|---|---|---|---|---|---|
| Unstable angina | Metoprolol | Placebo | Recurrent ischaemia at 48 h | 21% | 53% (–3% to 78%) | 9 (4 to 380) |

**Diltiazem reduces myocardial infarction and refractory angina better than nitroglycerin**

| Patient [A]60 | Treatment | Comparator | Outcome | CER | RRR | NNT |
|---|---|---|---|---|---|---|
| Unstable angina | iv diltiazem | iv nitroglycerin | MI or refractory angina at 2 days | 41% | 51% (12% to 73%) | 5 (3 to 20) |
| | | | Refractory angina at 2 days | 30% | 55% (4% to 79%) | 6 (3 to 54) |
| | | | Serious headache requiring analgesia at 2 days | 25% | 80% (33% to 94%) | 5 (3 to 13) |
| | | | AV conduction abnormalities at 2 days | 0% | | –12 (–75 to –7) |

**Verapamil or diltiazem reduces MI**

| Patient [A]56 [A]57 | Treatment | Comparator | Outcome | CER | OR | NNT |
|---|---|---|---|---|---|---|
| Unstable angina or MI | Verapamil or diltiazem | Placebo | MI at 2 days to 6 weeks | 7.5% | 0.79% (0.67% to 0.94%) | 68 (43 to 240) |

**Cardiovascular disease: verapamil reduces non-fatal MI**

| Patient [A]58 | Treatment | Comparator | Outcome | CER | OR | NNT |
|---|---|---|---|---|---|---|
| MI, angina or hypertension | Verapamil | Placebo | Non-fatal MI at ?months | 7.4% | 0.79% (0.65% to 0.97%) | 64 (38 to 450) |

**Note**
- Beta-blockers, calcium antagonists and nitrates are not clearly different in reducing MI or death from heart disease **[D]**[59] **[D]**[61] **[D]**[62], but more patients stop beta-blockers than calcium-channel blockers due to side-effects **[A]**[61].
- There is no clear benefit from starting beta-blockers and calcium-channel blockers together compared with beta-blockers alone **[A]**[55].
- Calcium-channel blockers do not clearly increase the risk of cancer **[A]**[63] **[B]**[64].
- There is no clear benefit in giving dihydropyridine calcium blockers (nifedipine and nicardipine) to patients with unstable angina or MI: they may well be harmful **[A]**[55–57]. Specifically, short-acting nifedipine increases mortality **[B]**[65].

**Short-acting nifedipine increases mortality**

| Patient **[B]**[65] | Treatment | Comparator | Outcome | CER | OR | NNH |
|---|---|---|---|---|---|---|
| MI or angina | Short-acting nifedipine | Placebo | Death at ?months | 6.6% | 1.16 (1.01 to 1.33) | 100 (51 to 1600) |

For patients already on a beta-blocker, add a calcium-channel blocker **[A]**[55].

**Why do this?**
- Adding a calcium-channel blocker reduces recurrent ischaemia **[A]**[67], MI, need for surgery and sudden death. **[A]**[66]

**Adding calcium-channel blockers to a beta-blocker reduces recurrent ischaemia and MI**

| Patient | Treatment | Comparator | Outcome | CER | RRR | NNT |
|---|---|---|---|---|---|---|
| Unstable angina on a beta-blocker **[A]**[55] | Nifedipine | Placebo | Recurrent ischaemia at 48 h | 31% | 46% (6% to 69%) | 7 (4 to 58) |
| Unstable angina on a beta-blocker and nitrates **[A]**[66] | Nifedipine | Placebo | MI, sudden death or need for surgey | 61% | 28% (1% to 48%) | 6 (3 to 110) |

For patients already on a calcium-channel blocker, add a beta-blocker **[A]**[67] if possible.

**Why do this?**
- Patients have fewer ischaemic attacks (roughly two fewer a day) and attacks are shorter (by approximately 17 min) **[A]**[67].

**More patients stop beta-blockers than calcium-channel blockers due to side-effects**

| Patient **[B]**[61] | Treatment | Comparator | Outcome | CER | RRR | NNH |
|---|---|---|---|---|---|---|
| Stable angina | Beta-blockers | Calcium-channel blockers | Withdrawal due to adverse effects at ?months | 8.5% | −34% (−57% to −14%) | 34 (22 to 75) |

Consider adding long-acting nitrates **[D]**[54] **[D]**[66].

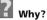

**Why?**
- Nitrates reduce recurrent ischaemia **[D]**[54], but there is no clear effect on mortality or MI **[C]**[66].

For patients with severe refractory unstable angina, consider:
- adding a glycoprotein IIb/IIIa inhibitor **[A]**[68]

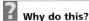

**Why do this?**
- Patients with unstable angina refractory to heparin and nitrates who receive a glycoprotein IIb/IIIa inhibitor are less likely to die, have a MI or require urgent revascularisation in the next 24 h **[A]**[68].

**Glycoprotein IIb/IIIa inhibitors reduce mortality and further ischaemia in refractory angina**

| Patient [A]68 | Treatment | Comparator | Outcome | CER | RRR | NNT |
|---|---|---|---|---|---|---|
| Refractory unstable angina | Glycoprotein IIb/IIIa inhibitor | Placebo | Death, MI, urgent revascularisation at 24 h | 23% | 86% (–9% to 98%) | 5 (3 to 28) |

- adding nicorandil **[A]**[69]

**Why do this?**
- Nicorandil reduces chest pain in patients with refractory unstable angina on aspirin, beta-blockers and diltiazem **[A]**[69].
- There is no clear effect on subsequent MI or death **[A]**[69].

**Nicorandil reduces recurrent chest pain in refractory unstable angina**

| Patient [A]69 | Treatment | Comparator | Outcome | CER | RRR | NNT |
|---|---|---|---|---|---|---|
| Unstable angina on aspirin, beta-blockers and diltiazem | Nicorandil | Placebo | Recurrent chest pain at 2 days | 36% | 43% (9% to 64%) | 6 (4 to 29) |

- thoracic epidural anaesthesia [A][70]

 **Why do this?**
- Thoracic epidural anaesthesia reduces the number of anginal attacks in patients with severe refractory unstable angina. Attacks are on average 16 min shorter [A][70].
- Side-effects are common (urinary retention and Horner's syndrome), but are reversible [A][70].

**Refractory angina: thoracic epidural anaesthesia reduces recurrent angina**

| Patient [A][70] | Treatment | Comparator | Outcome | CER | RRR | NNT |
|---|---|---|---|---|---|---|
| Severe refractory unstable angina | Thoracic epidural anaesthesia | Maximal medical therapy | Recurrent angina at 48 h | 55% | 93% (55% to 99%) | 1 (1 to 2) |
| | | | Side-effects at 48 h | 0.0% | | −2 (−3 to −1) |

- adding *N*-acetylcysteine to nitrates [A][54] [B][71]

 **Why?**
- Fewer patients have persistent angina requiring revascularisation, but severe headaches are common, and many patients stop therapy [A][54].

**Adding *N*-acetylcysteine to nitrates reduces persistent angina, but can cause severe headaches**

| Patient | Treatment | Comparator | Outcome | CER | RRR | NNT |
|---|---|---|---|---|---|---|
| Unstable angina [A][54] | *N*-acetylcysteine and topical nitrate | Topical nitrate | Persistent angina requiring revascularisation at 4 months | 33% | 67% (21% to 86%) | 5 (3 to 17) |
| | | | Severe headache at 4 months | 4.4% | −610% (−2800% to −73%) | −4 (−8 to −2) |
| | | | Treatment withdrawal at 4 months | 8.7% | −280% (−930% to −37%) | −4 (−11 to −3) |
| Refractory unstable angina [B][71] | *N*-acetylcysteine and iv nitrates | iv nitrates | MI at 1 day | 46% | 73% (13% to 91%) | 3 (2 to 12) |

- angiography and revascularisation [A].

UNIVERSITY COLLEGE CHESTER
JET LIBRARY

There is no clear benefit from:
- thrombolysis [A]⁷² [A]⁷³

**Why?**
- Patients who receive tissue plasminogen activator compared with placebo are not clearly less likely to die, have an MI or require revascularisation at 6 weeks or 1 year [A]⁷² [A]⁷³.

- urgent revascularisation (within 48 h) [A]⁷² [A]⁷³.

**Why?**
- Patients who have angioplasty within 48 h followed by bypass surgery if required, compared with angioplasty alone after failure of medical therapy, are less likely to be readmitted in the next 6 weeks, and fewer require antianginal medication.
- However, more patients have a revascularisation procedure at 1 year. There is no clear effect on death, non-fetal MI or episodes of ischaemia [A]⁷² [A]⁷³.

**Early angioplasty followed by CABG reduces readmission and antianginal drug use at 6 weeks**

| Patient [A]⁷² [A]⁷³ | Treatment | Comparator | Outcome | CER | RRR | NNT |
|---|---|---|---|---|---|---|
| Unstable angina or non-Q wave MI | Angioplasty within 48 h followed by CABG if required | Angioplasty if failure of medical therapy | Use of 1 or fewer antianginal drugs at 6 weeks | 46% | 15% (4% to 28%) | 14 (8 to 53) |
| | | | Readmission to hospital at 6 weeks | 14% | 46% (26% to 60%) | 16 (11 to 32) |
| | | | Revascularisation at 1 year | 58% | –10% (–20% to –2%) | –16 (–91 to –9) |

## Angioplasty

Offer angioplasty to patients with: single-vessel disease [B]⁷⁴.

**Why do this?**
- Patients with angiographically proven coronary artery disease who have angioplasty compared with medical therapy have less angina and require less medication or further revascularisation [A]⁷⁵.
- However, more die or have an MI [A]⁷⁵.
- There is no clear effect on recurrence of unstable angina [A]⁷⁵.
- Between 70% and 80% of patients post-angioplasty are symptom-free at 5 years, but 20% of patients require repeat angioplasty and 10% require CABG during that time [B]⁷⁴.

**Angioplasty reduces symptoms, but increases death and MI compared with medical therapy**

| Patient | Treatment | Comparator | Outcome | CER | RRR | NNT |
|---|---|---|---|---|---|---|
| Coronary artery disease with >50% stenosis in at least one vessel [A]⁷⁵ | Angioplasty +/– stent | Medical therapy | On 1 or fewer antianginal drugs at 3 years | 47c | –60% (–90% to –35%) | 4 (3 to 5) |
| | | | Revascularisation at 3 years | 25% | 21% (0 to 37%) | 19 (10 to 990) |
| | | | Death or non-fatal MI at 3 years | 3.3% | –92% (–241% to –8%) | –33 (–240 to –1) |

Assess your patient for risk of complications (Table 4) **[B]**[76] before deciding on angioplasty.

Look for:
- aortic valve disease **[A]**[76]
- shock **[A]**[76] **[A]**[79]
- acute MI within 24 h of coronary angioplasty **[A]**[76]
- unstable angina **[A]**[76] **[B]**[78]
- complex lesion on coronary angioplasty **[A]**[76] **[A]**[79] **[B]**[78]
- left main coronary artery lesions **[A]**[76]
- multivessel disease **[A]**[76] **[A]**[78].

**Table 4  Risk of angioplasty complications**

| Risk factors **[A]**[76] | Risk of major complications |
|---|---|
| >3 | Very high |
| 3 | High |
| 1–2 | Moderate |
| 0 | Low |

**Note**
- 4 to 10% of patients having angioplasty have an acute complication: half have an MI, a quarter require emergency bypass **[B]**[77] **[B]**[78].
- 8% of patients have acute coronary artery occlusion **[B]**[78].
- One in 30 die in hospital following angioplasty (3.4%; 95% CI: 2.5% to 4.3%) **[A]**[79].

**Why do this?**
**A clinical prediction rule can help identify patients at risk for angioplasty complications**

| Risk factors **[A]**[76] | % with major complications (95% CI) | NNF (95% CI) |
|---|---|---|
| >3 | 17% (5.4% to 28%) | 6 (4 to 19) |
| 3 | 5.4% (2.2% to 8.7%) | 18 (11 to 46) |
| 1–2 | 2.5% (1.9% to 3.1%) | 40 (33 to 52) |
| 0 | 1.3% (0.82% to 1.8%) | 76 (55 to 120) |

Give a glycoprotein IIb/IIIa antagonist (e.g. abciximab) [A][80].

 **Why do this?**
- Abciximab reduces death, MI and need for urgent revascularisation [A][81] [A][82] [A][83] . It is more effective than stenting at reducing death or MI [A][80] [A][84].
- Combining abciximab and stenting is more effectie than stenting alone [A][80] [A][84]; the combination is probably better than abciximab [A][84].
- There is no clear effect on major bleeding [A][80].

**Abciximab reduces death and MI with or without stenting**

| Patient | Treatment | Comparator | Outcome | CER | RRR | NNT |
|---|---|---|---|---|---|---|
| Urgent or elective angioplasty [A][82] | Abciximab | Placebo | Death, MI or urgent revascularisation at 12 months | 16% | 41% (25% to 54%) | 15 (10 to 28) |
| Urgent or elective angioplasty [A][84] | Abciximab | Stent | Death or MI at 6 months | 11% | 51% (31% to 66%) | 17 (12 to 32) |
| | Abciximab and stent | Stent | Death or MI at 6 months | 11% | 32% (7.0% to 50%) | 28 (15 to 140) |
| | Abciximab and stent | Abciximab | Death or MI at 6 months | 7.8% | 29% (–3% to 51%) | 44 (NNT = 21 to infinity; NNH = 500 to infinity) |

Insert a stent in new [A][85–89] and chronic occlusions [A][90–92].

 **Why do this?**
- Stent insertion reduces restenosis [A][85–91], and recurrent ischaemia [A][89] [A][90], but increases the risk of bleeding or vascular complications [A][86] [A][90] [A][93].
- Patients spend on average 5 days longer in hospital [A][86].
- Fewer patients require repeat angiography [A][85] [A][86].

**Stent insertion reduces restenosis, recurrent ischaemia, but increases the risk of complications**

| Patient | Treatment | Comparator | Outcome | CER | RRR | NNT |
|---|---|---|---|---|---|---|
| Stable angina and a single new lesion [A][85] | Stent insertion | No stent | Repeat angiography at 12 months | 21% | 51 (25% to 69%) | 9 (6 to 23) |
| Stable angina and new proximal left artery descending coronary artery lesion [A][89] | Stent insertion | No stent | Restenosis at 12 months | 40% | 54% (15% to 75%) | 5 (3 to 17) |
| | | | Death, MI or recurrence of angina at 12 months | 30% | 56% (6 to 79%) | 6 (3 to 45) |
| Angina with chronic coronary artery occlusion [A][90] | Stent insertion | No stent | Restenosis at 9 months | 69% | 53% (29% to 69%) | 3 (2 to 5) |
| | | | Recurrent ischaemia at 9 months | 46% | 69% (38% to 85%) | 3 (2 to 6) |
| | | | Bleeding and vascular complications at 9 months | 0.0% | | –14 (–250 to –7) |

Following stent insertion, give ticlopidine 250 mg for 1 month [A][94] [A][95].

**Why do this?**
- Adding ticlopidine to aspirin following stenting is more effective than anticoagulation and aspirin at reducing occlusion of the stented vessel, bleeding and MI or death [A][94].
- Using aspirin alone is not clearly as safe as using aspirin and ticlopidine [D][96].
- Adverse effects from ticlopidine severe enough to discontinue therapy are common (particularly neutropenia) [A][97] [A][98].

**Ticlopidine reduces death, MI and bleeding better than anticoagulation**

| Patient [A][94] | Treatment | Comparator | Outcome | CER | RRR | NNT |
|---|---|---|---|---|---|---|
| Recent MI: angiography with insertion of stent | Ticlopidine and aspirin | Anticoagulation and aspirin | Occlusion of stent vessel at 30 days | 9.7% | 100% | 10 (6 to 43) |
| | | | Bleeding at 30 days | 13% | 100% | 8 (5 to 22) |
| | | | Death of recurrent MI at 6 months | 9.7% | 100% | 10 (6 to 43) |

Consider giving:
- probucol [A][99].

**Why do this?**
- Patients who take probucol following angioplasty are less likely to die, have an MI or require revascularisation, but side-effects (particularly diarrhoea) are common [A][99].

**Angioplasty: probucol reduces death, MI and revascularisation**

| Patient | Treatment | Comparator | Outcome | CER | RRR | NNT [A][99] |
|---|---|---|---|---|---|---|
| Angioplasty | Probucol | Placebo | Death, MI or revascularisation at 6 months | 30% | 47% (3% to 71%) | 7 (4 to 86) |
| | | | Side-effects at 6 months | 1.3% | −1100% (−8800% to −58%) | −7 (−18 to −5) |

There is no clear benefit from:
- atherectomy [A][100]

**Why?**
- Atherectomy is not more effective than angioplasty at reducing death, MI or revascularisation [A][100].

- multivitamins [A][99]

> **?** **Why?**
> - There is no clear reduction in mortality, MI or revascularisation [A][99].

- routine angioplasty for patients with non-Q wave MI [D][101]

> **?** **Why?**
> - Patients with a non-Q wave MI who receive routine coronary revascularisation compared with more conservative management are not clearly less likely to die or have another MI [D][101].

## Coronary artery bypass surgery

Offer coronary artery bypass surgery to patients with:
- 3-vessel disease or left main artery disease [A][102]
- poor left ventricular function [A][102]
- severe angina [A][102]
- an abnormal exercise tolerance test [A][102].

> **?** **Why do this?**
> - Patients with multivessel disease, poor left ventricular function, severe angina or an abnormal exercise tests are less likely to die if they have coronary artery bypass surgery [A][102–105].
> - Patients at low risk of dying (1- or 2-vessel disease and ejection fraction > 58%) are more likely to die [A][103–105].
>
> **CABG reduces mortality with multivessel disease and poor LV function**
>
> | Patient [A][102] | Treatment | Comparator | Outcome | CER | OR | NNT |
> |---|---|---|---|---|---|---|
> | Stable coronary artery disease (CAD) | CABG | Medical therapy | Death at 10 years | 31% | 0.83 (0.70 to 0.98) | 26 (14 to 230) |
> | Stable CAD and abnormal exercise test | | | | 17% | 0.52 (0.37 to 0.72) | 14 (10 to 24) |
> | Stable CAD and 3-vessel disease | | | | 178% | 0.58 (0.42 to 0.80) | 15 (11 to 33) |
> | Stable CAD and left anterior descending disease | | | | 37% | 0.32 (0.15 to 0.70) | 5 (4 to 13) |
> | Stable CAD and normal LV function | | | | 13% | 0.61 (0.46 to 0.81) | 21 (15 to 44) |
> | Stable CAD and poor LV function | | | | 25% | 0.59 (0.39 to 0.91) | 12 (7 to 58) |
> | Stable CAD and mild angina | | | | 13% | 0.63 (0.46 to 0.87) | 24 (16 to 69) |
> | Stable CAD and severe angina | | | | 22% | 0.57 (0.40 to 0.81) | 12 (8 to 29) |

**? Why?**

**CABG reduces mortality in high-risk patients, but increases it in low-risk patients**

| Patient [A][103–105] | Treatment | Comparator | Outcome | CER | RRR | NNT |
|---|---|---|---|---|---|---|
| Unstable angina and 3-vessel disease or ejection fraction <58% | CABG | Medical therapy | Death at 8 years | 35% | 32% (1% to 53%) | 9 (5 to 140) |
| Unstable angina and 1- or 2-vessel disease and ejection fraction > 58% | | | Death at 8 years | 17% | –93% (–240% to –3%) | –6 (–33 to –4) |

■ Patients given CABG compared with angioplasty have less angina and require less antianginal medication or revascularisation. There is no clear difference in mortality and myocardial infarction [A][106–108].

**Fewer patients with multivessel disease who have a CABG require revascularisation or have further angina**

| Patient [A][106] | Treatment | Comparator | Outcome | CER | OR | NNT |
|---|---|---|---|---|---|---|
| Multivessel coronary artery disease | CABG | Angioplasty | Angina-free at 1–3 years | 73% | 1.57 (1.32 to 1.87) | 13 (10 to 20) |
| | | | CABG at 1–3 years | 20% | 0.04 (0.02 to 0.07) | 5 (5 to 6) |
| | | | Angioplasty at 1–3 years | 23% | 0.21 (0.16 to 0.27) | 5 (5 to 6) |

However, the procedure is more risky than angioplasty [A][108].

**? Why?**

■ Patients take roughly 5 weeks longer to return to work [A][109] and are at increased risk of an MI before discharge [A][108].
■ One in 30 die within 1 month of CABG (3.2%; 95% CI: 2.2% to 4.2%) [A][102].

**CABG causes more procedural MI than percutaneous transluminal coronary angioplasty (PTCA)**

| Patient [A][108] | Treatment | Comparator | Outcome | CER | RRR | NNT |
|---|---|---|---|---|---|---|
| Severe angina | CABG | Angioplasty | Myocardial infarction at discharge | 2.1% | –120% (–270% to –26%) | –42 (–130 to –25) |

Consider giving acadesine perioperatively [A][110].

> ### ❓ Why do this?
> ■ It reduces perioperative myocardial infarction and cardiac death [A][110].
>
> **Acadesine reduces perioperative MI and death**
>
> | Patient | Treatment | Comparator | Outcome | CER | OR | NNT |
> |---------|-----------|------------|---------|-----|-----|-----|
> | CABG [A][110] | Acadesine | Placebo | Perioperative MI at 4 days | 4.9% | 0.69 (0.51 to 0.95) | 68 (43 to 430) |
> | | | | Cardiac death at 4 days | 1.3% | 0.52 (0.27 to 0.98) | 120 (78 to 2900) |

Offer spinal cord stimulation surgery to patients with severe angina but at high risk for CABG [A][111].

> ### ❓ Why do this?
> **Spinal cord surgery causes less mortality in surgically high-risk patients than CABG**
>
> | Patient [A][111] | Treatment | Comparator | Outcome | CER | RRR | NNT |
> |------------------|-----------|------------|---------|-----|-----|-----|
> | Severe angina, at high risk for surgery but unsuitable for angioplasty | Spinal cord stimulation surgery | CABG | Death at 6 months | 14% | 86% (−8% to 98%) | 8 (5 to 59) |
>
> ■ Spinal cord stimulation is as effective at controlling symptoms as CABG in patients with severe angina who would only benefit symptomatically from CABG but are at increased risk of surgical complications [A][111].
> ■ Fewer patients given spinal cord stimulation die [A][111].

## PREVENTION

Lower cholesterol levels [A][112], even for patients with average levels (cholesterol 4.0–6.2 mmol/l) [A][113] [A][114].

> ### ❓ Why do this?
> ■ Patients with coronary artery disease who have cholesterol lowering therapy are less likely to die, particularly from heart disease [A][112].
>
> **Lowering cholesterol reduces mortality**
>
> | Patient [A][112] | Treatment | Comparator | Outcome | CER | RRR | NNT |
> |------------------|-----------|------------|---------|-----|-----|-----|
> | Coronary artery disease | Cholesterol lowering therapy | No therapy | Death at >2 years | 10% | 16% (12% to 19%) | 63 (51 to 81) |
> | | | | Death from coronary heart disease at > 2 years | 6.4% | 28% (24% to 32%) | 56 (48 to 67) |
>
> ■ Patients with cholesterol levels <6.2 mmol/l who take pravastatin are less likely to have another MI or die from heart disease, or require invasive therapy [A][112].

using
- diet modification [A][115]: encourage patients to eat less fat [A][116] (particularly cholesterol [A][117]) and more oats [A][118], fish [A][119] and soy protein [B][120]

> **? Why do this?**
> - Diet modification can lower cholesterol levels slightly, but there is no clear effect on blood pressure levels [A][115].
> - Low-fat diets help reduce cholesterol levels [A][116] – on average by 0.6 mmol/1. Triglycerides fall on average by 0.2 mmol/l [A][117].
> - Patients who eat oat products have a small fall in cholesterol levels (0.13 mmol/l; 95% CI: 0.017 to 0.19) [A][118].
> - Eating around 50 g of soy protein a day reduces cholesterol level by roughly 0.6 mmol/l, and triglyceride levels by 0.2 mmol/l [A][119].

- a statin [A][121] [A][122], particularly for patients revascularised following post-infarct angina [A][123]

> **? Why do this?**
> - Statins reduces mortality, particularly from myocardial infarction [A][114].
>
> **Pravastatin reduces MI or invasive therapy in patients with cholesterol levels <6.2 mmol/l**

| Patient | Treatment | Comparator | Outcome | CER | RRR | NNT |
|---|---|---|---|---|---|---|
| MI or unstable angina and cholesterol levels 4.0–7.0 mmol/l [A][114] | Pravastatin | Placebo | Death at 6 years | 14% | 22% (12% to 30%) | 33 (23 to 60) |
| | | | Hospitalisation with unstable angina at 6 years | 25% | 9% (2% to 16%) | 44 (25 to 180) |

> - Patients with cholesterol levels <6 mmol/l and revascularisation following an MI who take pravastatin compared with placebo are less likely to die, have an MI or a stroke [A][123].
>
> **Revascularisation: pravastatin reduces death, MI and stroke with average cholesterol levels**

| Patient | Treatment | Comparator | Outcome | CER | RRR | NNT |
|---|---|---|---|---|---|---|
| Post-MI, cholesterol <6 mmol/l, following PTCA or CABG [A][123] | Pravastatin | Placebo | Death from heart disease or non-fatal MI at 1 year | 12% | 34% (15% to 48%) | 24 (15 to 60) |
| | | | Stroke | 4.1% | 37% (1% to 60%) | 65 (33 to 1800) |

> - Statin therapy becomes more cost-effective as the number of cardiovascular risk factors present increase [A][124] [B][125].

- gemfibrozil for patients with a low HDL level [A][126].

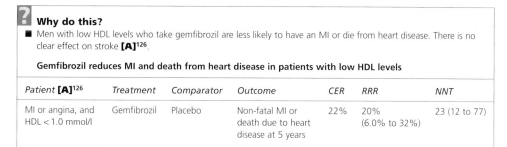

**Why do this?**

■ Men with low HDL levels who take gemfibrozil are less likely to have an MI or die from heart disease. There is no clear effect on stroke [A][126].

**Gemfibrozil reduces MI and death from heart disease in patients with low HDL levels**

| Patient [A][126] | Treatment | Comparator | Outcome | CER | RRR | NNT |
|---|---|---|---|---|---|---|
| MI or angina, and HDL < 1.0 mmol/l | Gemfibrozil | Placebo | Non-fatal MI or death due to heart disease at 5 years | 22% | 20% (6.0% to 32%) | 23 (12 to 77) |

Consider giving patients:
- vitamin E supplements (alpha-tocopherol) [A][127].

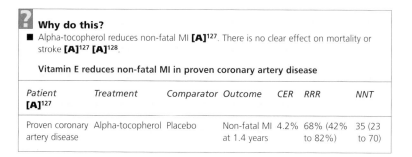

**Why do this?**

■ Alpha-tocopherol reduces non-fatal MI [A][127]. There is no clear effect on mortality or stroke [A][127] [A][128].

**Vitamin E reduces non-fatal MI in proven coronary artery disease**

| Patient [A][127] | Treatment | Comparator | Outcome | CER | RRR | NNT |
|---|---|---|---|---|---|---|
| Proven coronary artery disease | Alpha-tocopherol | Placebo | Non-fatal MI at 1.4 years | 4.2% | 68% (42% to 82%) | 35 (23 to 70) |

There is no clear benefit from:
- giving postmenopausal women oestrogen and progestin [D][129].

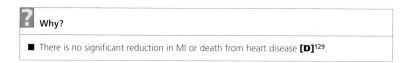

**Why?**

■ There is no significant reduction in MI or death from heart disease [D][129].

Treat hypertension [A][130].

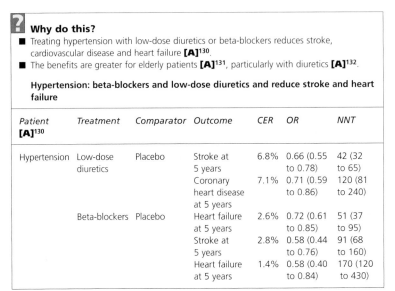

**Why do this?**

- Treating hypertension with low-dose diuretics or beta-blockers reduces stroke, cardiovascular disease and heart failure [A][130].
- The benefits are greater for elderly patients [A][131], particularly with diuretics [A][132].

**Hypertension: beta-blockers and low-dose diuretics and reduce stroke and heart failure**

| Patient [A][130] | Treatment | Comparator | Outcome | CER | OR | NNT |
|---|---|---|---|---|---|---|
| Hypertension | Low-dose diuretics | Placebo | Stroke at 5 years | 6.8% | 0.66 (0.55 to 0.78) | 42 (32 to 65) |
| | | | Coronary heart disease at 5 years | 7.1% | 0.71 (0.59 to 0.86) | 120 (81 to 240) |
| | Beta-blockers | Placebo | Heart failure at 5 years | 2.6% | 0.72 (0.61 to 0.85) | 51 (37 to 95) |
| | | | Stroke at 5 years | 2.8% | 0.58 (0.44 to 0.76) | 91 (68 to 160) |
| | | | Heart failure at 5 years | 1.4% | 0.58 (0.40 to 0.84) | 170 (120 to 430) |

Encourage patients to stop smoking [A][133] [A][134], and ask nurses [A][135] and other staff [C][136] to provide further advice.

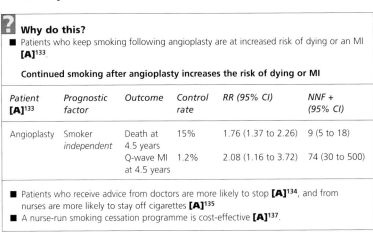

**Why do this?**

- Patients who keep smoking following angioplasty are at increased risk of dying or an MI [A][133].

**Continued smoking after angioplasty increases the risk of dying or MI**

| Patient [A][133] | Prognostic factor | Outcome | Control rate | RR (95% CI) | NNF + (95% CI) |
|---|---|---|---|---|---|
| Angioplasty | Smoker independent | Death at 4.5 years | 15% | 1.76 (1.37 to 2.26) | 9 (5 to 18) |
| | | Q-wave MI at 4.5 years | 1.2% | 2.08 (1.16 to 3.72) | 74 (30 to 500) |

- Patients who receive advice from doctors are more likely to stop [A][134], and from nurses are more likely to stay off cigarettes [A][135]
- A nurse-run smoking cessation programme is cost-effective [A][137].

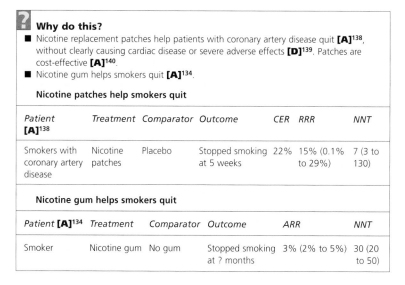

**Why?**

**Physician advice helps patients stop smoking**

| Patient [A]134 | Treatment | Comparator | Outcome | ARR | NNT |
|---|---|---|---|---|---|
| MI | Physician advice | No advice | Stopped smoking at ? months | 36% (23% to 48%) | 3 (2 to 4) |

**Nursing advice helps smokers stop smoking in the long term**

| Patient [A]135 | Treatment | Comparator | Outcome | CER | OR | NNT |
|---|---|---|---|---|---|---|
| Adult smoker | Nursing advice | No advice | Sustained smoking cessation at ? | 13% | 1.43 (1.24 to 1.66) | 22 (15 to 39) |

- Two-thirds of men with an MI who receive repeated advice to stop smoking will quit (63%; 95% CI: 55% to 72%). A sixth will continue smoking at the same rate (15%; 95% CI: 8.9% to 22%) [C]136.

Offer nicotine patches [A]138 or gum [A]134.

**Why do this?**

- Nicotine replacement patches help patients with coronary artery disease quit [A]138, without clearly causing cardiac disease or severe adverse effects [D]139. Patches are cost-effective [A]140.
- Nicotine gum helps smokers quit [A]134.

**Nicotine patches help smokers quit**

| Patient [A]138 | Treatment | Comparator | Outcome | CER | RRR | NNT |
|---|---|---|---|---|---|---|
| Smokers with coronary artery disease | Nicotine patches | Placebo | Stopped smoking at 5 weeks | 22% | 15% (0.1% to 29%) | 7 (3 to 130) |

**Nicotine gum helps smokers quit**

| Patient [A]134 | Treatment | Comparator | Outcome | ARR | NNT |
|---|---|---|---|---|---|
| Smoker | Nicotine gum | No gum | Stopped smoking at ? months | 3% (2% to 5%) | 30 (20 to 50) |

There is no clear benefit from:

- a vigorous exercise programme [D]141

**Why?**

- Women who undergo a vigorous exercise programme are not clearly less likely to stop smoking [D]141.

## PROGNOSIS

Death or an MI are uncommon [A][142–144] [B][145] [B][146], but many will require coronary revascularisation [A][144] [A][147].

> **? Why?**
> - 3% have an MI within 3 weeks (95% CI: 0.0% to 6.1%) [A][143].
> - 2–6% are dead within 6 weeks [B][145] [B][146].
> - A fifth to a third will require coronary revascularisation within 3 years [A][144] [A][147].
>
> **A clinical prediction rule may help indicate patients at risk of death or infarction**
>
> | [B][148] | Risk group | Intractable angina at discharge | MI at discharge | Death at discharge |
> |---|---|---|---|---|
> | Ia | Acceleration of previously chronic stable angina without new ECG changes | 0.0% | 2.7% | 0.0% |
> | Ib | Acceleration of previously chronic stable angina with new ECG changes | 3.5% | 5.6% | 0.0% |
> | II | Exertional angina of new onset | 3.9% | 5.7% | 0.0% |
> | III | New-onset resting angina | 11% | 8.8% | 1.5% |
> | IV | Protracted chest pain > 20 min duration per episode with persistent abnormalities of subendocardial ischaemia | 19% | 18% | 6.4% |

Patients are at increased risk of dying, having an MI or requiring revascularisation with:

- male sex [A][144]
- increasing age [A][142] [B][145]
- diabetes mellitus [A][142]

> **? Why?**
> **Male sex, increasing age and diabetes increase the risk of dying or infarction**
>
> | Patient | Prognostic factor | Outcome | Control rate | OR (95% CI) | NNF + (95% CI) |
> |---|---|---|---|---|---|
> | Unstable angina [A][144] | Male *independent* | Death, MI or revascularisation at 6 months | 42% | 2.7 (1.8 to 4.1) | 10 (6 to 20) |
> | Unstable angina or non-Q wave MI [B][145] | Age ≥ 65 years *independent* | Death at 6 weeks | 2.1% | 2.34 (1.11 to 4.96) | 38 (14 to 450) |
> | Unstable angina [A][142] | Diabetes mellitus *independent* | Death or MI at 6 months | 7.6% | 2.19 (1.25 to 3.83) | 13 (6 to 58) |

- an MI within the previous 14 days **[A]**[142] or angina at rest within the previous 48 h **[A]**[144]

---

**?** **Why?**
Recent angina at rest or a myocardial infarction increases the risk of dying or infarction

| Patient | Prognostic factor | Outcome | Control rate | OR (95% CI) | NNF + (95% CI) |
|---|---|---|---|---|---|
| Unstable angina **[A]**[142] | MI within last 14 days *independent* | Death or MI at 6 months | 7.6% | 5.72 (1.92 to 16.97) | 4 (2 to 16) |
| Unstable angina **[A]**[144] | Angina at rest in the previous 48 h *independent* | Death, MI or revascularisation at 6 months | 42% | 3 (2.1 to 4.3) | 9 (6 to 15) |

---

- ST depression on ECG **[A]**[142] **[A]**[149] **[B]**[150], particularly within 24 h of admission **[B]**[145]
- elevated troponin T **[A]**[143] **[A]**[147] **[B]**[146]

---

**?** **Why?**
ST depression and old age increase the risk of dying

| Patient | Prognostic factor | Outcome | Control rate | OR (95% CI) | NNF + (95% CI) |
|---|---|---|---|---|---|
| Unstable angina **[A]**[142] | Baseline ST depression *independent* | Death or MI at 6 months | 7.6% | 2.81 (1.45 to 5.47) | 9 (4 to 33) |

Elevated troponin T increases the risk of an MI

| Patient | Prognostic factor | Outcome | Control rate | RR (95% CI) | NNF + (95% CI) |
|---|---|---|---|---|---|
| Unstable angina **[A]**[143] | Elsevated troponin T *independent* | MI at 3 weeks | 2.9% | 14 (3.4 to 58) | 3 (1 to 14) |

Elevated troponin T increases the risk of requiring coronary revascularisation

| Patient | Prognostic factor | Outcome | Control rate | OR (95% CI) | NNF + (95% CI) |
|---|---|---|---|---|---|
| Unstable angina **[A]**[147] | Elevated troponin T within 24 h *independent* | Coronary revascularisation at 3 years | 22% | 3.18 (1.37 to 7.37) | 4 (2 to 17) |

---

**Note**
■ Elevated troponin I is not clearly associated with increased mortality **[B]**[145].

- requirement for iv nitrates on admission [A][142]
- not on a beta-blocker or rate-lowering calcium-channel blocker [A][142].

## Why?

**Need for iv nitrates and no beta-blocker or calcium-channel blocker medication increases the risk of dying**

| Patient | Prognostic factor | Outcome | Control rate | OR (95% CI) | NNF + (95% CI) |
|---|---|---|---|---|---|
| Unstable angina [A][144] | Requiring iv nitrates | Death or MI at 6 months | 42% | 2.1 (1.5 to 3.1) | 15 (8 to 31) |
| | No beta-blocker or rate-lowering calcium-channel blocker | | 7.6% | 3.83 (1.55 to 9.42) | 6 (3 to 27) |

**Guideline writers:** Christopher Ball, Nick Shenker
**CAT writers:** Nick Shenker, Clare Wotton, Christopher Ball, Robert Phillips

## REFERENCES

| No | Level | Citation |
|---|---|---|
| 1 | 1b | Solomon CG et al. Comparison of clinical presentation of acute myocardial infarction in patients older than 65 years of age to younger patients: the multicenter chest pain study experience. Am J Cardiol 1989; 63: 772–6 |
| 2 | 1b | Lee TH et al. Acute chest pain in the emergency room: identification and examination of low-risk patients. Arch Intern Med 1985; 145: 65–9 |
| 3 | 2a | Diamond GA Forrester JS. Analysis of probability as an aid in the clinical diagnosis of coronary-artery disease. N Engl J Med 1979; 300: 1350–8 |
| 4 | 1a | Goldman L et al. A computer protocol to predict myocardial infarction in emergency department patients with chest pain. N Engl J Med 1988; 318: 797–803 |
| 5 | 2a | Panju AA et al. Is this patient having a myocardial infarction? JAMA 1998; 280: 1256–63 |
| 6 | 2b | Tierney WM et al. Physicians' estimates of the probability of myocardial infarction in the emergency room patient with chest pain. Med Decis Making 1986; 6: 12–7 |
| 7 | 2b | Zalenski RJ et al. Evaluation of a chest pain diagnostic protocol to exclude acute cardiac ischemia in the emergency department. Arch Intern Med 1997; 157: 1085–91 |
| 8 | 1a | Lee TH, Juarez G, Cook EF et al. Ruling out acute myocardial infarction: prospective multicenter validation of a 12-hour strategy for patients at low risk. N Engl J Med 1991; 324: 1239–46 |
| 9 | 1b – | Gomez MA et al. An emergency department-based protocol for rapidly ruling out myocardial ischaemia decreases hospital time and expense: results of a randomised study (ROMIO). J Am Coll Cardiol 1996; 28: 25–33 |
| 10 | 1b | Roberts RR, Zalenski RJ, Mensah EK et al. Costs of an emergency department-based accelerated diagnostic protocol vs hospitalization in patients with chest pain: a randomized controlled trial. JAMA 1997; 278: 1670–6 |

| No | Level | Citation |
|----|-------|----------|
| 11 | 1a | Goldman L, Cook F, Johnson PA, et al. Prediction of the need for intensive care in patients who come to emergency departments with acute chest pain. New England Journal of Medicine 1996; 334: 1498–1504 |
| 12 | 4 | Berger JP et al. Right arm involvement and pain extension can help to differentiate coronary disease from chest pain of other origin: a prospective emergency ward study of 278 consecutive patients admitted for chest pain. J Intern Med 1990; 227: 165–72 |
| 13 | 1b | Solomon CG et al. Comparison of clinical presentation of actue myocardial infarction in patients older than 65 years of age to younger patients: the multicenter chest pain study experience: Am J Cardiol 1989; 63: 772–6 |
| 14 | 2b | Thomsen SP, Gibbons RJ, Smars PA et al. Incremental value of the leukocyte differential and the creatine kinase-MB isoenzyme for the early diagnosis of myocardial infarction. Ann Intern Med 1995; 122: 335–41 |
| 15 | 4 | de Winter RJ et al. Value of myoglobin, troponin T and CK-MB(mass) in ruling out an acute myocardial infarction in the emergency room. Circulation 1995; 92: 3401–7 |
| 16 | 4 | Zimmerman J, Fromm R, Meyer D et al. Diagnostic Marker Cooperative Study for the diagnosis of myocardial infarction. Circulation 1999; 99: 1671–77 |
| 17 | 1b | Antman EM et al. Evaluation of a rapid bedside assay for detection of serum cardiac troponin T. JAMA 1995; 273: 1279–82 |
| 18 | 2b | Sayre MR et al. Measurement of cardiac troponin T is an effective method for predicting complications among emergency department patients with chest pain. Ann Emerg Med 1998; 31: 539–49 |
| 19 | 4 | Smith AF. Diagnostic value of serum-creatine-kinase in a coronary-care unit. Lancet 1967; (i): 178–182 |
| 20 | 1b | Lee TH, Rouan GW, Weisberg MC et al. Sensitivity of routine clinical criteria for diagnosing myocardial infarction within 24 hours of hospitalization. Ann Intern Med 1987; 106: 181–6 |
| 21 | 1b | Jayes RL, Larsen GC, Beshansky JR et al. Physician electrocardiogram reading in the emergency department. Accuracy and effect on triage decisions: findings from a multicenter study. J Gen Intern Med 1992; 7: 387–92 |
| 22 | 1b | Fesmire FM et al. Usefulness of automated serial 12-lead ECG monitoring during initial emergency department evaluation of patients with chest pain. Ann Emerg Med 1998; 31: 3–11 |
| 23 | 4 | Stark JL, Vacek JL. The initial electrocardiogram during admission for myocardial infarction: use as a predictor of clinical course and facility utilization. Arch Intern Med 1987; 147: 843–6 |
| 24 | 1b | Froelicher VF et al. The electrocardiographic exercise test in a population with reduced workup bias: diagnostic performance, computerized interpretation and multivariate prediction. Ann Intern Med 1998; 128: 965–74 |
| 25 | 1a | Fleischmann KE, Hunink MGM, Kuntz KM et al. Exercise echocardiography or exercise SPECT imaging? A meta-analysis of diagnostic test performance. JAMA 1998; 280: 913–920 |
| 26 | 1a | Khattar RS. Assessment of myocardial perfusion and contractile dysfunction by inotropic stress Tc-99 m SPECT imaging and echocardiography for optimal detection of multivessel coronary artery disease. Heart 1998; 79: 274–280 |

| No | Level | Citation |
| --- | --- | --- |
| 27 | 1b | Garber AM. Solomon NA. Cost-effectiveness of alternative test strategies for the diagnosis of coronary artery disease. Ann Intern Med 1999; 130: 719–28 |
| 28 | 1b – | Boden WE et al. Outcomes in patients with acute non-G wave myocardial infarction randomly assigned to an invasive as compared with a conservative management strategy. N Engl J Med 1998; 338: 1785–92 |
| 29 | 2c | Yusuf S et al. Variations between countries in invasive cardiac procedures and outcomes in patients with suspected unstable angina or myocardial infarction without initial ST elevation. Lancet 1998; 352: 507–14 |
| 30 | 4 | Bar FW et al. Coronary angiographic findings do not predict clinical outcome in patients with unstable angina. J Am Coll Cardiol 1994; 24: 1453–9 |
| 31 | 1b – | Farkouh ME, Smars PA, Reeder GS et al. A clinical trial of a chest-pain observation unit for patients with unstable angina. N Engl J Med 1998; 339: 1882–8 |
| 32 | 1b – | Rogers WJ et al. Asymptomatic cardiac ischemia pilot (ACIP) study: outcome at 1 year for patients with asymptomatic cardiac ischemia randomised to medical therapy or revascularization. J Am Coll Cardiol 1995; 26: 594–605 |
| 33 | 1a | Antiplatelet Trialists' Collaboration. Collaborative overview of randomised trials of antiplatelet therapy I: Prevention of death, MI and stroke by prolonged antiplatelet therapy in various categories of patients. BMJ 1994; 308: 81–106 |
| 34 | 1b | RISC group. Risk of myocardial infarction and death during treatment with low dose aspirin and intravenous heparin in men with unstable coronary artery disease: Lancet 1990; 336: 827–30 |
| 35 | 1b | Balsano F, Rizzon P, Violi F et al. Antiplatelet treatment with ticlopidine in unstable angina: a controlled multicenter clinical trial. Circulation 1990; 82: 17–26 |
| 36 | 1b | Gent M, Blakely JA, Easton JD et al. The Canadian American ticlopidine study (CATS) in thromboembolic stroke. Lancet 1989; (i): 1215–1220 |
| 37 | 1b | Hass WK, Easton JD, Adams HP et al. A randomized trial comparing ticlopidine hydrochloride with aspirin for the prevention of stroke in high-risk patients. N Engl J Med 1989; 321: 501–7 |
| 38 | 1b | Theroux P et al. Aspirin versus heparin to prevent myocardial infarction during the acute phase of unstable angina. Circulation 1993; 88: 2045–8 |
| 39 | 1b | Aspirin plus low-molecular-weight heparin was effective for unstable angina: ACP J Club 1996 Mar–Apr; 124:39. Summary of Gurfinkel EP et al. Low molecular weight heparin versus regular heparin or aspirin in the treatment of unstable angina and silent ischaemia. J Am Coll Cardiol 1995; 26: 313–8 |
| 40 | 1b | Cohen M et al. A comparison of low-molecular weight heparin with unfractionated heparin for unstable coronary disease. N Engl J Med 1997; 337: 447–52 |
| 41 | 1b | Antman EM, McCabe CH, Gurfinkel EP et al. Enoxaparin prevents death and cardiac ischemic events in unstable angina/non-Q-wave myocardial infarction: results of the Thrombolysis in Myocardial Infarction (TIMI) IIB trial. Circulation 1999; 100: 1593–1601 |
| 42 | 1b | Low-molecular-weight heparin prevented new cardiac events unstable angina. ACP J Club 1996 July-Aug) 125:1 Summary of Fragmin during instability in Coronary Artery Disease (FRISC) Study Group Low molecular weight during instability in coronary artery disease. Lancet 1996; 347: 561–8 |

| No | Level | Citation |
|---|---|---|
| 43 | 1b | Mark DB, Cowper PA, Berkowitz SD et al. Economic assessment of low-molecular-weight heparin (enoxaparin) versus unfractionated heparin in acute coronary syndrome patients: results from the ESSENCE randomized trial. Circulation 1998; 97: 1702–7 |
| 44 | 1b | Discontinuation of heparin in patients with angina. ACP J Club 1993 Jan. Feb; 118:5. Summary of Theroux P et al. Reactivation of unstable angina after the discontinuation of heparin. N Engl J Med 1993; 327: 141–5 |
| 45 | 1b | Organisation to Assess Strategies for Ischaemic Syndromes (OASIS-2) Investigators. Effects of recombinant hirudin (lepirudin) compared with heparin on death, myocardial infarction, refractory angina, and revascularisation procedures in patients with acute myocardial ischaemia without ST elevation: a randomised trial. Lancet 1999; 353: 429–38 |
| 46 | 1b | GUSTO-IIb Investigators. A comparison of recombinant hirudin with heparin for the treatment of acute coronary syndromes. N Engl J Med 1996; 335: 775–82 |
| 47 | 1a − | Oler A et al. Adding heparin to aspirin reduces the incidence of myocardial infarction in patients with unstable angina: a meta-analysis. JAMA 1996; 276: 811–15 |
| 48 | 1b | The PURSUIT Trial Investigators. Inhibition of platelet glycoprotein IIb/IIIa with eptifibatide in patients with acute coronary syndromes. N Engl J Med 1998; 339: 436–43 |
| 49 | 1b | The Platelet Receptor Inhibition in Ischemic Syndrome Management in Patients Limited by Unstable Signs and Symptoms (PRISM-PLUS) Study Investigators. Inhibition of the platelet glycoprotein IIb/IIIa receptor with tirofiban in unstable angina and non-Q-wave myocardial infarction. N Engl J Med 1998; 338: 1488–97 |
| 50 | 1b | The Platelet Receptor Inhibition in Ischemic Syndrome Management (PRISM) study investigators: a comparison of aspirin plus tirofiban with aspirin plus heparin for unstable angina. N Engl J Med 1998; 1498–505 |
| 51 | 1b | Anand SS, Yusuf S, Pogue J et al. Long-term oral anticoagulant therapy in patients with unstable angina or suspected non-Q-wave myocardial infarction: organization to assess strategies for ischemic syndromes (OASIS) pilot study results. Circulation 1998; 98: 1064–70 |
| 52 | 1b | Karlberg KK et al. Intravenous nitroglycerin reduces ischaemia in unstable angina pectoris: a double-blind placebo-controlled trial. J Intern Med 1998; 243: 25–31 |
| 53 | 1b | Dellborg M et al. Buccal versus intravenous nitroglycerin in unstable angina pectoris. Eur J Clin Pharmacol 1991; 41: 5–9 |
| 54 | 1b | Ardissino D et al. Effect of transdermal nitroglycerin or N-acetylcysteine, or both, in the long-term treatment of unstable angina pectoris. J Am Coll Cardiol 1997; 29: 941–7 |
| 55 | 1b | HINT Research Group. Early treatment of unstable angina in the CCU: a randomised, double-blind, placebo controlled comparison of recurrent ischaemia in patients treated with nifedipine or metoprolol or both. Br Heart J 1986; 56: 400–13 |
| 56 | 1a | Held PH et al. Calcium channel blockers in acute myocardial infarction and unstable angina: an overview. BMJ 1989; 299: 1187–92 |
| 57 | 1a | Yusuf S et al. Update of effects of calcium antagonists in myocardial infarction or angina in light of the second Danish Verapamil Infarction Trial (DAVIT-II) and other recent studies. Am J Cardiol 1991; 67: 1295–7 |
| 58 | 1a | Pepine CJ, Faich G, Makuch R. Verapamil use in patients with cardiovascular disease: an overview of randomized trials. Clin Cardiol 1998; 21: 633–41 |
| 59 | 1b − | Theroux P et al. A randomised study comparing propranolol and diltiazem in the treatment of unstable angina. J Am Coll Cardiol 1985; 5: 717–22 |

| No | Level | Citation |
|----|-------|----------|
| 60 | 1b | Gobel EJ et al. Randomised double-blind trial of intravenous diltiazem versus glyceryl trinitrate for unstable angina pectoris. Lancet 1995; 346: 1653–57 |
| 61 | 1a | Heidenreich PA, McDonald KM, Hastie T et al. Meta-analysis of trials comparing β-blockers, calcium antagonists, and nitrates for stable angina. JAMA 1999; 281: 1927–1936 |
| 62 | 1b – | Andre-Fouet X et al. Comparision of short-term efficacy of diltiazem and propranolol in unstable angina at rest: a randomised trial in 70 patients. Euro Heart 1983; 4(10): 691–8 |
| 63 | 1b | Braun S et al. Calcium channel blocking agents and risk of cancer in patients with coronary artery disease. J Am Coll Cardiol 1998; 31: 804–8 |
| 64 | 3b | Rosenberg L et al. Calcium channel blockers and the risk of cancer. JAMA 1998; 279: 1000–4 |
| 65 | 2a | Furberg CD et al. Nifedipine: dose-related increase in mortality in patients with coronary heart disease: Circulation 1995; 92: 1326–1331 |
| 66 | 1b | Gerstenblith G et al. Nifedipine in unstable angina: a double-blind randomised controlled trial. N Engl J Med 1982; 306: 885–9 |
| 67 | 1b | Gottlieb SO et al. Effect of the addition of propranolol to therapy with nifedipine for unstable angina pectoris: a randomised double-blind, placebo-controlled trial. Circulation 1986; 73: 331 |
| 68 | 1b | Simoons ML et al. Randomised trial of GPIIb/IIIa platelet receptor blocker in refractory unstable angina. Circulation 1994; 89: 596–603 |
| 69 | 1b | Patel DJ et al. Cardioprotection by opening of the $K_{ATP}$ channel in unstable angina. Is this a clinical manifestation of myocardial preconditioning? Results of a randomized study with nicorandil. Eur Heart J 1999; 20: 51–7 |
| 70 | 1b | Olausson K et al. Anti-ischemic and anti-anginal effects of thoracic epidural anesthesia versus those of conventional medical therapy in the treatment of severe refractory unstable angina pectoris. Circulation 1997; 96: 2178–82 |
| 71 | 2b | Horowitz JD et al. Combined use of nitroglycerin and N-acetylcysteine in the management of unstable angina pectoris. Circulation 1988; 77: 787–94 |
| 72 | 1b | TIMI III-B Investigators. Effects of tissue plasminogen activator and a comparison of early invasive and conservative strategies in unstable angina and non-Q-wave myocardial infarction. Results of the TIMI III-B Trial. Circulation 1994; 89: 1545–56 |
| 73 | 1b | Anderson HV et al. One-year results of the thrombolysis in myocardial infarction (TIMI) IIIb trial: a randomised comparison of tissue-type plasminogen activator versus placebo and early invasive versus early conservative strategies in unstable angina and non-Q wave myocardial infarction. J Am Coll Cardiol 1995; 26: 1643–50 |
| 74 | 2a | de Feyter P J, Keane D, Deckers J W et al. Medium and long-term outcome after coronary balloon angioplasty. Progress in Cardiovascular Diseases (1994) 36(5): 385–396 |
| 75 | 1b | RITA participants. Coronary angioplasty versus medical therapy for angina: the second randomised intervention treatment for angina (RITA-2). Lancet 1997; 350: 461–8 |
| 76 | 1a | Kimmel SE, Berlin JA, Strom BL et al. Development and validation of a simplified predictive index for major complications in contemporary percutaneous transluminal coronary angioplasty practice. J Am Coll Cardiol 1995; 26: 931–8 |

| No | Level | Citation |
|---|---|---|
| 77 | 2b | Coronary restenosis was greater in diabetic patients than in nondiabetic patients after atherectomy but not after angioplasty. ACP J Club 1997 Sep. Oct; 127: 33. Levine GN, Jacobs AK, Keeler GP et al. for the CAVEAT-I Investigators. Impact of diabetes mellitus on percutaneous revascularization (CAVEAT-I). Am J Cardiol 1997; 79: 748–55 |
| 78 | 3b | de Feyter PJ, van den Brand M, Jaarman G et al. Acute coronary artery occlusion during and after percutaneous transluminal coronary angioplasty: frequency, prediction, clinical course, management, and follow-up. Circulation 1991; 83: 927–36 |
| 79 | 1a | Moscucci M, O'Connor GT, Ellis SG et al. Validation of risk adjustment models for in-hospital percutaneous transluminal coronary angioplasty mortality on an independent data set. Am Coll Cardiol 1999; 34: 692–7 |
| 80 | 1b | EPISTENT investigators. Randomised placebo-controlled and balloon-angioplasty-controlled trial to assess safety of coronary stenting with use of platelet glycoprotein-IIb/IIIa blockage. Lancet 1998; 352: 87–92 |
| 81 | 1b | The CAPTURE Investigators. Randomised placebo-controlled trial of abciximab before and during coronary intervention in refractory unstable angina: the CAPTURE study. Lancet 1997; 349: 1429–35 |
| 82 | 1b | Lincoff AM, Tcheng JE, Califf RM et al. Sustained suppression of ischemic complications of coronary intervention by platelet GP IIb/IIIa blockade with abciximab: one-year outcome in the EPILOG trial. Circulation 1999; 99: 1951–8 |
| 83 | 1b | The EPIC Investigators. Use of a monoclonal antibody directed against the platelet protein IIb/IIIa receptor in high-risk coronary angioplasty. N Eng J Med 1994; 330: 956–961 |
| 84 | 1b | Lincoff A-M, Califf RM, Moliterno DJ et al. Complementary clinical benefits of coronary-artery stenting and blockade of platelet glycoprotein IIb/IIIa receptors. N Eng J Med 1999; 341: 319–27 |
| 85 | 1b | Stent implantation reduced repeat angioplasty at 1 year in patients with stable angina. Evidence-Based Med 1996 July Aug; 1: 137. Macaya C, Serruys PW, Ruygrok P et al. for the Benestent Study Group. Continued benefit of coronary stenting versus balloon angioplasty: one-year clinical follow-up of Benestent trial. J Am Coll Cardiol 1996; 27: 255–61 |
| 86 | 1b | Benefit-risk trade-off was found for stent vs. balloon coronary angioplasty. ACP J Club 1995 Jan. Feb; 122:11. Serruys PW, de Jaegere P, Kiemeneij F et al. A comparison of balloon-expandable-stent implantation with balloon angioplasty in patients with coronary artery disease. N Engl J Med 1994; 331: 489–95 |
| 87 | 1b | Benefit-risk trade-off was found for stent vs. balloon coronary angioplasty. ACP J Club. 1995 Jan. Feb;122:10. Fischman DL, Leon MB, Baim DS et al. A randomized comparison of coronary-stent placement and balloon angioplasty in the treatment of coronary artery disease. N Engl J Med 1994; 331: 496–501 |
| 88 | 1b | Sievert H, Rohde S, Utech A et al. Stent or angioplasty after recanalization of chronic coronary occlusions? (The SARECCO Trial). Am J Cardiol 1999; 84: 386–90 |
| 89 | 1b | Stenting improves clinical outcomes in patients with isolated stenosis. ACP J Club 1997 Sep. Oct; 127: 32. Summary of Versaci F, Gaspardone A, Tomai F et al. A comparison of coronary-artery stenting with angioplasty for isolated stenosis of the proximal left anterior descending coronary artery. N Engl J Med 1997; 336: 817–22 |
| 90 | 1b | Rubartelli P, Niccoli L, Verna E et al. Stent implantation versus balloon angioplasty in chronic coronary occlusions: results from the GISSOC trial. J Am Coll Cardiol 1998; 32: 90–6 |

| No | Level | Citation |
|----|-------|----------|
| 91 | 1b | Hoher M, Wohrle J, Grebe OC et al. A randomized trial of elective stenting after balloon recanalization of chronic total occlusions. J Am Coll Cardiol 1999; 34: 722–9 |
| 92 | 1b | Sirnes PA, Golf S, Myreng Y et al. Stenting in chronic coronary occlusion (SICCO): a randomized, controlled trial of adding stent implantation after successful angioplasty. J Am Coll Cardiol 1996; 28: 1444–51 |
| 93 | 1b | Savage MP, Douglas JS, Fischman DL et al. Stent placement compared with balloon angioplasty for obstructed coronary bypass grafts. N Eng J Med 1997; 337: 740–7 |
| 94 | 1b | Antiplatelet therapy was better than anticoagulant therapy after coronary stenting. ACP J Club 1997 Jul. Aug; 127: 4. Schömig A, Neumann FJ, Walter H et al. Coronary stent placement in patients with acute myocardial infarction: comparison of clinical and angiographic outcome after randomization to antiplatelet or anticoagulant therapy. J Am Coll Cardiol 1997 29: 28–34 |
| 95 | 1b | Antiplatelet therapy reduced cardiac and noncardiac events after placement of coronary artery stents. ACP J Club 1996 Sep. Oct; 125: 31. Schömig A, Neumann FJ, Kastrati A et al. A randomized comparison of antiplatelet and anticoagulant therapy after the placement of coronary-artery stents. N Engl J Med 1996; 334: 1084–9 |
| 96 | 1b – | Hall P et al. A randomised comparison of combined ticlopidine and aspirin therapy versus aspirin therapy alone after successful intravascular ultrasound-guided stent implantation. Circulation 1996; 93: 215–22 |
| 97 | 1b | Gent M, Blakely JA, Easton JD et al. The Canadian American ticlopidine study (CATS) in thromboembolic stroke. Lancet 1989; (i): 1215–1220 |
| 98 | 1b | Hass WK, Easton JD, Adams HP, et al: A randomized trial comparing ticlopidine hydrochloride with aspirin for the prevention of stroke in high-risk patients. New England Journal of Medicine 1989; 321: 501–507 |
| 99 | 1b | Tardif JC et al. Probucol and multivitamins in the prevention of restenosis after coronary angioplasty. N Engl J Med 1997; 337: 365–72 |
| 100 | 1b | Topol EJ, Leya F, Pinkerton CA et al. A comparison of directional atherectomy with coronary angioplasty in patients with coronary artery disease. N Eng J Med 1993; 329: 221–7 |
| 101 | 1b – | Boden WE et al. Outcomes in patients with acute non-G wave myocardial infarction randomly assigned to an invasive as compared with a conservative mangement strategy. N Engl J Med 1998; 338: 1785–92 |
| 102 | 1a | Early coronary bypass graft surgery lowers mortality. ACP J Club 1995 Mar. April; 122: 29. Summary of Yusuf S, Zucker D, Peduzzi R et al. Effect of coronary artery bypass graft surgery on survival: overview of 10-year results from randomised trials by the Coronary Artery Bypass Graft Surgery Trialists Collaboration. Lancet 1994; 344: 563–70 |
| 103 | 1b | Lughi RJ et al. Comparison of medical and surgical treatment for unstable angina pectoris: results of a Veterans Administration Cooperative Study. N Engl J Med 1987; 316: 977–84 |
| 104 | 1b | Parisi AF et al. Medical compared with surgical management of unstable angina: 5 year mortality and morbidity study in the Veterans Administration Study. Circulation 1989; 89: 1176–89 |
| 105 | 1b | Sharma GV et al. Identification of unstable angina patients who have favorable outcome with medical or surgical therapy (eight-year follow-up of the Veterans Administration Co-operative Study). Am J Cardiol 1994; 74: 454–8 |

| No | Level | Citation |
|----|-------|----------|
| 106 | 1a | Sim I et al. A meta-analysis of randomised trials comparing coronary artery bypass grafting with percutaneous transluminal coronary angioplasty in multivessel coronary artery disease. Am J Cardiol 1995; 76: 1025–9 |
| 107 | 1a | CABG leads to less angina and less reintervention than PTCA, but mortality and subsequent MI are the same. ACP J Club 1996 Mar. April; 124: 43. Evidence-Based Med 1996 Mar. April; 1: 84. Summary of Pocock SJ, Henderson RA, Rickards AF et al. Meta-analysis of randomised trials comparing coronary angioplasty with bypass surgery. Lancet 1995; 346: 1184–9 |
| 108 | 1b | Bypass surgery and angioplasty led to similar 5-year mortality rates in multivessel coronary artery disease. ACP J Club 1997 Jan. Feb; 126: 12. Evidence-Based Med 1997 Jan. Feb;2:21. Summary of the Bypass Angioplasty Revascularization Investigation (BARI) Investigators. Comparison of coronary bypass surgery with angioplasty in patients with multivessel disease. N Engl J Med 1996; 335: 217–25 |
| 109 | 1b | The 5-year cost of coronary angioplasty was lower than that of bypass surgery only in patients with 2-vessel coronary disease. ACP J Club 1997 Jul. Aug; 127: 25. Summary of Hlatky MA, Rogers WJ, Johnstone I, et al., for the Bypass Angioplasty Revascularization Investigation (BARI) Investigators. Medical care costs and quality of life after randomization to coronary angioplasty or coronary bypass surgery. N Engl J Med 1997; 336: 92–9. |
| 110 | 1b | Mangano DT et al. Effects of acadesine on myocardial infarction, stroke and death following surgery: a meta-analysis of 5 international randomized trials. JAMA 1996; 277: 325–32 |
| 111 | 1b | Mannheimer C et al. Electrical stimulation versus coronary artery bypass surgery in severe angina pectoris: the ESBY study. Circulation 1998; 97: 1157–63 |
| 112 | 1a | Gould AL, Rossouw JE, Santanello NC et al. Cholesterol reduction yields clinical benefit: impact of statin trials. Circulation 1998; 97: 946–52 |
| 113 | 1b | Sacks FM et al. The effect of pravastatin on coronary events after myocardial infarction in patients with average cholesterol levels. N Engl J Med 1996; 335: 1001–9 |
| 114 | 1b | The Long-term Intervention with Pravastatin in Ischaemic Disease (LIPID) Study Group. Prevention of cardiovascular events and death with pravastatin in patients with coronary heart disease and a broad range of initial cholesterol levels. N Engl J Med 1998; 339: 1349–57 |
| 115 | 1a | Brunner E, White I, Thorogood M et al. Can dietary interventions change diet and cardiovascular risk factors? A meta-analysis of randomized controlled trials. Am J Public Health 1997; 87: 1415–22 |
| 116 | 1a | Tang JL, Armitage JM, Lancaster T et al. Systematic review of dietary intervention trials to lower blood cholesterol in free-living subjects. BMJ 1998; 316: 1213–20 |
| 117 | 1a | Yu-Poth S, Zhao G, Etherton T et al. Effects of the national cholesterol education program's step I and step II dietary intervention programs on cardiovascular disease risk factors: a meta-analysis. Am J Clin Nutr 1999; 69: 632–46 |
| 118 | 1a | Ripsin CM, Keenan JM, Jacobs DR et al. Oat products and lipid lowering: a meta-analysis. JAMA 1992; 267: 3317–25 |
| 119 | 1b | Burr ML, Fehily AM, Gilbert JF et al. Effects of changes in fat, fish and fibre intakes on death and myocardial infarction: diet and reinfarction trial (DART). Lancet 1989; ii: 757–761 |
| 120 | 2a | Anderson JW, Johnstone BM, Cook-Newall ME. Meta-analysis of the effects of soy protein intake on serum lipids. N Engl J Med 1995; 333: 276–82 |
| 121 | 1a | Rembold CM. Number-needed-to-treat analysis of the prevention of myocardial infarction and death by antidyslipidemic therapy. J Fam Pract 1996; 42: 577–86 |

| No | Level | Citation |
|----|-------|----------|
| 122 | 1a | Ross SD, Allen IE, Connelly JE et al. Clinical outcomes in statin trials. Arch Inten Med 1999; 159: 1793–802 |
| 123 | 1b | Flaker GC, Warnica JW, Sacks FM et al. Pravastatin prevents clinical events in revascularized patients with average cholesterol concentrations. J Am Coll Cardiol 1999; 34: 106–12 |
| 124 | 1b | Johannesson M, Jonsson B, Kjekshus J et al. Cost effectiveness of simvastatin treatment to lower cholesterol levels in patients with coronary heart disease. N Engl J Med 1997; 336: 332–6 |
| 125 | 2b | Pharoah PDP, Hollingworth W. Cost effectiveness of lowering cholesterol concentration with statins in patients with and without pre-existing coronary heart disease: life table method applied to a health authority population. BMJ 1996; 312: 1443–8 |
| 126 | 1b | Rubins HB, Robins SJ, Collins D et al. Gemfibrozil for the secondary prevention of coronary heart disease in men with low levels of high-density lipoprotein cholesterol. N Engl J Med 1999; 341: 410–18 |
| 127 | 1b | Stephens NG, Parsons A, Schofield PM et al. Randomised controlled trial of vitamin E in patients with coronary disease: Cambridge Heart Antioxidant Study (CHAOS). Lancet 1996; 347: 781–6 |
| 128 | 1b | GISSI-Prevenzione Investigators. Dietary supplementation with n-3 polyunsaturated fatty acids and vitamin E after myocardial infarction: results of the GISSI-Prevenzione trial. Lancet 1999; 354: 447–55 |
| 129 | 1b – | Hulley S, Grady D, Bush T et al. Randomized trial of estrogen plus progestin for secondary prevention of coronary heart disease in postmenopausal women. JAMA 1998; 280: 605–13 |
| 130 | 1a | Psaty BM, Smith NL, Siscovick DS et al. Health outcomes associated with antihypertensive therapies used as first-line agents: a systematic review and meta-analysis. JAMA 1997; 277: 739–45 |
| 131 | 1a | Mulrow CD, Cornell JA, Herrera CR et al. Hypertension in the elderly; implications and generalizability of randomized trials. JAMA 1994; 272: 1932–8 |
| 132 | 1a | Messerli FH, Grossman E, Goldbourt U. Are β-blockers efficacious as first-line therapy for hypertension in the elderly? A systematic review. JAMA 1998; 279: 1903–7 |
| 133 | 1b | Smoking increased the risk for death and MI after percutaneous revascularization. ACP J Club 1997 Sep. Oct; 127: 52. Evidence-Based Med 1997 Sep. Oct; 2: 157. Summary of Hasdai D, Garratt KN, Grill DE, Lerman A, Holmes DR Jr. Effect of smoking status on the long-term outcome after successful percutaneous coronary revascularization. N Engl J Med 1997; 336: 755–61 |
| 134 | 1a | Law M, and Tang JL. An analysis of the effectiveness of interventions intended to help people stop smoking. Archives of Internal Medicine 1995; 155: 1933–1941 |
| 135 | 1a | Rice VH, and Stead LF. Nursing interventions for smoking cessation (Cochrance Review). The Cochrane Library, Issue 3. Oxford: Update Software 1999; 3 |
| 136 | 2c | Burt A, Thornley P, Illingworth D, et al. Stopping smoking after myocardial infarction. Lancet 1974; 304–306 |
| 137 | 1b | Krumholz HM, Cohen BJ, Tsevat J et al. Cost-effectiveness of a smoking cessation program after myocardial infarction. J Am Coll Cardiol 1993; 22: 1697–702 |
| 138 | 1b | Working Group for the Study of Transdermal Nicotine. Nicotine replacement therapy for patients with coronary artery disease. Arch Intern Med 1994; 154: 989–95 |

| No | Level | Citation |
|---|---|---|
| 139 | 1b- | Joseph AM, Norman SM, Ferry LH et al. The safety of transdermal nicotine as an aid to smoking cessation in patients with cardiac disease. N Engl J Med 1996; 335: 1792–8 |
| 140 | 1b | Stapleton JA, Lowin A, Russell MAH. Prescription of transdermal nicotine patches for smoking cessation in general practice: evaluation of cost-effectiveness. Lancet 1999; 354: 210–15 |
| 141 | 1b- | Marcus BH, Albrecht AE, King TK et al. The efficacy of exercise as an aid for smoking cessation in women: a randomized controlled trial. Arch Intern Med 1999; 159: 1229–34. |
| 142 | 1b | Calvin JE et al. Risk stratification in unstable angina: prospective validation of the Braunwald Classification. JAMA 1995; 273: 136–41 |
| 143 | 1b | Wu A et al. Prognostic value of cardiac troponin T in unstable angina pectoris. Am J Cardiol 1995; 76: 970–2 |
| 144 | 1b | van Miltenburg-van Zijl AJ et al. Incidence and follow-up of Braunwald subgroups in unstable angina pectoris. J Am Coll Cardiol 1995; 25: 1286 |
| 145 | 2b | Antman EM et al. Cardiac-specific troponin I levels to predict the risk of mortality in patients with acute coronary syndromes. N Engl J Med 1996; 335: 1342–9 |
| 146 | 2b | Ohman EM and the GUSTO-IIA Investigators. Cardiac troponin T levels for risk stratification in acute myocardial ischaemia. N Engl J Med 1996; 335: 1333–41 |
| 147 | 1b | Stubb P et al. Prospective study of the role of cardiac troponin T in patients admitted with unstable angina. BMJ 1996; 313: 262–4 |
| 148 | 2a | Rizik DG et al. A new clinical classification for hospital prognosis of unstable angina pectoris. Am J Cardiol 1995; 75: 993–7 |
| 149 | 1b | Moss AJ et al. Detection and significance of myocardial ischemia in stable patients after recovery from an acute coronary event. JAMA 1993; 269: 2379–85 |
| 150 | 2b | Patel DJ et al. Early continuous ST segment monitoring in unstable angina: prognostic value additional to the clinical characteristics and the admission electrocardiogram. Heart 1996; 75: 222–8 |

Be cautious about starting anticoagulation and seek advice if there is [D]:

- known drug hypersensitivity
- cerebral haemorrhage
- acute gastric or duodenal ulceration
- known bleeding diathesis
- uncontrolled severe hypertension
- injuries or recent surgery to eyes, ears or central nervous system
- severely disturbed liver or renal function.

## LOW-MOLECULAR-WEIGHT HEPARIN

### Indications
Use LMWH rather than heparin for the following conditions:

**Why?**
- It has a more predictable dose-response [D].
- No monitoring is required [D].
- It is given subcutaneously, so patients are more mobile and can be discharged sooner or even not admitted [A][1] [A][2].
- It is more cost-effective [A][3] [A][4].
- It is as effective as heparin, and often more so [A][5] [D][6] [D][7] [A][8].
- It causes less bleeding [A][9-11] and thrombocytopenia [A][12].

**LMWH is less likely to cause thrombocytopenia than heparin**

| Patient [A][12] | Treatment | Comparator | Outcome | CER | RRR | NNT |
|---|---|---|---|---|---|---|
| Hip surgery | LMWH for 14 days | Heparin for 14 days | Heparin-induced thrombocytopenia at 5 days | 2.7% | 100% | 37 (22 to 100) |

- unstable angina [A][5] [A][8]
- deep vein thrombosis [A][9-11]
- pulmonary embolism [D][6]
- cardioversion for atrial fibrillation [D][13]

**Why?**

- In unstable angina, LMWH reduces recurrent angina, myocardial infarction, need for revascularisation and death more effectively than heparin, although causes slightly more minor bleeds **[A]**[5] **[A]**[8].

**Angina: LMWH reduces recurrent angina, myocardial infarction and death compared with heparin**

| Patient | Treatment | Comparator | Outcome | CER | RRR | NNT |
|---|---|---|---|---|---|---|
| Unstable angina **[A]**[8] | Enoxaparin | Heparin | Death, MI or recurrent angina at 30 days | 23% | 15% (3% to 26%) | 29 (16 to 160) |
| | | | Revascularisation at 30 days | 32% | 16% (7% to 25%) | 19 (12 to 49) |
| | | | Minor bleed at 30 days | 7.0% | −66% (−108% to −33%) | −21 (−38 to −15) |

- In deep vein thrombosis, LMWH reduces deaths and major bleeds, and is probably as effective as heparin at preventing recurrent venous thromboembolism **[A]**[9–11].
- In pulmonary embolism, tinzaparin or reviparin is as effective as heparin at preventing recurrent venous thromboembolism and death, without clearly increasing the rate of major bleeding **[D]**[6].

**Deep vein thrombosis: LMWH reduces death and major bleeding compared with heparin**

| Patient | Treatment | Comparator | Outcome | CER | OR | NNT |
|---|---|---|---|---|---|---|
| Deep vein thrombosis **[A]**[11] | LMWH | Heparin | Death at 3–6 months | 6.9% | 0.74 (0.57 to 0.98) | 59 (35 to 780) |
| | | | Major bleed at 3 to 6 months | 2.0% | 0.55 (0.34 to 0.89) | 120 (78 to 470) |

- Anticoagulation reduces embolic events following DC cardioversion for atrial fibrillation or flutter **[C]**[13]

**Atrial fibrillation: anticoagulation reduces embolic events following cardioversion**

| Patient | Treatment | Comparator | Outcome | CER | RRR | NNT |
|---|---|---|---|---|---|---|
| Atrial fibrillation undergoing cardioversion **[C]**[13] | Anticoagulation | No anticoagulation | Embolic events at 3 to 6 months | 2.2% | 100% | 45 (25 to 220) |

## LMWH is probably safe to use in pregnant women

 **Why?**
- It does not appear to cross the placenta **[C]**[14].

## Dosing and monitoring

- Use any LMWH: no clinically significant difference between current drugs has been noted **[D]**.
- Dose according to the patient's weight and give subcutaneously **[A]**.
- Monitoring is not required **[D]**.
- Check the platelet count after 5 days. If it is <150 × 10⁹/l, then repeat the test. If true, treat for heparin-induced thrombocytopenia **[A]**[8] **[A]**[12].

**Why?**
- Around 2% of patients on LMWH for 5 days or more develop heparin-induced thrombocytopenia **[A]**[8].
- Heparin-induced thrombocytopenia increases the risk of venous thromboembolism **[A]**[12].

## Complications

### Major bleeds

- Stop LMWH **[A]**.
- Protamine sulphate (1 mg inhibits 100 units of dalteparin). Maximum dose 50 mg by slow iv infusion **[D]**.

**Note**
- Note Fresh-frozen plasma does not reverse the anticoagulant effect of LMWH.

### Minor bleeds
- Stop LMWH **[D]**

**Note**
- Bleeding occurs rarely: around 1% of patients have a major bleed (fall in haemoglobin >2.0 g/dl, need for blood transfusion or intracranial or retroperitoneal bleed) **[A]**[11].

### Heparin-induced thrombocytopenia

- Stop LMWH **[A]**.
- An alternative is danaparoid **[D]**[15].

**Why?**
- Danaparoid may cause less thrombocytopenia than heparin (based on animal studies), and is probably as effective as heparin for treating venous thromboembolism **[D]**[15].

### Other complications

- Subcutaneous haematoma at site of injection **[D]**.
- Osteopenia in prolonged administration **[C]**[16] **[C]**[17].

**Note**
- Women who take heparin during pregnancy have a significant decrease in bone density at the end. Whether the risk is lower for LMWH is unclear **[C]**[16] **[C]**[17].

## HEPARIN

### Indications
Use this if LMWH is not available or is contraindicated.
The indications are the same as those for LMWH.

### Dosing and monitoring

● Give heparin subcutaneously **[A]**[18] using a weight-based regimen **[C]**[19]
(Tables 1 and 2)

**Table 1  Heparin: bolus and first dose**

| Body weight (kg) **[C]**[19] | iv bolus (units) | sc dose (units) |
|---|---|---|
| < 50 | 4000 | 12 500 |
| 50–70 | 5000 | 15 000 |
| >70 | 6000 | 17 500 |

**Table 2  Heparin subcutaneous dosing regimen**

| apTT (s) **[C]**[19] | Adjustment of heparin dose | Time to next aPTT (hours) |
|---|---|---|
| < 50 | One step up | After 6 |
| 50–90 | Same step | After 6 |
| 91–120 | One step down | After 6 |
| > 120 | Withhold heparin therapy, perform aPTT and proceed as follows: | |
| | <50 s: same step | After 6 |
| | 50–90 s: one step down | After 6 |
| | 91–120 s: two steps down | After 6 |
| | >120 s: withhold heparin therapy | After 3 |

Steps: 10 000–12 500–15 000–17 500–21 250–25 000–30 000 units

### ? Why?

■ Subcutaneous heparin reduces recurrence or extension of venous thromboembolism compared with intravenous heparin without clearly affecting the number of major bleeds.

**Subcutaneous heparin prevents more recurrent venous thromboembolism than intravenous heparin**

| Patient **[A]**[18] | Treatment | Comparator | Outcome | CER | OR (95% CI) | NNT (95% CI) |
|---|---|---|---|---|---|---|
| PE or DVT | Subcutaneous heparin | Intravenous heparin | Extension/recurrence of venous thromboembolism at 14 days | 11% | 0.62 (0.39 to 0.98) | 27 (16 to 530) |

If giving heparin intravenously, use a weight-based regimen **[A]**[20] (Table 3).

| Table 3 | Heparin: intravenous dosing regimen |
|---|---|
| aPTT(s) [A][20] | Dose change |
| Initially | 80 unit/kg bolus, then 18 units/kg per hour |
| <1.2 | 80 unit/kg bolus, then increase by 4 units/kg per hour |
| 1.2–1.5 | 80 unit/kg bolus, then increase by 2 units/kg per hour |
| 1.5–2.5 | No change |
| 2.3–3.0 | Decrease rate by 2 units/kg per hour |
| >3.0 | Stop infusion for 1 hour, then decrease rate by 3 units/kg per hour |

**Why?**

- It produces therapeutic levels or higher sooner than the standard method [A][20] without clearly affecting bleeding rates.
- Fewer recurrent DVTs occur [A][20].

**A weight-based regimen reduces recurrent DVT**

| Patient [A][20] | Treatment | Comparator | Outcome | CER | RRR | NNT |
|---|---|---|---|---|---|---|
| Acquiring heparin therapy | Weight-based regimen | Fixed-dose regimen | aPTT ratio > 1.5 at 24 hours | 77% | −25% (−46% to −7%) | 5 (3 to 14) |
| | | | Recurrent DVT | 25% | 80% (14% to 96%) | 5 (3 to 12) |

- Use aPTT to monitor: check the levels 6 h after initial infusion then check daily [B][21].
- Aim for an aPTT ratio of 1.5 to 2.5 [D].

**Note**

- Using an anti-factor Xa heparin assay is probably no better than aPTT for monitoring heparin dosing in patients requiring large amounts of heparin [D][22].
- There is no clear evidence to suggest that patients on iv heparin with subtherapeutic aPTT levels are at increased risk for recurrent venous thromboembolism [A][23].

- Check the platelet count after 5 days. If it is $< 150 \times 10^9/l$, then repeat the test. If true, treat for heparin-induced thrombocytopenia [A][8] [A][12].

**Why?**

- Around 3% of patients on heparin for 5 days or more develop heparin-induced thrombocytopenia [A][8].
- Heparin-induced thrombocytopenia increases the risk of venous thromboembolism [A][12].

## Complications

**Major bleeds**

Major bleeding is uncommon [B][24].

The risk is increased with:

- age > 72 [B][25]
- increasing aPTT levels [A][26].

**Note**
- 16% of patients on heparin will have a minor bleed (95% CI: 14% to 18%) **[B]**[24].
- 6% of patients have a major bleed (95% CI: 4% to 8%) **[B]**[24].

**Old age increases the risk of bleeding on heparin**

| Patient | Prognostic factor | Outcome | Control rate | OR (95% CI) | NNF + (95% CI) |
|---------|-------------------|---------|--------------|-------------|----------------|
| Proximal DVT | Aged > 72 *independent* | Bleed at 10 days | 7.1% | 1.61 (1.03 to 2.53) | 53 (21 to 1100) |

- Stop heparin **[A]**.
- Protamine sulphate. Maximum dose 50 mg by slow iv infusion **[D]**.
- *Note* Fresh-frozen plasma does not reverse the anticoagulant effect of LMWH.

## Minor bleeds

- Stop LMWH **[D]**.

**Note**
- Bleeding occurs rarely: around 2% of patients have a major bleed (fall in haemoglobin > 2.0 g/dl, need for blood transfusion, or intracranial or retroperitoneal bleed) **[A]**[11].

## Heparin-induced thrombocytopenia

- Stop heparin **[A]**.
- An alternative is danaparoid **[D]**[15].

**Why?**
- Danaparoid may cause less thrombocytopenia than heparin (based on animal studies), and is probably as effective as heparin for treating venous thromboembolism **[D]**[15].

## Other complications

- Subcutaneous haematoma at site of injection **[D]**.
- Osteopenia in prolonged administration **[D]**[16] **[D]**[17].

**Note**
- Women who take heparin during pregnancy have a significant decrease in bone density at the end; however, the risks are still low: vertebral fractures (2%) and bleeds (1%) are uncommon **[D]**[27] **[D]**[28] **[D]**[29].

# WARFARIN

## Indications

Give warfarin for the following conditions:

- venous thromboembolism **[A]**[30]

- atrial fibrillation [A][31]
- heart valves [C][32]
- antiphospholipid syndrome [C][33].

## Why?

■ Pulmonary embolism: anticoagulation reduces death and recurrent PE [A][30].

**Pulmonary embolism: anticoagulation reduces recurrent and fatal pulmonary embolism**

| Patient [A][30] | Treatment | Comparator | Outcome | CER | RRR | NNT |
|---|---|---|---|---|---|---|
| Pulmonary embolism | Warfarin | Placebo | Death from PE at 12 months | 26% | 100% | 4 (2 to 15) |
| | | | Recurrent PE at 12 months | 32% | 100% | 3 (2 to 9) |

■ Atrial fibrillation: anticoagulation reduces death and stroke [A][31].

**Atrial fibrillation: anticoagulation reduces death and stroke**

| Patient [A][38] | Treatment | Comparator | Outcome | CER | RRR | NNT |
|---|---|---|---|---|---|---|
| Atrial fibrillation | Warfarin | Placebo | Stroke at 1–2 years | 6.6% | 66% (48% to 78%) | 23 (17 to 36) |
| | | | Death at 1–2 years | 8.0% | 30% (5% to 48%) | 42 (23 to 260) |

■ Mechanical heart valves: warfarin reduces embolic events [C][32].
■ Antiphospholipid syndrome: warfarin reduces recurrent thrombosis [C][33].

**Antiphospholipid syndrome: anticoagulation reduces recurrent thrombosis**

| Patient [C][33] | Treatment | Comparator | Outcome | CER | RRR | NNT |
|---|---|---|---|---|---|---|
| Antiphospholipid syndrome | Warfarin | Nothing | Recurrent thrombosis at 10 years | 48% | 90% (70% to 97%) | 2 (2 to 3) |

**Table 4 Warfarin: use the following therapeutic ranges shown**

| Therapeutic range | INR |
|---|---|
| Venous thromboembolism [B][34] [B][35] | 2.0–3.0 |
| Venous thromboembolism with INR 2.0–3.0 [D] | 3.0–4.5 |
| Atrial fibrillation [B][36] | 2.0–3.0 |
| Biological heart valves [A][37] | 2.0–3.0 |
| Mechanical heart valves [C][32] | 3.0–4.5 |

**Why?**
- A therapeutic range of 2.0–3.0 for first or recurrent episodes of DVT or PE is effective **[B]**[34] **[B]**[35].
- Patients with AF on warfarin are at increased risk for a stroke, TIA or a major bleed if their INR ≥ 4.0 **[B]**[36].
- Patients with mechanical heart valves on warfarin have the fewest thromboembolic events or major bleeds when their INR is between 2.5 and 4.9 **[C]**[32].
- Patients with biological heart valves have fewer major bleeds with an INR 2.0–2.25 and no clear increase in embolic events than with an INR 2.5–4.0 **[A]**[37].

**Biological heart valves: a lower INR reduces the risk of major bleeding**

| Patient [A][34] | Treatment | Comparator | Outcome | CER | RRR | NNT |
|---|---|---|---|---|---|---|
| Biological heart valve | INR 2.0–2.25 | INR 2.5–4.0 | Major bleed at 3 months | 4.6% | 100% | 22 (12 to 150) |

- Determine your patient's potential risk of bleeding when anticoagulated before deciding if it is worthwhile **[D]**.

Score one point for each of the following risk factors **[A]**[38]:

- aged 65 or more
- history of stroke
- history of gastrointestinal bleed
- recent myocardial infarction, Hct < 30%, Cr > 133 μmol/l or diabetes mellitus.

Determine your patient's risk of bleeding **[A]**[38] (Table 5).

**Table 5   Risk of major bleeding on anticoagulation therapy**

| Score | Risk of major bleeding |
|---|---|
| 0 | Low |
| 1 or 2 | Medium |
| 3 or 4 | High |

**Why?**
- This bleeding index helps predict outpatients at high risk for major bleeding when anticoagulated **[A]**[38].

**Half of patients classified at high risk have a major bleed within 4 years**

| Risk [A][38] | % with major bleeding at 48 months | NNF (95% CI) |
|---|---|---|
| High | 53% (11% to 97%) | 2 (1 to 9) |
| Medium | 12% (5% to 19%) | 8 (5 to 20) |
| Low | 3% (0% to 8%) | 40 (13 to infinity) |

If warfarin is contraindicated consider:
- a vena caval filter for deep vein thrombosis.

> **Why?**
> ■ Vena caval filters are not a useful addition to warfarin **[A]**[39] but may offer some protection **[D]**.

- long-term subcutaneous heparin **[D]**[40] or LMWH **[D]**[41] **[D]**[42].

> **Why?**
> ■ Both are probably as effective as warfarin for long-term anticoagulation of patients with deep vein thrombosis **[D]**[42].
> ■ There is less bleeding with heparin than warfarin **[A]**[43].
> ■ However patients are at risk of osteopenia and thrombocytopenia on long-term heparin or LMWH, although there are fewer vertebral fractures with LMWH **[A]**[44].
>
> **Long-term heparin causes fewer bleeds than warfarin, but vertebral fractures are common**
>
> | Patient | Treatment | Comparator | Outcome | CER | RRR | NNT |
> |---|---|---|---|---|---|---|
> | Proximal DVT **[A]**[43] | Subcutaneous heparin | Warfarin | Any bleed at 12 weeks | 17% | 89% (15% to 99%) | 7 (4 to 23) |
> | Venous thromboembolism **[A]**[44] | Daltiparin | Heparin | Vertebral fracture at 6 months | 15% | 83% (3% to 100%) | 8 (4 to 240) |

## Dosing and monitoring

- Start warfarin as soon as possible **[A]**[45] and monitor its effect using INR **[A]**.

> **Why?**
> ■ Starting warfarin within 48 h of heparin reduces hospital stays (by around 4 days) and occurrence of infusion phlebitis compared with starting warfarin after 96 h **[A]**[45]
> ■ The effect on major bleeds or recurrent venous thromboembolism is unclear **[A]**[45]
>
> **Starting warfarin within 48 h reduces infusion phlebitis**
>
> | Patient **[A]**[45] | Treatment | Comparator | Outcome | CER | RRR | NNT |
> |---|---|---|---|---|---|---|
> | Thromboembolism | Warfarin started within 48 h | Warfarin started after 96 h | Infusion phlebitis at discharge | 18% | 91% (33% to 99%) | 6 (4 to 17) |

- In patients with venous thromboembolism, give LMWH or heparin while awaiting satisfactory oral anticoagulation **[A]**[46].

> **Why?**
> ■ It reduces symptomatic DVT recurrence without clearly increasing the risk of major bleeding **[A]**[46].
>
> **Adding heparin to warfarin reduces symptomatic recurrence of DVT**
>
> | Patient | Treatment | Comparator | Outcome | CER | RRR | NNT |
> |---|---|---|---|---|---|---|
> | Proximal **[A]**[46] DVT | Heparin and warfarin | Warfarin | Symptomatic recurrence of DVT at 6 months | 32% | 200% (3% to 780%) | 8 (4 to 71) |

Give heparin **[A]**[47] and LMWH **[D]** for longer than 5 days and
continue for 2 days after the INR is within therapeutic range **[D]**.

**Why?**

■ More patients die who have heparin for 5 days, and start warfarin on the first day, than patients who have heparin
for 10 days, and start warfarin on the fifth day **[A]**[47].

**Using heparin for 10 days compared with 5 days reduces mortality**

| Patient **[A]**[47] | Treatment | Comparator | Outcome | CER | RRR | NNH |
|---|---|---|---|---|---|---|
| Proximal DVT | Heparin for 5 days, and warfarin started on day 1 | Heparin for 10 days and warfarin started on day 5 | Death at 3 months | 32% | −30% (−1800% to −12%) | 16 (8 to 1900) |

● Use a set dosing regimen (preferably by computer **[A]**[48]) and seek
expert advice when indicated **[A]**[49].

**Why?**

■ Dosing using a computer program reaches a therapeutic and stable INR faster than using physicians' predictions (on
average 4 days) **[A]**[48]
■ Patients leave hospital a week sooner, and are more likely to have a therapeutic INR after 2 weeks **[A]**[48].

**Computer dosing of warfarin increases the chance of a therapeutic INR after 2 weeks**

| Patient **[A]**[48] | Treatment | Comparator | Outcome | CER | RRR | NNT |
|---|---|---|---|---|---|---|
| Venous thromboembolism, atrial fibrillation | Computer dosing of warfarin | Physician dosing of warfarin | Therapeutic PT at 10–14 days | 31% | −135% (−299% to −38%) | 2 (2 to 5) |

■ Guideline-based consultation reduces anticoagulant-related bleeding and venous thromboembolism **[A]**[49].

**Guideline-based consultation reduces bleeding and venous thromboembolism**

| Patient **[A]**[49] | Treatment | Comparator | Outcome | CER | RRR | NNT |
|---|---|---|---|---|---|---|
| Starting anticoagulation and considered moderate or high risk for bleeding | Guideline-based consultation | Usual care | Any bleeding at 3 months | 31% | 58% (2% to 82%) | 6 (3 to 45) |
| | | | New or recurrent PE or DVT at 3 months | 16% | 73% (17% to 94%) | 8 (4 to 160) |

Box 1 gives an example of a dosing regimen to achieve a therapeutic range of INR 2.0–3.0 [C][50].
Give the warfarin at 5 to 6 p.m. and measure the INR at 9 a.m. the next day.

### Box 1 Wafarin: example of dosing regimen

| Day 1 [C][50] | | Day 2 | | Day 3 | | Day 4 | | Day 5 | |
|---|---|---|---|---|---|---|---|---|---|
| INR | Dose (mg) | INR | Dose (mg) | INR | Dose (mg) | INR | Dose (mg) | INR | Dose (mg) |
| < 1.4 | 10 | < 1.8 | 10 | < 2.0 | 10 | < 1.4 | Refer to haematology | > 4.0 | 0.0 |
| | | 1.8 | 1.0 | 2.0–2.1 | 5.0 | 1.4 | 8.0 | | |
| | | > 1.8 | 0.5 | 2.2–2.3 | 4.5 | 1.5 | 7.5 | | |
| | | | | 2.4–2.5 | 4.0 | 1.6–1.7 | 7.0 | | |
| | | | | 2.6–2.7 | 3.5 | 1.8 | 6.5 | | |
| | | | | 3.0–3.1 | 3.0 | 1.9 | 6.0 | | |
| | | | | 3.2–3.3 | 2.5 | 2.0–2.1 | 5.5 | | |
| | | | | 3.4 | 2.0 | 2.2–2.3 | 5.0 | | |
| | | | | 3.5 | 1.5 | 2.4–2.6 | 4.5 | | |
| | | | | 3.6–4.0 | 1.0 | 2.7–3.0 | 4.0 | | |
| | | | | > 4.0 | 0.0 | 3.1–3.5 | 3.5 | | |
| | | | | | | 3.6–4.0 | 3.0 | | |
| | | | | | | 4.1–4.5 | Miss 1 day then 2.0 | | |
| | | | | | | > 4.5 | Miss 2 days then 1.0 | | |

Monitor INR daily until in range and stable.
Use lower loading doses: they are more effective [A][51] [A][53].

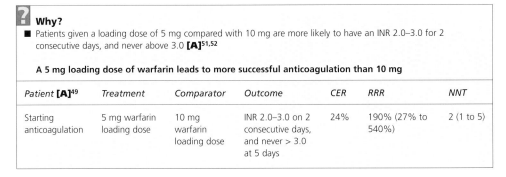

**? Why?**
- Patients given a loading dose of 5 mg compared with 10 mg are more likely to have an INR 2.0–3.0 for 2 consecutive days, and never above 3.0 [A][51,52]

**A 5 mg loading dose of warfarin leads to more successful anticoagulation than 10 mg**

| Patient [A][49] | Treatment | Comparator | Outcome | CER | RRR | NNT |
|---|---|---|---|---|---|---|
| Starting anticoagulation | 5 mg warfarin loading dose | 10 mg warfarin loading dose | INR 2.0–3.0 on 2 consecutive days, and never > 3.0 at 5 days | 24% | 190% (27% to 540%) | 2 (1 to 5) |

## Follow-up

- Patients should have their INR level checked regularly [A].
- Advise patients:
  - about the risk of bleeding, but indicate that serious bleeds are rare [B][24]

**Note**

■ 10% of patients on warfarin have one bleed per year (95% CI: 8.7 to 10%); 3% of patients have a major bleed (2.5 to 3.5%) **[B]**[24]

**Major bleeding and intracranial haemorrhage are uncommon**

| Indication | Regimen | Duration of anticoagulation | Major bleed/ year | Intracranial haemorrhage/ year |
|---|---|---|---|---|
| Atrial fibrillation **[A]**[31] **[A]**[53] **[B]**[54] **[B]**[55] | Warfarin | Indefinite | ~2–3% | ~1% |
| First DVT **[B]**[56] | Heparin and warfarin | 6 months | ~3% | |
| Recurrent DVT **[B]**[57] | Heparin and warfarin | Indefinitely | ~2% | |

– most patients on warfarin feel as healthy as patients who are not **[A]**[58]

**Note**

■ Patients on warfarin score no differently from control patients on a questionnaire asking about functional status, well-being and health perception. Only patients who have had a bleed on warfarin become more concerned about their health **[A]**[58].

– many drugs and foods interact with warfarin and patients should check that any new medication they take is safe **[B]**[59].

**Note**

■ Anticoagulation is potentiated by **[B]**[59]:
  – antibiotics and antifungals: co-trimoxazole, erythromycin, fluconazole, isoniazid, metronidazole, miconázole
  – cardiac drugs: amiodarone, statins, clofibrate, propafenone, propranolol, sulfinpyrazone
  – analgesics: piroxicam, phenylbutazone, paracetamol
  – alcohol (only with concomitant liver disease)
  – cimetidine and omeprazole.
■ Anticoagulation is inhibited by **[B]**[59]:
  – antibiotics and antifungals: griseofulvin, rifampicin, nafcillin
  – CNS drugs: barbiturates, carbemazepine, chlordiazepoxide
  – cholestyramine
  – sucralfate
  – foods and enteral feeds high in vitamin K, and large amounts of avocado.

- Monitor patients with the following conditions more carefully; they are at increased risk of having a supratherapeutic INR **[B]**[60]:
  - on > 2.5 g of paracetamol a week
  - recently started warfarin-potentiating medication
  - taking more warfarin than prescribed
  - advanced cancer
  - decreased oral intake in the last week
  - acute diarrhoeal illness in the last week.

| **Why?** Cancer and paracetamol use increase the risk of an INR > 6.0 | | | | |
| --- | --- | --- | --- | --- |
| Outcome **[B]**[60] | Risk factor | PEER | OR (95% CI) | NNH (95% CI) |
| INR > 6.0 | Advanced malignancy *independent* | 6% | 16.4 (2.4 to 111) | 2 (1 to 15) |
| | Newly-started potentiating medication *independent* | 4% | 8.5 (2.9 to 24.7) | 4 (2 to 11) |
| | Warfarin dose > prescribed *independent* | 3% | 8.1 (2.2 to 30) | 4 (2 to 17) |
| | Decreased oral intake *independent* | 6% | 3.6 (1.3 to 9.7) | 8 (3 to 64) |
| | Acute diarrhoeal illness *independent* | 8% | 3.5 (1.4 to 8.6) | 9 (4 to 48) |
| | Paracetamol dose > 9.1 g per week *independent* | 3% | 10.0 (2.6 to 37.9) | 3 (2 to 13) |
| | Paracetamol dose 4.6 to 9.0 g per week *independent* | 5% | 6.9 (2.2 to 21.9) | 4 (2 to 17) |
| | Paracetamol dose 2.2 to 4.5 g per week *independent* | 5% | 3.5 (1.2 to 10.0) | 9 (3 to 96) |

- Monitor the following patients closely; they are at increased risk of having a major bleed:
  - high therapeutic range **[B]**[61]
  - supratherapeutic INR (> 4.5) **[A]**[53] **[B]**[36] **[B]**[61]
  - recently started warfarin **[A]**[53]
  - old age **[A]**[53]
  - arterial disease **[A]**[53]
  - comorbid conditions **[B]**[26] **[B]**[36] (stroke, serious heart, liver or renal disease)
  - previous GI bleed **[A]**[62]
  - on NSAIDs **[B]**[24]

**Why?**
High anticoagulation and recent onset of warfarin increase the risk of major bleeding

| Patient | Prognostic factor | Outcome | Control rate | RR (95% CI) | NNF+ (95% CI) |
|---|---|---|---|---|---|
| Elderly on anticoagulation **[B]**[61] | INR range 3.0–4.0 *independent* | Severe bleed at 2–3 years *independent* | 9.8% | 1.55 (1.17 to 2.06) | 19 (10 to 63) |
| Anticoagulation **[A]**[53] | INR > 4.5 *independent* | Major bleed at 9 months | 1.0% | 5.96 (3.68 to 9.67) | 20 (11 to 37) |
| | < 90 days since commencing therapy *independent* | Major bleed at 9 months | 1.0% | 2.5 (1.4 to 3.3) | 65 (43 to 250) |
| | Aged ≥ 70 *independent* | Major bleed at 9 months | 0.7% | 1.69 (1.21 to 2.37) | 140 (72 to 470) |
| | Arterial disease requiring anticoagulation *independent* | Major bleed at 9 months | 1.0% | 1.72 (1.17 to 2.54) | 140 (64 to 580) |

- The following features increase the risk of an intracranial bleed **[A]**[63]:
  - supratherapeutic INR (> 4.0)
  - previous stroke
  - prosthetic heart valves
  - old age.

**Why?**
Previous strokes and prosthetic heart valves increase the risk of intracranial bleeding

| Outcome | Risk factor | PEER | OR (95% CI) | NNH (95% CI) |
|---|---|---|---|---|
| Intracranial haemorrhage | History of cerebrovascular disease *independent* | 0.8% | 2.3 (1.4 to 3.7) | 100 (50 to 330) |
| | Prosthetic heart valve *independent* | 0.8% | 2.1 (1.2 to 3.8) | 120 (48 to 660) |

Around half of intracranial bleeds are fatal, and few patients make a full recovery **[A]**[63].

**Note**
- In one study, 64% of cases had an intracerebral bleed (of which 46% were fatal); the rest were subdural (of which 20% were fatal). The risk of intracranial bleed increased sharply when INR > 4.0 **[A]**[63].

## Complications

### Life-threatening bleed

- Give 5 mg vitamin K by slow (5 min) iv infusion **[A].**
- Give a concentrate of factors II, VII, IX and X at a dose of 50 units of factor IX/kg body weight **[C]**[64].

**Why?**

■ It is better than fresh-frozen plasma at lowering INR ≤ 2.0 within 15 min **[C]**[64].

**Factor concentrate reverses INR faster than fresh-frozen plasma**

| Patient | Treatment | Comparator | Outcome | CER | RRR | NNT |
|---------|-----------|------------|---------|-----|-----|-----|
| Urgent reversal of INR required **[C]**[64] | Factor concentrate | Fresh frozen plasma | INR ≤ 2.0 at 15 min | 58% | 66% (2% to 168%) | 3 (1 to 10) |

- If no concentrate is available, give fresh-frozen plasma (~ 1 liter for an adult) **[D].**
- Stop warfarin **[C]**[65].

### Major bleed (e.g. haematuria or epistaxis)

- Stop warfarin for 1 or more days **[C]**[65].
- Consider giving 0.5–2.0 mg vitamin K iv (clinical response takes 4–6 h) **[C]**[66].

**Why?**

■ Few patients on steady-state warfarin dosing have normal INRs within 3 days of stopping. Most have normal INRs within 8 days. The INR declines more slowly in older patients **[C]**[65].

■ Vitamin K lowers INR effectively **[C]**[66].

### INR > 5.0 without haemorrhage

- Continue warfarin and give 2 mg of vitamin K orally.

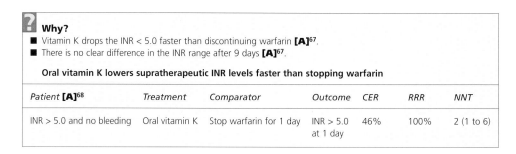

**Why?**

■ Vitamin K drops the INR < 5.0 faster than discontinuing warfarin **[A]**[67].

■ There is no clear difference in the INR range after 9 days **[A]**[67].

**Oral vitamin K lowers supratherapeutic INR levels faster than stopping warfarin**

| Patient **[A]**[68] | Treatment | Comparator | Outcome | CER | RRR | NNT |
|---------|-----------|------------|---------|-----|-----|-----|
| INR > 5.0 and no bleeding | Oral vitamin K | Stop warfarin for 1 day | INR > 5.0 at 1 day | 46% | 100% | 2 (1 to 6) |

Unexpected bleeding at therapeutic levels of INR

- Investigate for underlying malignancy (look for gastrointestinal and genitourinary especially).

 **Why?**

- Diagnostic evaluation of GI bleeding and gross haematuria may lead to the diagnosis of previously unknown lesions in one third of patients; half have malignancy **[B]**[24].
- The most common sites of bleeding for patients on heparin or warfarin are the GI tract, the urinary tract, soft tissues, the oropharynx **[B]**[24].

**Soft tissue or wounds are the commonest bleeding sites**

| Site **[B]**[24] | Heparin | Warfarin |
|---|---|---|
| Soft tissue/wound | 31% | 21% |
| GI tract | 27% | 15% |
| Urinary tract | 19% | 15% |
| Nasopharynx | 6% | 35% |
| Intracranial | 2% | 4% |
| Retroperitoneal | 3% | 1% |

Other complications

- Warfarin-induced skin necrosis; this is very rare.

**Note**

- It is said to be associated with protein C or protein S deficiency **[D]**.

**Guideline writer**: Christopher Ball
**CAT writer**: Christopher Ball

**With thanks to Drs David Keeling, John Reynolds, David Sackett, Sharon Straus and Alan Townsend for use of their anticoagulation guide on which this one is based.**

## REFERENCES

| No. | Level | Citation |
|---|---|---|
| 1 | 1b | Low-molecular-weight heparin at home was as effective as unfractionated heparin in the hospital in proximal DVT. ACP J Club 1996 July–Aug; 125: 3. Evidence-Based Med 1996 July Aug; 1: 141. Summary of: Levine M, Gent M, Hirsh J et al. A comparison of low-molecular-weight heparin administered primarily at home with unfractionated heparin administered in the hospital for proximal deep-vein thrombosis. N Engl J Med 1996; 334: 677–81 |
| 2 | 1b | Low-molecular-weight heparin at home was as effective as unfractionated heparin in the hospital in proximal DVT. ACP J Club 1996 July–Aug; 125: 2. Evidence-Based Med 1996 July–Aug; 1: 140. Summary of: Koopman MM et al. Treatment of venous thrombosis with intravenous unfractionated heparin administered in the hospital as compared with subcutaneous low-molecular-weight heparin administered at home. N Engl J Med 1996; 334: 682–7 |

| No. | Level | Citation |
|---|---|---|
| 3 | 1b | Hull RD et al. Treatment of proximal vein thrombosis with subcutaneous LMWH versus intravenous heparin: an economic perspective: Arch Intern Med 1997; 157: 289–94 |
| 4 | 1b | van den Belt AG et al. Replacing inpatient care by outpatient care in the treatment of DVT: an economic evaluation. Thromb Haemost 1998; 79: 259–63 |
| 5 | 1b | Aspirin plus low-molecular-weight heparin was effective for unstable angina. ACP J Club 1996 Mar–Apr; 124: 39. Summary of: Gurfinkel EP et al. Low molecular weight heparin versus regular heparin or aspirin in the treatment of unstable angina and silent ischamia. J Am Coll Cardiol 1995; 26: 313–8 |
| 6 | 1b | Simoneau S et al. A comparison of low-molecular-weight heparin and unfractionated heparin for acute pulmonary embolism. N Engl J Med 1997; 337: 663–9 |
| 7 | 1b | Columbus Investigators. Low-molecular-weight heparin in the treatment of patients with venous thromboembolism. N Engl J Med 1997; 337: 657–62 |
| 8 | 1b | Cohen M et al. A comparison of low-molecular weight heparin with unfractionated heparin for unstable coronary disease. N Engl J Med 1997; 337: 447–52 |
| 9 | 1a | Lensing A et al. Treatment of deep venous thrombosis with low-molecular-weight heparins: a meta-analysis. Arch Intern Med 1995; 155: 601–7 |
| 10 | 1a | Meta-analysis: LMWH is effective in reducing recurrent thromboembolism, bleeding, and death in acute DVT. ACP J Club 1996 Sept–Oct; 125: 30. Summary of: Siragusa S et al. Low-molecular-weight heparins and unfractionated heparin in the treatment of patients with acute venous thromboembolism: results of a meta-analysis. Am J Med 1996; 100: 269–77 |
| 11 | 1a | van den Belt AGM et al. Fixed dose subcutaneous low molecular weight heparins versus adjusted dose unfractionated heparin for venous thromboembolism (Cochrane Review). In: The Cochrane Library, Issue 2, 1998; Oxford: Update Software. |
| 12 | 1b | Warkentin TE et al. Heparin-induced thrombocytopenia in patients treated with LWMH or unfractionated heparin. N Engl J Med 1995; 332: 1330–5 |
| 13 | 4 | Zeiler Arnold A et al. Role of prophylactic anticoagulation for direct current cardioversion in patients with atrial fibrillation or atrial flutter. J Am Coll Cardiol 1992; 19: 851–5 |
| 14 | 4 | Melissari E et al. Use of low-molecular weight heparin in pregnancy. Thromb Haemost 1992; 68: 652–6 |
| 15 | 1b– | de Valk HW et al. Comparing subcutaneous danaparoid with intravenous unfractionated heparin for the treatment of venous thromboembolism. Ann Intern Med 1995; 123: 1–9 |
| 16 | 4 | Barbour LA et al. A prospective study of heparin-induced osteoporosis in pregnancy using bone densimetry. Am J Obstet Gynecol 1994; 170: 862–9 |
| 17 | 4 | Ginsberg JS et al. Heparin effect on bone density. Thromb Haemost 1990; 64: 286–9 |
| 18 | 1a | Hommes DW et al. Subcutaneous heparin compared with continuous intravenous heparin administered in the initial treatment of DVT: a meta-analysis. Ann Intern Med 1992; 116: 279–284 |
| 19 | 4 | Prandoni P et al. Use of an algorithm for administering subcutaneous heparin in the treatment of deep vein thrombosis. Ann Intern Med 1998; 129: 299–302 |
| 20 | 1b | Raschke RA et al. The weight-based heparin dosing nomogram compared with a standard care nomogram: a randomised controlled trial. Ann Intern Med 1993; 119: 874–81 |

| No. | Level | Citation |
|-----|-------|----------|
| 21 | 2b | Raschke RA et al. The weight-based heparin dosing nomogram compared with a standard care nomogram: a randomised controlled trial. Ann Intern Med 1993; 119: 874–81 |
| 22 | 1b– | Levine MD et al. Randomised trial comparing activated thromboplastin time with heparin assay in patients with acute venous thromboembolism requiring large daily doses of heparin. Arch Intern Med 1994; 154: 49–56 |
| 23 | 1a | Anand S et al. The relation between aPTT response and recurrence in patients with venous thrombosis treated with continuous intravenous heparin. Arch Intern Med 1996; 156: 1677–81 |
| 24 | 2a | Risk for anticoagulant-related bleeding: a meta-analysis. ACP J Club 1994 Mar–April 120: 52. Summary of: Landfeld CS, Beyth RJ. Anticoagulant-related bleeding: clinical epidemiology, prediction, and prevention. Am J Med 1993; 95: 315–28 |
| 25 | 2b | Campbell HR et al. Aging and heparin-related bleeding. Arch Intern Med 1996; 156: 857–60 |
| 26 | 1a | Landfeld CS et al. A bleeding risk index for estimating the probability of major bleeding in hospitalised patients starting anticoagulant therapy. Am J Med 1990; 89: 569–77 |
| 27 | 4 | Barbour L A et al. A prospective study of herparin-induced osteoporosis in pregnancy using bone densimetry. Am J Obstet Gynecol; 170: 862–9 |
| 28 | 4 | Ginsberg J S et al Heparin effect on bone density. Thromb Haemost 1990: 64: 286–9 |
| 29 | 4 | Dahlman T. Osteoporotic fractures and the recurrence of thromboembolism during pregnancy and puerperium in 184 women undergoing thromboprophylaxis with heparin. Am J Obstet Gynecol 1993; 168: 1265–70 |
| 30 | 1b | Barritt DW, Jordan SC. Anticoagulant drugs in the treatment of pulmonary embolism: a controlled trial. Lancet 1960; June 18: 1309–12 |
| 31 | 1a | Atrial Fibrillation Investigators et al. Risk factors for stroke and efficacy of antithrombotic therapy in atrial fibrillation: analysis of pooled data from five randomised controlled trials. Arch Intern Med 1994; 154: 1449–57 |
| 32 | 4 | Cannegieter S et al. Optimal oral anticoagulation therapy in patients with mechanical heart valves. N Engl J Med 1995; 333: 11–17 |
| 33 | 4 | Khamashta MA et al. Management of thrombosis in the antiphospholipid antibody syndrome. N Engl J Med 1995; 332: 993–7 |
| 34 | 2c | Schulman S and the Duration of Anticoagulation Trial Study Group. The duration of oral anticoagulation after a second episode of venous thromboembolism. N Engl J Med 1997; 336: 393–8 |
| 35 | 2b | Fewer venous thromboembolism recurrences occurred with 6 months than with 6 weeks of anticoagulant therapy. ACP J Club 1996 Jan–Feb; 124: 9. Evidence-Based Med 1996 Jan Feb; 1: 42. Summary of: Schulman S, Rhedin AS, Lindmarker P et al and the Duration of Anticoagulation Trial Study Group. A comparison of six weeks with six months of oral anticoagulant therapy after a first episode of venous thromboembolism. N Engl J Med 1995; 332: 1661–5 |
| 36 | 2b | European Atrial Fibrillation Trial Study Group. Optimal oral anticoagulation therapy in patients with non-rheumatic atrial fibrillation and recent cerebral ischemia. N Engl J Med 1995; 333: 5–10 |
| 37 | 1b | Turpie AA et al. Randomised comparison of two intensities of oral anticoagulant therapy after tissue heart valve replacement. Lancet 1988; i: 1242–5 |

| No. | Level | Citation |
|-----|-------|----------|
| 38 | 1a | Beyth RJ, Quinn LM, Landefeld CS. Prospective evaluation of an index for predicting the risk of major bleeding in outpatients treated with warfarin. Am J Med 1998; 105: 91–99 |
| 39 | 1b | Decousus H et al. A clinical trial of vena caval filters in the prevention of pulmonary embolism in patients with proximal deep venous thrombosis. N Engl J Med 1998; 338: 409–15 |
| 40 | 1b | Hull RD et al. Injected subcutaneous heparin versus warfarin in the long-term treatment of venous thrombosis. N Engl J Med 1982; 306: 189–99 |
| 41 | 1b | Monreal M et al. Comparison of subcutaneous unfractionated heparin with a low-molecular-weight heparin (Fragmin) in patients with venous thromboembolism and a contraindication to coumarin. Thromb Haemost 1994; 71: 7–11 |
| 42 | 1b– | Pini M et al. LMWH versus warfarin in the prevention of recurrences after DVT. Thromb Haemost 1994; 72: 191–7 |
| 43 | 1b | Hull R D, et al. Injected subscutaneous heparin versus warfarin in the long-term treatment of venous thrombosis. NEJM 1982; 306: 189–99 |
| 44 | 1b | Monreal M, et al. Comparison of subcutaneous unfractionated heparin with a low molecular weight heparin (Fragmin) in patients with venous tromboembolism and a contraindication to coumarin. Thromb Haemost 1994; 71: 7–11 |
| 45 | 1b | Mohiuddin SM et al. Efficacy and safety of early versus late initiation of warfarin during heparin therapy in acute thromboembolism. Am Heart J 1992; 123: 729–32 |
| 46 | 1b | Brandjes DP et al. Acencoumarol and heparin compared with acencoumarol alone in the initial treatment of proximal vein thrombosis. N Engl J Med 1992; 327: 1485 |
| 47 | 1b | Hull RD et al. Heparin for 5 days compared with ten days in the initial treatment of proximal venous thrombosis. N Engl J Med 1990; 322: 1260–4 |
| 48 | 1b | White RH et al. Initiation of warfarin therapy: comparison of physician dosing with computer-assisted dosing. J Gen Intern Med 1987; 2: 141–8 |
| 49 | 1b | Consultation and guidelines to reduce anticoagulant-related bleeding. ACP J Club 1992 Sept Oct; 117: 61. Summary of: Landfeld CS, Anderson PA. Guideline-based consultation to prevent anticoagulant-related bleeding. A randomized, controlled trial in a teaching hospital. Ann Intern Med 1992; 116: 829–37 |
| 50 | 4 | Fennerty A et al. Flexible induction dose regimen for warfarin and prediction of maintenance dose. BMJ 1984; 288: 1268–70 |
| 51 | 1b | Crowther MA, Ginsberg JB, Kearon C et al. A randomized trial comparing 5-mg and 10-mg warfarin loading doses. Arch Intern Med 1999; 159: 46–8 |
| 52 | 1b | Crowther MA et al. A randomised comparison of a 5 mg and 10 mg loading dose for the initiation of warfarin therapy. Thromb Haemost 1997; 583 |
| 53 | 1b | Palareti G et al. Bleeding complications of oral anticoagulant treatment: an inception-cohort, prospective collaborative study (ISCOAT). Lancet 1996; 348: 423–8 |
| 54 | 2b | Stroke prevention in Atrial Fibrillation Investigators. Adjusted-dose warfarin versus low intenstiy fixed-dose warfarin and aspirin for high-risk patients with atrial fibrillation. Lancet 1996; 348: 633–8 |
| 55 | 2b | Stroke prevention in Atrial Fibrillation Investigators. Bleeding during antithrombotic therapy in patients with atrial fibrillation. Arch Intern Med 1996; 156: 409–16 |

| No. | Level | Citation |
|-----|-------|----------|
| 56 | 2b | Fewer venous thrombembolism recurrences occurred with 6 months than with 6 weeks of anticoagulant therapy. ACP Journal Club 1996 Jan–Feb; 124:9. Evidence Based Medicine 1996 Jan–Feb; 1: 42. Summary of Schulan S, Rhedin A S, Lindmarker P, et al and the Duration of Anticoagulation Trial Study Group. A comparison of six weeks with six months of oral anticoagulant therapy after a first episode of venous thromboembolism. N Engl J Med 1997; 332: 1661–5 |
| 57 | 2b | Schulman S, et al. and the Duration of Anticoagulation Trial Study Group. The duration of oral anticoagulation after a second episode of venous thromboembolism. N Engl J Med 1997; 336: 393–8 |
| 58 | 1b | Lancaster TR et al. Impact of long-term warfarin therapy on quality of life: evidence from a randomised trial. Arch Intern Med 1991; 151: 1944–9 |
| 59 | 2a | Many drugs and foods interact with warfarin. ACP J Club 1995 Mar–April; 122: 44. Summary of: Wells PS, Holbrook AM, Crowther NR, Hirsh J. Interactions of warfarin with drugs and food. Ann Intern Med 1994; 121: 676–83 |
| 60 | 3b | Hylek EM et al. Acetominophen and other risk factors for excessive warfarin anticoagulation. JAMA 1998; 279: 657–62 |
| 61 | 2b | Fihn SD et al. The risk for and severity of bleeding complications in elderly patients treated with warfarin. Ann Intern Med 1996; 124: 970–9 |
| 62 | 1a | Landfeld CS et al. Major bleeding in outpatients treated with warfarin: incidence and prediction by factors known at the start of outpatient therapy. Am J Med 1989; 87: 144–51 |
| 63 | 1b | Hylek EM, Singer DE. Risk factors for intracranial haemorrhage in outpatients taking warfarin. Ann Intern Med 1994; 120: 897–902 |
| 64 | 4 | Makris M et al. Emergency oral anticoagulant reversal: the relative efficacy of infusions of fresh frozen plasma and clotting factor concentrate on correction of the coagulopathy. Thromb Haemost 1997; 77: 477–80 |
| 65 | 4 | White RH et al. Temporary discontinuation of warfarin therapy: changes in international normalised ratio. Ann Intern Med 1995; 122: 40–2 |
| 66 | 4 | Shetty HG et al. Effective reversal of warfarin-induced excessive anticoagulation with low dose vitamin K. Thromb Haemost 1992; 67: 13–15 |
| 67 | 1b | Pengo V et al. Reversal of excessive effect of regular anticoagulation: low oral dose of phytonadione (vitamin $K_1$) compared with warfarin discontinuation. Blood Coagul Fibrinolysis 1993; 4: 739–41 |

## PREVALENCE

Aortic dissection is uncommon [B][1] except in patients with Marfan syndrome [C][2];

> **Note**
> - 0.1% of medical emergencies are patients with aortic dissection (95% CI: 0.0% to 0.29%) [B][1].
> - 27% to 48% of patients with Marfan syndrome die from aortic dissection or rupture [C][2] [C][3].

however, it is common in patients if clinicians are suspicious enough to order an angiogram [A][4].

> **Note**
> - 55% of patients referred for angiogram due to a possible aortic dissection have one (95% CI: 45% to 64%) [A][4].
>   - Roughly 50% of these are proximal (starting above the aortic valve) [A][4].
>   - Roughly 50% are distal (starting beyond the origin of the left subclavian artery) [A][4].
>   - Around 30% to 40% are subacute (> 2 weeks old) [A][4].

## CLINICAL FEATURES

No individual sign or symptom is very helpful in diagnosing aortic dissection.
Consider it in all patients with chest or upper abdominal pain especially if they have:

- a history of hypertension [C][5] [C][6]

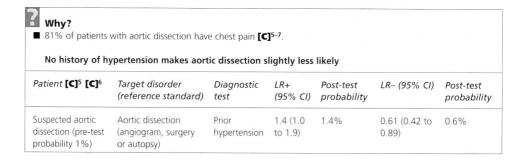

> **? Why?**
> - 81% of patients with aortic dissection have chest pain [C][5–7].
>
> **No history of hypertension makes aortic dissection slightly less likely**
>
> | Patient [C][5] [C][6] | Target disorder (reference standard) | Diagnostic test | LR+ (95% CI) | Post-test probability | LR− (95% CI) | Post-test probability |
> |---|---|---|---|---|---|---|
> | Suspected aortic dissection (pre-test probability 1%) | Aortic dissection (angiogram, surgery or autopsy) | Prior hypertension | 1.4 (1.0 to 1.9) | 1.4% | 0.61 (0.42 to 0.89) | 0.6% |

- chest pain [C][5–7]

> **Why?**
> ■ 90% to 94% of patients with aortic dissection have chest pain **[C]**[5–7]

- Marfan syndrome **[C]**[2] **[C]**[3]

> **Why?**
> ■ 27% to 48% of patients with Marfan syndrome die from aortic dissection or rupture **[C]**[2] **[C]**[3].

- pregnancy **[D]**[8].

Ask about:

- chest pain **[C]**[5–7] and if it has moved **[C]**[5] **[C]**[6]
- onset of symptoms **[C]**[5] **[C]**[6].

> **Why?**
> Symptoms lasting longer than 24 h makes aortic dissection slightly less likely

| Patient **[C]**[5] **[C]**[6] | Target disorder (reference standard) | Diagnostic test | LR + (95% CI) | Post-test probability | LR– (95% CI) | Post-test probability |
|---|---|---|---|---|---|---|
| Suspected aortic dissection undergoing angiography (pre-test probability 1%) | Aortic dissection (angiography, surgery or autopsy) | Prior hypertension | 1.4 (1.0 to 1.9) | 1.4% | 0.61 (0.42 to 0.89) | 0.61% |
| | | Symptoms for < 24 h | 1.5 (1.2 to 2.0) | 1.5% | 0.42 (0.27 to 0.67) | 0.42% |
| | | Pain migration | 1.3 (1.0 to 1.8) | 1.3% | 0.64 (0.43 to 0.93) | 0.64% |

> **Note**
> ■ Neither of the following are helpful in diagnosing aortic dissection or its location **[C]**[5] **[C]**[6]:
> - history of excitement triggering the pain
> - position of pain.

Look for:

- hypertension or hypotension **[C]**[5] **[C]**[6]
- absent or reduced pulses **[C]**[5] **[C]**[6]
- aortic regurgitation **[C]**[5] **[C]**[6]

**Why?**
Hypertension on initial examination makes a distal aortic dissection slightly more likely but a proximal one less

| Patient [C][5] [C][6] | Target disorder (reference standard) | Diagnostic test | LR+ (95% CI) | Post-test probability | LR– (95% CI) | Post-test probability |
|---|---|---|---|---|---|---|
| Suspected aortic dissection undergoing angiography (pre-test probability 1%) | Distal aortic dissection (angiography, surgery or autopsy) | Hypertension on initial examination (≥150/90 mmHg) | 2.5 (1.5 to 3.6) | 1.4% | 0.47 (0.33 to 0.66) | 0.47% |
| | Proximal aortic dissection (angiography, surgery or autopsy) | Hypertension on initial examination (≥150/90 mmHg | 0.19 (0.089 to 0.42) | 0.19% | 2.0 (1.6 to 2.5) | 2.0% |

Aortic regurgitation, hypotension and pulse deficits make a proximal aortic dissection more likely

| Patient [C][5] [C][6] | Target disorder (reference standard) | Diagnostic test | LR+ (95% CI) | Post-test probability | LR– (95% CI) | Post-test probability |
|---|---|---|---|---|---|---|
| Suspected aortic dissection undergoing angiography (pre-test probability 1%) | Proximal aortic dissection (angiography, surgery or autopsy) | Aortic regurgitation | 5.7 (3.3 to 9.6) | 5.7% | 0.39 (0.27 to 0.56) | 0.39% |
| | | Hypotension on initial examination (systolic < 100 mmHg) | 5.3 (2.0 to 14) | 5.3% | 0.82 (0.71 to 0.94) | 0.82% |
| | | pulse deficits | 3.9 (2.3 to 6.6) | 3.9% | 0.57 (0.43 to 0.74) | 0.57% |

- evidence of a stroke or paralysis [B][9].

**Why?**
- Dissection complications at presentation (pulse loss, renal or visceral ischaemia, myocardial infarction, stroke, renal failure or paralysis) increase the risk of death [B][9].
- Neurological problems (stroke, ischaemic peripheral neuropathy, ischaemic spinal cord damage, altered consciousness) are not helpful in diagnosing aortic dissection or its location; 19% to 26% of cases have syncope, stroke, leg weakness or reduced consciousness [C][5] [C][6].

## DIFFERENTIAL DIAGNOSIS

Think about other possible causes – these include [C][5] [C][6]:
- myocardial infarction
- aortic regurgitation

- thoracic non-dissecting aneurysm
- musculoskeletal pain
- mediastinal cyst or tumour
- pericarditis
- gallstones
- pleuritis
- pulmonary embolism.

---

**? Why?**

**Myocardial infarction and aortic regurgitation are alternative causes**

| Differential diagnosis in patients having an angiogram [C][5] [C][6] | % (95% CI) |
|---|---|
| Myocardial infarction | 5.1% (1.9% to 8.6%) |
| Aortic regurgitation | 2.8% (0.4% to 5.3%) |
| Thoracic non-dissecting aneurysm | 2.2% (0.1% to 4.4%) |
| Musculoskeletal pain | 2.2% (0.1% to 4.4v) |
| Mediastinal cyst or tumour | 2.2% (0.1% to 4.4%) |
| Pericarditis | 1.7% (0.0% to 3.6%) |
| Gallstones | 1.1% (0.0% to 2.7%) |
| Pleuritis | 0.6% (0.0% to 1.7%) |
| Pulmonary embolism | 0.6% (0.0% to 1.7%) |
| Unknown | 8.0% (4.0% to 12%) |

---

## INVESTIGATIONS

- ECG – look for:
  - myocardial infarction [D]
  - left ventricular hypertrophy [C][5] [C][6].

---

**? Why?**

**Left ventricular hypertrophy makes an aortic dissection slightly more likely**

| Patient [C][5] [C][6] | Target disorder (reference standard) | Diagnostic test | LR+ (95% CI) | Post-test probability | LR− (95% CI) | Post-test probability |
|---|---|---|---|---|---|---|
| Suspected aortic dissection undergoing angiography (pre-test probability 1%) | Aortic dissection (angiography, surgery or autopsy) | Hypertension on initial examination (≥150/90 mmHg) | 2.1 (1.2 to 3.8) | 2.1% | 0.73 (0.59 to 0.89) | 0.73% |

---

- Blood count [D].
- Cardiac enzymes [B][9].
- Urea and electrolytes, creatinine [B][9].

**Why?**
■ Dissection complications at presentation (pulse loss, renal or visceral ischaemia, myocardial infarction, stroke, renal failure or paralysis) increase the risk of death **[B]**[9].

● Group and save **[D].**
● Chest X-ray – look for **[B]**[10]:
  – widening of the
      aorta (particularly the aortic knob)
      mediastinum
  – pleural effusion
  – tracheal shift.

**Why?**

**An abnormal chest X-ray makes aortic dissection more likely**

| Patient **[B]**[10] | Target disorder (reference standard) | Diagnostic test | LR+ (95% CI) | Post-test probability | LR− (95% CI) | Post-test probability |
|---|---|---|---|---|---|---|
| Suspected aortic dissection | Aortic dissection (angiography) | Radiologist's conclusion of the chest X-ray | 7.3 | 7.3% | 0.21 | 0.21% |

**Note**
■ Radiologists guess at most features on a chest radiograph for a patient with suspected aortic dissection **[B]**[10].

**Radiologists agree most often about widening of the aorta or mediastinum**

| Radiological feature **[B]**[10] | $K_{interobserver}$ |
|---|---|
| Widening of aortic knob | 0.33 |
| Widening of mediastinum | 0.28 |
| Widening of descending aorta | 0.28 |
| Pleural effusion | 0.27 |
| Tracheal shift | 0.27 |
| Widening of ascending aorta | 0.26 |

Perform further imaging if aortic dissection still possible **[D]**, in consultation with cardiothoracic centre **[D]**:

● MRI **[A]**[4]

**Why?**
MRI can diagnose and exclude aortic dissection

| Patient [A][4] | Target disorder (reference standard) | Diagnostic test | LR+ (95% CI) | Post-test probability | LR− (95% CI) | Post-test probability |
|---|---|---|---|---|---|---|
| Suspected aortic dissection (pre-test probability 55%) | Aortic dissection (aortography, surgery, or autopsy) | MRI | 45 (6.5 to 310) | 98% | 0.017 (0.013 to 0.022) | 2% |

**Note**
- MRI takes longer than echocardiography (on average 10 min longer) [A][4].
- MRI may not be practical in ventilated patients or patients requiring extensive monitoring [D].

- transoesophageal echocardiography (TOE) [A][4]

**Why?**
TEE can diagnose and exclude aortic dissection

| Patient [A][4] | Target disorder (reference standard) | Diagnostic test | LR+ (95% CI) | Post-test probability | LR− (95% CI) | Post-test probability |
|---|---|---|---|---|---|---|
| Suspected aortic dissection (pre-test probability 55%) | Aortic dissection (aortography, surgery, or autopsy) | TOE | 4.2 (2.1 to 8.6) | 84% | 0.030 (0.004 to 0.20) | 4% |

**Note**
- TOE can be performed at the bedside [D].

If these are not available:
- CT thorax [A][4]
- transthoracic echocardiography (TTE) [A][4].

**Why?**
Abnormal CT and TTE make aortic dissection more likely, but cannot safely exclude it

| Patient [A][4] | Target disorder (reference standard) | Diagnostic test | LR+ (95% CI) | Post-test probability | LR− (95% CI) | Post-test probability |
|---|---|---|---|---|---|---|
| Suspected aortic dissection (pre-test probability 55%) | Aortic dissection (aortography, surgery, or autopsy) | CT thorax | 7.3 (2.9 to 18) | 90% | 0.071 (0.023 to 0.22) | 8% |
| | | TTE | 4.2 (2.1 to 8.6) | 84% | 0.030 (0.004 to 0.20) | 4% |

## THERAPY

- Give analgesia **[D]**, e.g. diamorphine 5 mg iv (in small or elderly patients 2.5 mg).
- Discuss with cardiothoracic surgeon (and cardiologist) and organise transfer to a cardiothoracic unit or intensive care unit **[D].**
- Meanwhile give antihypertensive therapy **[D]**[8]. Options include:
  - labetolol iv
  - nitroprusside and propranolol iv
  - trimetaphan iv.
- Consider inserting:
  - an intra-arterial line for constant BP montioring if using nitroprusside or trimetaphan **[D]**
  - a urinary catheter **[D]**.

Aim for systolic BP of 100–120 mmHg, provided the urine output is
> 30 ml/h **[D].**

- Consider surgery **[A]** for patients with **[D]**[8]:
  - acute dissection of ascending aorta
  - acute dissection of descending aorta with
      signs of impending rupture (persisting pain, hypotension, left-sided haemothorax)
      Marfan syndrome
  - chronic dissection, if aorta >5–6 cm in diameter or symptoms.
- Consider medical therapy (long-term antihypertensive therapy) for patients with:
  - acute or chronic dissection of descending aorta **[D]**[11].

**Why?**
- Patients who receive medical therapy are not clearly more likely to die than those who receive surgery **[D]**[11].

## PREVENTION

- Give propranolol to patients **[C]**[12] particularly with Marfan syndrome **[A]**[13]: initially 10 mg four times a day, and after 2–4 weeks titred so that heart rate is < 100 beats/min during exercise, or systolic interval increased by less than 30%.

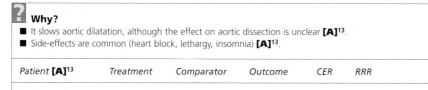

**Why?**
- It slows aortic dilatation, although the effect on aortic dissection is unclear **[A]**[13].
- Side-effects are common (heart block, lethargy, insomnia) **[A]**[13].

| Patient **[A]**[13] | Treatment | Comparator | Outcome | CER | RRR | NNH |
|---|---|---|---|---|---|---|
| Marfan syndrome | Propranolol | No therapy | Side-effects | 0% | 87% (27% to 100%) | 3 (2 to 7) |

## PROGNOSIS

Around a sixth of patients with aortic dissection die before surgery, many from aortic rupture [C][14].
Most survive surgery, and long-term survival is reasonable, although further surgery may be required [B][9], especially for rupture [C][15].

> **Note**
> - 18% of patients are dead within 30 days (95% CI: 12% to 25%), half are dead within 10 years [C][16] [C][17].
> - 10% require further surgery in the next 7 years (95% CI: 5% to 15%) [B][9].
> - Patients with dissecting aneurysms are more likely to have a rupture than patients with other types of aneurysm. The type of dissection has no effect on the chance of rupture.
>
> **A dissecting aneurysm increases the risk of subsequent rupture**
>
> | Patient [C][15] | Prognostic factor | Outcome | Control rate | RR (95% CI) | NNF (95% CI) |
> |---|---|---|---|---|---|
> | Aortic aneurysm | Dissecting aneurysm *not independent* | Rupture at 7 years | 40% | 3.3 (1.5 to 7.2) | 3 (2 to 10) |

Patients are at increased risk of dying if they have [B][9]:

- a pleural rupture
- complications of dissection at presentation
- increasing age
- cardiac disease.

**Guideline writer**: Chris Ball
**CAT writers**: Chris Ball, Clare Wotton

## REFERENCES

| No. | Level | Citation |
|---|---|---|
| 1 | 2c | Zampaglione B et al. Hypertensive urgencies and emergencies: prevalence and clinical presentation. Hypertension 1996; 27: 144–7 |
| 2 | 4 | Lamont Murdoch J et al. Life expectancy and causes of death in the Marfan syndrome. N Engl J Med 1972; 286: 804–8 |
| 3 | 4 | Marsalese DL et al. Marfan syndrome: natural history and long-term follow-up of cardiovascular involvement. J Am Coll Cardiol 1989; 14: 422–8 |
| 4 | 1b | Noninvasive detection of thoracic aortic dissection. ACP J Club 1992 May–June; 116: 85. Summary of: Nienaber CA, Spielmann RP, von Kodolitsch Y et al. Diagnosis of thoracic aortic dissection. Magnetic resonance imaging versus transeosphageal echocardiography. Circulation 1992; 85: 434–47 |
| 5 | 4 | Slater EE, DeSanctis RW. Clinical recognition of dissecting aortic aneurysm. Am J Med 1976; 60: 625–31 |
| 6 | 4 | Eagle KA et al. Spectrum of conditions initially suggestive of acute aortic dissection but with negative aortograms. Am J Cardiol 1986; 57: 322–6 |

| No. | Level | Citation |
|---|---|---|
| 7 | 4 | Lindsay J, Hurst JW. Clinical features and prognosis in dissecting aneurysm of the aorta: a reappraisal. Circulation 1967; 35: 880–7 |
| 8 | 5 | DeSanctis RW et al. Aortic dissection. N Engl J Med 1987; 317: 1060–7 (narrative review) |
| 9 | 2b | Glower DD, Fann JI, Speier RH et al. Comparison of medical and surgical therapy for uncomplicated descending aortic dissection (supplement IV). Circulation 1990; 82: 39–46 |
| 10 | 2b | Jagannath AS et al. Aortic dissection: a statistical analysis of the usefulness of plain chest radiographic findings. Am J Radiol 1986; 147: 1123–6 |
| 11 | 2b– | Glower DD, Fann JI, Speier RH, et al. Comparison of medical and surgical therapy for uncomplicated descending aortic dissection (supplement IV). Circulation 1990; 82: 39–46 |
| 12 | 2b | Glower DD, Fann JI, Speier RH, et al. Comparison of medical and surgical therapy for uncomplicated descending aortic dissection (supplement IV). Circulation 1990; 82: 39–46 |
| 13 | 1b | Shores J et al. Progression of aortic dilatation and benefit of long-term beta-adrenergic blockade in Marfan syndrome. N Engl J Med 1994; 330: 1335–41 |
| 14 | 4 | Chirillo F et al. Outcome of 290 patients with aortic dissection: a 12 year multicentre experience. Eur Heart J 1990; 11: 311–9 |
| 15 | 4 | Perko MJ et al. Unoperated aortic aneurysms: a survey of 170 patients. Ann Thorac Surg 1995; 59: 1204–9 |
| 16 | 4 | Miller DC et al. Independent determinants of operative mortality for patients with aortic dissection. Circulation 1984; 70 (SI): I-153–63 |
| 17 | 4 | Haverich A et al. Acute and chronic aortic dissection: determinants of long-term outcome for operative survivors. Circulation 1985; 72 (SII): II-22–33 |

## PREVALENCE

Asthma attacks are common **[B]**[1].

**Note**
- Asthma causes 33% of cases of dyspnoea requiring hospital admission **[B]**[1].

Watch out for hypercapnia **[C]**[2] and respiratory failure **[C]**[3].

**Note**
- 9% of acute severe attacks have respiratory failure (defined as $Po_2 < 8$ kPa and/or $Pco_2 > 6$ kPa) **[C]**[3].
- A quarter of patients have $Pco_2 > 5$ kPax **[C]**[2].

## CLINICAL FEATURES

Ask about:
- a previous history of asthma **[B]**[1]
- severity of asthma:
  - normal peak expiratory flow rate **[D]** and whether it feels worse than normal **[C]**[4]

**Why?**
- Patients are not very good at assessing changes in their peak flows over time, although they are better at guessing when it is much worse **[C]**[4].

  - any life-threatening asthma attacks (e.g. respiratory arrests or intubations)

**Why?**
- Previous life-threatening attacks increase the risk of dying **[B]**[5]

**Life-threatening asthma attacks increase the risk of death from asthma**

| Outcome **[B]**[5] | Risk factor | PEER (%) | OR (95% CI) | NNF + (95% CI) |
|---|---|---|---|---|
| Death following asthma attack | ≥ 1 life-threatening asthma attacks *independent* | 0.0057 | Infinity (4.9 to infinity) | <180 (1 to 4500) |

- number of emergency department visits in the last 6 months **[A]**[6] **[A]**[7]
- any hospital admission within 12 months **[B]**[8]
- recent discharge from hospital **[A]**[6]

---

**Note**

■ Patients who have three or more emergency department visits within 6 months **[A]**[6] **[A]**[7] or have a hospital admission within 12 months **[B]**[5] **[B]**[8] are at increased risk of having a relapse.

■ Leaving hospital within 24 h without achieving 50% predicted PEFR increases the risk of relapse **[A]**[6].

**Frequent ED visits and early discharge without improvement increase the risk of asthma relapse**

| Patient | Prognostic factor | Outcome | Control rate | OR (95% CI) | NNF + (95% CI) |
|---|---|---|---|---|---|
| Severe asthma exacerbation | ≥ 3 ED visits within last 6 months *independent* **[A]**[6] **[A]**[7] | Relapse at 8 weeks | 45% | 2.3 (1.6 to 3.4) | 5 (4 to 9) |
| | Left before 24 h without achieving 50% predicted PEFR *independent* **[A]**[6] | Relapse at 8 weeks | 45% | 2.6 (1.6 to 4.1) | 4 (3 to 9) |

**Previous hospital admissions in the last year are associated with asthma relapse**

| Outcome | Risk factor | PEER | OR (95% CI) | NNH (95% CI) |
|---|---|---|---|---|
| Asthma relapse | Admission in last year *independent* **[B]**[8] | 30% | 3.0 (1.0 to 9.3) | 4 (2 to infinity) |

---

- recent symptoms
  - wheezing **[B]**[9]
  - cough **[B]**[1] **[B]**[9]
  - any dyspnoea
  - exertional dyspnoea

---

**Why?**

**Symptoms help predict airflow limitation**

| Patient | Target disorder (reference standard) | Diagnostic test | LR+ (95% CI) | Post-test probability | LR− (95% CI) | Post-test probability |
|---|---|---|---|---|---|---|
| Suspected airflow limitation (pre-test probability 33%) | Airflow limitation ($FEV_1$ and FVC by spirometry) | Wheezing **[B]**[9] | 3.8 | 65% | 0.66 | 25% |
| | | Cough **[B]**[1] **[B]**[9] | 1.8 | 47% | 0.69 | 25% |
| | | Any dyspnoea **[B]**[1] **[B]**[9] | 1.2 | 37% | 0.55 | 21% |
| | | Exertional dyspnoea **[C]**[9] | 3.0 | 60% | 0.98 | 33% |

– difficulty performing work or other activities due to physical health within last 4 weeks [A][6]

> **?  Why?**
> **Problems with breathing in the last 4 weeks increase the risk of asthma relapse**
>
> | Patient | Prognostic factor | Outcome | Control rate | OR (95% CI) | NNF + (95% CI) |
> |---|---|---|---|---|---|
> | Severe asthma exacerbation | Difficulty performing work or other activities due to physical health within last 4 weeks [A][6] | Relapse at 8 weeks | 45% | 2.7 (1.6 to 4.3) | 4 (3 to 9) |

● current medication and its use [B][5]

> **?  Why?**
> ■ Patients who have started three or more new types of medication in the last year are at increased risk of dying [B][5].
> ■ Irregular or infrequent use increases the risk of dying. [B][5]
>
> **Poor compliance and multiple medications started in the last year are associated with asthma death**
>
> | Outcome [B][5] | Risk factor | PEER | OR (95% CI) | NNH (95% CI) |
> |---|---|---|---|---|
> | Death from asthma | ≥ 3 categories of asthma drug prescribed in last year *independent* | 0.0057% | 3.0 (1.04 to 10.5) | 8800 (1900 to 440 000) |
> | | Non-compliance with treatment *independent* | 0.0057% | Infinity (5.2 to infinity) | <180 (1 to 4200) |

● triggers for attacks [D]
● any psychosocial problems [B][5].

> **?  Why?**
> **Psychosocial problems are associated with asthma relapse**
>
> | Outcome [B][5] | Risk factor | PEER | OR (95% CI) | NNH (95% CI) |
> |---|---|---|---|---|
> | Asthma relapse | Psychosocial problems *independent* | 30% | 3.5 (1.004 to 13.7) | 400 (80 to 250 000) |

Look for:
● signs of severity [B][10]
    – moderate-severe dyspnoea
    – pulse ≥ 120 beats/min
    – respiratory rate ≥ 30/min

- evidence of airway obstruction **[B]**[9]
  - wheezing
  - barrel chest
  - hyperresonance

| **? Why?** Clinical signs help predict airflow limitation | | | | | | |
|---|---|---|---|---|---|---|
| Patient **[B]**[9] | Target disorder (reference standard) | Diagnostic test | LR+ (95% CI) | Post-test probability | LR– (95% CI) | Post-test probability |
| Suspected airflow limitation (pre-test probability 33%) | Airflow limitation (FEV$_1$ and FVC by spirometry) | Wheezing | 36 | 95% | 0.85 | 30% |
| | | Barrel chest | 10 | 83% | 0.90 | 31% |
| | | Hyperresonance | 4.8 | 70% | 0.73 | 26% |

- forced expiratory time

| **? Why?** A long forced expiratory time increases the chance of airflow limitation | | | | |
|---|---|---|---|---|
| Patient **[B]**[9] | Target disorder (reference standard) | Diagnostic test | LR+(95% CI) | Post-test probability |
| Suspected airflow limitation (pre-test probability 33%) | Airflow limitation (FEV$_1$ and FVC by spirometry) | Forced expiratory time >9 s | 4.8 | 70% |
| | | 6–9 s | 2.7 | 57% |
| | | <6 s | 0.45 | 18% |

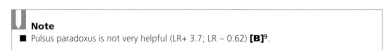

**Note**
- Pulsus paradoxus is not very helpful (LR+ 3.7; LR – 0.62) **[B]**[9].

- evidence of hypercapnia; **[C]**[2] this is more likely with:
  - a quiet chest
  - too dyspnoeic to talk
  - cyanosis
  - requiring supplemental oxygen

  and less likely with:
  - patient on beta-agonists
  - use of accessory muscles
  - no previous visit to emergency department within 2 weeks

**Why?**

Clinical signs can help rule hypercapnia in or out

| Patient [C][2] | Target disorder (reference standard) | Diagnostic test | LR+ (95% CI) | Post-test probability | LR– (95% CI) | Post-test probability |
|---|---|---|---|---|---|---|
| Admitted with acute asthma (pre-test probability 27%) | Hypercapnia (arterial blood gas $P_{CO_2}$>5 kPa) | Quiet chest | 13 (4.6 to 37) | 83% | 0.71 (0.59 to 0.84) | 20% |
| | | Too dyspnoeic to talk | 6.0 (3.1 to 12) | 69% | 0.65 (0.53 to 0.80) | 19% |
| | | Cyanosis | 5.1 (2.1 to 12) | 65% | 0.82 (0.72 to 0.94) | 23% |
| | | Requiring supplemental oxygen | 5.1 (3.0 to 9.0) | 65% | 0.59 (0.47 to 0.75) | 18% |
| | | On beta-agonists | 1.2 (1.1 to 1.4) | 31% | 0.32 (0.13 to 0.77) | 10% |
| | | Use of accessory muscles | 1.2 (1.1 to 1.3) | 30% | 0.11 (0.015 to 0.76) | 4% |
| | | No previous visit to emergency department within 2 weeks | 1.2 (1.1 to 1.3) | 30% | 0.40 (0.15 to 0.90) | 12% |

- psychiatric symptoms or denial [C][11].

 **Why?**

■ Psychiatric symptoms are common in patients with near-fatal asthma attacks. Many patients are in denial of their symptoms [C][11].

## INVESTIGATIONS

- Peak expiratory flow rate [C][4] [C][12]
  Admit patients with a PEFR [C][12]:
  - <100 l/min before therapy
  - <300 l/min after therapy.

**Why?**
- Neither clinicians nor patients accurately judge peak flows **[C]**[4].
- PEFR correlates reasonably well with $FEV_1$ in patients with acute asthma **[C]**[12].
- Both PEFR and $FEV_1$ can predict which patients will require admission or have continuing symptoms **[C]**[12–14].

**Peak expiratory flow rate helps predict patients who required admission**

| Patient | Prognostic factor | Outcome | Control rate | RR (95% CI) | NNF (95% CI) |
|---|---|---|---|---|---|
| Acute asthma **[C]**[12] | Pre-treatment PEFR <100 l/min *not independent* | Admitted to hospital or failed discharge at 48 h | 41% | 1.86 (1.32 to 2.61) | 3 (2 to 8) |
| | Post-treatment PEFR <300 l/min *not independent* | Admitted to hospital or failed discharge at 48 h | 14% | 5.43 (2.55 to 11.56) | 2 (1 to 5) |

- Pulse oximetry **[C]**[3] **[C]**[15].

 **Why?**
- Patients with an oxygen saturation >92% are less likely to be hypoxic **[C]**[3].
- Significant hypoxia produces minimal changes in vital signs in healthy people **[C]**[15].

**Pulse oximetry can help rule out hypoxia, but further tests may be required**

| Patient **[C]**[3] | Target disorder (reference standard) | Diagnostic test | LR+ (95% CI) | Post-test probability | LR− (95% CI) | Post-test probability |
|---|---|---|---|---|---|---|
| Acute severe asthma (pre-test probability 9%) | Hypoxia ($Po_2$<8 kPa arterial blood gas) | $Sao_2 \leq 92\%$ | 6.7 (3.2 to 13) | 38% | 0.3 (0.08 to 0.94) | 2% |

- Arterial blood gases **[C]**[16] **[C]**[17], using local anaesthetic **[A]**[18] **[A]**[19], if $Sao_2 \leq 92\%$ or signs of hypercapnia.

 **Why?**
- PEFR or $FEV_1$ alone cannot safely exclude hypercapnia or hypoxia **[C]**[16] **[C]**[17].

**Peak expiratory flow rate cannot safely rule out hypercapnia or hypoxia**

| Patient **[C]**[16] | Target disorder (reference standard) | Diagnostic test | LR+ (95% CI) | Post-test probability | LR− (95% CI) | Post-test probability |
|---|---|---|---|---|---|---|
| Acute asthma (pre-test probability 18%) | Hypoxia ($Po_2$ < 8 kPa on arterial blood gas) | PEFR ≤ 25% predicted | 1.3 (0.92 to 1.8) | 22% | 0.59 (0.24 to 1.4) | 11% |
| Acute asthma (pre-test probability 4.5%) | Hypercapnia ($Pco_2$ > 6 kPa on arterial blood gas) | PEFR ≤ 25% predicted | 1.2 (0.64 to 2.1) | 5% | 0.71 (0.13 to 4.0) | 3% |

- Arterial blood gas sampling is more painful than venous sampling: local anaesthetic before sampling reduces pain. Moreover, injecting local anaesthetic is not clearly more painful than saline **[A]**[18] **[A]**[19].
- The procedure takes around 40 s longer to perform **[A]**[18].

After therapy repeat:
- PEFR [C][20]
- arterial blood gases [C][17].

**Why?**
- Improvement in signs and symptoms in patients with asthma does not correlate well with improvement in PEFR. When 90% of patients feel better, 40% still have expiratory wheeze. When other clinical signs have gone, PEFR can be as low as 55% predicted [C][20].
- Blood gas levels of many patients improve following treatment; however, improvement in FEV$_1$ does not predict improvement in blood gas levels [C][17].

Consider a chest X-ray for complicated cases [C][21] to exclude a pneumothorax [D].

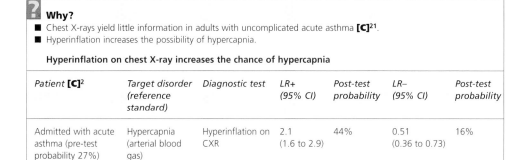
**Why?**
- Chest X-rays yield little information in adults with uncomplicated acute asthma [C][21].
- Hyperinflation increases the possibility of hypercapnia.

**Hyperinflation on chest X-ray increases the chance of hypercapnia**

| Patient [C][2] | Target disorder (reference standard) | Diagnostic test | LR+ (95% CI) | Post-test probability | LR– (95% CI) | Post-test probability |
|---|---|---|---|---|---|---|
| Admitted with acute asthma (pre-test probability 27%) | Hypercapnia (arterial blood gas) | Hyperinflation on CXR | 2.1 (1.6 to 2.9) | 44% | 0.51 (0.36 to 0.73) | 16% |

## THERAPY

- Give oxygen 40–60% [D].
- Give a beta-agonist [A] (e.g. salbutamol 2.5–5 mg) via an inhaler and holding chamber or a nebuliser [A][22] regularly [A][23–25] (and continuously if possible [A][26]) using air or oxygen [D][27].
- Add an anticholinergic [A][28] (e.g. ipratropium 500 µg).

**Why do this?**

■ The combination of ipratropium and beta-agonists given together reduces hospital admissions and improves $FEV_1$ (on average 100 ml) and PEFR (on average 32 l/min) better than beta-agonists alone **[A]**[28].

■ Combination treatment is more effective in severe over moderate/mild cases (in children) **[A]**[29].

**Ipratropium and beta-agonists together reduce hospital admissions**

| Patient [A][28] | Treatment | Comparator | Outcome | CER | OR | NNT |
|---|---|---|---|---|---|---|
| Asthma exacerbation | Ipratropium and beta-agonists | Beta-agonists | Hospitalisation at 60 min | 20% | 0.73 (0.53 to 0.99) | 19 (11 to 500) |

| Patient [A][29] | Treatment | Comparator | Outcome | CER | OR | NNT |
|---|---|---|---|---|---|---|
| Children with severe exacerbation of asthma | Ipratropium and beta-agonists | Beta-agonists | Hospitalisation at 2.5 h | 53% | 29 (7 to 46) | 7 (4 to 30) |

■ Beta-agonists delivered by holding chamber are as effective as wet nebulisation. There is no clear increase in hospital admissions, time spent in the emergency department or need for more steroids **[A]**[22].

■ Multiple doses of anticholinergics added to beta-agonists improve $FEV_1$ (on average 14 ml) and **reduce** hospital admissions, without clearly increasing side-effects **[A]**[23–25].

**Multiple doses of anticholinergics reduce hospital admissions**

| Patient [A][25] | Treatment | Comparator | Outcome | CER | OR | NNT |
|---|---|---|---|---|---|---|
| Asthma exacerbation | Multiple doses of ipratropium | No ipratropium | Hospitalisation at 60 min | 34% | 0.62 (0.39 to 0.98) | 10 (6 to 220) |

■ Continuous nebulisers lead to a greater improvement in $FEV_1$ at 2 h than intermittent nebulisers. Low-dose continuous nebulisers (2.5 mg salbutamol) appear to give the same benefit as high-dose intermittent nebulisers (5.0 mg salbutamol) **[A]**[26].

■ Salbutamol nebulisers are probably equally effective whether oxygen or air is used as the driving gas. Children who receive oxygen-driven nebulisers only have a rise in oxygen saturation while the nebuliser is working **[D]**[27].

● Give steroids **[A]** immediately **[A]**[30–32] in doses of equivalent to 40 mg prednisolone daily **[A]**[33]. The best route is unclear **[A]**[31] **[A]**[34].

**? Why do this?**

■ Steroids improve symptoms **[A]**[30] and reduce hospital admissions if given early **[A]**[31].

■ Oral corticosteroids are statistically, though not clinically, more effective than iv corticosteroids at improving PEFR and shortening hospital stay; however, there is no clear difference in the number of patients developing respiratory failure **[A]**[31] **[A]**[34].

**Early steroids reduce hospital admissions**

| Patient | Treatment | Comparator | Outcome | CER | OR | NNT |
|---|---|---|---|---|---|---|
| Asthma exacerbation **[A]**[25] | Steroids in the emergency department | No steroids | Hospitalisation at 6 h | 40% | 0.47 (0.27 to 0.79) | 6 (4 to 18) |

**Early steroids reduce wheezing**

| Patient | Treatment | Comparator | Outcome | CER | RRR | NNT |
|---|---|---|---|---|---|---|
| Admitted with an asthma exacerbation **[A]**[30] | iv hydrocortisone | Placebo | Wheezing at 24 h | 100% | 73% (28%to 90%) | 1 (1 to 2) |

■ Doses of intravenous methylprednisolone $\geq 40$ mg given 6-hourly are more effective at improving $FEV_1$ than 15 mg 6-hourly. There appears to be little difference between 40 mg and 125 mg **[A]**[33].

**Low-dose steroids are less effective in improving symptoms**

| Patient | Treatment | Comparator | Outcome | CER | RBI | NNT |
|---|---|---|---|---|---|---|
| Admitted with an asthma exacerbation | Methylprednisolone $\geq 40$ mg every 6 h | Methylprednisolone 15 mg every 6 h | > 50% predicted $FEV_1$ at 3 days | 50% | 100% (0% to 300%) | 2 (1 to 7) |

If patients are not improving, inform ITU **[D]** and consider using the following:

● aminophylline iv **[A]**[35] **[A]**[36] (e.g. a loading dose of 5.6 mg/kg over 20 min (not if patient has taken theophyllines within the last 24 h), followed by continuous infusion 0.9 mg/kg per hour)

**Why do this?**
- It reduces hospital admissions **[A]**[35] and relapses **[B]**[37].
- It reduces need for intubation or iv salbutamol in children with severe asthma **[A]**[36].
- Patients require fewer nebulisers (on average six fewer at 48 h) **[A]**[38], but there is no clear effect on pulmonary function tests for up to 2 h **[A]**[35] **[A]**[39].
- However, side-effects (tremor, nausea or vomiting, and palpitations) are common, and children on aminophylline are more likely to stop therapy due to adverse effects **[A]**[36].

**Aminophylline reduces hospital admissions and need for intubation but causes side-effects**

| Patient | Treatment | Comparator | Outcome | CER | RRR | NNT |
|---|---|---|---|---|---|---|
| Asthma or COPD exacerbation **[A]**[35] | iv aminophylline | Placebo | Hospital admission at 2 h | 21% | 70% (14% to 90%) | 7 (4 to 31) |
| Children with acute severe asthma **[A]**[36] | iv aminophylline | Placebo | iv salbutamol required at 48 h | 32% | 42% (−2% to 67%) | 8 (4 to 2800) |
| | | | Intubation required at 48 h | 6.1% | 100% | 16 (9 to 110) |
| | | | Therapy stopped due to side-effects at 48 h | 4.9% | −558% (−1700% to −140%) | −4 (−6 to −3) |

**Aminophylline reduces relapse in children**

| Patient | Treatment | Comparator | Outcome | CER | OR | NNT |
|---|---|---|---|---|---|---|
| Children with acute asthma **[B]**[37] | Theophyllines in emergency department | No theophyllines | Relapse at 10 days | 55% | 0.4 (0.2 to 0.8) | 5 (3 to 18) |

- salbutamol iv **[A]**[40] **[A]**[41] (e.g. 5 µg/min initially, adjusted to response up to 20 µg/min)

 **Why do this?**
- Children with severe asthma who have iv salbutamol in addition to nebulisers are more likely to improve than those who do not, **and** are less likely to be on continuous oxygen. Children come off nebulisers faster. **[A]**[42]
- Intravenous salbutamol alone is effective in adults, though not much better alone than nebulised salbutamol. Tachycardia is common **[A]**[40] **[A]**[41].

**Intravenous salbutamol improves symptoms and the need for oxygen in children with severe asthma**

| Patient | Treatment | Comparator | Outcome | CER | RRR | NNT |
|---|---|---|---|---|---|---|
| Children with acute severe asthma **[A]**[42] | Intravenous salbutamol | Placebo | Moderate-to-severe asthma at 2 h | 93% | 62% (22% to 81%) | 2 (1 to 3) |
| | | | On continuous oxygen at 2 h | 53% | 73% (−5% to 93%) | 3 (1 to 13) |

- epinephrine (adrenaline) sc **[A]**[43] (0.3 ml 1:1000)

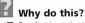

**Why do this?**
- More patients with severe asthma who receive subcutaneous epinephrine compared with inhaled metaproterenol **improve after** 1 h (increase in PEFR > 20%) but side-effects (palpitations, tremor, tachycardia, arrhythmia, nervousness) **are common [A]**[43].

**Adrenaline helps improve PEFR in severe cases**

| Patient | Treatment | Comparator | Outcome | CER | RRR | NNT |
|---|---|---|---|---|---|---|
| Acute severe asthma **[A]**[43] | Subcutaneous epinephrine | No therapy | No PEFR improvement at 1 h | 39% | 72% (34% to 88%) | 4 (2 to 9) |
| | | | Side-effects at 1 h | 72% | −24% (−52% to 1%) | −6 (−60 to −3) |

- magnesium sulphate (1.0–1.2 g iv over 30 min) **[A]**[44]

**Why do this?**
- It reduces hospital admissions and improves predicted PEFR (on average by 17%) in severe cases, though not in mild-moderate ones **[A]**[44].

**Magnesium sulphate helps prevent hospital admissions in severe cases**

| Patient | Treatment | Comparator | Outcome | CER | OR | NNT |
|---|---|---|---|---|---|---|
| Acute severe asthma **[A]**[44] | Magnesium sulphate | Placebo | Hospital admission at ? hours | 91% | 0.10 (0.04 to 0.27) | 2 (2 to 5) |

- heliox (helium/oxygen) **[A]**[45] or other anaesthetic drugs **[A]**.

**Why do this?**
- Paediatric patients with status asthmaticus who receive heliox compared with air have improved respiratory symptoms and a 70% improvement in PEFR after 15 min **[A]**[45]

Patients with the following should be considered for intubation and ventilation **[D]**:
- worsening peak flows
- worsening hypoxia or hypercapnia
- exhaustion or confusion
- coma or respiratory arrest.

Patients who improve can be discharged if:
- PEFR > 300 l/min and >60% predicted and improving **[C]**[12–14] **[C]**[46]
- they are symptom-free **[D]**.

Give steroids and advice (see Prevention)

There is no clear benefit from:
- antibiotics **[D]**[47].

## PREVENTION

- Give oral [A]⁴⁸ steroids for 7–10 days (e.g. 40 mg prednisolone daily, and inhaled budesonide 800 μg twice daily). These can be stopped abruptly without tapering [A]⁴⁹.
- Combine this with inhaled [A]⁵⁰ steroids.

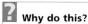

**Why do this?**

- A short course of steroids reduces relapse and hospital admissions, and patients use less beta-agonists [A]⁴⁸.
- Combining oral and inhaled steroids prevents relapse better than oral steroids alone. There is no clear effect on hospital admissions [A]⁵⁰.
- Side-effects (sore throat, hoarse voice or nausea) are more common on the combination.
- Abrupt termination of oral steroids, rather than tapered, does not cause a significant worsening of PEFR on stopping or a greater risk of acute exacerbations [A]⁴⁹.

**Steroids reduce asthma relapse and hospital admission**

| Patient | Treatment | Comparator | Outcome | CER | OR | NNT |
|---------|-----------|------------|---------|-----|-----|-----|
| Acute asthma | Steroids for 7–10 days | No therapy | Relapse at 21 days | 44% | 0.34 (0.14 to 0.82) | 4 (3 to 21) |
| | | | Admission to hospital at 21 days | 14% | 0.34 (0.13 to 0.89) | 11 (8 to 74) |
| Acute asthma | Oral and inhaled steroids | Oral steroids | Relapse at 21 days | 24% | 48 (1 to 72) | 9 (4 to 140) |
| | | | Side-effects at 21 days | 52% | 29 (1 to 48) | 7 (3 to 120) |

- Provide information on asthma for high-risk patients.

**Why do this?**

- Limited asthma education (information only) programmes reduce emergency department visits in high-risk adults (on average two fewer a year) [A]⁵¹

- Provide an action plan and a peak flow meter [A]⁵²
  If the PEFR is:
  - ≤ 70% or ≥ 20% diurnal variation – double inhaled steroid dose
  - ≤ 50% – steroid course
  - ≤ 30% – seek urgent treatment.

**Why do this?**

- A peak flow-based action plan reduces the need for urgent treatment. There is no clear effect on number of hospital admissions [A]⁵².
- A symptom-based action plan is not clearly better than giving no advice [A]⁵².

| Patient | Treatment | Comparator | Outcome | CER | OR | NNT |
|---------|-----------|------------|---------|-----|-----|-----|
| Acute asthma | PEFR action plan | No plan | Urgent treatment | 40% | 73 (33 to 89) | 3 (2 to 8) |

- Check the patient's inhaler technique [D].
- If the patient has confirmed severe gastro-oesophageal reflux, consider treatment [C][53].

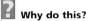
**Why do this?**
■ Surgery for reflux in asthmatics improved asthma as well as reflux symptoms [C][53].

## PROGNOSIS

Relapse is common [A][54].

**Note**
■ 45% of patients with acute severe asthma exacerbations relapse within 8 weeks [A][54].

The risk is increased if the patient has:
- ≥ 3 emergency department visits within the last 6 months [A][7] [A][54]
- difficulty performing work or other activities due to physical health within the last 4 weeks [A][54]
- left hospital within 24 h without achieving 50% predicted PEFR [A][54]
- hospital admission within 12 months [B][8].

The more risk factors present, the greater is the risk of relapse [A][54].

**Why?**
The higher the number of risk factors, the greater the risk of relapse

| Patient [A][54] | Prognostic factor | Outcome | Control rate | OR (95% CI) | NNF+ (95% CI) |
|---|---|---|---|---|---|
| Severe asthma exacerbation | ≥3 ED visits within last 6 months *independent* [A][54] [B][55] | Relapse at 8 weeks | 45% | 2.3 (1.6 to 3.4) | 5 (4 to 9) |
| | Left before 24 h without achieving 50% predicted PEFR *independent* [A][54] | Relapse at 8 weeks | 45% | 2.6 (1.6 to 4.1) | 4 (3 to 9) |
| | Difficulty performing work or other activities due to physical health within last 4 weeks *independent* [A][54] | Relapse at 8 weeks | 45% | 2.7 (1.6 to 4.3) | 4 (3 to 9) |

| Number of risk factors [B][56] | % relapse (95% CI) |
|---|---|
| 3 | 100% (79% to 100%) |
| 2 | 63% (53% to 73%) |
| 1 | 32% (24% to 39%) |
| 0 | 14% (3.8% to 26%) |

Death is rare **[B]**[57].

> **Note**
> ■ 1% of patients have fatal/near fatal attacks a year **[B]**[57].

The risk is increased in patients attending hospital with **[B]**[5]:
- ≥1 life-threatening asthma attacks
- psychosocial problems.

The risk is increased in patients in the community with:
- non-compliance with treatment **[B]**[5]
- ≥1 life-threatening asthma attacks **[B]**[5]
- ≥1 previous respiratory arrests **[B]**[5]
- ≥1 hospital admission with asthma in last year **[B]**[5] **[B]**[8]
- ≥1 attendance to an emergency department with asthma in last year **[B]**[5] **[B]**[8]
- ≥3 categories of asthma drug prescribed in last year **[B]**[5] **[B]**[8]
- regular beta-agonist use **[B]**[58].

> **Note**
> **Clinical features can help predict death from asthma**
>
> | Outcome | Risk factor **[B]**[5] | PEER | OR (95% CI) | NNH (95% CI) |
> |---|---|---|---|---|
> | Death from asthma (community) | ≥3 categories of asthma drug prescribed in last year *independent* | 0.0057% | 3.0 (1.04 to 10.5) | 8800 (1900 to 440 000) |
> | | Non-compliance with treatment *independent* | 0.0057% | >100 (5.2 to inf) | <180 (1 to 4200) |
> | | ≥1 life-threatening asthma attacks *independent* | 0.0057% | >100 (4.9 to inf) | <180 (1 to 4500) |
> | | ≥1 previous respiratory arrests *independent* | 0.0057% | >100 (1.4 to inf) | <180 (1 to 44000) |
> | | ≥1 hospital admission with asthma in last year *independent* | 0.0057% | 16.0 (2.5 to 665.7) | 1200 (27 to 12 000) |
> | | ≥1 attendance to an emergency department with asthma in last year *independent* | 0.0057% | 8.5 (2.0 to 75.9) | 2300 (240 to 18 000) |
> | Death from asthma (attending hospital) | ≥1 life-threatening asthma attacks *independent* | 0.0057% | 3.8 (1.2 to 15.5) | 360 (70 to 5000) |
> | | Psychosocial problems *independent* | 0.0057% | 3.5 (1.004 to 13.7) | 400 (80 to 250 000) |

Most patients who are ventilated do well.

> **Note**
> ■ Deaths are uncommon in patients who go to ITU (0.0%; 95% CI: 0.0% to 3.4%) **[B]**[59].
> ■ Patients who are mechanically ventilated are at increased risk of pulmonary barotrauma, hypotension and cardiac arrhythmias **[B]**[59].

**Guideline writers**: Ben Wong, Christopher Ball
**CAT writers**: Ben Wong, Christophher Ball

## REFERENCES

| No. | Level | Citation |
| --- | --- | --- |
| 1 | 2a | History and physical examination for dyspnoea: a review. ACP Journal Club. 1993 Nov-Dec; 119: 90. Summary of Mulrow CD et al. Discriminating causes of dyspnoea through clinical examination. J Gen Intern Med 1993; 8: 383–92 |
| 2 | 4 | Mountain RD, Sahn SA. Clinical features and outcome in patients with acute asthma presenting with hypercapnia. Am Rev Respir Dis 1988; 138: 535–9 |
| 3 | 4 | Carruthers DM, Harrison BD. Arterial blood gas analysis or oxygen saturation in the assessment of acute asthma? Thorax 1995; 50: 186–8 |
| 4 | 4 | Shim CS, Williams MH. Evaluation of the severity of asthma; patients versus physicians. Am J Med 1980; 68: 11–13 |
| 5 | 3b | Rea HH et al. A case-control study of deaths from asthma. Thorax 1986; 41: 833–9 |
| 6 | 1b | McCarren M et al. Prediction of relapse within eight weeks after an acute asthma exacerbation in adults. J Clin Epidemiol 1998; 51: 107–18 |
| 7 | 1b | Ducharme FM, Kramer MS. Relapse following emergency treatment for acute asthma: can it be predicted or prevented? J Clin Epidemiol 1993; 46: 1395–402 |
| 8 | 3b | Crane J et al. Markers of risk of asthma death or readmission in the 12 months following a hospital admission for asthma. Int J Epidemiol 1992; 21: 737–44 |
| 9 | 2a | Holleman DR, Simel DL. Does the clinical examination predict airflow limitation? JAMA 1995; 275: 313–9 |
| 10 | 2a | Fischl MA et al. Index predicting relapse and need for hospitalisation in patients with acute bronchial asthma. N Engl J Med 1981; 305: 783–9 |
| 11 | 4 | Campbell DA et al. Psychiatric and medical features of near-fatal asthma. Thorax 1995; 50: 254–9 |
| 12 | 4 | Nowak RM et al. Comparison of peak expiratory flow and $FEV_1$ admission criteria for acute bronchial asthma. Ann Emerg Med 1982; 11: 64–9 |
| 13 | 4 | Nowak RM et al. Spirometric evaluation of acute bronchial asthma. Journal of the American College of Experimental Physiology 1979; 8: 9–12 |
| 14 | 4 | Worthington JR, Ahuja J. The value of pulmonary function tests in the management of asthma. Can Med Assoc J 1989; 149: 153–6 |
| 15 | 4 | Thrush DN et al. Does significant arterial hypoxemia alter vital signs? J Clin Anesth 1997; 9: 355–7 |
| 16 | 4 | Martin TG et al. Use of peak expiratory flow rates to eliminate unnecessary arterial blood gases in acute asthma. Ann Emerg Med 1982; 11: 70–3 |

| No. | Level | Citation |
|-----|-------|----------|
| 17 | 4 | Nowak RM et al. Arterial blood gases and pulmonary function testing in acute bronchial asthma: predicting patient outcomes. JAMA 1983; 249: 2043–6 |
| 18 | 1b | Giner J et al. Pain during arterial puncture. Chest 1996; 110: 1443–5 |
| 19 | 1b | Lightowler JV, Elliott MW. Local anaesthetic infiltration prior to arterial puncture for blood gas analysis: a survey of current practice and a randomised double-blind placebo-controlled trial. J R Coll Physicians 1997; 31: 645–6 |
| 20 | 4 | McFadden E et al. Acute bronchial asthma: correlations between clinical and physiologic manifestations. N Engl J Med 1973; 288: 221–5 |
| 21 | 4 | Findley LJ, Sahn SA. The value of chest roentgenograms in acute asthma in adults. Chest 1981; 80: 535–6 |
| 22 | 1a | Cates CJ. Comparison of holding chambers and nebulisers for beta-agonists in acute asthma (Cochrane Review). In: The Cochrane Library, Issue 3, 1998. Oxford: Update Software |
| 23 | 1b | Rebuck AS et al. Nebulised anticholinergic and sympathomimetic treatment of asthma and chronic obstructive airways disease in the emergency room. Am J Med 1987; 82: 59–64 |
| 24 | 1b | Bryant DH. Nebulized ipratropium bromide in the treatment of acute asthma. Chest 1985; 88: 24–9 |
| 25 | 1a | Plotnick LH, Ducharme FM. Efficacy and safety of combined inhaled anticholinergics and beta-2-agonists in the initial management of acute pediatric asthma (Cochrane Review). In: The Cochrane Library, Issue 3, 1998. Oxford: Update Software |
| 26 | 1b | Shrestha M et al. Continuous vs intermittent albuterol at high and low doses in the treatment of severe acute asthma in adults. Chest 1996; 110: 42–7 |
| 27 | 1b- | Gleeson JG et al. Air or oxygen as a driving gas for nebulised salbutamol. Arch Dis Child 1988; 63: 900–4 |
| 28 | 1a | Stoodley RG, Aaron SD, Dales RE. The role of ipratropium bromide in the emergency management of acute asthma exacerbation: a meta-analysis of randomized clinical trials. Ann Emerg Med 1999; 34: 8–18 |
| 29 | 1b | Qureshi F, Pestian J. Effect of nebulized ipratropium on the hospitalization rates of children with asthma. N Engl J Med 1998; 339: 1030–5 |
| 30 | 1b | Fanta CH et al. Glucocorticoids in acute asthma: a critical controlled trial. Am J Med 1983; 74: 845–51 |
| 31 | 1a | Rowe BH et al. Effectiveness of steroid therapy in acute exacerbations of asthma: a meta-analysis. Am J Emerg Med 1992; 10: 301–10 |
| 32 | 1a | Rodrigo G, Rodrigo C. Corticosteroids in the emergency department therapy of acute adult asthma: an evidence-based evaluation. Chest 1999; 116: 285–95 |
| 33 | 1b | Haskell RJ et al. A double-blind, randomised clinical trial of methylprednisolone in status asthmaticus. Arch Intern Med 1983; 143: 1324–7 |
| 34 | 1b | Ratto D et al. Are intravenous corticosteroids required in status asthmaticus. JAMA 1988; 260: 527–9 |
| 35 | 1b | Wrenn K et al. Aminophylline therapy for acute bronchospastic disease in the emergency room. Ann Intern Med 1991; 115: 241–7 |
| 36 | 1b | Yung M, South M. Randomised controlled trial of aminophylline for severe acute asthma. Arch Dis Child 1998; 79: 405–10 |

| No. | Level | Citation |
|-----|-------|----------|
| 37 | 2b | Ducharme FM, Kramer MS. Relapse following emergency treatment for acute asthma: can it be predicted or prevented? J Clin Epidemiol 1993; 46: 1395–1402 |
| 38 | 1b | Huang D et al. Does aminophylline benefit adults admitted to the hospital for an acute exacerbation of asthma? Ann Intern Med 1993; 119: 1155–60 |
| 39 | 1a | Littenberg B. Aminophylline treatment in severe, acute asthma; a meta-analysis. JAMA 1988; 259: 1678–84 |
| 40 | 1b | Cheong B et al. Intravenous beta-agonists in acute severe asthma. BMJ 1988; 297: 448–50 |
| 41 | 1b | Salmeron S et al. Nebulized versus intravenous albuterol in hypercapnic acute asthma: a multicenter double-blind randomized study. Am J Respir Crit Care Med 1994; 149: 1466–70 |
| 42 | 1b | Browne GJ et al. Randomised trial of intravenous salbutamol in early management of acute severe asthma in children. Lancet 1997; 349: 301–5 |
| 43 | 1b | Appel D et al. Epinephrine improves expiratory flow rates in patients with asthma who do not respond to inhaled metaproterenol sulfate. J Allergy Clin Immunol 1989; 84: 90–8 |
| 44 | 1a | Rowe BH et al. Magnesium sulfate for acute asthma exacerbations treated in the emergency department (Cochrane Review). In: The Cochrane Library, Issue 3, 1999. Oxford: Update Software |
| 45 | 1b | Kudukis TM et al. Inhaled helium–oxygen revisited: effect of inhaled helium–oxygen during the treatment of children with status asthmaticus. J Pediatr 1997; 130: 217–24 |
| 46 | 4 | McDermott MF et al. A comparison between emergency diagnostic and treatment unit and inpatient care in the management of acute asthma. Arch Intern Med 1997; 157: 2055–62 |
| 47 | 1b- | Graham VA et al. Routine antibiotics in hospital management of acute asthma. Lancet 1982; i: 418–20 |
| 48 | 1a | Rowe BH, Spooner CH, Ducharme FM et al. The effectiveness of corticosteroids in the treatment of acute exacerbations of asthma: a meta-analysis of their effect on relapse following acute assessment (Cochrane Review). In: The Cochrane Library, Issue 3, 1998. Oxford: Update Software |
| 49 | 1b | O'Driscoll BR et al. Double-blind trial of steroid tapering in acute asthma. Lancet. 1993; 341: 324–7 |
| 50 | 1b | Rowe BH et al. Inhaled budesonide in addition to oral corticosteroids to prevent asthma relapse following discharge from the emergency department: a randomised controlled trial. JAMA 1999; 281: 2119–26 |
| 51 | 1a | Gibson PG et al. The effects of limited (information only) patient education programs on the health outcomes of adults with asthma (Cochrane Review). In: The Cochrane Library, Issue 4, 1998. Oxford: Update Software |
| 52 | 1b | Cowie RL et al. The effect of a peak flow-based action plan in the prevention of exacerbations of asthma. Chest 1997; 112: 1534–38 |
| 53 | 3b | Field SK, Gelfand AJ, McFadden SD. The effects of antireflux surgery on asthmatics with gastroesophageal reflux. Chest 1999; 116: 766–74 |
| 54 | 1b | McCarren M et al. Prediction of relapse within eight weeks after an acute asthma exacerbation in adults. J Clin Epidemiol 1998; 51: 107–18 |
| 55 | 2a | Ducharme FM & Kramer MS: relapse following emergency treatment for acute asthma: can it be predicted or prevented?: J Clin Epidemiol (1993); 46: 1395–1402 |

| No. | Level | Citation |
|-----|-------|----------|
| 56 | 2a | McCarren M et al: prediction of relapse within eight weeks after an acute asthma exacerbation in adults: J Clin Epidemiol 1998; 51: 107–118 |
| 57 | 3b | Spitzer WO et al. The use of beta-agonists and the risk of death and near death from asthma. N Engl J Med 1992; 326: 501–6 |
| 58 | 2a | Mullen M et al. The association between beta-agonist use and death from asthma: a meta-analytic integration of case-control studies. JAMA 1993; 270: 1842–5 |
| 59 | 4 | Williams IJ et al. Risk factors for morbidity in mechanically ventilated patients in acute severe asthma. Am Rev Respir Dis 1992; 146: 607–15 |

## PREVALENCE

Atrial fibrillation is relatively common **[A]**[1], especially in:
- the elderly **[A]**[2]
- patients with permanent pacemakers **[C]**[3].

---

**Note**
- 8–12% of people develop AF **[A]**[1]**[A]**[4].
- 10% of patients with permanent pacemakers are in chronic AF (95% CI: 6 to 14%) **[C]**[3].

**The risk of developing AF increases with age**

| Age **[A]**[2] (years) | Prevalence of AF |
|---|---|
| 50 to 59 | 0.5% |
| 60 to 69 | 1.8% |
| 70 to 79 | 4.8R |
| 80 to 89 | 8.8% |

---

## CAUSES

The risk of atrial fibrillation is increased with:
- cardiomyopathy **[A]**[4]
- ischaemic heart disease **[A]**[1] **[A]**[4]
- congestive heart failure **[A]**[1] **[A]**[4]
- valvular heart disease **[A]**[1] **[A]**[4]
- other arrhythmias **[A]**[4]
- hypertension **[A]**[4]
- obesity **[A]**[4]
- low TSH levels **[A]**[5].

---

**Why?**
**Cardiomyopathy, ischaemic heart disease, heart failure and valvular heart disease increase the risk of AF**

| Patient | Prognostic factor | Outcome | Control rate | OR (95% CI) | NNF+ (95% CI) |
|---|---|---|---|---|---|
| Healthy men **[A]**[4] | Cardiomyopathy *independent* | Atrial fibrillation at 44 years | 7.4% | 4.07 (1.45 to 11.45) | 4 (1 to 30) |
| | Myocardial infarction *independent* | | 5.8% | 3.62 (2.59 to 5.07) | 7 (4 to 11) |
| | Congestive heart failure *independent* | | 6.4% | 3.37 (2.29 to 4.96) | 7 (4 to 12) |
| | Valvular heart disease *independent* | | 6.9% | 3.15 (1.99 to 5.00) | 7 (4 to 15) |
| | Angina *independent* | | 6.5% | 2.84 (1.91 to 4.21) | 8 (5 to 17) |
| | Palpitations *independent* | | 6.9% | 2.22 (1.24 to 2.97) | 12 (7 to 60) |
| | Supraventricular arrhythmia *independent* | | 5.5% | 2.28 (1.74 to 2.98) | 14 (9 to 25) |

**? Why?** *(continued)*

**Cardiomyopathy, ischaemic heart disease, heart failure and valvular heart disease increase the risk of AF**

| Patient | Prognostic factor | Outcome | Control rate | OR (95% CI) | NNF+ (95% CI) |
|---------|-------------------|---------|--------------|-------------|---------------|
| | ST or T wave changes *independent* | | 3.7% | 2.21 (1.62 to 3.00) | 22 (14 to 44) |
| | Ventricular rhythm disturbance *independent* | | 5.4% | 1.37 (1.06 to 1.78) | 50 (24 to 310) |
| | Hypertension *independent* | | 3.5% | 1.42 (1.10 to 1.84) | 68 (34 to 290) |
| | Obesity *independent* | | 3.4% | 1.28 (1.02 to 1.62) | 110 (47 to 1500) |
| Elderly **[A]**[5] | Low TSH (≤ 0.1 min/l) *independent* | Atrial fibrillation at 10 years | 21% | 3.1 (1.7 to 5.5) | 6 (3 to 17) |

Common causes of acute onset atrial fibrillation include **[B]**[6]:
- alcohol
- valvular heart disease
- pulmonary disease
- ischaemic heart disease or cardiomyopathy
- hypertension.

**? Why?**

**Alcohol, valvular disease and pulmonary disease are common causes of acute AF**

| Causes of AF **[B]**[6] | % (95% CI) |
|-------------------------|------------|
| Alcohol | 28% (13% to 42%) |
| Valve disease | 19% (6.5% to 32%) |
| Pulmonary disease | 17% (4.5% to 29%) |
| Heart muscle disease | 8.3% (0.0% to 17%) |
| Hypertension | 5.6% (0.0% to 13%) |
| Coronary artery disease | 5.6% (0.0% to 13%) |

## CLINICAL FEATURES

Measure the rate using the apical pulse **[D]**[7].

**? Why do this?**
- Measuring the apical pulse is more accurate than measuring the radial pulse (on average by 10 beats/min). Both however underestimate the true rate **[D]**[7].
- Measuring the pulse for 60 s is slightly more accurate than 15 or 30 s, but only by 2 beats/min **[D]**[7].

Look for evidence of:
- ischaemic heart disease **[A]**[1]**[A]**[4]

- congestive heart failure [A][1] [A][4]
- valvular heart disease [A][1] [A][4]
- cardiomyopathy [A][4]
- other arrhythmias [A][4]
- hypertension [A][4]
- obesity [A][4]
- thyrotoxicosis [A][5].

## INVESTIGATIONS

- Urea and electrolytes [D].
- Thyroid function tests [A][5].

 **Why?**
■ 5% of patients admitted as an acute medical emergency with AF have thyrotoxicosis, but only 0.5% of patients on acute medical wards [B][8].

**Note**
**A low TSH level alone is insufficient to diagnose hyperthyroidism**

| Patient | Target disorder (reference standard) | Diagnostic test | LR (95% CI) | Post-test probability |
|---|---|---|---|---|
| Suspected hyperthyroidism (pre-test probability 5%) | Hyperthyroidism (?) | TSH <0.1 miu/ml | 7.7 (5.6 to 11) | 29% |
| | | TSH 0.1–0.6 miu/ml | 0.0 (0.0 to 1.6) | 0% |
| | | TSH >0.6–6.7 miu/ml | 0.0 (0.0 to 1.9) | 0% |

- ECG [A].
- Chest X-ray [D]. '
- Consider performing an echocardiography, looking for:
  - global left ventricular dysfunction [A][9] [A][10], an enlarged left atrium [A][9] [A][10]
  - occult mitral stenosis [D].

 **Why?**
**Global LV dysfunction or an enlarged atrium may increase the risk of stroke**

| Patient | Prognostic factor | Outcome | Control rate | RR (95% CI) | NNF+ (95% CI) |
|---|---|---|---|---|---|
| AF | Global LV dysfunction [A][9] [A][10] *independent* | Stroke or systemic embolism at 1.5 years | 6.0% | 2.0 (1.0 to 4.0) | 17 (6 to infinity) |
| | Enlarged left atrium [A][9] [A][10] *independent* | | 3.9% | 1.0 (1.0 to 2.5) | Infinity (17 to infinity) |
| AF | LV dysfunction (including atrial diameter and overall function) | Stroke or systemic embolism at 2.0 years | 33% | Not independent | |

## THERAPY

### Acute-onset atrial fibrillation

- Control the ventricular rate **[D]** using:
  - digoxin **[A]**[12].

 **Why?**
- It slows the ventricular rate (on average by 25 beats/min) **[A]**[12], but has no clear effect on the rate of cardioversion **[D]**[6] **[D]**[13] **[D]**[14].
- Bolus doses are not clearly more effective than intravenous infusions **[D]**[15].

Alternatives include:
- calcium-channel blockers: verapamil **[A]**[16] **[A]**[17] or diltiazem **[A]**[18]
- beta-blockers: esmolol **[A]**[19] or sotalol **[A]**[20]
- clonidine **[B]**[21].

 **Why?**
- Verapamil slows the ventricular rate (on average by 40 beats/min) **[A]**[17] **[A]**[18] but has no clear effect on cardioversion **[A]**[22] **[A]**[23].
- Diltiazem slows the ventricular rate (on average by 20 beats/min) **[A]**[18].
- Esmolol **[A]**[19] or sotalol **[A]**[20] slow the ventricular rate, but neither has any clear effect on cardioversion.
- Clonidine slows the ventricular rate **[B]**[21].

**Clonidine slows the ventricular rate**

| Patient | Treatment | Comparator | Outcome | CER | RRR | NNT |
|---------|-----------|------------|---------|-----|-----|-----|
| Fast AF **[B]**[21] | Oral clonidine | Placebo | >20% fall in ventricular rate at 15 min | 11% | 500% (−11% to 3900%) | 2 (1 to 5) |

- Consider cardioversion to sinus rhythm **[A]** if your patient fails to revert spontaneously **[D]**.

 **Note**
- Half of patients with acute AF revert spontaneously within 18 h **[B]**[6].

Options include:

- DC cardioversion **[A]**. Cardioversion is more likely to be successful if **[A]**[24]:
  - the onset of this episode of arrhythmia is recent
  - your patient is young.

Anticoagulate the patient before and after cardioversion **[C]**[25]**[C]**[26].

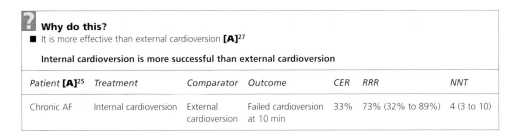

**Why do this?**
■ Anticoagulation preceding and up to a month after cardioversion reduces thromboembolism **[C]**[25]

**Anticoagulation reduces thromboembolism following cardioversion**

| Patient | Treatment | Comparator | Outcome | CER | RRR | NNT |
|---|---|---|---|---|---|---|
| Undergoing DC cardioversion for AF or flutter **[C]**[25] | Anticoagulation | No anticoagulation | Thromboembolism at 6 weeks | 2.2% | 100% | 45 (25 to 220) |

Consider:
● internal cardioversion **[A]**[27]

**Why do this?**
■ It is more effective than external cardioversion **[A]**[27]

**Internal cardioversion is more successful than external cardioversion**

| Patient **[A]**[25] | Treatment | Comparator | Outcome | CER | RRR | NNT |
|---|---|---|---|---|---|---|
| Chronic AF | Internal cardioversion | External cardioversion | Failed cardioversion at 10 min | 33% | 73% (32% to 89%) | 4 (3 to 10) |

● giving an infusion of ibutilide before cardioversion **[A]**[28].

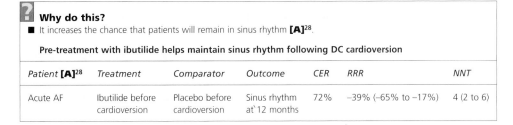

**Why do this?**
■ It increases the chance that patients will remain in sinus rhythm **[A]**[28].

**Pre-treatment with ibutilide helps maintain sinus rhythm following DC cardioversion**

| Patient **[A]**[28] | Treatment | Comparator | Outcome | CER | RRR | NNT |
|---|---|---|---|---|---|---|
| Acute AF | Ibutilide before cardioversion | Placebo before cardioversion | Sinus rhythm at 12 months | 72% | −39% (−65% to −17%) | 4 (2 to 6) |

There is no clear benefit from:
● transoesophageal echocardiography **[B]**[29]

**Why?**
■ Using transoesophageal echocardiography to predict which patients require anticoagulation **[B]**[29] or when cardioversion should occur **[D]**[30], has no clear effect on subsequent embolic events.

● using propafenone before DC cardioversion **[D]**[31]
● different pad **[D]**[32] or electrode positions **[D]**[33]

**Why?**
- Cardioversion using anteroposterior pads compared with anteroanterior pads is not clearly more successful **[D]**[32].
- Electrode position has no clear effect on the success of internal cardioversion **[D]**[33].

## Pharmacological cardioversion

**Note**
- No one method of pharmacological cardioversion is definitively better than another – studies are small and have short follow-up, so some of the differences noted below may be due to chance. In addition, adverse effects from cardioversion and effects on mortality are unclear.

- flecainide **[A]**[34]**[A]**[35]**[A]**[36]

**Why do this?**
- Flecainide is more effective at cardioversion than procainamide **[A]**[34], digoxin **[A]**[35] or verapamil **[A]**[36].
- Watch for severe hypotension **[A]**[37].

**Flecainide is more effective at cardioversion than procainamide, digoxin or verapamil**

| Patient | Treatment | Comparator | Outcome | CER | RRR | NNT |
|---|---|---|---|---|---|---|
| Acute AF **[A]**[34] | Flecainide | Procainamide | Sinus rhythm at 1 h | 62% | 32% (13% to 48%) | 3 (2 to 8) |
| Recent-onset AF **[A]**[35] | Flecainide | Digoxin | Sinus rhythm at 6 h | 35% | 32 (13% to 50%) | 3 (2 to 8) |
| Recent-onset AF **[A]**[37] | Flecainide | Digoxin | Severe hypotension at 6 h | 5.9% | –270% (–110%0 to –9%) | –6 (–37 to –3) |
| Paroxysmal AF **[A]**[36] | Flecainide | Verapamil | Sinus rhythm at 1 h | 5.0% | 1300% (100% to 9600%) | 2 (1 to 2) |

- ibutilide **[A]**[38]

**Why do this?**
- Ibutilide is more effective at cardioversion than procainamide **[A]**[39] sotalol **[A]**[40] or placebo **[A]**[38].
- However, it increases the risk of ventricular tachycardias **[A]**[38], but still causes fewer overall adverse effects than procainamide **[A]**[39].

**Ibutilide is effective at cardioversion, but causes ventricular tachycardia**

| Patient | Treatment | Comparator | Outcome | CER | RRR | NNT |
|---|---|---|---|---|---|---|
| Recent-onset AF or flutter **[A]**[38] | Ibutilide | Placebo | Sinus rhythm at 1.5 h | 2.5% | 1800% (380% to 7400%) | 2 (2 to 3) |
| | | | Polymorphic VT at 24 h | 0.0% | | –11 (–21 to –7) |
| Recent-onset AF or flutter **[A]**[39] | Ibutilide | Procainamide | Sinus rhythm at 24 h | 18% | 220% (79% to 4705%) | 3 (2 to 4) |
| | | | Adverse effects | 47% | 39% (1% to 63%) | 5 (3 to 76) |
| Recent-onset AF or flutter **[A]**[40] | Ibutilide | Sotalol | Sinus rhythm at 1 h | 11% | 65% (33% to 82%) | 5 (3 to 9) |

- procainamide [A][41][A][42]

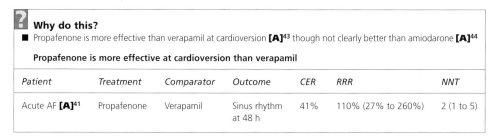

**Why do this?**

■ Procainamide is more effective at cardioversion than propafenone [A][4] or digoxin [A][42].

**Procainamide is more effective at cardioversion than propafenone or digoxin**

| Patient | Treatment | Comparator | Outcome | CER | RRR | NNT |
|---|---|---|---|---|---|---|
| Acute or chronic AF [A][41] | Procainamide | Propafenone | Sinus rhythm at 48 h | 47% | 36% (5% to 56%) | 4 (2 to 19) |
| Acute fast AF [A][42] | Procainamide and digoxin | Digoxin | Sinus rhythm at 1 h | 28% | 81% (11% to 195%) | 4 (2 to 19) |

- propafenone [A][43]

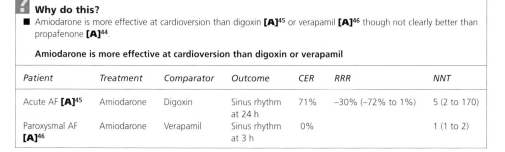

**Why do this?**

■ Propafenone is more effective than verapamil at cardioversion [A][43] though not clearly better than amiodarone [A][44]

**Propafenone is more effective at cardioversion than verapamil**

| Patient | Treatment | Comparator | Outcome | CER | RRR | NNT |
|---|---|---|---|---|---|---|
| Acute AF [A][41] | Propafenone | Verapamil | Sinus rhythm at 48 h | 41% | 110% (27% to 260%) | 2 (1 to 5) |

- amiodarone [A][45]

**Why do this?**

■ Amiodarone is more effective at cardioversion than digoxin [A][45] or verapamil [A][46] though not clearly better than propafenone [A][44].

**Amiodarone is more effective at cardioversion than digoxin or verapamil**

| Patient | Treatment | Comparator | Outcome | CER | RRR | NNT |
|---|---|---|---|---|---|---|
| Acute AF [A][45] | Amiodarone | Digoxin | Sinus rhythm at 24 h | 71% | −30% (−72% to 1%) | 5 (2 to 170) |
| Paroxysmal AF [A][46] | Amiodarone | Verapamil | Sinus rhythm at 3 h | 0% | | 1 (1 to 2) |

- quinidine and verapamil [A][47].

**Why do this?**

■ Quinidine and verapamil leads to faster cardioversion than digoxin and quinidine and more patients are discharged home **[A]**[47]

**Quinidine and verapamil speed cardioversion compared with quinidine and digoxin**

| Patient | Treatment | Comparator | Outcome | CER | RRR | NNT |
|---|---|---|---|---|---|---|
| Acute fast AF **[A]**[47] | Quinidine and verapamil | Quinidine and digoxin | Sinus rhythm at 3 h | 46% | 85% (13% to 205%) | 3 (2 to 8) |
| | | | Sinus rhythm at 24 h | 73% | 23% (–9% to 66%) | 6 (NNT = 3 to inf; NNH = 13 to inf) |
| | | | Discharged home at 6 h | 27% | 132% (8% to 400%) | 3 (2 to 14) |

### Chronic atrial fibrillation
- Control the ventricular rate **[A]** using digoxin **[D]**.
- Consider conversion to sinus rhythm **[A]**[48] using DC cardioversion **[C]**[49] followed by amiodarone **[B]**[56].

See **Acute atrial fibrillation** chapter for more details.

**Why do this?**

■ Most patients with chronic AF who receive DC cardioversion will revert to sinus rhythm immediately (86%; 95% CI: 79% to 93%). At 2 years, 41% will still be in sinus rhythm (95% CI: 31% to 51%), though most require repeat cardioversions **[C]**[49].

■ 60% of patients who receive DC cardioversion followed by amiodarone are still in sinus rhythm at 12 months (95% CI: 51% to 69%). Around 10% stop due to side-effects **[B]**[50].

■ The most cost-effective strategies for treating patients with non-valvular AF are (in decreasing cost and decreasing effectiveness) **[A]**[48]:
  ■ DC cardioversion, amiodarone and warfarin
  ■ DC cardioversion, amiodarone and aspirin, charging to warfarin if AF recurs
  ■ DC cardioversion and aspirin, changing to warfarin if AF recurs.
  ■ If patients have few or no AF symptoms: DC cardioversion followed by aspirin or warfarin alone, if AF recurs is best.
  ■ If patients are at high-risk of amiodarone pulmonary toxicity or adverse effects: DC cardioversion followed by warfarin if AF recurs is best.

Cardioversion is less likely to be successful in the long term if patients:
- have had AF for more than 3 months **[A]**[51]
- have severe heart failure **[A]**[51][A][52]
- are old **[A]**[51]

and more likely if they have
- non-rheumatic mitral valve disease **[A]**[52].

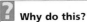

**Why?**
The duration of AF, severe heart failure and increasing age reduce the long-term success of cardioversion

| Patient | Prognostic factor | Outcome | Control rate | OR (95% CI) | NNF+ (95% CI) |
|---|---|---|---|---|---|
| Cardioverted out of chronic AF | AF for 3–35 months *independent* | Chronic AF at 4 years | 21% | 2.1 (1.3 to 3.4) | 7 (4 to 21) |
| | AF for ≥ 36 months *independent* | | 3.0% | 5.0 (3.0 to 8.3) | 10 (6 to 18) |
| | NYHA class III *independent* | | 27% | 1.8 (1.3 to 2.6) | 8 (5 to 18) |
| | Aged > 56 years *independent* | | 18% | 1.5 (1.0 to 2.2) | 15 (7 to inf) |

Alternatives to amiodarone include:
- flecainide **[B]**[50]

**Why do this?**
- 34% of patients who take flecainide are in sinus rhythm at 12 months (95% CI: 27% to 42%); 9% discontinue therapy owing to side-effects (95% CI:4% to 13%) **[B]**[50].

- disopyramide **[A]**[53]

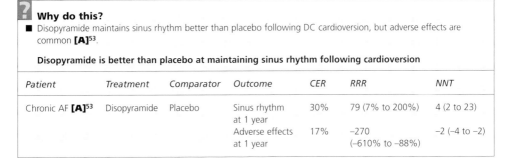

**Why do this?**
- Disopyramide maintains sinus rhythm better than placebo following DC cardioversion, but adverse effects are common **[A]**[53].

**Disopyramide is better than placebo at maintaining sinus rhythm following cardioversion**

| Patient | Treatment | Comparator | Outcome | CER | RRR | NNT |
|---|---|---|---|---|---|---|
| Chronic AF **[A]**[53] | Disopyramide | Placebo | Sinus rhythm at 1 year | 30% | 79 (7% to 200%) | 4 (2 to 23) |
| | | | Adverse effects at 1 year | 17% | −270 (−610% to −88%) | −2 (−4 to −2) |

Consider pharmacological cardioversion if your patient is unsuitable for DC cardioversion **[D]**, using one of:
- amiodarone **[A]**[54]
- propafenone **[A]**[54].

**Why do this?**

■ Both amiodarone and propafenone are better at cardioversion than placebo **[A]**[52].

**Chronic AF: amiodarone or propafenone are better than placebo at cardioversion**

| Patient | Treatment | Comparator | Outcome | CER | RRR | NNT |
|---------|-----------|-----------|---------|-----|-----|-----|
| Chronic AF | Amiodarone | Placebo | Still in AF at 4 weeks | 100% | 47% (2%7 to 61%) | 2 (2 to 3) |
|  | Propafenone | Placebo | Still in AF at 4 weeks | 100% | 59% (38% to 73%) | 2 (1 to 2) |

Avoid using:
- quinidine **[A]**[55]
- sotalol **[D]**[56].

 **Why do this?**

■ Although long-term quinidine reduces relapse following cardioversion, it increases mortality **[A]**[55]; 18% of patients on quinidine experience side-effects (diarrhoea, syncope and pyrexia and 9% have to stop it **[A]**[55].
■ Sotalol is less effective than quinidine for achieving cardioversion **[A]**[57], and is not clearly more effective or safer than quinidine for maintenance of sinus rhythm**[D]**[56].

**Chronic AF: sotalol is less effective than quinidine at cardioversion**

| Patient | Treatment | Comparator | Outcome | CER | RRR | NNT |
|---------|-----------|-----------|---------|-----|-----|-----|
| Chronic AF **[A]**[57] | Sotalol | Quinidine | Sinus rhythm at 7 days | 40% | −40% (−65% to −15%) | −3 (−7 to −2) |

**Chronic AF: quinidine helps maintain sinus rhythm following DC cardioversion, but increases mortality**

| Patient | Treatment | Comparator | Outcome | CER | OR | NNT |
|---------|-----------|-----------|---------|-----|-----|-----|
| Chronic AF **[A]**[57] | Quinidine following DC cardioversion | Placebo or no medication following DC cardioversion | Sinus rhythm at 1 year | 25% | — | 4 (3 to 7) |
|  |  |  | Death at 3 months | 0.3% | 2.98 (1.07 to 8.33) | 67 (19 to 1900) |

For patients with symptomatic chronic AF resistant to medication, consider:
- radiofrequency AV node modulation **[C]**[58]

 **Why do this?**

■ AV node modulation controls symptoms in 92% of patients (95% CI:85% to 99%), but AV block is common (16%; 95% CI: 8% to 25%) **[C]**[58]

- atriotomy **[C]**[59].

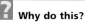
**Why do this?**

- Atriotomy controls symptoms in 93% of patients (95% CI: 89% to 97%); 2% die during surgery (95% CI:0.1% to 4.4%) and 0.6% require a permanent pacemaker (95% CI:0.0% to 1.8%) **[C]**[59].

## PREVENTION

Anticoagulate patients who remain in, or are at risk of relapsing back into, atrial fibrillation **[A]**.
For patients with one or more other risk factors for stroke **[A]**[60] **[A]**[61] **[A]**[61]
- give warfarin, adjusted **[A]**[62] so INR 2.0–3.0 **[A]**[63].
See **Anticoagulation** chapter for more details on warfarin therapy.

**Why do this?**

- It reduces the risk of stroke and death, but causes more major bleeds than placebo **[A]**[62].
- It prevents more strokes than aspirin **[A]**[62], but causes more major bleeds **[A]**[64]. There is no clear effect on mortality. **[A]**[62]
- Warfarin is more cost-effective than aspirin at preventing stroke in elderly patients with one or more risk factors for stroke **[A]**[60] **[A]**[61].
- Low-dose or fixed-dose warfarin is not as effective as adjusted-dose warfarin **[A]**[62] **[A]**[65].
- Patients with AF on warfarin are at increased risk for a stroke, TIA or a major bleed if their INR ≥ 4.0 **[B]**[63].

**Adjusted-dose warfarin reduces stroke and death, but increases the risk of major bleeds**

| Patient | Treatment | Comparator | Outcome | CER | OR | NNT |
|---------|-----------|------------|---------|-----|-----|-----|
| AF | Adjusted-dose warfarin **[A]**[62] | Placebo | Stroke at 1.6 years | 9.2% | 0.38 (0.28 to 0.52) | 18 (16 to 24) |
| | | | Death at 1.6 years | | 0.74 (0.57 to 0.96) | 63 (to) |
| | | | Major extracranial bleed at 1.6 years | | 2.4 (1.2 to 4.6) | −33 (to) |
| | Adjusted-dose warfarin **[A]**[62] | Aspirin | Stroke at 2.2 years | 8.7% | 0.64 (0.40 to 0.73) | 34 (20 to 46) |

**Warfarin causes more major bleeds than aspirin**

| Patient | Treatment | Comparator | Outcome | CER | RRR | NNH |
|---------|-----------|------------|---------|-----|-----|-----|
| AF **[A]**[64] | Warfarin | Aspirin | Major bleed at 2.6 years | 2.9% | −110% (−270% to −17%) | 31 (18 to 140) |

**Adjusted-dose warfarin prevents more strokes than fixed-dose warfarin and aspirin**

| Patient | Treatment | Comparator | Outcome | CER | RRR | NNH |
|---------|-----------|------------|---------|-----|-----|-----|
| AF **[A]**[65] | Adjusted-dose warfarin | Fixed-dose warfarin and aspirin | Ischaemic stroke or systemic emboli at 1 year | 2.1% | −300% (−670% to −110%) | 16 (11 to 27) |

For patients at low-risk of stroke (<1% per year), at high-risk for a major bleed, or who particularly dislike the thought of taking warfarin **[A]**[60] **[A]**[61]:

● give aspirin **[A]**[62].

See **Anticoagulation** chapter for more details on calculating your patient's risk of bleeding.

**Why do this?**

■ Aspirin is more cost-effective than warfarin for low-risk elderly patients or patients at high-risk of major haemorrhage **[A]**[65].

■ Let patients who are at low or medium risk for stroke, make the choice — it is more cost-effective than giving all patients warfarin **[A]**[66].

**Aspirin reduces stroke compared with placebo**

| Patient | Treatment | Comparator | Outcome | CER | OR | NNT |
|---------|-----------|------------|---------|-----|-----|-----|
| AF | Aspirin **[A]**[62] | Placebo | Stroke at 1.6 years | 13% | 0.78 (0.62 to 0.98) | 39 (22 to 440) |

**Note**

■ In one decision analysis, a patient's risk of falling had no effect on treatment option determined on the basis of the risk of bleeding or stroke **[A]**[61].

**Paroxysmal atrial fibrillation**

Consider long-term antiarrhythmic therapy in symptomatic cases **[D]**.
Start medication in hospital **[C]**[67].

**Why do this?**

■ Cardiac adverse events are common (13%; 95% CI: 11% to 16%), particularly bradyarrhythmias (8%; 95% CI: 6% to 10%), though symptomatic bradyarrhythmias, ventricular arrhythmias and cardiac emboli are rare **[C]**[67].

■ Starting antiarrhythmic medication in hospital is more cost-effective than in the outpatient clinic **[A]**[68].

Consider using one of:

● amiodarone **[A]**[69]

**Why?**

- It prevents reversion to AF better than sotalol following DC cardioversion **[A]**[69].

**Paroxysmal AF: amiodarone prevents recurrence of AF better than sotalol**

| Patient | Treatment | Comparator | Outcome | CER | RRR | NNT |
|---|---|---|---|---|---|---|
| Cardioverted paroxsymal or chronic AF **[A]**[69] | Amiodarone | Sotalol | Recurrence of AF at 1 year | 60% | 52 (14% to 74%) | 3 (2 to 11) |

- However, adverse effects are common and often lead to patients stopping therapy **[A]**[68].

**Many patients on long-term low-dose amiodarone discontinue medication due to adverse effects**

| Patient [A][70] | Treatment | Comparator | Outcome | CER | RR (95% CI) | NNH |
|---|---|---|---|---|---|---|
| On oral amiodarone | Low-dose amiodarone | No amiodarone | Drug discontinued at 12 months | 15.4% | 1.60 (1.22 to 2.09) | 14 (8 to 36) |
| | | | Neurological disturbance at 12 months | 1.9% | 2.00 (1.09 to 3.70) | 54 (21 to 590) |
| | | | Bradycardia at 12 months | 1.4% | 2.18 (1.11 to 4.27) | 63 (24 to 670) |
| | | | Thyroid disease at 12 months | 0.4% | 4.23 (2.04 to 8.75) | 76 (32 to 240) |
| | | | Skin rash at 12 months | 0.7% | 2.48 (1.05 to 6.17) | 100 (29 to 2900) |
| | | | Visual complaints at 12 months | 0.1% | 3.43 (1.22 to 9.64) | 300 (85 to 3300) |

 **Note**

- Arrhythmias due to amiodarone are uncommon (2.8%; 95% CI: 2.1% to 3.5%), particularly torsades de pointes (0.7%; 95% CI: 0.5% to 1.4%) **[B]**[71].
- High doses of amiodarone increase the risk of developing pulmonary toxicity (5.8% of patients on 50–800 mg daily; 95% CI: 3.9% to 7.7%) **[C]**[72].

- flecainide – at least 100 mg twice daily

 **Why?**

- Flecainide reduces symptomatic arrhythmias better than placebo **[A]**[73]. In addition, the interval between attacks is longer (on average 17 days longer) **[A]**[74].
- Fewer patients on flecainide withdraw than do those on quinidine **[A]**[75].

**Paroxysmal AF: flecainide prevents symptomatic attacks and causes fewer side-effects than quinidine**

| Patient | Treatment | Comparator | Outcome | CER | RRR | NNT |
|---|---|---|---|---|---|---|
| Paroxysmal AF **[A]**[76] | Flecainide 100 mg twice daily | Placebo | No attacks at ? | 7.1% | –600% (–2700% to 75%) | 2 (2 to 5) |
| Symptomatic paroxysmal AF or flutter **[A]**[75] | Flecainide | Quinidine | Discontinued medication due to adverse effects at 1 year | 30% | 40% (4% to 62%) | 8 (4 to 88) |

- propafenone **[A]**[77]**[A]**[78], 600 mg **[A]**[78] daily by mouth

 **Why?**
■ It reduces symptomatic arrhythmias compared with placebo **[A]**[77] **[A]**[78] or quinidine without clearly causing adverse effects at doses up to 600 mg daily **[A]**[78]
■ It is not clearly more effective than flecainide **[D]**[79] **[D]**[80] or sotalol **[D]**[81].

**Paroxysmal AF: propafenone reduces symptomatic episodes better than quinidine or placebo**

| Patient | Treatment | Comparator | Outcome | CER | RRR | NNT |
|---|---|---|---|---|---|---|
| Paroxysmal AF **[A]**[77] | Oral propafenone | Placebo | Free from symptomatic arrhythmias at 6 months | 34% | −96% (−220% to −22%) | 3 (2 to 7) |
| Paroxysmal AF and frequent attacks **[A]**[80] | Oral propafenone | Quinidine | >75% reduction in attacks at 6 months | 46% | −90% (−170% to −36%) | 2 (2 to 4) |

- sotalol – at least 120 mg twice daily **[A]**[82].

 **Why?**
■ Sotalol reduces recurrent symptomatic episodes compared with placebo, but only at doses of at least 120 mg twice daily **[A]**[82].

**Paroxysmal AF: sotalol reduces recurrent symptomatic episodes**

| Patient | Treatment | Comparator | Outcome | CER | RRR | NNT |
|---|---|---|---|---|---|---|
| Symptomatic AF or flutter **[A]**[82] | Sotalol 120 mg twice daily | Placebo | Recurrent symptomatic episodes at 1 year | 70% | 27% (3% to 4%5) | 5 (3 to 43) |

There is no clear benefit from digoxin **[D]**[83].

 **Why?**
■ Digoxin has no clear effect on reducing recurrent symptomatic episodes **[D]**[83].

For patients with intolerable paroxysmal AF resistant to antiarrhythmic medication, consider:
- ablation of AV node and insertion of a DDDR permanent pacemaker **[A]**[84]

**Why do this?**

- Ablation and pacemaker insertion compared with drug therapy reduces symptoms, hospital admissions or need for DC cardioversion **[A]**[84]
- However, more patients go into permanent AF **[A]**[84]
- Patients have fewer symptoms with AV junction ablation than with AV junction modification **[A]**[85].

**Resistant paroxysmal AF: AV node ablation and pacemaker insertion improves symptoms**

| Patient | Treatment | Comparator | Outcome | CER | RRR | NNT |
|---------|-----------|------------|---------|-----|-----|-----|
| Intolerable paroxysmal AF resistant to antiarrhythmic medication **[A]**[84] | AV node ablation and insertion of pacemaker | Drug therapy | Permanent AF at 6 months | 0% | 87% (27 to 100) | −4 (−18 to −2) |
| | | | Subjective perception of AF tachyarrhythmia at 6 months | 89% | 79% (47% to 91%) | 1 (1 to 2) |
| | | | Hospitalisation or DC cardioversion at 6 months | 33% | 86% (−8% to 98%) | 4 (2 to 20) |

- an implantable atrial defibrillator **[C]**[86].

**Why do this?**

- The defibrillator will cardiovert 80% of patients (95% CI: 70% to 91%) who develop AF; however, recurrent episodes are common (41%; 95% CI: 28% to 55%) **[C]**[86].

## PROGNOSIS

- Half of patients with acute AF revert spontaneously to sinus rhythm within 18 h **[B]**[6].
- Recurrent symptomatic attacks are common in patients with paroxysmal AF **[B]**[87–91].

**Note**

- A third to a half of patients will have a recurrent symptomatic episode within a year **[B]**[88–92].

- Few patients with chronic AF remain in sinus rhythm long-term following cardioversion **[A]**[93].

**Note**

- 42% are in sinus rhythm at 4 years following serial cardioversions, but only 10% who had one cardioversion (95% CI 6.2% to 14%) **[A]**[93].

Patients are more likely to revert to AF if they:
- had AF for more than 3 months **[A]**[93]
- have severe heart failure **[A]**[93] **[A]**[94]
- are old **[A]**[93]

and less likely if they have
- non-rheumatic mitral valve disease **[A]**[94].

**Why?**
The duration of AF, severe heart failure and increasing age reduce the long-term success of cardioversion

| Patient | Prognostic factor | Outcome | Control rate | OR (95% CI) | NNF+ (95% CI) |
|---|---|---|---|---|---|
| Cardioverted out of chronic AF | AF for 3–35 months *independent* | Chronic AF at 4 years | 21% | 2.1 (1.3 to 3.4) | 7 (4 to 21) |
| | AF for ≥ 36 months *independent* | | 3.0% | 5.0 (3.0 to 8.3) | 10 (6 to 18) |
| | NYHA class III *independent* | | 27% | 1.8 (1.3 to 2.6) | 8 (5 to 18) |
| | Aged > 56 years *independent* | | 18% | 1.5 (1.0 to 2.2) | 15 (7 to inf) |

- Antiarrhythmic side-effects are common **[A]**[93].

**Note**
- One in 20 suffer antiarrhythmic drug adverse effects (4.7%; 95% CI: 2.0% to 7.4%) **[A]**[93]
- A fifth develop congestive heart failure (19%; 95% CI: 14% to 24%) **[A]**[93].

Atrial fibrillation is an important risk factor for stroke **[A]**[2].

**Why?**
AF increases the risk of stroke, especially with other risk factors

| Strokes per year **[A]**[95] | No other risk factors (95% CI) | 1 + other risk factor (95% CI) |
|---|---|---|
| Aged < 65 years | 1.0% (0.%3 to 3.1%) | 4.9% (3.0% to 8.1%) |
| Aged 65–75 years | 4.3% (2.7% to 7.1%) | 5.7% (3.9% to 8.3%) |
| Aged > 75 years | 3.5% (1.6% to 7.7%) | 8.1% (4.7% to 14%) |

**The risk of stroke increases with increasing numbers of risk factors**

| Number of prognostic factors **[A]**[9] **[A]**[10] | Rate of thromboembolism (%) |
|---|---|
| ≥3 | 19% (12% to 30%) |
| 1 or 2 | 6.0% (4.1% to 8.8%) |
| 0 | 1.0% (0.2% to 4.0%) |

The risk of stroke is increased further with:
- a history of hypertension **[A]**[2]
- previous TIA or stroke **[A]**[95]
- ischaemic heart disease **[A]**[2] **[B]**[63]
- diabetes mellitus **[A]**[95]
- recent heart failure **[A]**[2]
- increasing age **[A]**[95]

and possibly
- markers of LV dysfunction **[A]**[9–11]
- cardiomegaly **[A]**[2].

---

**?** **Why?**
Hypertension, heart failure, ischaemic heart disease and previous strokes increase the risk of stroke

| Patient | Prognostic factor | Outcome | Control rate | RR (95% CI) | NNF+ (95% CI) |
|---|---|---|---|---|---|
| AF | History of hypertension **[A]**[9]**[A]**[10] *independent* | Stroke or systemic embolism at 1.5 years | 4.4% | 1.9 (1.0 to 3.9) | 25 (8 to 23) |
| | Previous TIA or stroke **[A]**[95] *independent* | Stroke | ? | 2.5 | ? |
| | Diabetes mellitus **[A]**[95] *independent* | Stroke | ? | 1.7 | ? |
| Non-rheumatic AF and minor stroke | Ischaemic heart disease **[B]**[63] *independent* | Stroke, TIA or major bleed at 2 years | 22% | 2.9 (1.4 to 5.9) | 3 (1 to 14) |
| AF | Increasing age (per decade) *independent* **[A]**[95] | Stroke | ? | 1.4 | ? |
| AF | LV dysfunction (including atrial diameter and overall function) **[A]**[11] *not independent* | Stroke or systemic embolism at mean 2.0 years | 3.3% | ? | ? |
| | Global LV dysfunction **[A]**[9] **[A]**[10] *independent* | | 6.0% | 2.0 (1.0 to 4.0) | 17 (6 to inf) |
| | Enlarged left atrium **[A]**[9] **[A]**[10] *independent* | | 3.9% | 1.0 (1.0 to 2.5) | Infinity (17 to inf) |
| Non-rheumatic AF and minor stroke | Cardiomegaly **[B]**[63] *independent* | | | 1.4 (1.3 to 1.5) | 14 (11 to 18) |

---

Patients with atrial fibrillation who have a stroke are at increased risk of having a severe stroke or dying **[A]**[96].

---

**?** **Why?**
Atrial fibrillation increases the risk of dying from a stroke

| Patient **[A]**[88] | Prognostic factor | Outcome | Control rate | OR (95% CI) | NNF+ (95% CI) |
|---|---|---|---|---|---|
| First stroke | AF *independent* | Severe stroke or death at 3 months | 14% | 1.84 (1.04 to 3.27) | 11 (5 to 210) |

---

**Guideline writers**: Christopher Ball, Nick Shenker
**CAT writers**: Christopher Ball, Nick Shenker, Clare Wotton

## REFERENCES

| No. | Level | Citation |
|---|---|---|
| 1 | 1b | Benjamin EJ et al. Independent risk factors for atrial fibrillation in a population-based cohort: the Framingham Heart Study: JAMA, 1994; 271: 840–844 |
| 2 | 1b | Wolf PA et al. Atrial fibrillation as an independent risk factor for stroke: the Framingham Study. Stroke 1991; 22: 983–8 |
| 3 | 4 | Mattioli AV, Castellani ET, Vivoli D et al. Prevalence of atrial fibrillation and stroke in paced patients without prior atrial fibrillation: a prospective study. Clin Cardiol 1998; 21: 117–22 |
| 4 | 1b | Krahn AD et al. The natural history of atrial fibrillation: incidence, risk factors and prognosis in the Manitoba follow-up study. Am J Med 1995; 98: 476–84 |
| 5 | 1b | Sawin CT et al. Low serum thyrotropin concentrations as a risk factor for atrial fibrillation in older persons. N Engl J Med 1994; 331: 1249–52 |
| 6 | 2b | Falk RH et al. Digoxin for converting recent-onset atrial fibrillation to sinus rhythm. Ann Intern Med 1987; 106: 503 |
| 7 | 5 | Sneed NV, Hollerbach AD. Accuracy of heart rate assessment in atrial fibrillation. Heart Lung 1992; 21: 427–33 |
| 8 | 2a | Attia J et al. Diagnosis of thyroid disease in hospitalised patients: a systematic review. Arch Intern Med 1999; 159: 658–65 |
| 9 | 1b | SPAF Investigators. Predictors of thrombembolism in atrial fibrillation: clinical features of patients at risk. Ann Intern Med 1992; 116: 1–5 |
| 10 | 1b | SPAF Investigators. Predictors of thromboemoblism in atrial fibrillation: echocardiographic features of patients at risk. Ann Intern Med 1992; 116: 6–12 |
| 11 | 1b | Hart RG et al. Factors associated with ischaemic stroke during aspirin therapy in atrial fibrillation. Analysis of 2012 participants in the SPAF I:III clinical trials. Stroke 1999; 30: 1223–39 |
| 12 | 1b | Digitalis in Acute Atrial Fibrillation Trial Group. Intravenous digoxin in acute atrial fibrillation: results of a randomized, placebo-controlled multicentre trial in 239 patients. Eur Heart J 1997; 18: 649–54 |
| 13 | 1b – | Digitalis in acute atrial fibrillation trial group: intravenous digoxin in acute atrial fibrillation: results of a randomized, placebo-controlled multicentre trial in 239 patients: Eur Heart J (1997): 18: 649–54 |
| 14 | 1b – | Jordaens L et al. Conversion of atrial fibrillation to sinus rhythm and rate control by digoxin in comparision with placebo. Eur Heart J 1997; 18: 643–8 |
| 15 | 1b – | Smit AJ, Scaf AHJ, van Essen LH et al. Digoxin infusion versus bolus injection in rapid atrial fibrillation: relation between serum levels and response. Eur J Clin Pharmacol 1990; 38: 335–41 |
| 16 | 1b | Platia EV et al. Esmolol versus verapamil in the acute treatment of atrial fibrillation or atrial flutter. Am J Cardiol 1989; 63: 925–9 |
| 17 | 1b | Tommaso C et al. Atrial fibrillation and flutter: immediate control and conversion with intravenously administered verapamil. Arch Intern Med 1983; 143: 877–81 |
| 18 | 1b | Salerno DM et al. Efficacy and safety of intravenous diltiazem for treatment of atrial fibrillation and flutter. Am J Cardiol 1989; 63: 1046–51 |

| No. | Level | Citation |
|-----|-------|----------|
| 19 | 1b | Platia EV et al. Esmolol versus verapamil in the acute treatment of atrial fibrillation or atrial flutter. Am J Cardiol 1989; 63: 925–9 |
| 20 | 1b | Sung RJ et al. Intravenous sotalol for the termination of supraventricular tachycardia and atrial fibrillation and flutter: a mulicenter randomized, double-blind, placebo-controlled trial. Am Heart J 1995; 129: 739–48 |
| 21 | 2b | Roth A et al. Clonidine for patients with rapid atrial fibrillation. Ann Intern Med 1992; 116: 388–90 |
| 22 | 1b | Platia EV et al. Esmolol versus verapamil in the acute treatment of atrial fibrillation or atrial flutter: Am J Cardiol 1989: 63: 925–929 |
| 23 | 1b – | Aronow WS, Ferlinz J. Verapamil versus placebo in atrial fibrillation and atrial flutter. Clin Invest Med 1980; 3: 35–9 |
| 24 | 1b | Van Gelder IC et al. Prediction of uneventful cardioversion and maintenance of sinus rhythm from direct-current electrical cardioversion of chronic atrial fibrillation and flutter. Am J Cardiol 1991; 68: 41–6 |
| 25 | 4 | Zeiler Arnold A et al. Role of prophylactic anticoagulation for direct current cardioversion in patients with atrial fibrillation or atrial flutter. J Am Coll Cardiol 1992; 19: 851–5 |
| 26 | 4 | Bjerkelund CJ, Orning OM. The efficacy of anticoagulant therapy for preventing embolism related to DC electrical conversion of atrial fibrillation. Am J Cardiol 1969; 23: 208–16 |
| 27 | 1b | Levy S et al. A randomized comparison of external and internal cardioversion of chronic atrial fibrillation. Circulation 1992; 86: 1415–20 |
| 28 | 1b | Oral H, Souza JJ, Michaud GF et al. Facilitating transthoracic cardioversion of atrial fibrillation with ibutilide pretreatment. N Engl J Med 1999; 340: 1849–54 |
| 29 | 2a | Moreyra E, Finkelhor RS, Cebul RD. Limitations of transesophageal echocardiography in the risk assessment of patients before nonanticoagulated cardioversion from atrial fibrillation and flutter: an analysis of pooled trials. Am Heart J 1995; 129: 71–5 |
| 30 | 1b – | Klein AL et al. Cardioversion guided by transoesophageal echocardiography: the ACUTE pilot study. Ann Intern Med 1997; 126: 200–9 |
| 31 | 1b – | Biaconi L et al. Effects of oral propafenone administration before electrical cardioversion of chronic atrial fibrillation: a placebo-controlled study. J Am Coll Cardiol 1996; 28: 700–6 |
| 32 | 1b – | Mathew TP, Moore A, McIntyre M et al. Randomised comparison of electrode positions for cardioversion of atrial fibrillation. Heart 1999; 81: 576–9 |
| 33 | 1b – | Alt E et al. Impact of electrode position on outcome of low-energy intracardiac cardioversion of atrial fibrillation. Am J Cardiol 1997; 79: 621–5 |
| 34 | 1b | Madrid AH et al. Comparison of flecainide and procainamide in cardioversion of atrial fibrillation. Eur Heart J 1994; 14: 1127–31 |
| 35 | 1b | Donovan KD et al. Reversion of recent-onset atrial fibrillation to sinus rhythm by intravenous flecainide. Am J Cardiol 1991; 67: 137–41 |
| 36 | 1b | Suttorp MJ et al. Intravenous flecainide versus verapamil for acute conversion of paroxysmal atrial fibrillation or flutter to sinus rhythm. Am J Cardiol 1989; 63: 693–6 |
| 37 | 1b | Donovan KD et al. Efficacy of flecainide for the reversion of acute onset atrial fibrillation. Am J Cardiol 1992; 70: 50A–55A |

| No. | Level | Citation |
|-----|-------|----------|
| 38 | 1b | Stambler BS et al. Efficacy and safety of repeated intravenous doses of ibutilide for rapid conversion of atrial flutter or fibrillation. Circulation 1996; 94: 1613–21 |
| 39 | 1b | Volgman AS et al. Conversion efficacy and safety of intravenous ibutilide compared with intravenous procainamide in patients with atrial flutter or fibrillation. J Am Coll Cardiol 1998; 31: 1414–19 |
| 40 | 1b | Vos MA et al. Superiority of ibutilide (a new class III agent) over DL-sotalol in converting atrial flutter and atrial fibrillation. Heart 1998; 79: 568–75 |
| 41 | 1b | Mattioli AV, Lucchi GR, Vivoli D et al. Propafenone versus procainamide for conversion of atrial fibrillation to sinus rhythm. Clin Cardiol 1998; 21: 763–6 |
| 42 | 1b | Kochiadakis GE, Igoumenidis NE, Solomou MC et al. Conversion of atrial fibrillation to sinus rhythm using acute intravenous procainamide infusion. Cardiovasc Drugs Therapy 1998; 12: 75–81 |
| 43 | 1b | Weiner P et al. Clinical course of recent-onset atrial fibrillation treated with oral propafenone. Chest 1994; 105: 1013–16 |
| 44 | 1b | Treglia A, Alfano C, Rossini E. Confronto tra propafenone ed amiodarone nella conversione al ritmo sinusale della fibrillazione atriale di recente insorgenza. Minerva Cardioangiol 1994; 42: 293–7 |
| 45 | 1b | Hou ZY. Acute treatment of recent-onset atrial fibrillation and flutter with a tailored dosing regimen of intravenous amiodarone: a randomised digoxin-controlled study. Eur Heart J 1995; 16: 521–8 |
| 46 | 1b | Noc M et al. Intravenous amiodarone versus verapamil for acute conversion of paroxysmal atrial fibrillation to sinus rhythm. Am J Cardiol 1990; 65: 679–80 |
| 47 | 1b | Innes GD, Vertesi L, Dillon EC et al. Effectiveness of verapamil-quinidine versus digoxin-quinidine in the emergency department; treatment of paroxysmal atrial fibrillation. Ann Emerg Med 1997; 29: 126–34 |
| 48 | 1b | Eckman MH et al. Cost-effectiveness of therapies for patients with nonvalvular atrial fibrillation. Arch Intern Med 1998; 158: 1669–77 |
| 49 | 4 | Lundstrom T, Ryden L. Chronic atrial fibrillation: long term results of direct current cardioversion. Acta Med Scand 1988; 223: 53–9 |
| 50 | 2a | Zarembski DG et al. Treatment of resistant atrial fibrillation: a meta-analysis comparing amiodarone and flecainide. Arch Intern Med 1995; 155: 1885–91 |
| 51 | 1b | Van Gelder IC et al. Chronic atrial fibrillation: success of serial cardioversion therapy and safety of oral anticoagulation. Arch Intern Med 1996; 156: 2585–92 |
| 52 | 1b | Van Gelder IC et al. Prediction of uneventful cardioversion and maintenance of sinus rhythm from direct-current electrical cardioversion of chronic atrial fibrillation and flutter. Am J Cardiol 1991; 68: 41–6 |
| 53 | 1b | Karlson BW et al. Disopyramide in the maintenance of sinus rhythm after electrocardioversion of atrial fibrillation. A placebo-controlled one-year follow-up study. Eur Heart J 1988; 9: 284–90 |
| 54 | 1b | Kochiadakis GE, Igoumenidis NE, Parthenakis FI et al. Amiodarone versus propafenone for conversion of chronic atrial fibrillation: results of a randomized controlled study. J Am Coll Cardiol 1999; 33: 966–71 |

| No. | Level | Citation |
|---|---|---|
| 55 | 1a | Coplen SE et al. Efficacy and safety of quinidine therapy for maintenance of sinus rhythm after cardioversion: a meta-analysis of randomised control trials. Circulation 1990; 82: 1106–16 |
| 56 | 1a – | Southworth MR, Zarembski D, Viana M et al. Comparison of sotalol versus quinidine for maintenance of normal sinus rhythm in patients with chronic atrial fibrillation. Am J Cardiol 1999; 83: 1629–32 |
| 57 | 1b | Hohnloser SH et al. Efficacy and proarrhythmic hazards of pharmacologic cardioversion of atrial fibrillation: prospective comparison of sotalol versus quinidine. J Am Coll Cardiol 1995; 26: 852–8 |
| 58 | 4 | Morady F et al. Long-term follow-up after radiofrequency modification of the atrioventricular node in patients with atrial fibrillation. J Am Coll Cardiol 1997; 27: 113–21 |
| 59 | 4 | Cox JL et al. An 8.5 year clinical experience with surgery for atrial fibrillation. Ann Surg 1996; 224(3): 267–73 |
| 60 | 1b | Gage BF, Cardinalli AG, Albers GW et al. Cost-effectiveness of warfarin and aspirin for prophylaxis of stroke in patients with nonvalvular atrial fibrillation. JAMA 1995; 274: 1839–45 |
| 61 | 1b | Man-Son-Hing M, Nichol G, Lau A, et al. Choosing antithrombotic therapy for elderly patients with atrial fibrillation who are at risk for falls. Archives of Internal Medicine 1999; 159: 677–685 |
| 62 | 1a | Hart RG, Benavente O, McBride R et al. Antithrombotic therapy to prevent stroke in patients with atrial fibrillation: a meta-analysis. Ann Intern Med 1999; 131: 492–501 |
| 63 | 2b | European Atrial Fibrillation Trial Study Group. Optimal oral anticoagulation therapy in patients with non-rheumatic atrial fibrillation and recent cerebral ischemia. N Engl J Med 1995; 333: 5–10 |
| 64 | 1b | Stroke Prevention in Atrial Fibrillation Investigators. Bleeding during antithrombotic therapy in patients with atrial fibrillation. Arch Intern Med 1996; 156: 409–16 |
| 65 | 1b | Stroke Prevention in Atrial Fibrillation Investigators. Adjusted-dose warfarin versus low intensity fixed-dose warfarin and aspirin for high-risk patients with atrial fibrillation. Lancet 1996; 348: 633–8 |
| 66 | 1b | Gage BF, Cardinalli AB, Owens DK. Cost-effectiveness of preference-based antithrombotic therapy for patients with nonvalvular atrial fibrillation. Stroke 1998; 29: 1083–91 |
| 67 | 4 | Maisel WH, Kuntz KM, Reimold SC et al. Risk of initiating antiarrhythmic drug therapy for atrial fibrillation in patients admitted to a university hospital. Ann Intern Med 1997; 127: 281–4 |
| 68 | 1b | Simons GR, Eisenstein EL, Shaw LJ et al. Cost effectiveness of inpatient initiation of antiarrhythmic therapy for supraventricular tachycardias. Am J Cardiol 1997; 80: 1551–7 |
| 69 | 1b | Kochiadakis GE et al: low-dose amiodarone versus sotalol for suppression of recurrent symptomatic atrial fibrillation: Am J Cardiol (1998): 81: 995–8 |
| 70 | 1a | Vorperian VR et al. Adverse effects of low-dose amiodarone: a meta-analysis. J Am Coll Cardiol 1997; 30: 791–8 |
| 71 | 2a | Hohnloser SH et al. Amiodarone-associated proarrhythmic effects: a review with special reference to torsades de pointes tachycardia. Ann Intern Med 1994; 121: 529–35 |

| No. | Level | Citation |
| --- | --- | --- |
| 72 | 4 | Dusman RE et al. Clinical features of amiodarone-induced pulmonary toxicity. Circulation 1990; 82: 51–9 |
| 73 | 1b | Pritchett ELC, Datorre SD, Platt ML et al. Flecainide acetate treatment of paroxysmal supraventricular tachycardia and paroxysmal atrial fibrillation: dose–response studies. J Am Coll Cardiol 1991; 17: 297–303 |
| 74 | 1b | Anderson JL et al. Prevention of symptomatic recurrences of paroxysmal atrial fibrillation in patients initially tolerating antiarrhythmic therapy: a multicenter, double-blind cross-over study of flecainide and placebo with transtelephonic monitoring. Circulation 1989; 80: 1557–70 |
| 75 | 1b | Naccarelli GV et al. Prospective comparison of flecainide and quinidine for the treatment of paroxysmal atrial fibrillation/flutter. Am J Cardiol 1996; 77: 53A–59A |
| 76 | 1b | Pritchett ELC, Datorre SD, Platt ML, et al: Flecainide acetate treatment of paroxysmal supraventricular tachycardia and paroxysmal atrial fibrillation: Dose-response studies. Journal of American College of Cardiology 1991; 17: 297–303 |
| 77 | 1b | Stroobandt R et al. Propafenone for conversion and prophylaxis of atrial fibrillation. Am J Cardiol 1997; 79: 418–23 |
| 78 | 1b | UK Propafenone PSVT Study Group. A randomized placebo-controlled trial of propafenone in the prophylaxis of paroxysmal supraventricular tachycardia and paroxysmal atrial fibrillation. Circulation 1995; 92: 2550–7 |
| 79 | 1b – | Aliot E et al. Comparison of the safety and efficacy of flecainide versus propafenone in hospital out-patients with symptomatic paroxysmal atrial fibrillation/flutter. Am J Cardiol 1996; 77: 66A–71A |
| 80 | 1b – | Lee SH et al. Comparisons of oral propafenone and quinidine as an initial treatment option in patients with symptoms of atrial fibrillation: a double-blind randomised trial. J Intern Med 1996; 239: 253–60 |
| 81 | 1b – | Reimold SC et al. Propafenone versus sotalol for suppression of recurrent atrial fibrillation. Am J Cardiol 1993; 71: 558–63 |
| 82 | 1b | Benditt DG, Williams JH, Jin J et al. Maintenance of sinus rhythm with oral d,l-sotalol therapy in patients with symptomatic atrial fibrillation and/or atrial flutter. Am J Cardiol 1999; 84: 270–7 |
| 83 | 1b – | Murgatroyd FD, Gibson SM, Baiyan X et al. Double-blind placebo-controlled trial of digoxin in symptomatic paroxysmal atrial fibrillation (CRAFT). Circulation 1999; 99: 2765–70 |
| 84 | 1b | Brignole M et al. Assessment of atriventricular junction ablation and DDDR mode-switching pacemaker versus pharmacological treatment in patients with severely symptomatic paroxysmal atrial fibrillation: a randomised controlled study. Circulation 1997; 96: 2617–24 |
| 85 | 1b | Lee S-H, Chen S-A, Tai C-T et al. Comparisons of quality of life and cardiac performance after complete atrioventricular junction ablation and atrioventricular junction modification in patients with medically refractory atrial fibrillation. J Am Coll Cardiol 1998; 31: 637–44 |
| 86 | 4 | Wellens HJJ, Lau C-P, Luderitz B et al. Atrioverter: an implantable device for the treatment of atrial fibrillation. Circulation 1998; 98: 1651–6 |
| 87 | 2b | Kochiadakis GE et al. Low-dose amiodarone versus sotalol for suppression of recurrent symptomatic atrial fibrillation: Am J Cardiol 1998: 81: 995–8 |

| No. | Level | Citation |
|---|---|---|
| 88 | 2b | Pritchett ELC, Datorre SD, Platt ML, et al. Flecainide acetate treatment of paroxysmal supraventricular tachycardia and paroxysmal atrial fibrillation: Dose-response studies. Journal of American College of Cardiology 1991; 17: 297–303 |
| 89 | 2b | Stroobandt R et al. Propafenone for conversion and prophylaxis of atrial fibrillation: Am J Cardiol 1997: 79: 418–23 |
| 90 | 2b | UK Propafenone PSVT Study Group,: a randomized placebo-controlled trial of propafenone in the prophylaxis of paroxysmal supraventricular tachycardia and paroxysmal atrial fibrillation. Circulation 1995; 92: 2550–2557 |
| 91 | 2b | Benditt DG, Williams JH, Jin J, et al. Maintenance of sinus rhythm with oral d,l-sotalol therapy in patients with symptomatic atrial fibrillation and/or atrial flutter. American Journal of Cardiology 1999; 84: 270–277 |
| 92 | 2b | Kochiadakis GE et al. Low-dose amiodarone versus sotalol for suppression of recurrent symptomatic atrial fibrillation. Am J Cardiol 1998: 81: 995–8 |
| 93 | 1b | Van Gelder IC et al. Chronic atrial fibrillation: success of serial cardioversion therapy and safety of oral anticoagulation. Arch Intern Med 1996; 156: 2585–92 |
| 94 | 1b | Van Gelder IC et al. Prediction of uneventful cardioversion and maintenance of sinus rhythm from direct-current electrical cardioversion of chronic atrial fibrillation and flutter. Am J Cardiol 1991; 68: 41–46 |
| 95 | 1a | Atrial Fibrillation Investigators et al. Risk factors for stroke and efficacy of antithrombotic therapy in atrial fibrillation: analysis of pooled data from five randomised controlled trials. Arch Intern Med 1994; 1449–57 |
| 96 | 1b | Lin H-J et al. Stroke severity in atrial fibrillation: the Framingham Study. Stroke 1996; 27: 1760–4 |

## CAUSES

Common causes include:
- myocardial infarction **[B]**[1]

**Note**
- 21% of MI patients have bradycardia within 4 h of symptom onset (95% CI: 17% to 25%); 9% have bradycardia after this (95% CI: 4.2% to 13%) **[B]**[1].

- sick sinus syndrome (symptomatic bradycardia <50 beats/min or symptomatic PRS pauses >2 s) **[D]**
- drugs **[D]**
- hypothermia **[C]**[2]

**Note**
- 36% of patients with hypothermia have sinus bradycardia (95% CI: 16% to 56%) **[C]**[2].

- fitness **[D]**.

## CLINICAL FEATURES

Common symptoms of bradycardia include **[C]**[3]:
- syncope
- palpitations
- light-headedness
- dyspnoea and oedema
- fatigue
- angina.

**Note**
Common symptoms of sick sinus syndrome include syncope and palpitations

| Symptom **[C]**[3] | Sensitivity (95% CI) |
| --- | --- |
| Symptomatic | 77% (66% to 88%) |
| Syncope | 45% (33% to 58%) |
| Light-headedness | 27% (15% to 38%) |
| Palpitations | 30 %(18% to 42%) |
| Dyspnoea + oedema | 16% (6.5% to 26%) |
| Angina | 11% (2.6% to 19%) |
| Fatigue | 11% (2.6% to 19%) |

**Note**
- Symptoms are not very helpful in diagnosing arrhythmias **[C]**[4].

## INVESTIGATIONS

- Temperature [C][2].
- Urea and electrolytes [D].
- Cardiac enzymes [B][1]
- Thyroid function test [D].
- ECG [A].

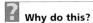

**Why?**

Conduction disturbances are common in sick sinus syndrome

| Sick sinus syndrome [C][3] | Sensitivity (95% CI) |
|---|---|
| Conduction disturbance | 59% (46% to 72%) |
| First-degree heart block | 34% (22% to 46%) |
| Bundle-branch block | 18% (7.8% to 28%) |

## THERAPY

- Give symptomatic patients (evidence of heart failure, chest pain or reduced consciousness) [D] atropine [C][5]

**Why do this?**
- It raises blood pressure and speeds up the heart (on average by 30 beats/min) [C][5].
- It controls ventricular arrhythmias in 87% of cases (95% CI: 75% to 99%) [C][5].
- It normalises blood pressure in 88% of hypotensive patients (95% CI: 73% to 100%) [C][5].

- Set up temporary pacing in patients who remain symptomatic [A].
  Use either:
  - transcutaneous pacing

**Why do this?**
- It increases survival [C][6].

Transcutaneous pacing increases survival

| Patient [C][6] | Treatment | Comparator | Outcome | CER | RRR | NNT |
|---|---|---|---|---|---|---|
| Haemodynamically compromised bradycardia | Transcutaneous pacing | No pacing | Survival at discharge | 0% | | 7 (4 to 71) |

or
  - transvenous pacing [A], preferably using balloon-flotation catheters.

**Why do this?**

■ It is faster than using a semirigid catheter (by roughly 4 min) and the catheter is more likely to be in a satisfactory position **[A]**[7].

**Balloon flotation catheters are easier to place correctly than are semirigid catheters**

| Patient **[A]**[7] | Treatment | Comparator | Outcome | CER | RRR | NNT |
|---|---|---|---|---|---|---|
| Requiring temporary ventricular-demand pacing | Balloon-flotation catheters | Semirigid catheter | Satisfactory catheter position | 10% | 600% (82% to 2600%) | 2 (1 to 3) |

**Note**

■ There is no clear benefit from antibiotic prophylaxis **[D]**[8].

● Consider giving potassium, glucose and insulin in second- or third-degree heart block if pacing not available.

**Why do this?**

■ It reduces death **[C]**[9].

**An infusion of insulin, glucose and potassium reduces mortality in heart block**

| Patient **[C]**[9] | Treatment | Comparator | Outcome | CER | RRR | NNT |
|---|---|---|---|---|---|---|
| 2nd or 3rd degree heart block | Potassium, glucose and insulin | Placebo | Death at 11–22 months | 63% | 82% (–22% to 97%) | 2 (1 to 8) |

● Stop any medication potentially causing bradycardia **[D]**, e.g. beta-blockers, digoxin, diltiazem.
● Insert a permanent pacemaker in patients with sick sinus syndrome **[A]**[10] or carotid sinus syndrome **[C]**[11].

**Why do this?**

■ It reduces syncope and heart failure **[A]**[10]

**Permanent pacemakers reduce syncope and heart failure**

| Patient **[A]**[10] | Treatment | Comparator | Outcome | CER | RRR | NNT |
|---|---|---|---|---|---|---|
| Symptomatic sick sinus syndrome | Permanent pacemaker | No treatment | Syncope at 4 years | 23% | 76% (–7.0% to 94%) | 6 (3 to 66) |
| | | | Overt heart failure at 4 years | 17% | 84% (–28% to 98%) | 7 (4 to 130) |

● Provide antibiotic prophylaxis during pacemaker insertion **[A]**[12].

**Why do this?**

■ Prophylaxis with penicillins or cephalosporins reduces infection **[A]**[12] and the need for repeat surgery **[A]**[13].

**Antibiotic prophylaxis reduces infection following permanent pacemaker insertion**

| Patient **[A]**[12] | Treatment | Comparator | Outcome | CER | OR | NNT |
|---|---|---|---|---|---|---|
| Permanent pacemaker insertion | Antibiotic prophylaxis | Placebo | Pacemaker or systemic infection | 3.7% | 0.26 (0.10 to 0.66) | 37(30 to 81) |

**Antibiotic prophylaxis reduces the need for further surgery**

| Patient **[A]**[13] | Treatment | Comparator | Outcome | CER | RRR | NNT |
|---|---|---|---|---|---|---|
| Permanent pacemaker insertion | Antibiotic prophylaxis | Placebo | Surgery required for infection | 3.6% | 100% | 28 (17 to 77) |

## Carotid sinus syndrome

● Use dual-chamber pacing **[A]**[11].

**Why do this?**

■ DDD-pacing controls symptoms (syncope, dizziness, heart failure) better than ventricular-inhibited pacing (VVI) **[A]**[11].

**DDD-pacing controls symptoms better than VVI-pacing**

| Patient **[A]**[11] | Treatment | Comparator | Outcome | CER | RRR | NNT |
|---|---|---|---|---|---|---|
| Carotid sinus syndrome | DDD-pacing | VVI-pacing | Symptoms at 2 months | 73% | 58% (22% to 77%) | 2 (1 to 6) |

## Sick sinus syndrome

● Use atrial pacing **[A]**[14] **[A]**[15].

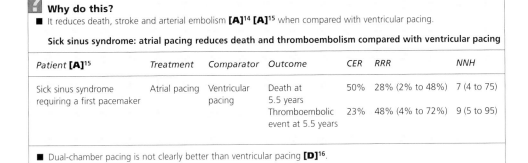

**Why do this?**

■ It reduces death, stroke and arterial embolism **[A]**[14] **[A]**[15] when compared with ventricular pacing.

**Sick sinus syndrome: atrial pacing reduces death and thromboembolism compared with ventricular pacing**

| Patient **[A]**[15] | Treatment | Comparator | Outcome | CER | RRR | NNH |
|---|---|---|---|---|---|---|
| Sick sinus syndrome requiring a first pacemaker | Atrial pacing | Ventricular pacing | Death at 5.5 years | 50% | 28% (2% to 48%) | 7 (4 to 75) |
| | | | Thromboembolic event at 5.5 years | 23% | 48% (4% to 72%) | 9 (5 to 95) |

■ Dual-chamber pacing is not clearly better than ventricular pacing **[D]**[16].

• Consider slow-release theophylline **[A]**[10].

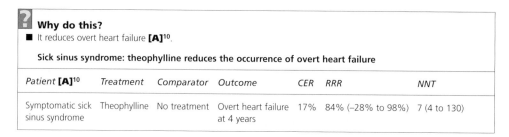

> **? Why do this?**
> ■ It reduces overt heart failure **[A]**[10].
>
> **Sick sinus syndrome: theophylline reduces the occurrence of overt heart failure**
>
> | Patient **[A]**[10] | Treatment | Comparator | Outcome | CER | RRR | NNT |
> |---|---|---|---|---|---|---|
> | Symptomatic sick sinus syndrome | Theophylline | No treatment | Overt heart failure at 4 years | 17% | 84% (–28% to 98%) | 7 (4 to 130) |

## PROGNOSIS

• Complete heart block increases the risk of dying after an inferior myocardial infarction **[A]**[17].

> **? Why?**
> **Complete heart block increases the risk of dying**
>
> | Patient **[A]**[17] | Prognostic factor | Outcome | Control rate | OR (95% CI) | NNF (95% CI) |
> |---|---|---|---|---|---|
> | Inferior myocardial infarction | Complete heart block *independent* | Death at 12 months | 16% | 2.7 (1.3 to 5.5) | 5 (3 to 25) |

• Untreated sick sinus syndrome probably increases the risk of dying **[C]**[45].

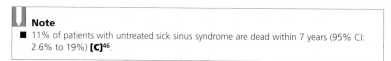

> **Note**
> ■ 11% of patients with untreated sick sinus syndrome are dead within 7 years (95% CI: 2.6% to 19%) **[C]**[46].

**Guideline writers**: Euan Ashley, Christopher Ball and information from Dave Sackett's Redbook version 7
**CAT writers**: Euan Ashley, Christopher Ball

## REFERENCES

| No | Level | Citation |
|---|---|---|
| 1 | 2c | Adgey AAJ, Geddes JS, Mulholland HC et al. Incidence, significance, and management of early bradyarrhythmia complicating acute myocardial infarction. Lancet 1968; ii: 1097–101 |
| 2 | 4 | Rankin AC, Rae AP. Cardiac arrhythmias during rewarming of patients with accidental hypothermia. BMJ 1984; 289: 874–7 |
| 3 | 4 | Rubenstein JJ et al. Clinical spectrum of the sick sinus syndrome. Circulation 72; 46: 5–11 |

| No | Level | Citation |
|----|-------|----------|
| 4 | 4 | Zeldis SM et al. Cardiovascular complaints: correlation with 24 hour electrocardiographic monitoring. Chest 1980; 78: 456–62 |
| 5 | 4 | Scheinman MM, Thorburn D, Abbott JA. Use of atropine in patients with acute myocardial infarction and sinus bradycardia. Circulation 1975; 52: 627–33 |
| 6 | 4 | Hedges JR, Ferro S, Shultz B et al. Prehospital transcutaneous cardiac pacing for symptomatic bradycardia. Pacing Clin Electrophysiol 1991; 14: 1473–1478 |
| 7 | 1b | Ferguson JD, Banning AP, Bashir Y. Randomised trial of temporary cardiac pacing with semirigid and balloon-flotation electrode catheters. Lancet 1997; 349: 1883 |
| 8 | 1b- | Patton RD, Kenamore B, Stein E. Antibiotic prophylaxis for temporary transvenous pacemakers. N Eng J Med 1966; 281: 1106–8 |
| 9 | 4 | Mittra B, et al. Potassium, glucose, and insulin in treatment of heart block after myocardial infarction. Lancet 1966; 1438–1441 |
| 10 | 1b | Alboni P, Menozzi C, Brignole M et al. Effects of permanent pacemaker and oral theophylline in sick sinus syndrome. The THEOPACE study: a randomized controlled trial. Circulation 1997; 96: 260–6 |
| 11 | 4 | Brignole M, Menozzi C, Lolli G et al. Validation of a method for choice of pacing mode in carotid sinus syndrome with or without sinus bradycardia. Pacing Clin Electrophysiol 1991; 14: 196–203 |
| 12 | 1a | Da Costa A et al. Antibiotic prophylaxis for permanent pacemaker implantation: a meta-analysis. Circulation 1998; 97: 1796–1801 |
| 13 | 1b | Mounsey JP, Griffith MJ, Tynan M et al. Antibiotic prophylaxis in permanent pacemaker implantation: a prospective randomised trial. Br Heart J 1994; 72: 339–43 |
| 14 | 1b | Andersen HR, Thuesen L, Bagger JP et al. Prospective randomised trial of atrial versus ventricular pacing in sick-sinus syndrome. Lancet 1994; 344: 1523–8 |
| 15 | 1b | Andersen HR, Nielsen JC, Thomsen PE et al. Long-term follow-up of patients from a randomised trial of atrial versus ventricular pacing for sick-sinus syndrome. Lancet 1997; 350: 1210–1216 |
| 16 | 1b- | Lamas GA, Orav EJ, Stambler BS et al. Quality of life and clinical outcomes in elderly patients treated with ventricular pacing as compared with dual-chamber pacing. N Engl J Med 1998; 338: 1097–104 |
| 17 | 1b | Moreno AM, Tomas JG, Alberola AG et al. Significacion pronostica del bloqueo auriculoventricular completo en pacientes con infarto agudo de miocardio inferior. Un estudio en la era trombolitica. Rev Esp Cardiol 1997; 50: 397–405 |

## PREVALENCE

Think about carbon monoxide (CO) poisoning in **[C]**[1] **[C]**[2]:
- victims of accidental or intentional CO exposure
- non-specific symptoms (e.g. headache, nausea)
- unconscious patients without a clear cause.

**Note**
- Suicide attempts are a common cause of CO poisoning: 69% of cases (excluding burns patients) **[C]**[2] (95% CI: 62% to 75%).
- Many patients present in a coma: 53% of cases **[C]**[2] (95% CI: 46% to 61%).

## CLINICAL FEATURES

Ask about:
- symptoms of carbon monoxide poisoning **[C]**[1] **[C]**[2]
  - headache
  - dizziness
  - GI dysfunction
  - difficulty in thinking
  - loss of consciousness
  - neurological symptoms (visual disturbances, focal neurological signs, seizures)

- exposure to carbon monoxide **[D]**
  - vehicle exhaust fumes in a contained environment
  - a combustion stove with a non-functioning exhaust system
  - fire exposure in a contained environment.

**Note**
**Headache and dizziness are common**

| **[C]**[1] **[C]**[2] | % (95% CI) |
|---|---|
| Headache | 84% (81% to 87%) |
| Dizziness and/or muscle weakness | 78% (75% to 81%) |
| GI dysfunction | 53% (49% to 56%) |
| Difficulty in thinking | 44% (36% to 51%) |
| Loss of consciousness | 34% (30% to 37%) |
| Acute confusional state | 16% (11% to 21%) |
| Coma | 13% (10% to 16%) |
| Paraesthesia | 8.9v (4.9% to 13%) |
| Focal neurological deficits | 7.9% (4.0% to 11.2%) |
| Visual disturbance | 6.8% (3.2% to 10%) |
| Palpitations | 5.8v (2.5% to 9.1%) |
| Seizures | 2.9% (1.6% to 4.2%) |

## INVESTIGATIONS

- Arterial blood gas.

*Note*
Do not use pulse oximetry alone – it can be deceptively wrong.

**Why?**
■ It is unable to distinguish HbCO from HbO$_2$, and may give false high ('normal') readings **[C]**[3] **[C]**[4].
■ The higher the carboxyhaemoglobin level, the greater the inaccuracy in pulse oximetry.

- Carboxyhaemoglobin (HbCO) level (arterial or venous sample acceptable) **[C]**[5] abnormal if >5% in non-smokers, >10% in smokers **[C]**[6].

**Why?**
■ Venous blood gas HbCO levels accurately reflect arterial HbCO values **[C]**[5].
■ Non-smokers have <3% HbCO normally. Smokers have <10% HbCO normally **[C]**[6].
■ There is no clear evidence to indicate toxic levels of HbCO; levels depend on the concentration and duration of CO exposure, subsequent therapy and time since exposure. Thus, persisting or even worsening neurocognitive status may occur at low levels of HbCO **[C]**[6].

- ECG monitoring **[C]**[2].

**Why?**
■ Roughly 5% of patients with CO poisoning develop arrhythmias **[C]**[2].
■ Myocardial ischaemia (unstable angina) may be precipitated by CO poisoning **[D]**.

- Chest X-ray **[C]**[7].

**Note**
■ 7.5% of patients with inhalation injury have an abnormal CXR **[C]**[7].

- Consider performing a Mini-Mental State Examination.

**Why?**
■ Early neurological impairment occurs in a third of patients with suspected CO poisoning **[C]**[1].

## THERAPY

- Assess airway, breathing, circulation **[D]**.
- Give 100% oxygen by rebreather mask for 6 h, and repeat for 100 min for at least 3 days (with simple high-flow oxygen in between) **[A]**[8].
- Avoid using hyperbaric oxygen **[A]**[8].

**Why do this?**
- It improves symptoms and CO levels better than normobaric oxygen at 2 h, but there is no difference after 12 h **[A]**[9].
- It is less effective than normobaric oxygen – more patients have continued mental retardation requiring further treatment after three sessions **[A]**[8].
- Patients are more likely to have delayed neurological sequelae (NNT = 17 at 1 month) and are not clearly less likely to die **[A]**[1] **[A]**[8].
- Chamber-related complications (ear barotrauma, oxygen toxicity, severe claustrophobia) are common **[A]**[8].
- It has not been shown to be clearly safe in pregnancy **[C]**[10].

| Patient **[A]**[8] | Treatment | Comparator | Outcome | CER | RRR | NNT |
|---|---|---|---|---|---|---|
| CO poisoning | Hyperbaric oxygen | Normobaric oxygen | Further treatment required after 3 days | 13% | 63% (3%2 to 79%) | 5 (3 to 11) |
| CO poisoning | Hyperbaric oxygen | Normobaric oxygen | Chamber complications at 3 days | 9.2% | 90% (18% to 99%) | 12 (7 to 53) |
| CO poisoning | Hyperbaric oxygen | Normobaric oxygen | Delayed neurological sequelae after 1 month | 5.8% | 100% | 17 (9 to 120) |

## PROGNOSIS

Early neurological complications are common (headache, nausea, lack of concentration).

**Note**
- Early neurological impairment occurs in a third of patients with suspected CO poisoning.
- Patients with a HCO > 10% are more likely to have neurological impairment at 10 days.

Late complications are uncommon, and are usually minor and transient, but are more common in patients who lose consciousness initially **[B]**[11].

**Note**
- A third of patients still have minor symptoms after 1 month **[B]**[11].
- Most patients with delayed neurological sequelae recover within a month, and many can continue normal daily activity in the meantime **[B]**[11].
- There is no good evidence to support long-term neuropsychiatric testing **[B]**[12].

In pregnancy, mild toxicity has little effect on the fetus; however, toxicity severe enough to cause maternal unconsciousness increases the risk of fetal death or anoxia.

**Note**
- In one study, no pregnant women who had mild symptoms had a stillbirth or a child who had fetal anoxia (0%: 95% CI: 0% to 9%) **[C]**[13].
- Around 30% of pregnant women exposed to CO who have hyperbaric oxygen will still have at least one symptom of poisoning after 1 month. Around 8% will have an abnormal birth **[C]**[10].

Death is uncommon **[C]**[1] **[C]**[8].

**Note**
- Around 4% of patients die before hospital discharge **[C]**[1] **[C]**[8].

**Guideline writers:** Joel Ray, Christopher Ball
**CAT writers**: Joel Ray, Christopher Ball

## REFERENCES

| No | Level | Citation |
|----|-------|----------|
| 1 | 4 | Raphael JC, Elkharrat D, Jars-Guincestre MC et al. Trial of normobaric and hyperbaric oxygen for acute carbon monoxide intoxication. Lancet 1989; ii: 414–18 |
| 2 | 4 | Hyperbaric oxygen did not reduce persistent neurologic sequelae of carbon monoxide poisoning. Evidence-Based Med 1999; 4: 124. Summary of Scheinkestel CD et al. Hyperbaric or normobaric oxygen for acute carbon monoxide poisoning: a randomized controlled clinical trial. Med J Aust 1999; 170: 203–10 |
| 3 | 4 | Bozeman WP, Myers RAM, Barish RA. Confirmation of the pulse oximetry gap in carbon monoxide poisoning. Ann Emerg Med 1997; 30: 608–11 |
| 4 | 4 | Buckley RG, Aks SE, Eshoum JL et al. The pulse oximetry gap in carbon monoxide intoxication. Ann Emerg Med 1994; 24: 252–5 |
| 5 | 4 | Touger M, Gallagher EJ, Tyrell J. Relationship between venous and arterial carboxyhaemoglobin levels in patients with suspected carbon monoxide poisoning. Ann Emerg Med 1995; 25: 481–3 |
| 6 | 4 | Stewart RD et al. Carboxyhaemoglobin levels in American blood donors. JAMA 1974; 229: 1187–95 |
| 7 | 4 | Clark WR, Bonaventura M, Myers W. Smoke inhalation and airway management at a regional burn unit: 1974–1983. Part I: diagnosis and consequences of smoke inhalation. J Burn Care Rehabil 1989; 10: 52–62 |
| 8 | 1b | Hyperbaric oxygen did not reduce persistent neurologic sequelae of carbon monoxide poisoning. Evidence-Based Med 1999; 4: 124. Summary of Scheinkestel CD et al: hyperbaric or normobaric oxygen for acute carbon monoxide poisoning: a randomized controlled clinical trial: Med J Aust 1999; 170: 203–10 |

| No | Level | Citation |
|---|---|---|
| 9 | 1b | Ducasse JL, Celsis P, Vergnes JPM. Non-comatose patients with acute carbon monoxide poisoning: hyperbaric or normobaric oxygenation? Undersea Hyperb Med 1995; 22: 9–15 |
| 10 | 4 | Elkharrat D, Raphael JC, Korach JM et al. Acute carbon monoxide intoxication and hyperbaric oxygen in pregnancy. Intensive Care Med 1991; 17: 289–92 |
| 11 | 2b | Raphael JC, Elkharrat D, Jars-Guincestre MC, Chastang C, Chasles V, Vercken JB, et al. Trial of normobaric and hyperbaric oxygen for acute carbon monoxide intoxication. Lancet 1989; 414–18 |
| 12 | 2b | Thom SR, Taber RL, Mendiguren II et al. Delayed neuropsychologic sequelae after carbon monoxide poisoning: prevention by treatment with hyperbaric oxygen. Ann Emerg Med 1995; 25: 474–80 |
| 13 | 4 | Koren G, Sharav T, Pastuszak A et al. A multicenter, prospective study of foetal outcome following accidental carbon monoxide poisoning in pregnancy. Reprod Toxicol 1991; 5: 397–403 |

## CAUSES

Think about potentially reversible causes **[D]**:

- hypoxia
- hypovolaemia
- hyper/hypokalaemia and other metabolic disorders
- hypothermia
- tension pneumothorax
- tamponade
- toxic/therapeutic disturbances
- thromboembolic/mechanical obstruction.

## THERAPY

- Go on a life support course before joining a cardiac arrest team **[A]**[1].

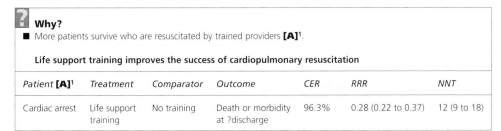

**?** **Why?**
- More patients survive who are resuscitated by trained providers **[A]**[1].

**Life support training improves the success of cardiopulmonary resuscitation**

| Patient **[A]**[1] | Treatment | Comparator | Outcome | CER | RRR | NNT |
|---|---|---|---|---|---|---|
| Cardiac arrest | Life support training | No training | Death or morbidity at ?discharge | 96.3% | 0.28 (0.22 to 0.37) | 12 (9 to 18) |

- Run to the arrest **[A]**[2].

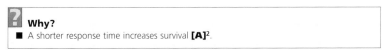

**?** **Why?**
- A shorter response time increases survival **[A]**[2].

- Assess the airway, breathing and circulation **[A]**.
- Perform a precordial thump **[A]**[3].

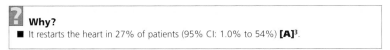

**?** **Why?**
- It restarts the heart in 27% of patients (95% CI: 1.0% to 54%) **[A]**[3].

- Start basic life support **[A]**.

Perform:

- active compression–decompression CPR using a cardiopump **[B]**[4] **[B]**[5]
- or interposed abdominal counterpulsation (compression over the umbilicus to coordinate with early relaxation of chest compression (rate 80–100 min) **[A]**[6].

**? Why?**

■ More patients are resuscitated and survive, particularly without neurological deficit, if given active compression–decompression CPR compared with standard CPR **[B]**[4] **[B]**[5].

■ More patients are resuscitated and survive if given interposed abdominal counterpulsation compared with standard CPR **[A]**[6].

**Active compression–decompression CPR saves lives**

| Patient [B][4] | Treatment | Comparator | Outcome | CER | RRR | NNT |
|---|---|---|---|---|---|---|
| Cardiac arrest | Active compression–decompression CPR | Standard CPR | Return of spontaneous circulation at ?minutes | 29% | 33.0% (9% to 63%) | 10 (6 to 34) |
| | | | Survival at 24 h | 14% | 68% (23% to 131%) | 11 (7 to 26) |
| | | | Survival at 7 days | 5.3% | 92% (14% to 224%) | 20 (11 to 94) |
| | | | Survival without neurological impairment at discharge | 1.9% | 200% (30% to 610%) | 27 (15 to 94) |
| | | | Survival at 12 months | 1.9% | 150% (3% to 485%) | 37 (19 to 550) |

**Interposed abdominal counterpulsation saves lives**

| Patient [A][6] | Treatment | Comparator | Outcome (%) | CER | RRR | NNT |
|---|---|---|---|---|---|---|
| Cardiac arrest | Interposed abdominal counterpulsation | Standard CPR | Return of spontaneous circulation at 3 min | 26% | 137% (43% to 294%) | 3 (2 to 6) |
| | | | Survival at 24 h | 13% | 162% (18% to 483%) | 5 (3 to 22) |
| | | | Survival at discharge | 7.2% | 244% (19% to 895%) | 6 (3 to 27) |

● Establish a definitive airway **[A].**
  – Insert a laryngeal mask if unfamiliar with endotracheal tubes **[B]**[7] **[B]**[8].

**? Why?**

■ Inexperienced users are more successful and faster (on average 3 min) at inserting laryngeal masks than endotracheal tubes **[B]**[7] **[B]**[9].

**Laryngeal masks are easier to insert than endotracheal tubes**

| Patient [B][7] | Treatment | Comparator | Outcome | CER | RRR | NNT |
|---|---|---|---|---|---|---|
| Elective surgery | Laryngeal mask | Endotracheal tube | Failed intubation at 5 min | 53% | 100% | 2 (1 to 3) |

■ Aspiration using laryngeal masks is very rare in elective surgery (0.023%, 95% CI: 0.0% to 0.050%) **[B]**[10].

- Attach an ECG monitor and assess the rhythm.

## Ventricular fibrillation or tachycardia

- Defibrillate **[A]** immediately **[B]**[11].

**Why?**
- Patients with an out-of-hospital cardiac arrest who receive defibrillation by basic life support providers are less likely to die **[B]**[11].

**Defibrillation by basic life support providers saves lives**

| Patient **[B]**[11] | Treatment | Comparator | Outcome | CER | RR | NNT |
|---|---|---|---|---|---|---|
| Out-of-hospital cardiac arrest | Defibrillation by basic life support providers | Standard basic life support care | Death at discharge | 80% | 0.915 (0.876 to 0.955) | 15 (10 to 28) |

**Note**
- The polarity of the defibrillator electrodes has no clear effect on resuscitation **[D]**[12].
- Apex-anterior chest pads or apex-posterior chest pads are probably equally effective **[C]**[13].
- High-energy shocks are not clearly better than low-energy shocks **[D]**[14] **[D]**[15].
- Automatic defibrillators may be worse than manual defibrillators: fewer patients are resuscitated but there is no clear effect on survival at discharge **[B]**[16].

**Automatic defibrillators are less successful than manual defibrillators**

| Patient **[B]**[16] | Treatment | Comparator | Outcome | CER | RRR | NNH |
|---|---|---|---|---|---|---|
| Out-of-hospital cardiac arrest | Automatic defibrillator | Manual defibrillators | Successful resuscitation | 35% | −30% (−50% to −1%) | 10 (5 to 300) |

There is no clear benefit from:

- adrenaline **[A]**[17] **[B]**[18].

**Why?**
- High-dose adrenaline compared with standard dose adrenaline **[A]**[17] or placebo **[D]**[19] has no effect on survival, but increases the risk of brain damage **[B]**[20].

**A high cumulative dose of adrenaline increases the risk of brain damage**

| Patient | Prognostic factor | Outcome | Control rate | OR (95% CI) | NNF+ (95% CI) |
|---|---|---|---|---|---|
| Cardiac arrest | Cumulative dose of adrenaline > 5 mg *independent* | Unfavourable neurological outcome at 6 months | 16% | 1.22 (1.01 to 1.46) | 36 (18 to 770) |

- amiodarone **[A]**[21]

**Why?**

■ It increases survival to hospital admission in out-of-hospital cardiac arrest, but has no clear effect on survival to discharge **[A]**[21].

**Amiodarone increases survival to hospital admission following out-of-hospital cardiac arrest**

| Patient **[A]**[21] | Treatment | Comparator | Outcome | CER | RRR | NNT |
|---|---|---|---|---|---|---|
| Out-of-hospital cardiac arrest | Amiodarone | Placebo | Survival to hospital admission | 35% | 27.0% (2% to 59.0%) | 11 (6 to 110) |

- vasopressin **[A]**[22]

**Why?**

■ More patients are resuscitated than patients given adrenaline, but there is no clear effect on survival to discharge **[A]**[22].

**Vasopressin increases successful resuscitation and survival at 24 h**

| Patient **[A]**[22] | Treatment | Comparator | Outcome | CER | RRR | NNT |
|---|---|---|---|---|---|---|
| Out-of-hospital cardiac arrest | Vasopressin | Adrenaline | Successful resuscitation | 35% | 100% (3.00% to 290%) | 3 (2 to 17) |
| | | | survival at 24 h | 20% | 200% (16% to 673%) | 3 (1 to 8) |

- atropine for brady-asystolic arrest **[B]**[18] **[D]**[23]
- external pacing for asystole or pulseless electrical activity **[D]**[24]
- calcium chloride **[B]**[18] **[D]**[25] **[D]**[26]
- buffer therapy **[D]**[27]
- magnesium **[D]**[28] **[D]**[29]
- bretylium sulphate **[B]**[18] **[D]**[30] **[C]**[31]
- lidocaine **[B]**[18]
- pneumatic trousers **[D]**[32]

**Why?**

■ Atropine **[B]**[18] **[D]**[23], pneumatic trousers **[D]**[32], magnesium **[D]**[28] **[D]**[29], and buffer therapy **[B]**[18] **[D]**[27] have no clear effect on resuscitation or survival.
■ Bretylium sulphate increases admission to hospital, but has no clear effect on survival to discharge **[B]**[18] **[D]**[30] **[C]**[31].
■ Calcium chloride **[D]**[25] **[D]**[26] and external pacing **[D]**[24] have no effect on resuscitation in refractory asystole or pulseless electrical activity.

- calcium antagonists (e.g. lidoflazine **[D]**[33] or nimodipine **[D]**[34]).

**Why?**

■ There is no clear effect on cerebral function or survival **[D]**[33].

Consider stopping resuscitation if all of the following are present [B][35]:

- >10 min since CPR started
- initial rhythm not VT or VF
- arrest not witnessed.

 **Why?**
- In one study no patients with these features survived to discharge (95% CI: 0.0% to 2.5%) [B][35].

## PREVENTION

- Ask patients on admission whether they want cardiopulmonary resuscitation [A][36] and educate them about the chance of survival [C][37].

**Why?**
- Most patients want to be resuscitated (88%; 95% CI: 81% to 96%) [A][36]. Information on chances of survival reduce the number of patients who want to be resuscitated [C][37].
- Neither physicians [C][38] nor clinical prediction rules [A][39] accurately predict which patients will survive in-hospital cardiac arrest using information available in the first 24 h.
- Neither physicians nor family members are good at guessing elderly patients' wishes [A][36].

**Elderly patients are less slightly likely to want CPR if family members predict this**

| Patient [A][36] | Target disorder (reference standard) | Diagnostic test | LR+ (95% CI) | Post-test probability | LR– (95% CI) | Post-test probability |
|---|---|---|---|---|---|---|
| Healthy elderly (pre-test probability 88%) | Desire resuscitation (patients' wishes) | Family member's prediction | 1.4 (0.8 to 2.5) | 92% | 0.18 (0.036 to 0.85) | 60% |

Consider the following:

- amiodarone [A][40]

**Why?**
- Fewer patients die [A][40].

**Amiodarone reduces the risk of dying suddenly**

| Patient [A][40] | Treatment | Comparator | Outcome | CER | OR | NNT |
|---|---|---|---|---|---|---|
| At risk of sudden death | Amiodarone | Placebo, sotalol, propranolol | Death at ?1 year | 26% | 0.81 (0.69 to 0.94) | 26 (16 to 86) |
| | | | Sudden death at ?1 year | 13% | 0.70 (0.58 to 0.85) | 28 (20 to 57) |

- implantable defibrillators [A][41].

**Why?**

- Implantable defibrillators reduce mortality in patients who had a VF or VT arrest following a myocardial infarction [A][41].
- However, implantable defibrillators are not clearly more effective than amiodarone and are less cost-effective [A][42].

**Implantable defibrillators reduce the risk of sudden death**

| Patient [A][41] | Treatment | Comparator | Outcome | CER | RRR | NNT |
|---|---|---|---|---|---|---|
| Previous VT/VF arrest following MI | Implantable defibrillators | Conventional therapy | Death at 2 years | 36% | 61% (8% to 86%) | 5 (2 to 150) |

## PROGNOSIS

- Watch out for post-arrest complications – rib fractures are common [B][43].

**Why?**

- Complications found on autopsy include rib fractures (32%), marrow emboli (11%), haemopericardium (5%) and liver (5%) or spleen lacerations (5%) [B][43].

- Few patients are discharged alive [A][44] [B][17] [B][43] [B][45] [B][46].
  Survival is worse in:
  - out-of-hospital arrests [B][17]
  - asystole or pulseless electrical activity [A][44] [B][17]
  - elderly patients [B][46].

**Why?**
**Survival is best in hospital and with VT/VF arrests**

| Survival to discharge [A][44] [B][17] [B][43] [B][45] [B][46] | Inpatients (95% CI) | Outpatients (95% CI) |
|---|---|---|
| All patients | 13% to 22% | |
| VF/VT arrest | 20% (18% to 22%) | 8% (5% to 10%) |
| Other rhythm | 10% (8% to 11%) | |
| Pulseless electrical activity (PEA) | | 4% (2% to 6%) |
| Asystole | | 1.3% (0.8% to 1.7%) |
| Elderly patients | 7% to 12% | 0.82% (0.0% to 2.0%) |

Patients are at increased risk of dying following a cardiac arrest if they have:

- previous disease [B][46]
  - stroke [A][44]
  - renal failure [A][44] [B][45]

- – cancer (particularly if metastatic) **[B]**[45]
- – diabetes **[B]**[47]
- current illness
  - – congestive heart failure **[A]**[44] **[B]**[47]
  - – sepsis **[B]**[45]
  - – pneumonia**[B]**[45]
- old age **[A]**[44] or a poor functional status **[B]**[45]
- fine ventricular fibrillation on admission ECG **[B]**[48]
- prolonged arrest or resuscitation attempt **[B]**[46] **[B]**[47]
- coma following the arrest **[C]**[49].

---

**? Why?**

**Previous and current illness, old age and prolonged resuscitation increase the risk of dying**

| Patient | Prognostic factor | Outcome | Control rate | OR (95% CI) | NNF+ (95% CI) |
|---|---|---|---|---|---|
| Post-cardiac arrest | Stroke before admission *independent* **[A]**[44] | Survival at discharge | 23% | 0.3 (0.1 to 0.7) | 7 (5 to 17) |
| | Renal failure before admission *independent* **[A]**[44] | Survival at discharge | 23% | 0.3 (0.1 to 0.8) | 7 (5 to 27) |
| | Cancer *independent* **[B]**[45] | Death at discharge | 84% | 3.08 (1.82 to 5.20) | 10 (8 to 15) |
| | Metastatic cancer *independent* **[B]**[45] | Death at discharge | 86% | 44.9 (9.53 to 212) | 8 (7 to 8) |
| | Diabetes *independent* **[B]**[47] | Death at 6 months | 81% | 1.38 (1.12 to 1.70) | 15 (8 to 46) |
| | Congestive heart failure during admission *independent* **[A]**[44] | Survival at discharge | 23% | 0.4 (0.2 to 0.9) | 8 (6 to 56) |
| | Sepsis *independent* **[B]**[45] | Death at discharge | 85% | 6.86 (2.51 to 18.8) | 8 (7 to 12) |
| | Pneumonia *independent* **[B]**[45] | Death at discharge | 83% | 2.86 (1.43 to 5.72) | 9 (7 to 22) |
| | Aged 70 or more *independent* **[A]**[44] | Survival at discharge | 25% | 0.6 (0.4 to 0.9) | 13 (8 to 56) |
| | Dependent functional status *independent* **[B]**[45] | Death at discharge | 81% | 4.99 (2.92 to 8.55) | 7 (6 to 8) |
| | Total arrest time > 5 min *independent* **[B]**[47] | Death at 6 months | 81% | 1.74 (1.47 to 2.06) | 3 (2 to 5) |
| | Resuscitation time > 20 min *independent* **[B]**[46] | Death at 6 months | 81% | 1.36 (1.12 to 1.64) | 9 (5 to 26) |

**Fine VF increases the risk of dying**

| Patient **[B]**[48] | Prognostic factor | Outcome | Control rate | RR (95% CI) | NNF (95% CI) |
|---|---|---|---|---|---|
| Out-of-hospital cardiac arrest | Fine VF *independent* | Death at discharge | 31% | 1.46 (1.32 to 1.62) | 3 (3 to 5) |

■ 4.2% of patients in a coma post-arrest survive 1 month (95% CI: 1.8% to 6.6%) **[C]**[49].

Patients are less likely to die following an in-hospital cardiac arrest if they have:

- a cardiac cause **[B]**[47]
  - ventricular dysrhythmias on admission **[A]**[44]
  - angina before admission **[A]**[44]
  - myocardial infarction **[B]**[45].

**? Why?**
**Cardiac causes reduce the risk of dying**

| Patient | Prognostic factor | Outcome | Control rate | OR (95% CI) | NNF+ (95% CI) |
|---------|-------------------|---------|--------------|-------------|----------------|
| Post-cardiac arrest | Ventricular dysrhythmia on admission *independent* **[A]**[44] | Survival at discharge | 20% | 11.0 (4.1 to 33.7) | −2 (−3 to −1) |
| | Angina before admission *independent* **[A]**[44] | Survival at discharge | 19% | 2.1 (1.3 to 3.3) | −7 (−23 to −4) |
| | Myocardial infarction *independent* **[B]**[45] | Death at discharge | 85% | 0.53 (0.36 to 0.79) | −10 (−31 to −6) |

- Recovery is good in patients who survive to be discharged, but further cardiac arrests are common **[C]**[50].

**? Why?**
**Most patients return to work, but further arrests and deaths are common**

| Out-of-hospital arrest **[C]**[50] | % (95% CI) |
|------------------------------------|------------|
| Returned to work at 12 months | 71% (66% to 76%) |
| Further cardiac arrest at 12 months | 14% (10% to 18%) |
| Death at 5 years | 24% (19% to 29%) |
| Death at 10 years | 82% (78% to 86%) |

The risk of cardiac arrest is increased with:

- a prolonged QTc interval **[B]**[51].

**? Why?**
**A prolonged QTc increases the risk of cardiac arrest**

| Patient **[B]**[51] | Prognostic factor | Outcome | Control rate | OR (95% CI) | NNF+ (95% CI) |
|---------------------|-------------------|---------|--------------|-------------|----------------|
| Undergoing ECG | Prolonged QTc interval (> 440:ms) *independent* | Sudden death due to cardiac arrest | 3.7% | 2.1 (1.4 to 3.1) | 17 (9 to 47) |

**Guideline writer**: Christopher Ball
**CAT writers**: Christopher Ball, Clare Wotton

## REFERENCES

| No. | Level | Citation |
|---|---|---|
| 1 | 1a | Jabbour M, Osmond MH, Klassen TP. Life support courses: are they effective? Ann Emerg Med 1996; 28: 690–8 |
| 2 | 1a | Nichol G, Detsky AS, Stiell IG, et al. Effectiveness of emergency medical services for victims of out-of- hospital cardiac arrest: a meta-analysis. Ann Emerg Med 1996; 27: 700–10 |
| 3 | 1c | Scherf D, Bornemann C. Thumping of the precordium in ventricular standstill. Am J Cardiol 1960; 1: 30–40 |
| 4 | 2b | Plaisance P et al. A comparison of standard cardiopulmonary resuscitation and active compression-decompression resuscitation for out-of-hospital cardiac arrest. N Engl J Med 1999; 341: 569–75 |
| 5 | 2b | Cohen TJ, Goldner BG, Maccaro PC et al. A comparison of active compression-decompression cardiopulmonary resuscitation with standard cardiopulmonary resuscitation for cardiac arrests occurring in the hospital. N Engl J Med 1993; 329: 1918–21 |
| 6 | 1b | Sack JB, Kesselbrenner MB, Bregman D. Survival from in-hospital cardiac arrest with interposed abdominal counterpulsation during cardiopulmonary resuscitation. JAMA 1992; 267: 379–85 |
| 7 | 2b | Reinhart DJ, Simmons G. Comparison of placement of laryngeal mask airway with endotracheal tube by paramedics and respiratory therapists. Ann Emerg Med 1994; 24: 260–3 |
| 8 | 2b | Davies PR, Tighe SQ, Greenslade GL et al. Laryngeal mask airway and tracheal tube insertion by unskilled personnel. Lancet 1990; 336: 977–9 |
| 9 | 2b | Davies PR, Tighe SQ, Greenslade GL et al. Laryngeal mask airway and tracheal tube insertion by unskilled personnel. Lancet 1990; 336: 977–9 |
| 10 | 2a | Brimacombe JR, Berry A. The incidence of aspiration associated with the laryngeal mask airway: a meta-analysis of the published literature. J Clin Anesth 1995; 7: 297–305 |
| 11 | 2a | Auble TE, Menegazzi JJ, Paris PM et al. Effect of out-of-hospital defibrillation by life support providers on cardiac arrest mortality: a meta-analysis. Ann Emerg Med 1995; 25: 642–8 |
| 12 | 1b– | Weaver WD et al. Influence of external defibrillator electrode polarity on cardiac resuscitation. PACE 1993; 16: 285–90 |
| 13 | 4 | Kerber RE, Martins JB, Kelly KJ et al. Self-adhesive preapplied electrode pads for defibrillation and cardioversion. J Am Coll Cardiol 1984; 3: 815–20 |
| 14 | 2b– | Morgan JP, Hearne SF, Raizes GS et al. High-energy versus low-energy defibrillation: experience in patients (excluding those in the intensive care unit) at Mayo Clinic-affiliated hospitals. Mayo Clin Proc 1984; 59: 829–34 |
| 15 | 2b– | Weaver WD, Cobb LA, Copass MK et al. Ventricular fibrillation: a comparative trial using 175-J and 320-J shocks. N Engl J Med 1982; 307: 1101–6 |
| 16 | 2b | Cummins RO, Eisenberg MS, Litwin PE. Automatic external defibrillators used by emergency medical technicians: a controlled clinical trial. JAMA 1987; 257: 1605–10 |

| No. | Level | Citation |
|-----|-------|----------|
| 17 | 1b | Gueugniaud P-Y, Mols P, Goldstein P et al. A comparison of repeated high doses and repeated standard doses of epinephrine for cardiac arrest outside the hospital. N Engl J Med 1998; 339: 1595–1601 |
| 18 | 2b | van Walraven C, Stiell IG, Wells GA et al. Do advanced cardiac life support drugs increase resuscitation rates for in-hospital cardiac arrest? Ann Emerg Med 1998; 32: 544–53 |
| 19 | 1b– | Woodhouse SP, Cox S, Boyd C et al. High dose and standard dose adrenaline do not alter survival, compared with placebo, in cardiac arrest. Resuscitation 1995; 30: 243–9 |
| 20 | 2b | Behringer W, Kittler H, Sterz F et al. Cumulative epinephrine dose during cardiopulmonary resuscitation and neurologic outcome. Ann Intern Med 1998; 129: 450–6 |
| 21 | 1b | Kudenchuk PJ, Cobb LA, Copass MK et al. Amiodarone for resuscitation after out-of-hospital cardiac arrest due to ventricular fibrillation. N Engl J Med 1999; 341: 871–8 |
| 22 | 1b | Lindner KH, Dirks B, Strohmenger H-U et al. Randomised comparison of epinephrine and vasopressin in patients with out-of-hospital ventricular fibrillation. Lancet 1997; 349: 535–7 |
| 23 | 2b– | Coon GA et al. Use of atropine for brady-asystolic prehospital cardiac arrest. Ann Emerg Med 1981; 10: 462–7 |
| 24 | 2b– | Barthell E et al. Prehospital external cardiac pacing: a prospective controlled clinical trial. Ann Emerg Med 1988; 17: 1221–6 |
| 25 | 1b– | Steuven HA, Thompson B, Aprahamian C et al. Lack of effectiveness of calcium chloride in refractory asystole. Ann Emerg Med 1985; 14: 630–2 |
| 26 | 1b– | Stueven HA, Thompson B, Aprahamian C et al. The effectiveness of calcium chloride in refractory electromechanical dissociation. Ann Emerg Med 1985; 14: 626–9 |
| 27 | 1b– | Dybvik T, Strand T, Steen PA. Buffer therapy during out-of-hospital cardiopulmonary resuscitation. Resuscitation 1995; 29: 89–95 |
| 28 | 1b– | Thel MC, Armstrong AL, McNulty SE et al. Randomised trial of magnesium in in-hospital cardiac arrest. Lancet 1997; 350: 1272–6 |
| 29 | 1b– | Fatovich DM, Prentice DA, Dobb GJ. Magnesium in cardiac arrest (the magic trial). Resuscitation 1997; 35: 237–41 |
| 30 | 2b– | Nowak RM, Bodnar TJ, Dronen S et al. Bretylium tosylate as initial treatment for cardiopulmonary arrest: randomized comparison with placebo. Ann Emerg Med 1981; 10: 404–7 |
| 31 | 4 | Stang JM, Washington SE, Barnes SA et al. Treatment of prehospital refractory ventricular fibrillation with bretylium tosylate. Ann Emerg Med 1984; 13: 234–6 |
| 32 | 1b– | Mahoney BD, Mirick MJ. Efficacy of pneumatic trousers in refractory prehospital cardiopulmonary arrest. Ann Emerg Med 1983; 12: 8–12 |
| 33 | 1b– | Brain Resuscitation Clinical Trial II Study Group et al. Randomized clinical study of a calcium-entry blocker (lidoflazine) in the treatment of comatose survivors of cardiac arrest. N Engl J Med 1991; 324: 1225–31 |
| 34 | 1b– | Roine RO, Kajaste S, Kaste M. Neuropsychological sequelae of cardiac arrest. JAMA 1993; 269: 237–42 |
| 35 | 2a | van Walraven C, Forster AJ, Stiell IG. Derivation of a clinical decision rule for the discontinuation of in-hospital cardiac arrest resuscitations. Arch Intern Med 1999; 159: 129–34 |

| No. | Level | Citation |
|---|---|---|
| 36 | 1b | Seckler AB, Meier DE, Mulvihill M et al. Substituted judgement: how accurate are proxy predictions? Ann Intern Med 1991; 115: 92–8 |
| 37 | 4 | Murphy DJ, Burrows D, Santilli S et al. The influence of the probability of survival on patients' preferences regarding cardiopulmonary resuscitation. N Engl J Med 1994; 330: 545–9 |
| 38 | 4 | Ebell MH, Bergus GR, Warbasse L et al. The inability of physicians to predict the outcome of in-hospital resuscitation. J Gen Intern Med 1996; 11: 16–22 |
| 39 | 1a | Ebell MH, Kruse JA, Smith M et al. Failure of three decision rules to predict the outcome of in-hospital cardiopulmonary resuscitation. Med Decis Making 1997; 17: 171–7 |
| 40 | 1a | Sim I, McDonald KM, Lavori PW et al. Quantitative overview of randomised trials of amiodarone to prevent sudden cardiac death. Circulation 1997; 96: 2823–9 |
| 41 | 1b | Wever EF, Hauer RN, van Capelle F et al. Randomized study of implantable defibrillator as first-choice therapy versus conventional strategy in postinfarct sudden death survivors. Circulation 1995; 91: 2195–203 |
| 42 | 1b | Owens DK, Sanders GD, Harris RA et al. Cost-effectiveness of implantable cardioverter defibrillators relative to amiodarone for prevention of sudden cardiac death. Ann Intern Med 1997; 126: 1–12 |
| 43 | 2a | Schneider AP, Nelson DJ, Brown DD. In-hospital cardiopulmonary resuscitation: a 30-year review. J Am Board Fam Pract 1993; 6: 91–101 |
| 44 | 1b | de Vos R, Koster RW, de Haan RJ et al. In-hospital cardiopulmonary resuscitation: prearrest morbidity and outcome. Arch Intern Med 1999; 159: 845–50 |
| 45 | 2a | Ebell M et al. Best predictors of survival following in-hospital cardiopulmonary resuscitation: a meta-analysis. J Fam Pract 1992; 34: 551–8 |
| 46 | 2b | Murphy DJ, Murray AM, Robinson BE et al. Outcomes of cardiopulmonary resuscitation in the elderly. Ann Intern Med 1989; 111: 199–205 |
| 47 | 2b | Rogove HJ, Safar P, Sutton-Tyrrell K et al. Old age does not negate good cerebral outcome after cardiopulmonary resuscitation: analyses from the brain resuscitation clinical trials. Crit Care Med 1995; 23: 18–25 |
| 48 | 2b | Weaver WD, Cobb LA, Dennis D et al. Amplitude of ventricular fibrillation waveform and outcome after cardiac arrest. Ann Intern Med 1985; 102: 53–5 |
| 49 | 4 | Edgren E, Hedstrand U, Kelsey S et al. Assessment of neurological prognosis in comatose survivors of cardiac arrest. Lancet 1990; 343: 1055–9 |
| 50 | 4 | Reid Graves J, Herlitz J, Bang A et al. Survivors of out of hospital cardiac arrest: their prognosis, longevity and functional status. Resuscitation 1997; 35: 117–21 |
| 51 | 2b | Algra A, Tijssen JG, Roelandt JR et al. QTc prolongation measured by standard 12-lead electrocardiography is an independent risk factor for sudden death due to cardiac arrest. Circulation 1991; 83: 1888–94 |

## PREVALENCE

Cellulitis is common **[D]** and can be serious in diabetes **[A]**[1].

>  **Note**
> ■ 6% of patients with suspected DVT have cellulitis **[A]**[2] **[A]**[3].
> ■ In diabetics with severe foot ulcers, osteomyelitis is present in 68% **[A]**[1].

Think about a differential diagnosis **[A]**[2] **[A]**[3]:
- deep vein thrombosis
- ruptured Baker's cyst.

## CLINICAL FEATURES

Most cases of cellulitis are obvious. Look for **[C]**[4]
- pain or tenderness
- erythema
- increased warmth
- swelling
- temperature $\geq 37.7°C$
- regional lymphadenopathy.

> **Note**
> Pain, erythema and swelling are common in cellulitis
>
> | Clinical features **[C]**[4] | Sensitivity (95% CI) |
> | --- | --- |
> | Pain or tenderness | 97% (90v to 100%) |
> | Erythema | 97% (90v to 100%) |
> | Increased warmth | 93% (84% to 100%) |
> | Swelling | 90% (79% to 100%) |
> | Temperature $\geq 37.7°C$ | 57% (39% to 74%) |
> | Regional adenopathy | 27% (11% to 43%) |

Look for a possible cause **[B]**[5]:
- a site of entry (e.g. leg ulcer, toe-web intertrigo, traumatic wound)
- lymphoedema, leg oedema or venous insufficiency
- obesity.

**Why?**
■ These clinical features increase the risk of cellulitis developing.
■ Diabetes, alcohol misuse and smoking are not significantly associated with an increased risk of cellulitis.

**Lymphoedema and a site of entry increase the risk of cellulitis**

| Outcome | Risk factor [B][5] | PEER | OR (95% CI) | NNF (95% CI) |
|---|---|---|---|---|
| Cellulitis | Lymphoedema *independent* | 0.1% | 71.2 (5.6 to 908) | 15 (2 to 220) |
| | Site of entry *independent* | 0.1% | 23.8 (10.7 to 52.5) | 45 (20 to 100) |
| | Leg oedema (excluding venous insufficiency) *independent* | 0.1% | 2.5 (1.2 to 5.1) | 670 (250 to 5000) |
| | Venous insufficiency *independent* | 0.1% | 2.9 (1.0 to 8.7) | 530 (130 to infinity) |
| | Overweight *independent* | 0.1% | 2.0 (1.1 to 3.7) | 1000 (370 to 10000) |

If a DVT is possible, further investigations are required, e.g ultrasound scanning.

**Why?**
■ Clinical examination cannot accurately diagnose or exclude DVT [A][6].

If a Baker's cyst is possible, look for [A][7]:
● crepitus on flexing knee
● history of arthritis
● a positive ultrasound scan.

**Why?**
**Arthritis or crepitus makes a Baker's cyst more likely**

| Patient [A][7] | Target disorder (reference standard) | Diagnostic test | LR+(95% CI) | Post-test probability | LR−(95% CI) | Post-test probability |
|---|---|---|---|---|---|---|
| Suspected DVT (pre-test probability 33%) | Baker's cyst (venography, arthroscopy) | Crepitus on flexing the knee | 3.0 (1.2 to 7.5) | 64% | 0.54 (0.30 to 0.96) | 24% |
| | | History of arthritis | 3.4 (1.2 to 9.4) | 67% | 0.59 (0.35 to 0.98) | 26% |
| | | Ultrasound scan | infinity (0.16 to infinity) | 100% | 0.88 (0.73 to 1.1) | 34% |

Remember the presence of a Baker's cyst (ruptured or not) does not exclude a DVT [A][7].

Think about necrotising fasciitis with [C][8]:

- crepitus
- sensation loss
- severe pain.

Think about osteomyelitis in patients with diabetes and foot ulcers and any of the following [A][1] [A][9]:

- clinical suspicion
- ulcer area > 2 cm$^2$
- bone exposed within ulcer
- bone palpable (by probe) in ulcer.

<table>
<tr><td colspan="7">? Why?<br>Clinical suspicion, large ulcers and detectable bone increase the chance of osteomyelitis</td></tr>
<tr><td>Patient<br>[A][1] [A][9]</td><td>Target disorder<br>(reference<br>standard)</td><td>Diagnostic<br>test</td><td>LR+(95% CI)</td><td>Post-test<br>probability</td><td>LR–(95% CI)</td><td>Post-test<br>probability</td></tr>
<tr><td>Diabetes and<br>infected foot<br>ulcer (pre-test<br>probability<br>68%)</td><td>Osteomyelitis<br>(histology)</td><td>Clinical<br>suspicion</td><td>Infinity (2.1<br>to infinity)</td><td>100%</td><td>0.83 (0.75<br>to 0.92)</td><td>64%</td></tr>
<tr><td></td><td></td><td>Ulcer area<br>> 2 cm$^2$</td><td>3.6 (1.2 to 11)</td><td>88%</td><td>0.76 (0.63<br>to 0.91)</td><td>62%</td></tr>
<tr><td></td><td></td><td>Bone<br>exposed<br>within ulcer</td><td>Infinity (2.1<br>to infinity)</td><td>100%</td><td>0.83 (0.75<br>to 0.92)</td><td>64%</td></tr>
<tr><td></td><td></td><td>Bone palpable<br>in ulcer</td><td>3.9 (1.5 to 10)</td><td>89%</td><td>0.63 (0.50<br>to 0.80)</td><td>58%</td></tr>
</table>

## INVESTIGATIONS

In unwell patients, consider:

- swabbing any skin breaks, wounds or ulcers [C][10] [C][11].

<table>
<tr><td colspan="2">? Why?<br>■ Swabbing of any breaks in the skin in patients with cellulitis frequently isolates a pathogen – around 40% are positive [C][10] [C][11].<br>■ More invasive techniques are not very helpful [C][10] [C][11] and contaminants are common [C][12].</td></tr>
<tr><td colspan="2">Culture techniques are not very sensitive for diagnosing the cause of cellulitis</td></tr>
<tr><td>[C][10]</td><td>% (95% CI)</td></tr>
<tr><td>Primary lesion swab</td><td>42% (28% to 56%)</td></tr>
<tr><td>Punch biopsy</td><td>20% (8.9% to 31%)</td></tr>
<tr><td>Needle aspiration</td><td>10% (1.7% to 18%)</td></tr>
<tr><td>Blood culture</td><td>4.0% (0.0% to 9.4%)</td></tr>
</table>

**Note**

■ Identification of an organism may reflect colonisation rather than infection **[D]**.

In patients with diabetes and serious infection, consider:

● blood count **[C]**[4].

**Note**

■ Sensitivity of a white cell count > 10: 50% (95% CI: 32% to 68%) **[C]**[4].

If osteomyelitis is a possibility consider **[A]**[1] **[A]**[9]:

● ESR
● a bone scan
● MRI.

**Why?**

**Grossly raised ESR is diagnostic**

| Patient [A][1] [A][9] | Target disorder (reference standard) | Diagnostic test | LR+(95% CI) | Post-test probability | LR–(95% CI) | Post-test probability |
|---|---|---|---|---|---|---|
| Diabetes and infected foot ulcer (pre-test probability 68%) | Osteomyelitis (histology) | ESR > 100 mm/hour [A][1] [A][9] | Infinity (1.3 to infinity) | 100% | 0.89 (0.83 to 0.97) | 66% |
| | | Bone scan [A][1] [A][9] | 0.52 (0.36 to 0.75) | 53% | 2.2 (1.3 to 3.8) | 82% |
| Diabetes and admitted with foot ulcer or cellulitis (pre-test probability 46%) | Deep infection (surgery or long-term antibiotics) | MRI [C][13] | 3.9 (1.4 to 11) | 77% | 0.12 (0.018 to 0.78) | 9% |

**Note**

■ X-rays and leucocyte scans are unhelpful. **[A]**[1] **[A]**[9]

**X-rays and leucocyte scans do not help diagnose or exclude osteomyelitis in diabetes**

| Patient [A][1] [A][9] | Target disorder (reference standard) | Diagnostic test | LR+(95% CI) | Post-test probability | LR–(95% CI) | Post-test probability |
|---|---|---|---|---|---|---|
| Diabetes and infected foot ulcer | Osteomyelitis (histology) | X-ray | 1.7 (0.51 to 5.7) | 79% | 0.93 (0.81 to 1.1) | 67% |
| | | 24 h leucocyte scans | 1.3 (0.75 to 2.3) | 74% | 0.86 (0.64 to 1.2) | 65% |

In suspected cases of necrotising fasciitis, consider:
- a frozen biopsy **[C]**[8] – 1% lidocaine anaesthesia, 2 cm × 1 cm elliptical biopsies (skin and deep soft tissue) of suspected necrotising area and at another area (leading edge of erythema, induration or necrosis)
- MRI **[C]**[14].

| **? Why?** |
|---|
| **Frozen punch biopsy and MRI can help exclude necrotising fasciitis** |

| Patient | Target disorder (reference standard) | Diagnostic test | LR+(95% CI) | Post-test probability | LR–(95% CI) | Post-test probability |
|---|---|---|---|---|---|---|
| Suspected necrotising fasciitis (pre-test probability 28%) **[C]**[8] | Necrotising fasciitis (surgery) | Frozen section biopsy | Infinity (11 to infinity) | 100% | 0.0 (0.0 to 0.22) | 0% |
| Suspected necrotising fasciitis (pre-test probability 65%) **[C]**[14] | Necrotising fasciitis (surgery/ autopsy) | MRI | 6.0 (1.0 to 36) | 92% | 0.00 (0.0 to 0.29) | 0% |

## THERAPY

- Give analgesia **[D]**.
- Give antibiotics **[A]** to cover *Staphylococcus* spp. and *Streptococcus* spp. **[C]**[12], e.g. flucloxacillin 500 mg qds for 7 days **[D]**[15].

| **? Why do this?** |
|---|
| ■ Oral antibiotics are effective for initial therapy of cellulitis in children **[A]**[16]. |
| ■ No one antibiotic regimen has been shown to be better than another **[D]**[15]. |
| **Prevalence of infecting organisms** |

| **[C]**[10] **[C]**[12] | Range of estimates |
|---|---|
| *Staphylococci* and *Streptococci* | 46% |
| *Staphylococci* alone | 13% to 53% |
| *Streptococci* alone | 24% to 29% |
| *Klebsiella* | 5.9% |
| Other (*Morganella morgani, Pseudomonas aeruginosa, Peptococcus*) | 8% to 12% |

Review the patient, as some are not cured **[C]**[17].

> **Why do this?**
> ■ Patients with skin and soft-tissue infections presenting to the emergency department
>   can be treated as out patients safely – around 3% of infections are not successfully
>   treated.

Admit patients with severe infections for parenteral antibiotics [D].

● Consider granulocyte colony-stimulating factor in patients with
  diabetes who require admission **[A]**[18].

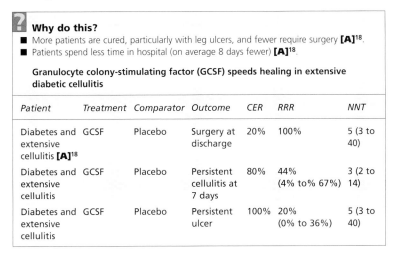

> **Why do this?**
> ■ More patients are cured, particularly with leg ulcers, and fewer require surgery **[A]**[18].
> ■ Patients spend less time in hospital (on average 8 days fewer) **[A]**[18].
>
> **Granulocyte colony-stimulating factor (GCSF) speeds healing in extensive
> diabetic cellulitis**

| Patient | Treatment | Comparator | Outcome | CER | RRR | NNT |
|---|---|---|---|---|---|---|
| Diabetes and extensive cellulitis **[A]**[18] | GCSF | Placebo | Surgery at discharge | 20% | 100% | 5 (3 to 40) |
| Diabetes and extensive cellulitis | GCSF | Placebo | Persistent cellulitis at 7 days | 80% | 44% (4% to% 67%) | 3 (2 to 14) |
| Diabetes and extensive cellulitis | GCSF | Placebo | Persistent ulcer | 100% | 20% (0% to 36%) | 5 (3 to 40) |

● Urgent surgery is required for necrotising fasciitis **[D]**.

## PREVENTION

Clean wounds with povidone-iodine **[B]**[19]. Check patients are not
allergic to iodine **[D]**.

> **Why do this?**
> **Wound cleaning of simple lacerations with povidone-iodine reduces wound infections [B][19].**

| Patient | Treatment | Comparator | Outcome | CER | RRR | NNT |
|---|---|---|---|---|---|---|
| Simple laceration | Wound cleaning with povidone-iodine | Saline | Infected wound at 14 days | 15% | 65% (31% to 82%) | 10 (6 to 25) |
| Simple laceration | Wound cleaning with povidone-iodine | Saline | Purulent wound at 14 days | 6.2% | 84% (29% to 96%) | 19 (11 to 65) |

Give prophylactic antibiotics for:
- dog bites [A][20]
- human bites [D] – remember to cover anaerobes (e.g. co-amoxiclav).

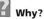 **Why do this?**
Prophylactic antibiotic administration for dog-bite wounds prevents wound infection [A][20]

| Patient [A][20] | Treatment | Comparator | Outcome | CER | RRR | NNT |
|---|---|---|---|---|---|---|
| Uninfected dog bite | Prophylactic antibiotics | No antibiotics | Infected wound at? | 16% | 0.58% (0.38% to 0.82%) | 15 (10 to 35) |

There is no clear benefit for:
- simple wounds [A][21]
- burns [D][22].

**Why?**
- Prophylactic antibiotics do not reduce wound infections in simple wounds [A][21].
- Patients with burns who receive penicillin prophylaxis are not clearly less likely to develop cellulitis or burns than those who do not [D][22].

**Guideline writers**: John Epling, Christopher Ball
**CAT writers:** John Epling, Christopher Ball

## REFERENCES

| No | Level | Citation |
|---|---|---|
| 1 | 1b | Unsuspected osteomyelitis in diabetic foot ulcers. ACP J Club 1992 Jan-Feb; 116–18. Review of Newman LG et al. Unsuspected osteomyelitis in diabetic foot ulcers. Diagnosis and monitoring by leukocyte scanning with indium-111 oxyquinolone. JAMA 1991; 266: 1246–51 |
| 2 | 1b | Wells PS et al. A simple clinical model for the diagnosis of DVT combined with impedence plethysmography: potential for an improvement in the diagnostic process. J Intern Med 1998; 243: 15–23 |
| 3 | 1b | Huisman MV et al. Serial impedance plethysmogram for suspected deep venous thrombosis in outpatients: Amsterdam General Practitioner Study. N Engl J Med 1986; 314: 823–8 |
| 4 | 4 | Newell PM, Norden CW. Value of needle aspiration in bacteriologic diagnosis of cellulitis in adults. J Clin Microbiol 1988; 26: 401–4 |
| 5 | 3b | Dupuy A et al. Risk factors for erysipelas of the leg (cellulitis): case-control study. BMJ 1999; 318: 1591–4 |
| 6 | 1a | Anand SS et al. The rational clinical exam: does this patient have deep vein thrombosis? JAMA 1998; 279: 1094–9 |
| 7 | 1b | Simpson FW et al. A prospective study of thrombophlebitis and 'pseudothrombophlebitis'. Lancet 1980; 1: 331–3 |
| 8 | 4 | Majeski J, Majeski E. Necrotising fasciitis: improved survival with early recognition by tissue biopsy and aggressive surgical treatment. South Med J 1997: 90: 1065–8 |

| No | Level | Citation |
|----|-------|----------|
| 9 | 1b | Probing diabetic pedal ulcers for bone detected osteomyelitis. ACP J Club 1995 Nov-Dec; 123:74. Review of Grayson et al. Probing to bone in infected pedal ulcers: a clinical sign of underlying osteomyelitis in diabetic patients. JAMA 1995; 273: 721–3 |
| 10 | 4 | Hook EW et al. Microbiologic evaluation of cutaneous cellulitis in adults. Arch Intern Med 1986; 146: 295–7 |
| 11 | 4 | Leppard BJ et al. The value of bacteriology and serology in the diagnosis of cellulitis and erysipelas: Br J Dermatol 1985; 112: 559–67 |
| 12 | 4 | Sigurdsson AF, Gudmundsson S. The etiology of bacterial cellulitis as determined by fine-needle aspiration. Scand J Infect Dis 1989; 21: 537–42 |
| 13 | 4 | Cook TA et al. Magnetic resonance imaging in the management of diabetic foot infection. Br J Surg 1996; 83: 245–8 |
| 14 | 4 | Schmid MR et al. Differentiation of necrotising fasciitis and cellulitis using MR imaging. Am J Radiol 1998; 170: 615–20 |
| 15 | 1b | Powers RD et al. Soft tissue infections in the emergency department: the case for the use of 'simple' antibiotics. South Med J 1991; 84: 1313–5 |
| 16 | 1c | Fleisher G et al. Cellulitis and prospective study. Ann Emerg Med 1980; 9: 246–9 |
| 17 | 4 | Powers RD et al. Soft tissue infections in the emergency department: the case for the use of 'simple' antibiotics: Southern Medical Journal 1991: Vol. 84, (11); 1313–1315. |
| 18 | 1b | Gough A et al. Randomised placebo-controlled trial of granulocyte-colony stimulating factor in diabetic foot infection. Lancet 1997; 350: 855–9 |
| 19 | 2b | Gravett A et al. A trial of povidone-iodine in the prevention of infection in sutured lacerations. Ann Emerg Med 1987; 16: 167–71 |
| 20 | 1a | Cummings P. Antibiotics to prevent infection in patients with dog bite wounds: a meta-analysis of randomized trials. Ann Emerg Med 1994; 23: 535–40 |
| 21 | 1a | Cumming P, Del Beccaro MA. Antibiotics to prevent infection of simple wounds: a meta-analysis of randomized studies. Am J Emerg Med 1995; 13: 396–400 |
| 22 | 2b | Durtschi MB et al. A prospective study of prophylactic penicllin in acutely burned hospitalized patients. J Trauma 1982; 22: 11–14 |

## DIFFERENTIAL DIAGNOSIS

Common causes of chest pain include [C][1]:

- myocardial infarction
- angina
- pulmonary embolism
- chest infection
- musculoskeletal pain
- pericarditis.

Rarer causes include [D]:

- aortic dissection
- oesophageal spasm.

---

**Note**

- One in six patients with anterior or left-sided chest pain has an MI (14%–20%) [A][2] [A][3].
- The risk is higher in elderly patients (20%; 95% CI: 19% to 22%) [A][2] and patients with a typical history [A][2].
- One in four patients with anterior or left-sided chest pain has unstable angina (24%; 95% CI: 21% to 27%) [A][3] – the risk is higher in elderly patients (44%; 95% CI: 42% to 45%) [A][2].

**MI, angina and PE are common causes of chest pain**

| Chest pain in emergency department [A][2] [A][3] [C][1] | (%) |
|---|---|
| MI | 12% to 20% |
| Unstable angina | 24% (21% to 27%) |
| Stable angina | 9.0% (5.6% to 12%) |
| PE | 5.8% (3.0% to 8.5%) |
| Other pulmonary disease | 5.8% (3.0% to 8.5%) |
| Chest wall pain | 5.4% (2.7% to 8.1%) |
| Pericarditis | 5.0% (2.5% to 7.6%) |
| Psychogenic | 2.9% (0.9% to 4.8%) |
| Other heart disease | 1.1% (0.0% to 2.3%) |
| Other disease | 1.1% (0.0% to 2.3%) |
| Unknown | 11% (7.5% to 15%) |

- Only 40% of cases of aortic dissection are diagnosed following history, physical, ECG and chest X-ray (14% mistaken for ischaemic heart disease, 14% for other aortic disease, 7% heart failure) [C][4].

---

Estimate your patient's risk of significant coronary artery disease (≥50% coronary artery stenosis in at least one major artery; Tables 1 and 2) using age [A][3] and the following symptoms [B][5]:

- retrosternal chest pain
- pain brought on by exertion
- pain relieved in <10 min by rest or nitroglycerin.

## Table 1  Men: probability (%) of ≥ 50% coronary artery stenosis in at least one major artery

| Symptoms [B][5] | Age (years) | | | |
| --- | --- | --- | --- | --- |
| | 30–39 | 40–49 | 50–59 | 60–69 |
| Asymptomatic (0 symptoms) | 2% | 6% | 10% | 12% |
| Non-anginal chest pain (1 symptom) | 5% | 14% | 22% | 28% |
| Atypical angina (2 symptoms) | 22% | 46% | 59% | 67% |
| Typical angina (all 3 symptoms) | 70% | 87% | 92% | 94% |

## Table 2  Women: probability (%) of ≥ 50% coronary artery stenosis in at least one major artery

| Symptoms [B][5] | Age (years) | | | |
| --- | --- | --- | --- | --- |
| | 30–39 | 40–49 | 50–59 | 60–69 |
| Asymptomatic (0 symptoms) | 0.3% | 1% | 3% | 8% |
| Non-anginal chest pain (1 symptom) | 1% | 3% | 8% | 19% |
| Atypical angina (2 symptoms) | 4% | 13% | 32% | 54% |
| Typical angina (all 3 symptoms) | 26% | 55% | 79% | 91% |

## ? Why?

### Increasing age increases the risk of having unstable angina or an MI

| Patient [A][3] | Target disorder (reference standard) | Diagnostic test | LR+ (95% CI) | Post-test probability |
| --- | --- | --- | --- | --- |
| Central or left-sided chest pain (pre-test probability 41%) | MI or unstable angina (ECG, cardiac enzymes, stress tests) | Aged > 80 years | 3.5 (1.9 to 6.4) | 71% |
| | | 70–79 years | 2.2 (1.4 to 3.4) | 61% |
| | | 60–69 years | 1.8 (1.3 to 2.4) | 56% |
| | | 50–59 years | 1.1 (0.83 to 1.5) | 44% |
| | | 40–49 years | 0.50 (0.34 to 0.72) | 26% |
| | | 30–39 years | 0.12 (0.047 to 0.28) | 8% |
| | | 25–29 years | 0.10 (0.024 to 0.42) | 7% |

### Men who have chest pain are more likely to have an MI or unstable angina

| Patient [A][3] | Target disorder (reference standard) | Diagnostic test | LR+ (95% CI) | Post-test probability | LR– (95% CI) | Post-test probability |
| --- | --- | --- | --- | --- | --- | --- |
| Central or left-sided chest pain (pre-test probability 41%) | MI or unstable angina (ECG, cardiac enzymes, stress tests) | Male | 1.3 (1.1 to 1.5) | 48% | 0.77 (0.65 to 0.91) | 35% |

## CLINICAL FEATURES

Ask about:

- Pain, specifically:
  - its position **[B]**[5] **[B]**[6] and if it has moved **[C]**[7] **[C]**[8]

| **Why?** | | | | |
|---|---|---|---|---|
| **Chest or left arm pain makes an MI more likely** | | | | |
| Patient **[B]**[6] | Target disorder (reference standard) | Diagnostic test | LR+ (95% CI) | Post-test probability |
| Attending emergency department with chest pain (pre-test probability 20%) | MI (ECG and cardiac enzyme changes) | Pain in chest or left arm | 2.7 | 40% |

| **Pain migration makes aortic dissection slightly more likely** | | | | | | |
|---|---|---|---|---|---|---|
| Patient **[C]**[7] **[C]**[8] | Target disorder (reference standard) | Diagnostic test | LR+ (95% CI) | Post-test probability | LR− (95% CI) | Post-test probability |
| Suspected aortic dissection undergoing angiography (pre-test probability 1%) | Aortic dissection (angiography, surgery or autopsy) | Pain migration | 1.3 (1.0 to 1.8) | 1.3% | 0.64 (0.43 to 0.93) | 0.64% |

  - its duration **[A]**[9] **[B]**[10] **[C]**[7] **[C]**[8] **[C]**[11]

| **Why?** | | | | | | |
|---|---|---|---|---|---|---|
| ■ Chest pain, which began 48 h or more ago makes an MI more likely**[A]**[9]. | | | | | | |
| **Episodes of chest pain for over 1 year makes coronary artery disease more likely** | | | | | | |
| Patient **[C]**[11] | Target disorder (reference standard) | Diagnostic test | LR+ (95% CI) | Post-test probability | LR− (95% CI) | Post-test probability |
| Intermittent chest pain referred for investigation (pre-test probability 67%) | Coronary artery disease (angiography and exercise test) | Chest pain for over 1 year | Infinity (3.5 to infinity) | 100% | 0.37 (0.23 to 0.59) | 43% |

| **Constant pain makes a myocardial infarction more likely** | | | | | | |
|---|---|---|---|---|---|---|
| Patient **[B]**[10] | Target disorder (reference standard) | Diagnostic test | LR+ (95% CI) | Post-test probability | LR− (95% CI) | Post-test probability |
| Anterior chest pain (pre-test probability 12%) | MI (cardiac enzymes, ECG) | Constant pain | 1.7 (1.3 to 2.1) | 19% | 0.58 (0.41 to 0.82) | 8% |

?

**Symptoms lasting longer than 24 hours make aortic dissection slightly less likely**

| Patient [C][7] [C][8] | Target disorder (reference standard) | Diagnostic test | LR+ (95% CI) | Post-test probability | LR– (95% CI) | Post-test probability |
|---|---|---|---|---|---|---|
| Suspected aortic dissection undergoing angiography (pre-test probability 1%) | Aortic dissection (angiography, surgery or autopsy) | Symptoms for <24 h | 1.5 (1.2 to 2.0) | 1.5% | 0.42 (0.27 to 0.67) | 0.42% |

–  its nature [A][3] [A][9] [B][6] [B][10]

?  **Why?**

**Pressure makes coronary artery disease more likely, but sharp or stabbing pain makes it less likely**

| Patient [A][3] | Target disorder (reference standard) | Diagnostic test | LR+ (95% CI) | Post-test probability | LR– (95% CI) | Post-test probability |
|---|---|---|---|---|---|---|
| Central or left-sided chest pain (pre-test probability 41%) | MI or unstable angina (ECG, cardiac enzymes, stress tests) | Pressure | 1.7 (1.4 to 2.0) | 54% | 0.67 (0.57 to 0.78) | 32% |
| | | Sharp or stabbing pain | 0.41 (0.29 to 0.63%) | 22% | 1.3 (1.2 to 1.5%) | 48% |

**A pleuritic chest pain makes unstable angina or a myocardial infarction unlikely**

| Patient [A][3] | Target disorder (reference standard) | Diagnostic test | LR+ (95% CI) | Post-test probability |
|---|---|---|---|---|
| Central or left-sided chest pain (pre-test probability 41%) | MI or unstable angina (ECG, cardiac enzymes, stress tests) | Pleuritic pain | 0.0 (0.0 to 0.12) | 0% |
| | | Partly pleuritic pain | 0.22 (0.13 to 0.39) | 14% |
| | | Pain not pleuritic | 1.4 (1.3 to 1.6) | 50% |

**Positional chest pain makes unstable angina or an MI less likely**

| Patient [A][3] | Target disorder (reference standard) | Diagnostic test | LR+ (95% CI) | Post-test probability |
|---|---|---|---|---|
| Central or left-sided chest pain (pre-test probability 41%) | MI or unstable angina (ECG, cardiac enzymes, stress tests) | Positional pain | 0.13 (0.030 to 0.54) | 8% |
| | | Pain partly positional | 0.31 (0.20 to 0.48) | 18% |
| | | Pain not positional | 1.4 (1.3 to 1.5) | 49% |

**Note**
- Aching or burning pain is not helpful at diagnosing or excluding MI or unstable angina **[A]**[3].
- Neither of the following are helpful in diagnosing aortic dissection or its locations **[C]**[7] **[C]**[8]:
  - history of excitement triggering the pain
  - position of pain.

– any radiation **[A]**[9] particularly to the right arm or shoulder **[B]**[6] **[B]**[10]

**Why?**
**Chest pain that radiates to the arms makes an MI more likely**

| Patient | Target disorder (reference standard) | Diagnostic test | LR+ (95% CI) | Post-test probability | LR– (95% CI) | Post-test probability |
|---|---|---|---|---|---|---|
| Anterior chest pain (pre-test probability 12%) **[B]**[10] | MI (cardiac enzymes, ECG) | Chest pain radiation to right shoulder | 2.9 (1.4 to 6.0) | 29% | 0.90 (0.81 to 1.0) | 11% |
| Attending emergency department with chest pain (pre-test probability 20%) **[B]**[6] | MI (ECG and cardiac enzyme changes) | Chest pain radiation to left arm | 2.3 (1.7 to 3.1) | 37% | | |
| | | Chest pain radiation to both left and right arms | 7.1 (3.6 to 14) | 64% | | |

– any similarity to previous infarcts on angina attacks **[A]**[9]

**Why?**
- Pain similar to previous MI or angina attacks makes an MI more likely **[A]**[9].

– any exacerbating or relieving factors **[B]**[52]

**Why?**
- Pain brought on by exertion, or relieved by nitrates or rest, makes significant coronary artery disease more likely **[B]**[5].

– any associated nausea or vomiting **[B]**[6] **[B]**[10]

**Why?**

**Nausea and vomiting make an MI more likely**

| Patient | Target disorder (reference standard) | Diagnostic test | LR+ (95% CI) | Post-test probability | LR– (95% CI) | Post-test probability |
|---|---|---|---|---|---|---|
| Attending emergency department with chest pain **[B]**[6] (pre-test probability 20%) | MI (ECG and cardiac enzyme changes) | Nausea or vomiting | 1.9 (1.7 to 2.3) | 32% | | |
| Anterior chest pain **[B]**[10] (pre-test probability 12%) | MI (cardiac enzymes, ECG) | History of associated nausea | 1.9 (1.4 to 2.4) | 21% | 0.63 (0.47 to 0.84) | 8% |

– any associated sweating **[B]**[10]

**Why?**

**Sweating makes an MI more likely**

| Patient **[B]**[10] | Target disorder (reference standard) | Diagnostic test | LR+ (95% CI) | Post-test probability | LR– (95% CI) | Post-test probability |
|---|---|---|---|---|---|---|
| Anterior chest pain (pre-test probability 12%) | MI (cardiac enzymes, ECG) | History of sweating | 2.5 (2.0 to 3.3) | 26% | 0.52 (0.38 to 0.71) | 7% |

**Note**
- Classic cardiac risk factors (smoking, hypertension, diabetes, etc.) are not clearly helpful at diagnosing an MI **[B]**[6].

● History of:
  – angina or MI **[A]**[9] **[B]**[6] **[B]**[10]

**Why?**

**Previous unstable angina or MI makes a further episode more likely**

| Patient **[A]**[3] | Target disorder (reference standard) | Diagnostic test | LR+ (95% CI) | Post-test probability | LR– (95% CI) | Post-test probability |
|---|---|---|---|---|---|---|
| Central or left-sided chest pain (pre-test probability 41%) | MI or unstable angina (ECG, cardiacnzymes, stress tests) | Previous history of MI or angina | 2.3 (1.9 to 2.7) | 62% | 0.37 (0.30 to 0.47) | 21% |

– hypertension

 **Why?**

A history of hypertension makes aortic dissection slightly more likely

| Patient [C][7] [C][8] | Target disorder (reference standard) | Diagnostic test | LR+ (95% CI) | Post-test probability | LR– (95% CI) | Post-test probability |
|---|---|---|---|---|---|---|
| Suspected aortic dissection undergoing angiography (pre-test probability 1%) | Aortic dissection (angiography, surgery or autopsy) | Prior hypertension | 1.4 (1.0 to 1.9) | 1.4% | 0.61 (0.42 to 0.89) | 0.61% |

– asthma [A][12]
– dementia [A][13]
– immunosuppression [A][13]

 **Why?**

Dementia and immunosuppression increase the risk of pneumonia

| Patient | Target disorder (reference standard) | Diagnostic test | LR+ (95% CI) | Post-test probability | LR– (95% CI) | Post-test probability |
|---|---|---|---|---|---|---|
| Suspected pneumonia (pre-test probability 5%) | Pneumonia (chest X-ray) | History of dementia | 3.4 | 15% | 0.94 | 5% |
| | | History of immunosuppression | 2.2 | 10% | 0.85 | 4% |

– Marfan syndrome [C][14] [C][15].

 **Why?**

■ 27% to 48% of patients with Marfan syndrome die from aortic dissection or rupture [C][14] [C][15].

Look for:

● a cough [A][16]
● fever [A][12] [A][16]
● respiratory rate >30/min [A][16]
● tachycardia [A][12] [A][16]

**Why?**

**No cough and normal vital signs make pneumonia less likely**

| Patient | Target disorder (reference standard) | Diagnostic test | LR+ (95% CI) | Post-test probability | LR– (95% CI) | Post-test probability |
|---|---|---|---|---|---|---|
| Suspected pneumonia (pre-test probability 5%) | Pneumonia (chest X-ray) | Cough | 1.8 | 9% | 0.31 | 2% |
| | | Fever | 2.1 (1.4 to 2.9) | 10% | 0.59 | 3% |
| | | Respiratory rate > 30/min | 2.6 | 12% | 0.80 | 4% |
| | | Any of respiratory rate >30/min, heart rate >100 beats/min, temperature >37.8°C | 1.2 | 6% | 0.18 (0.07 to 0.46) | 0.9% |

- hypertension [C][7] [C][8] or hypotension [B][10] [C][7] [C][8]

**Why?**

**Hypotension with chest pain makes an MI more likely**

| Patient | Target disorder (reference standard) | Diagnostic test | LR+ (95% CI) | Post-test probability |
|---|---|---|---|---|
| Attending emergency department with chest pain [B][6] (pre-test probability 20%) | MI (ECG and cardiac enzyme changes) | Hypotension (systolic BP ≤ 80 mmHg) | 3.1 (1.8 to 5.2) | 44% |

**Hypertension on initial examination makes a distal aortic dissection slightly more likely but a proximal one less**

| Patient [C][7] [C][8] | Target disorder (reference standard) | Diagnostic test | LR+ (95% CI) | Post-test probability | LR– (95% CI) | Post-test probability |
|---|---|---|---|---|---|---|
| Suspected aortic dissection undergoing angiography (pre-test probability 1%) | Distal aortic dissection (angiography, surgery or autopsy) | Hypertension on initial examination (≥150/90 mmHg) | 2.5 (1.5 to 3.6) | 1.4% | 0.47 (0.33 to 0.66) | 0.47% |
| | Proximal aortic dissection (angiography, surgery or autopsy) | Hypertension on initial examination (≥150/90 mmHg) | 0.19 (0.089 to 0.42) | 0.19% | 2.0 (1.6 to 2.5) | 2.0% |
| | | Hypotension on initial examination (systolic <100 mmHg) | 5.3 (2.0 to 14) | 5.3% | 0.82 (0.71 to 0.94) | 0.82% |

● sweating [B]10

| | | | | | | |
|---|---|---|---|---|---|---|
| **?** **Why?** Sweating makes an MI more likely | | | | | | |
| Patient [B]10 | Target disorder (reference standard) | Diagnostic test | LR+ (95%) CI) | Post-test probability | LR– (95% CI) | Post-test probability |
| Anterior chest pain (pre-test probability 12%) | MI (cardiac enzymes, ECG) | Sweating | 4.6 (2.7 to 8.0) | 40% | 0.77 (0.66 to 0.90) | 10% |

● absent or reduced pulses [C]7 [C]8

| | | | | | | |
|---|---|---|---|---|---|---|
| **?** **Why?** Absent or reduced pulses make proximal aortic dissection more likely | | | | | | |
| Patient [C]7 [C]8 | Target disorder (reference standard) | Diagnostic test | LR+ (95% CI) | Post-test probability | LR– (95% CI) | Post-test probability |
| Suspected aortic dissection undergoing angiography (pre-test probability 1%) | Proximal aortic dissection (angiography, surgery or autopsy) | Pulse deficits | 3.9 (2.3 to 6.6) | 3.9% | 0.57 (0.43 to 0.74) | 0.57% |

● a third heart sound [B]10

| | | | | | | |
|---|---|---|---|---|---|---|
| **?** **Why?** A third heart sound make an MI more likely | | | | | | |
| Patient [B]10 | Target disorder (reference standard) | Diagnostic test | LR+ (95% CI) | Post-test probability | LR– (95% CI) | Post-test probability |
| Anterior chest pain (pre-test probability 12%) | MI (cardiac enzymes, ECG) | Third heart sound on auscultation | 3.2 (1.6 to 6.5) | 31% | 0.88 (0.79 to 0.99) | 11% |

● aortic regurgitation [C]7 [C]8

**?  Why?**
**Aortic regurgitation makes a proximal aortic dissection more likely**

| Patient [C][7] [C][8] | Target disorder (reference standard) | Diagnostic test | LR+ (95% CI) | Post-test probability | LR– (95% CI) | Post-test probability |
|---|---|---|---|---|---|---|
| Suspected aortic dissection undergoing angiography (pre-test probability 1%) | Proximal aortic dissection (angiography, surgery or autopsy) | Aortic regurgitation | 5.7 (3.3 to 9.6) | 5.7% | 0.39 (0.27 to 0.56) | 0.39% |

- chest pain that is reproduced on palpation **[A]**[3] **[A]**[9] **[B]**[6] **[B]**[10]

**?  Why?**
**Pain reproduced on palpation makes unstable angina or a myocardial infarction less likely**

| Patient [A][3] | Target disorder (reference standard) | Diagnostic test | LR+ (95% CI) | Post-test probability |
|---|---|---|---|---|
| Central or left-sided chest pain (pre-test probability 41%) | MI or unstable angina (ECG, cardiac enzymes, stress tests) | Pain reproduced by chest wall palpation | 0.11 (0.057 to 0.21) | 7% |
| | | Pain partially reproduced by chest wall palpation | 0.43 (0.20 to 0.94) | 24% |
| | | Pain not reproduced by chest wall palpation | 1.6 (1.4 to 1.7) | 53% |

- asymmetric respiration **[A]**[16]
- chest dullness on percussion **[A]**[16]
- decreased breath sounds **[A]**[12] **[A]**[16]
- bronchial breathing **[A]**[16]
- crackles **[A]**[12] **[B]**[10]
- egophony **[A]**[16]

**Why?**

**Abnormal chest findings make pneumonia more likely**

| Patient [A][16] | Target disorder (reference standard) | Diagnostic test | LR+ (95% CI) | Post-test probability | LR– (95% CI) | Post-test probability |
|---|---|---|---|---|---|---|
| Suspected pneumonia (pre-test probability 5%) | Pneumonia (chest X-ray) | Asymmetric respiration | Infinity (3.2 to infinity) | 100% | 0.96 | 5% |
| | | Dullness to percussion | 2.2 | 10% | 0.92 | 5% |
| | | Decreased breath sounds | 2.3 | 11% | 0.78 | 4% |
| | | Bronchial breath sounds | 3.5 | 16% | 0.90 | 5% |
| | | Crackles | 1.6 | 8% | 0.83 | 4% |
| | | Egophony | 2.0 | 10% | 0.96 | 5% |

**Pulmonary crackles with chest pain make an MI more likely**

| Patient | Target disorder (reference standard) | Diagnostic test | LR+ (95% CI) | Post-test probability | LR– (95% CI) | Post-test probability |
|---|---|---|---|---|---|---|
| Attending emergency department with chest pain [B][6] (pre-test probability 20%) | MI (ECG and cardiac enzyme changes) | Pulmonary crackles on auscultation | 2.1 (1.5 to 3.1) | 23% | 0.76 (0.62 to 0.92) | 10% |

- evidence of a stroke or paralysis [B][17].

**Why?**

- Dissection complications at presentation (pulse loss, renal or visceral ischaemia, MI, stroke, renal failure or paralysis) increase the risk of death [B][17].
- Neurological problems (stroke, ischaemic peripheral neuropathy, ischaemic spinal cord damage, altered consciousness) are not helpful in diagnosing aortic dissection or its location; 19–26% of cases have syncope, stroke, leg weakness or reduced consciousness [C][7] [C][8].

**Note**

- In the elderly, the following features are less helpful at diagnosing an MI [A][2]:
  - male sex
  - pain location and similarity to previous MI or angina
  - ECG changes in the emergency department.

## INVESTIGATIONS

Consider performing simple investigations (ECG, cardiac enzymes), even in low-risk patients **[A]**[18].

---

 **Why?**

- Physicians are good at predicting which patients are at high risk for acute MI, but are less good at excluding it. **[B]**[10] **[C]**[19].
- Patients at low-risk for ischaemic heart disease who have an ECG and cardiac enzymes measured feel better, and have improved activity at 3 weeks **[A]**[18].

**Basic investigations make patients feel better**

| Patient **[A]**[18] | Treatment | Comparator | Outcome | CER | RRR | NNT |
|---|---|---|---|---|---|---|
| Chest pain at low risk for ischaemic heart disease | Basic investigations | No basic investigations | Activity same or less than before at 3 weeks | 20% | 120% (37% to 260%) | 4 (3 to 9) |
| | | | 'Feel sick all the time' at 3 weeks | 11% | 130% (10% to 370%) | 7 (4 to 44) |

---

Perform:

- a blood count **[B]**[20]

---

 **Why?**

**A high leucocyte count or low relative lymphocyte percentage makes an MI more likely**

| Patient **[B]**[20] | Target disorder (reference standard) | Diagnostic test | LR+ (95% CI) | Post-test probability | LR– (95% CI) | Post-test probability |
|---|---|---|---|---|---|---|
| Central or left-sided chest pain (pre-test probability 18%) | MI (CK-MB at 24 h) | Elevated leucocyte count | 6.8 (4.3 to 11) | 60% | 0.56 (0.45 to 0.70) | 11% |
| | | Decreased relative lymphocyte percentage | 6.3 (4.2 to 9.4) | 58% | 0.46 (0.35 to 0.61) | 9% |

---

- urea, electrolytes and creatinine **[D]**
- glucose **[D]**
- lipid levels **[D]**
- serial cardiac enzymes, ideally CK-MB **[C]**[19] **[C]**[21].

## Why?
**Early CK-MB rise diagnoses an MI, and normal levels at 20 h rule it out**

| Patient [C][19] | Target disorder (reference standard) | Diagnostic test | LR+ (95% CI) | Post-test probability | LR– (95% CI) | Post-test probability |
|---|---|---|---|---|---|---|
| Suspected MI (pre-test probability 18%) | MI (history, ECG, CK-MB$_{act}$) | Elevated CK-MB$_{mass}$ at 3 h after symptom onset | Infinity (16 to infinity) | 100% | 0.68 (0.61 to 0.75) | 13% |
| | | at 4 h | 28 (19 to 42) | 86% | 0.45 (0.39 to 0.52) | 9% |
| | | at 6 h | 29 (19 to 44) | 86% | 0.13 (0.11 to 0.16) | 3% |
| | | at 8 h | 19 (13 to 27) | 81% | 0.063 (0.053 to 0.076) | 1% |
| | | at 12 h | 14 (11 to 18) | 75% | 0.032 (0.027 to 0.039) | 0.7% |
| | | at 20 h | 11 (8 to 16) | 71% | 0.00 (0.0 to 0.020) | 0% |

Less helpful alternatives include:

- troponin T [A][22] [B][23] [C][19] [C][21] or troponin I [C][21]

## Why?
**A normal troponin T at 20 h makes an MI unlikely**

| Patient [C][19] | Target disorder (reference standard) | Diagnostic test | LR+ (95% CI) | Post-test probability | LR– (95% CI) | Post-test probability |
|---|---|---|---|---|---|---|
| Suspected MI (pre-test probability 18%) | MI (history, ECG, CK-MB$_{act}$) | Elevated troponin T at 3 h after symptom onset | 6 (4 to 9) | 57% | 0.67 (0.59 to 0.76) | 13% |
| | | at 4 h | 11 (7 to 16) | 71% | 0.59 (0.52 to 0.67) | 9% |
| | | at 6 h | 7 (4 to 10) | 61% | 0.37 (0.31 to 0.43) | 8% |
| | | at 8 h | 9 (6 to 13) | 66% | 0.23 (0.19 to 0.27) | 5% |
| | | at 12 h | 9 (7 to 12) | 66% | 0.078 (0.064 to 0.094) | 2% |
| | | at 20 h | 9 (6 to 13) | 66% | 0.022 (0.019 to 0.027) | 0.5% |

**Normal CK-MB and troponin I can help rule out MI**

| Patient [C][21] | Target disorder (reference standard) | Diagnostic test | LR+ (95% CI) | Post-test probability | LR– (95% CI) | Post-test probability |
|---|---|---|---|---|---|---|
| Chest pain lasting for at least 15 min within previous 24 h [C][21] (pre-test probability 37%) | MI (CK-MB$_{mass}$ at 24 h) | Troponin I at 6 h | 10 (7.3 to 14) | 59% | 0.45 (0.37 to 0.56) | 6% |
| | | Troponin I at 18 h | 15 (11 to 19) | 67% | 0.045 (0.019 to 0.11) | 1% |

- myoglobin [C][19]

**Why?**

An elevated myoglobin helps diagnose a myocardial infarction, but normal levels cannot safely rule it out

| Patient [C][19] | Target disorder (reference standard) | Diagnostic test | LR+ (95% CI) | Post-test probability | LR− (95% CI) | Post-test probability |
|---|---|---|---|---|---|---|
| Suspected MI (pre-test probability 18%) | MI (history, ECG, CK-MB$_{act}$) | Elevated myoglobin at 3 h after symptom onset | 34 (23 to 49) | 88% | 0.33 (0.28 to 0.38) | 7% |
| | | at 4 h | 26 (17 to 38) | 85% | 0.24 (0.20 to 0.28) | 5% |
| | | at 6 h | 26 (17 to 39) | 85% | 0.23 (0.19 to 0.27) | 5% |
| | | at 8 h | 25 (17 to 36) | 85% | 0.26 (0.22 to 0.30) | 5% |
| | | at 12 h | 23 (16 to 31) | 83% | 0.33 (0.28 to 0.39) | 7% |
| | | at 20 h | 13 (8 to 20) | 74% | 0.63 (0.56 to 0.71) | 12% |

- serial creatine kinase (CK) [B][20] [C][24] aspartate transaminase (AST) [A][3], lactate dehydrogenase (LDH) [A][3] taken over 24 h [A][25]

**Why?**

■ 96% of MIs can be diagnosed at 24 h using CK-MB, LDH, CK and ECG changes (95–98%) [A][25].

**Elevated CK levels diagnose MI**

| Patient [C][24] | Target disorder (reference standard) | Diagnostic test | LR+ (95% CI) | Post-test probability |
|---|---|---|---|---|
| Suspected MI (pre-test probability: 64%) | MI (ECG changes) | Highest CK ≥ 280 iu/l | 54 (7.7 to 380) | 99% |
| | | CK 80–279 iu/l | 4.5 (2.7 to 7.3) | 89% |
| | | CK 40–79 iu/l | 0.30 (0.16 to 0.56) | 35% |
| | | CK < 40 iu/l | 0.013 (0.0032 to 0.051) | 2.0% |

**Elevated AST levels taken 12 h or more after symptom onset help diagnose MI**

| Patient [A][3] | Target disorder (reference standard) | Diagnostic test | LR+ (95% CI) | Post-test probability |
|---|---|---|---|---|
| Central or left-sided chest pain (pre-test probability 41%) | MI (ECG, cardiac enzymes, stress tests) | AST taken more than 12 h after chest pain onset: | | |
| | | ≥ 100 iu/l | 30 | 89% |
| | | 80 iu/l | 2.3 | 39% |
| | | 60 iu/l | 5.6 | 60% |
| | | 50 iu/l | 0.40 | 10% |
| | | 40 iu/l | 0.59 | 14% |
| | | 30 iu/l | 0.32 | 8% |
| | | < 30 iu/l | 0.078 | 2% |

> **?** **Why?**
>
> ■ CK **[A]**[3] **[B]**[20], AST **[A]**[3] or LDH **[A]**[3] taken within 12 h of symptom onset cannot safely exclude an MI.
>
> **Cardiac enzymes taken in the emergency department cannot diagnose or exclude an MI**
>
> | Patient **[A]**[3] | Target disorder (reference standard) | Diagnostic test | LR+ (95% CI) | Post-test probability | LR– (95% CI) | Post-test probability |
> |---|---|---|---|---|---|---|
> | Central or left-sided chest pain (pre-test probability 17%) | MI (ECG, cardiac enzymes) | CK > 180 iu/l | 1.8 (1.3 to 2.5) | 27% | 0.77 (0.65 to 0.91) | 14% |
> | | | AST > 60 iu/l | 6.1 (3.5 to 10) | 56% | 0.43 (0.29 to 0.64) | 8% |
> | | | AST > 47 iu/l | 3.4 (2.3 to 5.1) | 41% | 0.44 (0.29 to 0.68) | 8% |
> | | | LDH > 200 iu/l | 2.0 | 29% | 0.59 | 11% |
> | | | CK or AST abnormal | 1.7 (1.3 to 2.2) | 26% | 0.65 (0.51 to 0.82) | 12% |
>
> **CK levels alone taken at 24 h cannot safely diagnose or exclude myocardial infarction**
>
> | Patient **[B]**[20] | Target disorder (reference standard) | Diagnostic test | LR+ (95% CI) | Post-test probability | LR– (95% CI) | Post-test probability |
> |---|---|---|---|---|---|---|
> | Central or left-sided chest pain (pre-test probability 18%) | MI (CK-MB at 24 h) | Elevated creatine kinase | 6.0 (3.7 to 9.8) | 57% | 0.62 (0.50 to 0.76) | 12% |

● a 12-lead ECG **[A]**[9] **[B]**[6] **[B]**[10] **[B]**[20] – read it carefully! **[A]**[26]

> **?** **Why?**
>
> **ECG features suggestive of an MI make an MI or unstable angina more likely**
>
> | Patient **[A]**[3] | Target disorder (reference standard) | Diagnostic test | LR+ (95% CI) | Post-test probability |
> |---|---|---|---|---|
> | Central or left-sided chest pain (pre-test probability 41%) | MI or unstable angina (ECG, cardiac ezymes, stress tests) | Probable MI | 13 (8.5 to 20) | 73% |
> | | | Ischaemia or strain not known to be old | 1.6 (1.1 to 2.3) | 25% |
> | | | Ischaemia or strain or infarction but changes known to be old | 0.34 (0.13 to 0.91) | 7% |
> | | | Abnormal but not diagnostic of ischaemia | 0.21 (0.66 to 0.64) | 4% |
> | | | Non-specific ST or T wave changes | 0.13 (0.049 to 0.34) | 3% |
> | | | Normal | 0.042 (0.0059 to 0.30) | 1% |
>
> ■ Emergency physicians can misread ECGs for patients with cardiac chest pain – missing 12% of ST elevation and 12% of T wave inversion **[A]**[26].

look for features suggestive of cardiac ischaemia:

– any ST elevation, particularly if in two or more leads or not known to be old **[A]**[9] **[B]**[6] **[B]**[10] **[B]**[20]
– any ST depression, particularly if not known to be old **[B]**[6] **[B]**[10]
– any Q waves, particularly if in two leads or more or not known to be old **[A]**[9] **[B]**[6] **[B]**[10]
– any T wave inversion, particularly if not known to be old **[B]**[6] **[B]**[10]
– any conduction defect, particularly if not known to be old **[B]**[6] **[B]**[10]

**? Why?**
**ST elevation or depression, Q waves and T wave inversion help diagnose MI**

| Patient | Target disorder (reference standard) | Diagnostic test | LR+ (95% CI) | Post-test probability | LR– (95% CI) | Post-test probability |
|---|---|---|---|---|---|---|
| Central or left-sided chest pain **[B]**[2] (pre-test probability 18%) | MI (CK-MB at 24 h) | ST elevation in two contiguous leads | 62 (15 to 250) | 93% | 0.61 (0.51 to 0.74) | 12% |
| Attending emergency department with chest pain **[B]**[6] (pre-test probability 20%) | MI (ECG and cardiac enzyme changes) | New ST segment elevation ≥ 1 mm | 5.7 to 54 | 59% to 93% | | |
| Anterior chest pain **[B]**[10] (pre-test probability 12%) | | Any ST segment elevation | 11 (7.1 to 18) | 61% | 0.45 (0.34 to 0.60) | 6% |
| Attending emergency department with chest pain **[B]**[6] (pre-test probability 20%) | | New ST depression | 3.0 to 5.2 | 43% | | |
| Anterior chest pain **[B]**[10] (pre-test probability 12%) | | Any ST segment depression | 3.2 (2.5 to 4.1) | 31% | 0.38 (0.26 to 0.56) | 5% |
| Attending emergency department with chest pain **[B]**[6] (pre-test probability 20%) | | New Q wave | 5.3 to 25 | 57% to 86% | | |
| Anterior chest pain **[B]**[10] (pre-test probability 12%) | | Any Q wave | 3.9 (2.7 to 5.7) | 36% | 0.60 (0.47 to 0.7) | 8% |
| | | T wave peaking and/or inversion ≥ 1 mm | 3.1 | 44% | | |
| | | New T wave inversion | 2.4 to 2.8 | 38% to 41% | | |
| Attending emergency department with chest pain **[B]**[6] (pre-test probability 20%) | | New conduction defect | 6.3 (2.5 to 16) | 61% | | |
| Anterior chest pain **[B]**[10] (pre-test probability 12%) | | Any conduction defect | 2.7 (1.4 to 5.4) | 28% | 0.89 (0.79 to 1.00) | 11% |
| | | Normal ECG | 0.1 to 0.3 | 2% to 7% | | |

- followed by serial ECGs **[A]**[27], looking for:
  - acute injury: ST elevation in ≥ 1 mm in two contiguous limb leads, or ≥ 2 mm in two contiguous precordial leads.
  - acute ischaemia: ST depression ≥ 1 mm in two contiguous leads or symmetrical T wave inversion of ≥ 3 mm in two contiguous leads,
  - in patients with bundle branch block: ST depression or elevation ≥ 1 mm towards deflection of main QRS deflection in two contiguous leads, or ≥ 7 mm away from QRS deflection and > 50% amplitude of T wave in two contiguous leads.

**Why?**

Abnormalities on serial ECGs help diagnose a myocardial infarction or unstable angina

| Patient **[A]**[27] | Target disorder (reference standard) | Diagnostic test | LR+ (95% CI) | Post-test probability | LR– (95% CI) | Post-test probability |
|---|---|---|---|---|---|---|
| Chest pain (pre-test probability 52%) | MI or unstable angina (ECG at 24 h, cardiac enzymes) | Initial ECG | 9.5 (5.6 to 16) | 91% | 0.75 (0.70 to 0.79) | 44% |
| | | Serial ECG | 55 (18 to 170) | 98% | 0.66 (0.62 to 070) | 41% |

**Note**

■ Few patients with a normal ECG go on to have life-threatening complications (1.3%; 95% CI: 0.0% to 3.0%) **[C]**[28].

- chest X-ray **[A]** looking for:
  - a lobar infiltrate **[C]**[29]

**Why?**

■ A lobar infiltrate makes pneumococcal pneumonia more likely **[C]**[29].

  - widening of the **[B]**[30]:
    aorta (particularly the aortic knob)
    mediastinum
  - pleural effusion **[B]**[30]
  - tracheal shift **[B]**[30]

## ? Why?

**An abnormal chest X-ray makes aortic dissection more likely**

| Patient [B][30] | Target disorder (reference standard) | Diagnostic test | LR+ (95% CI) | Post-test probability | LR– (95% CI) | Post-test probability |
|---|---|---|---|---|---|---|
| Suspected aortic dissection (pre-test probability 1%) | Aortic dissection (angiography) | Radiologist's conclusion of the chest X-ray | 7.3 | 7.3% | 0.21 | 0.21% |

## Note

- Radiologists guess at most features on a CXR for a patient with suspected aortic dissection [B][30].

**Radiologists agree most often about widening of the aorta or mediastinum**

| Radiological feature [B][30] | $K_{interobserver}$ |
|---|---|
| Widening of aortic knob | 0.33 |
| Widening of mediastinum | 0.28 |
| Widening of descending aorta | 0.28 |
| Pleural effusion | 0.27 |
| Tracheal shift | 0.27 |
| Widening of ascending aorta | 0.26 |

Use the clinical prediction rule in Table 3 to rank your patient for risk of an MI [A][9].

| Table 3  Table 3 Ranking a patient for risk of an MI | | | | |
|---|---|---|---|---|
| If clinical finding not present, go on to next question [A][9] | | | LR (95% CI) | Probability of MI (%) (95% CI) |
| ST elevation or Q waves in ≥ 2 leads, not known to be old ⇓ | | | 22 (17 to 27) | 75% (70% to 79%) |
| Chest pain began ≥ 48 h ago | ⇒ | ST-T changes of ischaemia or strain, not known to be old ⇓ | 2.0 (1.5 to 2.9) | 22% (15% to 28%) |
| ⇓ | | No changes or old | 0.12 (0.076 to 0.19) | 1.6% (0.9% to 2.4%) |
| Previous history of angina or MI | ⇒ | ST-T changes of ischaemia or strain, not known to be old | 2.6 (2.0 to 3.2) | 26% (21% to 31%) |
| | | longest pain episode < 1 h ⇓ | 0.30 (0.18 to 0.49) | 4.0% (2.1% to 5.9%) |
| ⇓ | | Pain worse than prior angina or the same as a prior MI ⇓ | 0.92 (0.65 to 1.3) | 11% (7.6% to 15%) |
| | | Pain not as bad | 0.076 (0.019 to 0.31) | 1.0% (0.0% to 2.5%) |
| Pain radiates to neck, left shoulder or left arm | ⇒ | Aged < 40 years | 0.18 (0.058 to 0.57) | 2.4% (0.0% to 5.1%) |
| | | ⇓ | | |
| | | Chest pain reproduced by palpation ⇓ | 0.093 (0.013 to 0.67) | 1.3% (0.0% to 3.7%) |
| ⇓ | | Pain radiates to back, abdomen or legs ⇓ | 0.60 (0.25 to 1.5) | 7.7% (1.2% to 14%) |
| | | Chest pain stabbing ⇓ | 0.13 (0.018 to 0.94) | 1.8% (0.0% to 5.2%) |
| | | Chest pain not stabbing | 1.5 (1.1 to 2.0) | 17% (13% to 22%) |
| ST-T changes of ischaemia or strain, not known to be old ⇓ | | | 2.3 (1.7 to 3.3) | 26% (19% to 33%) |
| No changes or old | | | 0.15 (0.099 to 0.22) | 2.0% (1.2% to 2.8%) |

**? Why do this?**
■ A third of patients can be classified as low risk (36%; 95% CI: 34% to 38%) – 1% will die in hospital (95% CI: 0.3% to 1.8%) and 0.4% have life-threatening complications (95% CI: 0.0% to 0.8%).

Patients at low-risk for an MI can be assessed in a rapid evaluation unit [B][31] by:

● CK-MB at 0, 4, 8, 12 h
● serial 12-lead ECGs
● clinical assessment at 0, 6, 12 h
● exercise ECG: if all the above negative.

> **Why?**
> Patients at low-risk for an MI who have no CK-MB rise or further pain within 12 h are unlikely to have one

| Patient [A][32] | Target disorder (reference standard) | Diagnostic test | LR+ (95% CI) | Post-test probability | LR– (95% CI) | Post test probability |
|---|---|---|---|---|---|---|
| Low-risk for MI (pre-test probability 7%) | MI (typical change in cardiac enzymes or cardiac arrest) | Cardiac enzyme rise or recurrent chest pain within 12 h | 6.8 (5.7 to 8.1) | 34% | 0.069 (0.027 to 0.18) | 0.5% |

- Patients admitted to [D][36] rapid assessment unit are not clearly less likely to be diagnosed with an MI or unstable angina [D][33], but spend on average 40 h less in hospital [D][33].
- Half of patients are still admitted to hospital (45%; 95% CI: 34% to 56%) [A][34].

Use the clinical prediction rule (Table 4) to help determine admission to coronary care units [A][35]. Look for the following risk factors:

- pain worse than prior angina or the same as the pain associated with a prior MI
- systolic blood pressure < 110 mmHg
- rales above the bases bilaterally
- ST elevation or Q waves, not known to be old, in two or more leads
- ST segment or T wave changes, not known to be old, indicative of myocardial ischaemia.

**Table 4 Risk of major complications**

| Group [A][35] | Risk of major complication at 4 days |
|---|---|
| Suspected MI on ECG or Suspected ischaemia on ECG and ≥ two risk factors | High |
| Suspected ischaemia on ECG and ≤ one risk factor | Moderate |
| One risk factor with no MI or ischaemia on ECG | Low |
| No risk factors | Very low |

> **Why do this?**
> A clinical prediction rule can help identify patients at risk of having major complications

| Group [A][35] | Risk of major complication at 4 days | % (95% CI) | NNF (95% CI) |
|---|---|---|---|
| Suspected MI on ECG or suspected ischaemia on ECG and ≥ two risk factors | High | 16% (12% to 20%) | 6 (5 to 8) |
| Suspected ischaemia on ECG and ≤ one risk factor | Moderate | 7.8% (6.0% to 9.6%) | 13 (11 to 17) |
| One risk factor with no MI or ischaemia | Low | 3.9% (2.7% to 5.2%) | 26 (19 to 37) |
| No risk factors | Very low | 0.58% (0.29% to 0.87%) | 170 (110 to 340) |

Avoid making decisions on further investigations based solely on your patient's style of presentation [A]36.

---

 **Why?**

■ Physicians are less likely to order non-invasive investigations for more emotional patients [A]36.

**Emotional patients with chest pain are less likely to receive non-invasive testing**

| Patient | Treatment | Comparator | Outcome | CER | RRR | NNT |
|---|---|---|---|---|---|---|
| Internists [A]36 | Emotional patient | Calm patient | Further non-invasive tests ordered at ?days | 93% | 43% (6% to 65%) | 3 (1 to 9) |

---

For patients with possible coronary artery disease, but no clear evidence, consider:
● adding three right precordial leads to the 12-lead ECG [A]37

---

 **Why?**

■ More patients are diagnosed with coronary artery stenosis > 70% using an additional three right precordial leads [A]37.

---

● stress testing, using any of:
　– exercise ECG [A]38 looking for [A]38:
　　i) horizontal or down-sloping ST slope and 1 mm or more of depression [B]5 in any lead
　　ii) angina during test

---

 **Why?**

**Abnormalities on exercise ECG make coronary artery disease more likely**

| Patient | Target disorder (reference standard) | Diagnostic test | LR+ (95% CI) | Post-test probability | LR– (95% CI) | Post-test probability |
|---|---|---|---|---|---|---|
| Probable or definite stable angina (pre-test probability 51%) [A]38 | Coronary artery stenosis (coronary angiography) | Exercise ECG | 3.0% (2.3% to 3.9%) | 76% | 0.65% (0.59% to 0.71%) | 40% |

**Why?**
**Exercise ECG: deepening ST segment depression makes coronary artery disease more likely**

| Patient [B][5] | Target disorder (reference standard) | Diagnostic test | LR+ (95% CI) | Post-test probability |
|---|---|---|---|---|
| Suspected coronary artery disease (pre-test probability 51%) | Coronary artery stenosis (coronary angiography) | Non-sloping ST segment depression exercise ECG: | | |
| | | ≥ 2.50 mm | 39 | 98% |
| | | 2.0–2.49 mm | 11 | 92% |
| | | 1.5–1.99 mm | 4.2 | 81% |
| | | 1.0–1.49 mm | 2.1 | 69% |
| | | 0.5–0.99 mm | 0.92 | 49% |
| | | < 0.5 mm | 0.23 | 19% |

– exercise echocardiography [A][39] [A][40]

**Why?**
**An abnormal exercise echocardiogram makes coronary artery disease more likely**

| Patient | Target disorder (reference standard) | Diagnostic test | LR+ (95% CI) | Post-test probability | LR– (95% CI) | Post-test probability |
|---|---|---|---|---|---|---|
| Suspected coronary artery disease (pre-test probability 64%) [A][39] | Coronary artery disease (coronary angiography) | Exercise echocardiography | 3.3 (2.9 to 3.6) | 85% | 0.16 (0.14 to 0.19) | 23% |

– scintigraphy [[A][40] [B][5]

look for a reversible perfusion defect [B][5]

**Why?**
**Scintigraphy makes multivessel coronary artery disease more likely**

| Patient | Target disorder (reference standard) | Diagnostic test | LR+ (95% CI) | Post-test probability | LR– (95% CI) | Post-test probability |
|---|---|---|---|---|---|---|
| Chest pain referred for further investigation (pre-test probability 52%) [A][40] | Multivessel coronary artery disease (coronary angiography) | Scintigraphy | 2.5 (1.5 to 4.2) | 76% | 0.44 (0.29 to 0.67) | 36% |

**Why?**

Scintigraphy: a reversible perfusion defect makes coronary artery disease more likely

| Patient [B][5] | Target disorder (reference standard) | Diagnostic test | LR+ (95% CI) | Post-test probability |
|---|---|---|---|---|
| Suspected coronary artery disease (pre-test probability 51%) | Coronary artery stenosis (coronary angiography) | Scintigraphy:<br>reversible perfusion defect<br>fixed perfusion defect<br>no perfusion defect | <br>12<br>1.4<br>0.18 | <br>93%<br>59%<br>16% |

- exercise SPECT (single-photon emission computerised tomography) [A][39].

**Why?**

An abnormal exercise SPECT makes coronary artery disease more likely

| Patient | Target disorder (reference standard) | Diagnostic test | LR+ (95% CI) | Post-test probability | LR– (95% CI) | Post-test probability |
|---|---|---|---|---|---|---|
| Suspected coronary artery disease (pre-test probability 76%) [A][39] | Coronary artery disease (coronary angiography) | Exercise SPECT | 2.2 (2.0 to 2.4) | 87% | 0.18 (0.16 to 0.20) | 36% |

- angiography [A][43]

**Why?**

- Few patients with normal or near-normal angiograms die in the next 7 years (2.0%; 95% CI: 1.5% to 2.4%) [A][41].

**Note**

- There is little difference in the cost-effectiveness of angiography, PET (positron emission tomography), SPECT, echocardiography or thallium scanning [A][42].

Consider performing oesophageal tests [C][11] [C][43] after coronary artery disease has been excluded [D]. Treat the results cautiously – they may suffer from observer bias [D][44] and may not indicate the true cause [C][43].

**Why?**
- Gastroesophageal reflux or motility disorder is common in patients both with and without coronary artery disease. **[C]**[11]
- Neither abnormal ambulatory oesophageal pressure and pH monitoring nor relief with nitrates clearly exclude coronary artery disease **[C]**[11]
- There are wide differences in patients reporting chest pain during oesophageal edrophonium testing depending on the clinician performing the test. These differences may be due to the manner of the clinician **[D]**[44].

**Abnormal oesophageal manometry makes coronary artery disease less likely but cannot rule it out**

| Patient **[C]**[45] | Target disorder (reference standard) | Diagnostic test | LR+ (95% CI) | Post-test probability | LR– (95% CI) | Post-test probability |
|---|---|---|---|---|---|---|
| Recurrent exertional chest pain (pre-test probability ? 40%) | Coronary artery disease (coronary angiography) | Normal oesophageal manometry | 1.6 (1.2 to 2.1) | 52% | 0.22 (0.056 to 0.83) | 13% |

- Patients with normal coronary arteries and chest pain can be found to have multiple potential causes on exhaustive testing – including psychiatric disorders **[C]**[43].

## THERAPY

See the relevant chapter for more information on the management of:
- aortic dissection
- bradyarrhythmias
- myocardial infarction
- pulmonary embolism
- tachycardias
- unstable angina.

There is no clear benefit from:

- prophylactic lidocaine **[D]**[46].

**Why?**
- Patients with chest pain who receive prophylactic lidocaine are not clearly less likely to die **[D]**[46].

Consider trying the following for patients with chest pain who continue to have symptoms, but have had cardiac disease excluded:

- a proton-pump inhibitor **[A]**[47]

**Why do this?**

■ Patients with non-cardiac retrosternal chest pain and gastro-oesophageal reflux on pH monitoring who take omeprazole have less chest pain **[A]**[47].

**Omeprazole reduces non-cardiac chest pain with gastro-oesophageal reflux**

| Patient **[A]**[47] | Treatment | Comparator | Outcome | CER | RRR | NNT |
|---|---|---|---|---|---|---|
| Non-cardiac chest pain and gastro-oesophageal reflux | Omeprazole | Placebo | Chest pain better at 2 months | 5.6% | −1400% (−9900% to −120%) | 1 (1 to 2) |
| | | | Fewer days with chest pain | 44% | −83% (−220% to −4%) | 3 (1 to 14) |

– imipramine **[A]**[43]

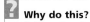

**Why do this?**

■ Patients with non-specific recurrent chest pain who take imipramine have 50% fewer episodes of chest pain after 3 weeks **[A]**[43].

● cognitive-behavioural therapy **[A]**[50].

**Why do this?**

■ Patients given 4–12 weeks of cognitive-behavioural therapy have fewer episodes of pain, which is less severe **[A]**[48].

**Cognitive-behavioural therapy reduces non-cardiac chest pain**

| Patient **[A]**[48] | Treatment | Comparator | Outcome | CER | RRR | NNT |
|---|---|---|---|---|---|---|
| Non-cardiac chest pain | Cognitive-behavioural therapy | No therapy | ≥ four episodes of chest pain per week at 1 year | 56% | 78% (43% to 92%) | 2 (2 to 4) |

## PROGNOSIS

Be cautious about discharging patients with even a low chance of an MI **[B]**[49].

**Why?**

■ Patients with an MI who are discharged from the emergency department are at increased risk of dying **[B]**[49].

Many patients die in the next few years **[A]**[50] **[A]**[51].

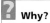 **Why?**
- One in five patients with acute chest pain is dead within 2.5 years (20%; 95% CI: 16% to 23%) **[A]**[50] **[A]**[51].

## The risk of dying is increased with:

- increasing age **[A]**[51]
- male sex **[A]**[51]

**Why?**
**Increasing age and male sex increase the risk of dying**

| Patient **[A]**[51] | Prognostic factor | Outcome | Control rate | RR (95% CI) | NNF+ (95% CI) |
|---|---|---|---|---|---|
| Symptoms suggestive of MI | Age (increase per year added) *independent* | Death at 5 years | 26% | 1.07 (1.06 to 1.08) | |
| | Female *independent* | | 26% | 0.73 (0.64 to 0.84) | −14 (−24 to −11) |

- cardiovascular risk factors **[A]**[51]
  - smoker
  - diabetes mellitus
  - hypertension

**Why?**
**Cardiovascular risk factors increase the risk of dying**

| Patient **[A]**[51] | Prognostic factor | Outcome | Control rate | RR (95% CI) | NNF+ (95% CI) |
|---|---|---|---|---|---|
| Symptoms suggestive of MI | Smoker *independent* | Death at 5 years | 26% | 1.65 (1.42 to 1.90) | 6 (4 to 9) |
| | Diabetes *independent* | | | 1.60 (1.35 to 1.90) | 6 (4 to 11) |
| | Hypertension *independent* | | | 1.20 (1.05 to 1.37) | 19 (11 to 78) |

- history of MI **[A]**[53]

**Why?**
**A history of MI or congestive heart failure increases the risk of dying**

| Patient **[A]**[51] | Prognostic factor | Outcome | Control rate | RR (95% CI) | NNF+ (95% CI) |
|---|---|---|---|---|---|
| Symptoms suggestive of MI | History of MI *independent* | Death | 26% | 1.28 (1.11 to 1.48) | 14 (8 to 35) |

- heart failure [A][52] [A][53]

| Why? Heart failure increases the risk of dying | | | | | |
|---|---|---|---|---|---|
| Patient [A][51] | Prognostic factor | Outcome | Control rate | RR (95% CI) | NNF+ (95% CI) |
| Symptoms suggestive of MI | History of congestive heart failure *independent* | Death at 5 years | 26% | 1.59 (1.36 to 1.84) | 7 (5 to 11) |
| | Acute severe heart failure on presentation *independent* | Death at 5 years | 26% | 1.63 (1.35 to 2.06) | 6 (4 to 11) |

- moderate to severe mitral regurgitation [A][50]

| Why? Mitral regurgitation increases the risk of dying | | | | | |
|---|---|---|---|---|---|
| Patient [A][50] | Prognostic factor | Outcome | Control rate | RR (95% CI) | NNF+ (95% CI) |
| Acute chest pain | Moderate to severe mitral regurgitation *independent* | Death at 2.5 years | 20% | 2.4 (1.5 to 3.7) | 4 (2 to 10) |

- ECG changes [A][51]

| Why? ECG changes increase the risk of dying | | | | | |
|---|---|---|---|---|---|
| Patient [A][51] | Prognostic factor | Outcome | Control rate | RR (95% CI) | NNF+ (95% CI) |
| Symptoms suggestive of MI | Signs of acute ischaemia on admission ECG *independent* | Death at 5 years | 26% | 2.24 (1.83 to 2.75) | 3 (2 to 5) |
| | Pathological but no sign of acute ischaemia on admission ECG *independent* | | | 1.90 (1.57 to 2.29) | 4 (3 to 7) |
| | Presence of Q waves on admission ECG *independent* | | | 1.47 (1.12 to 1.92) | 8 (4 to 32) |

- an elevated CK-MB or troponin T [A][23].

| ? Why? | | | | | |
|---|---|---|---|---|---|
| **Elevated cardiac enzymes increase the risk of dying or having cardiovascular complications** | | | | | |
| *Patient* **[A]**[23] | *Prognostic factor* | *Outcome* | *Control rate* | *RR (95% CI)* | *NNF+ (95% CI)* |
| Chest pain suggestive of ischaemic heart disease | Troponin T ≥ 2 μg/l within 24 h *independent* | MI, revascularisation, heart failure, death at 2 months | 5.2% | 6.9 (3.4 to 13.9) | 4 (3 to 10) |

Use the clinical prediction rule (Tables 5 and 6) to rank your patient for risk of dying **[A]**[52].

Sum the following:
- duration of exercise in minutes
- minus (5 × maximal net ST segment deviation during or after exercise, mm)
- minus (4 × treadmill angina index)

**Table 5  Treadmill angina index**

| Angina during stress test | Score |
|---|---|
| No angina during exercise | 0 |
| Non-limiting angina | 1 |
| Stopped due to angina | 2 |

**Table 6  Exercise ECG score**

| Total score | Risk of dying |
|---|---|
| < −10 | High |
| −10 to 4 | Moderate |
| ≥ 5 | Low |

| ? Why? | | | | |
|---|---|---|---|---|
| **Exercise ECG: a clinical prediction rule can help predict mortality** | | | | |
| *Patient* **[A]**[52] | *Prognostic factor* | *Outcome* | *Control rate* | *NNF (95% CI)* |
| Suspected coronary artery disease | Score < −10 Score −10 to 4 Score ≥ 5 | Death at 4 years | 22% (4.9% to 39%) 5.2% (2.2% to 8.2%) 1.1% (0.0% to 2.1%) | 5 (3 to 20) 19 (12 to 45) 95 (48 to 3800) |

**Guideline writer**: Christopher Ball
**CAT writers**: Clare Wotton, Christopher Ball, Nick Shenker, Robert Phillips

## REFERENCES

| No. | Level | Citation |
| --- | --- | --- |
| 1 | 4 | Berger JP et al. Right arm involvement and pain extension can help to differentiate coronary disease from chest pain of other origin: a prospective emergency ward study of 278 consecutive patients admitted for chest pain. J Intern Med 1990; 227: 165–72 |
| 2 | 1b | Solomon CG et al. Comparison of clinical presentation of acute myocardial infarction in patients older than 65 years of age to younger patients: the multicenter chest pain study experience. Am J Cardiol 1989; 63: 772–6 |
| 3 | 1b | Lee TH et al. Acute chest pain in the emergency room: identification and examination of low-risk patients. Arch Intern Med 1985; 145: 65–9 |
| 4 | 4 | Spittell PC et al. Clinical features and differential diagnosis of aortic dissection: experience of 236 cases (1980 to 1990). Mayo Clin Proc 1993; 68: 642–51 |
| 5 | 2a | Diamond GA, Forrester JS. Analysis of probability as an aid in the clinical diagnosis of coronary artery disease. N Engl J Med 1979; 300: 1350–8 |
| 6 | 2a | Panju AA et al. Is this patient having a myocardial infarction? JAMA 1998; 280: 1256–63 |
| 7 | 4 | Slater EE, DeSanctis RW. Clinical recognition of dissecting aortic aneurysm. Am J Med 1976; 60: 625–31 |
| 8 | 4 | Eagle KA et al. Spectrum of conditions initially suggestive of acute aortic dissection but with negative aortograms. Am J Cardiol 1986; 57: 322–6 |
| 9 | 1a | Goldman L et al. A computer protocol to predict myocardial infarction in emergency department patients with chest pain. N Engl J Med 1988; 318: 797–803 |
| 10 | 2b | Tierney WM et al. Physicians' estimates of the probability of myocardial infarction in the emergency room patient with chest pain. Med Decis Making 1986; 6: 12–17 |
| 11 | 4 | Lux G et al. Ambulatory pressure, pH and ECG recording in patients with normal and pathological coronary angiography and intermittent chest pain. Neurogastroenterol Motil 1995; 7: 23–30 |
| 12 | 1a | Heckerling PS, Tape TG, Wigton RS et al. Clinical prediction rule for pulmonary infiltrates. Ann Intern Med 1990; 113: 664–70 |
| 13 | 1a | Metlay JP, Kapoor WN, Fine MJ et al. Does this patient have community-acquired pneumonia? Diagnosing pneumonia by history and physical examination. JAMA 1997; 278: 1440–5 |
| 14 | 4 | Lamont Murdoch J et al. Life expectancy and causes of death in the Marfan syndrome. N Engl J Med 1972; 286: 804–8 |
| 15 | 4 | Marsalese DL et al. Marfan syndrome: natural history and long-term follow-up of cardiovascular involvement. J Am Coll Cardiol 1989; 14: 422–8 |
| 16 | 1a | Metlay JP, Kapoor WN, Fine MJ et al. Does this patient have community-acquired pneumonia? Diagnosing pneumonia by history and physical examination. JAMA 1997; 278: 1440–5 |
| 17 | 2b | Glower DD, Fann JI, Speier RH et al. Comparison of medical and surgical therapy for uncomplicated descending aortic dissection (supplement IV). Circulation 1990; 82: 39–46 |
| 18 | 1b | Sox HC et al. Psychologically-mediated effects of diagnostic tests. Ann Intern Med 1981; 95: 680–5 |

| No. | Level | Citation |
|-----|-------|----------|
| 19 | 4 | de Winter RJ et al. Value of myoglobin, troponin T and CK-MB (mass) in ruling out an acute myocardial infarction in the emergency room. Circulation 1995; 92: 3401–7 |
| 20 | 2b | Thomsen SP, Gibbons RJ, Smars PA et al. Incremental value of the leukocyte differential and the creatine kinase-MB isoenzyme for the early diagnosis of myocardial infarction. Ann Intern Med 1995; 122: 335–41 |
| 21 | 4 | Zimmerman J, Fromm R, Meyer D et al. Diagnostic Marker Cooperative Study for the diagnosis of myocardial infarction. Circulation 1999; 99: 1671–7 |
| 22 | 1b | Antman EM et al. Evaluation of a rapid bedside assay for detection of serum cardiac troponin T. JAMA 1995; 273: 1279–82 |
| 23 | 2b | Sayre MR et al. Measurement of cardiac troponin T is an effective method for predicting complications among emergency department patients with chest pain. Ann Emerg Med 1998; 31: 539–49 |
| 24 | 4 | Smith AF. Diagnostic value of serum-creatine-kinase in a coronary-care unit. Lancet 1967; i: 178–182 |
| 25 | 1b | Lee TH, Rouan GW, Weisberg MC et al. Sensitivity of routine clinical criteria for diagnosing myocardial infarction within 24 hours of hospitalization. Ann Intern Med 1987; 106: 181–6 |
| 26 | 1b | Jayes RL, Larsen GC, Beshansky JR et al. Physician electrocardiogram reading in the emergency department. Accuracy and effect on triage decisions: findings from a multicenter study. J Gen Intern Med 1992; 7: 387–92 |
| 27 | 1b | Fesmire FM et al. Usefulness of automated serial 12-lead ECG monitoring during initial emergency department evaluation of patients with chest pain. Ann Emerg Med 1998; 31: 3–11 |
| 28 | 4 | Stark JL, Vacek JL. The initial electrocardiogram during admission for myocardial infarction: use as a predictor of clinical course and facility utilization. Arch Intern Med 1987; 147: 843–6 |
| 29 | 4 | Farr BM, Kaiser DL, Harrison BD et al. Prediction of microbial aetiology at admission to hospital for pneumonia from the presenting clinical features. Thorax 1989; 44: 1031–5 |
| 30 | 2b | Jagannath AS et al. Aortic dissection: a statistical analysis of the usefulness of plain chest radiographic findings. Am J Radiol 1986; 147: 1123–6 |
| 31 | 2b | Zalenski RJ et al. Evaluation of a chest pain diagnostic protocol to exclude acute cardiac ischemia in the emergency department. Arch Intern Med 1997; 157: 1085–91 |
| 32 | 1a | Lee TH, Juarez G, Cook EF et al. Ruling out acute myocardial infarction: prospective multicenter validation of a 12-hour strategy for patients at low risk. N Engl J Med 1991; 324: 1239–46 |
| 33 | 1b– | Gomez MA et al. An emergency department-based protocol for rapidly ruling out myocardial ischaemia decreases hospital time and expense: results of a randomised study (ROMIO). J Am Coll Cardiol 1996; 28: 25–33 |
| 34 | 1b | Roberts RR, Zalenski RJ, Mensah EK et al. Costs of an emergency department-based accelerated diagnostic protocol vs hospitalization in patients with chest pain: a randomized controlled trial. JAMA 1997; 278: 1670–6 |
| 35 | 1a | Goldman L, Cook F, Johnson PA et al. Prediction of the need for intensive care in patients who come to emergency departments with acute chest pain. N Engl J Med 1996; 334: 1498–504 |

| No. | Level | Citation |
|-----|-------|----------|
| 36 | 1b | Birdwell BG et al. Evaluating chest pain: the patient's presenting style alters the physician's diagnostic approach. Arch Intern Med 1993; 153: 1991–5 |
| 37 | 1b | Michaelides AP, Psomadaki ZD, Dilaveris PE et al. Improved detection of coronary artery disease by exercise electrocardiography with the use of right precordial leads. N Engl J Med 1999; 340: 340–5 |
| 38 | 1b | Froelicher VF et al. The electrocradiographic exercise test in a population with reduced workup bias; diagnostic performance, computerized interpretation and multivariate prediction. Ann Intern Med 1998; 128: 965–74 |
| 39 | 1a | Fleischmann KE, Hunink MGM, Kuntz KM et al. Exercise echocardiography or exercise SPECT imaging? A meta-analysis of diagnostic test performance. JAMA 1998; 280: 913–20 |
| 40 | 1a | Khattar RS. Assessment of myocardial perfusion and contractile dysfunction by inotropic stress Tc-99m SPECT imaging and echocardiography for optimal detection of multivessel coronary artery disease. Heart 1998; 79: 274–80 |
| 41 | 1b | Kemp HG et al. Seven year survival of patients with normal or near normal coronary arteriograms: a CASS registry study. J Am Coll Cardiol 1986; 7: 479–83 |
| 42 | 1b | Garber AM, Solomon NA. Cost-effectiveness of alternative test strategies for the diagnosis of coronary artery disease. Ann Intern Med 1999; 130: 719–28 |
| 43 | 4 | Cannon RO et al. Imipramine in patients with chest pain despite normal coronary angiography. N Engl J Med 1994; 330: 1411–7 |
| 44 | 1b– | Rose S et al. Interaction between patient and test administrator may influence the results of edrophonium provocative testing in patients with noncardiac chest pain. Am J Gastroenterol 1993; 88: 20–4 |
| 45 | 4 | Schofield PM et al. Oesophageal function in patients with angina pectoris: a comparison of patients with normal coronary angiograms and patients with coronary artery disease. Digestion 1989; 42: 70–8 |
| 46 | 1b– | Hargarten KM, Aprahamian C, Stueven HA et al. Prophylactic lidocaine in the prehospital patients with chest pain of suspected cardiac origin. Ann Emerg Med 1986; 15: 881–5 |
| 47 | 1b | Achem SR et al. Effects of omeprazole versus placebo in treatment of noncardiac chest pain and gastroesophageal reflux. Dig Dis Sci 1997; 42: 2138–45 |
| 48 | 1b | van Peski-Oosterbaan AS, Spinhoven P, van Rood Y et al. Cognitive-behavioural therapy for noncardiac chest pain: a randomized trial. Am J Med 1999; 106: 424–9 |
| 49 | 3b | Lee TH et al. Clinical characteristics and natural history of patients with acute myocardial infarction sent home from the emergency room. Am J Cardiol 1987; 60: 219–24 |
| 50 | 1b | Fleischmann KE, Goldman L, Robiolio PA et al. Echocardiographic correlates of survival in patients with chest pain. J Am Coll Cardiol 1994; 23: 1390–6 |
| 51 | 1b | Herlitz J et al. Predictors and mode of death over 5 years amongst patients admitted to the emergency department with acute chest pain or other symptoms raising suspicion of acute myocardial infarction. J Intern Med 1998; 243: 41–8 |
| 52 | 1a | Mark DB, Shaw L, Harrell FE et al. Prognostic value of a treadmill exercise score in outpatients with suspected coronary artery disease. N Engl J Med 1991; 325: 849–53 |

## CAUSES

Common causes of coma include:
- overdose
- trauma
- shock [C][1]
- cardiac arrest [C][1]
- stroke or cerebral haemorrhage
- hepatic encephalopathy
- hypoglycaemia.

Exclude rare but important causes:
- infection
- brain tumours
- uraemia and other metabolic disorders
- psychogenic.

> **? Why?**
> Hypoxia-ischaemia, cardiac arrest or stroke are common causes of non-traumatic coma
>
> | Causes of non-traumatic coma [C][1] | % (95% CI) |
> | --- | --- |
> | Hypoxia-ischaemia | 42% (38% to 46%) |
> | Cardiac arrest | 30% (26% to 34%) |
> | Brain infarct | 15% (12% to 18%) |
> | Brain haemorrhage | 13% (10% to 16%) |
> | Hepatic encephalopathy | 10% (7.5% to 13%) |
> | Subarachnoid haemorrhage | 7.6% (5.3% to 9.9%) |
> | Other metabolic disturbances | 3.8% (2.1% to 5.5%) |
> | Infection | 3.2% (1.7% to 4.7%) |
> | Isolated disorders like hypoglycaemia | 2.4% (1.1% to 3.7%) |
> | Mass lesions | 2.2% (0.9% to 3.5%) |
>
> - 10% of patients with an altered level of consciousness have an opiate overdose: 10% (95% CI: 6.4% to 14%) [B][2].

## IMMEDIATE MANAGEMENT

- Assess the airway and breathing.
  - Clear airway [A] and stabilise the cervical spine if there is a history of head or neck trauma [A].
  - Ventilate with a bag-valve-mask and 100% oxygen [A].
  - Consider intubation [D].
- Assess the circulation [D].
  - Correct any hypovolaemia or arrhythmias [D].
  - Obtain large bore iv access and consider CVP monitoring [D].
- Look for evidence of hypoglycaemia [C][3].

**Note**

Altered mental state: absence of hypoglycaemia symptoms does not exclude hypoglycaemia

| Patient [C][3] | Target disorder (reference standard) | Diagnostic test | LR+ (95% CI) | Post-test probability | LR– (95% CI) | Post-test probability |
|---|---|---|---|---|---|---|
| Altered mental state (pre-test probability 9%) | Hypoglycaemia (blood glucose or clinical diagnosis) | Any of tachycardia, sweating or available history of diabetes mellitus | 1.7 (1.3 to 2.1) | 14% | 0.45 (0.23 to 0.86) | 4% |

● Measure glucose rapidly using reagent strips **[A]**[4] **[B]**[5] or a capillary blood glucose in triage. **[A]**[6]

**Why?**

Normoglycaemia on a reagent strip makes hypoglycaemia unlikely

| Patient [A][7] | Target disorder (reference standard) | Diagnostic test | LR+ (95% CI) | Post-test probability | LR– (95% CI) | Post-test probability |
|---|---|---|---|---|---|---|
| Altered mental status (pre-test probability 7%) | Hypoglycaemia (blood glucose) | Reagent strip | 12.1 (6.8 to 21) | 48% | 0.090 (0.014 to 0.6) | 0.68% |

■ Immediate blood glucose measurement reduces time to definitive care (mean 2 h to nursing care, 1 h to medical care) **[A]**[6].

● Measure blood glucose **[A]**.

Remember patients with diabetes may experience hypoglycaemia at 'normoglycaemic levels'.

**Why?**

■ Patient with diabetes experience symptoms of hypoglycaemia at higher blood glucose levels than patients without diabetes (on average 1.4 mmol/l higher) **[D]**[8].

● If you believe hypoglycaemia is present, try a test dose of 50% glucose iv **[C]**[3].

**Why?**

**A full recovery following 50% glucose diagnosing hypoglycaemia**

| Patient [C][3] | Target disorder (reference standard) | Diagnostic test | LR+ (95% CI) | Post-test probability |
|---|---|---|---|---|
| Altered mental consciousness (pre-test probability 9%) | Hypoglycaemia (blood glucose or clinical diagnosis) | Complete response to 50% glucose | 43 (18 to 110) | 80% |
| | | Partial response to 50% glucose | 1.2 (0.47 to 3.2) | 10% |
| | | No response to 50% glucose | 0.20 (0.089 to 0.44) | 1.8% |

- Give thiamine 100 mg **[D]** iv **[C]**[9] to alcoholics or malnourished patients **[D]**.

**Note**

■ Few patients develop adverse effects when given thiamine iv (0.1%, 95%, CI: 0.0% to 0.3%) **[C]**[9].

- Look for status epilepticus **[C]**[10].
  Signs can be subtle. Look for twitching of extremities, mouth and eyes, but these may be absent.

**Why?**

■ Patients in a coma who have rhythmic clonic movements are at increased risk of having status epilepticus **[A]**[11].
■ Patients in a coma may display no clinical signs of status epilepticus, but still have it **[A]**[11].
■ A fifth of patients with status epilepticus may not be convulsing **[C]**[10].

- Give lorazepam **[A]**[12] 0.1 mg/kg iv at 2 mg/min.

**Why do this?**

■ It is faster than diazepam, phenobarbital (10 min faster) or phenytoin (25 min faster) at terminating seizures **[A]**[12].
■ It is better than phenytoin at terminating seizures, but is not clearly different from diazepam with or without phenytoin, or phenobarbital **[D]**[13] **[D]**[14].

**Lorazepam stops more seizures than phenytoin**

| Patient | Treatment | Comparator | Outcome | CER | RBI | NNT |
|---|---|---|---|---|---|---|
| Status epilepticus **[A]**[12] | Lorazepam | Phenytoin | Termination of seizures at 60 min | 42% | 29% (1% to 64%) | 8 (4 to 160) |

- Correct hypothermia or hyperthermia **[D]**.
- Assess the level of consciousness using the Glasgow Coma Scale (Box 1): maximum score = 15; minimum score = 3.

 **Why?**
- Clinic staff agree better using GCS than using simple descriptions **[A]**[15].
- It helps predict mortality **[A]**[16] **[B]**[17].

**BOX 1 Glasgow Coma Scale**

| Response | Score |
|---|---|
| **Eye opening** | |
| ● spontaneous | 4 |
| ● on your verbal command ('Open your eyes') | 3 |
| ● in response to painful stimulus | 2 |
| ● no response | 1 |
| **Motor response** | |
| ● correct response to 'Show me two fingers' | 6 |
| ● localises painful stimulus and tries to stop it | 5 |
| ● withdraws from painful stimulus to fingernail | 4 |
| ● abnormal flexor response of forearms, wrists and fingers | 3 |
| ● abnormal extensor response of arms and legs | 2 |
| ● no response | 1 |
| **Verbal response** to the question: 'What year is this?' | |
| ● correct year | 5 |
| ● wrong year | 4 |
| ● words but no year | 3 |
| ● incomprehensible sounds | 2 |
| ● no response | 1 |

## CLINICAL FEATURES

Ask ambulance crews, family, friends and clinicians who know the patient about:
- known allergies **[D]**
- recent symptoms **[D]**
- recent head injury **[D]**
- speed of onset of coma **[D]**
- previous episodes of coma **[D]**
- medical history **[D]**
- drug use **[D]**.

If you suspect an opiate overdose, ask about **[B]**[2]:
- drug paraphernalia where the patient was found
- needle track marks on skin
- history of iv drug use by bystanders.

Look for evidence of:
- head injury [D]
- drug overdose [D]
- uraemia or other metabolic derangement [D]
- malignancy [C][1]
- stroke or cerebral haemorrhage [C][1]
- infection (brain, meninges, sepsis) [C][1]
- hypertension [C][1].

If you suspect an opiate overdose, look for [B][2]:
- a reduced respiratory rate
- pinpoint pupils.

**? Why?**
A reduced respiratory rate, pinpoint pupils and evidence of drug misuse make opiate overdose more likely

| Patient [B][2] | Target disorder (reference standard) | Diagnostic test | LR+ (95% CI) | Post-test probability | LR– (95% CI) | Post-test probability |
|---|---|---|---|---|---|---|
| Altered mental state (pre-test probability 10%) | Opiate overdose (physician review of hospital chart) | Respiration <13 breaths/min | 14 (7.8 to 24) | 61% | 0.21 (0.097 to 0.47) | 2.3% |
| | | Pinpoint pupils | 5.1 (to) | 37% | 0.28 (0.14 to 0.57) | 3.1% |
| | | Circumstantial evidence • drug paraphemalia where found • needle track marks on skin • history of iv drug use by bystanders | 14 (7.2 to 26) | 61% | 0.34 (0.19 to 0.60) | 3.7% |
| | | Any of the above | 3.8 (3.0 to 5.0) | 30% | 0.11 (0.028 to 0.40) | 1.2% |

Look for raised intracranial pressure by assessing the fundi. Look for:
- papilloedema [D]
- retinal vein pulsation [C][18]

**? Why?**
Retinal vein pulsation makes raised intracranial pressure unlikely

| Patient [C][18] | Target disorder (reference standard) | Diagnostic test | LR+ (95% CI) | Post-test probability | LR– (95% CI) | Post-test probability |
|---|---|---|---|---|---|---|
| Suspected raised intracranial pressure (pre-test probability 23%) | Raised intracranial pressure (lumbar puncture or follow-up) | Absence of retinal vein pulsation | 8.1 (5.3 to 13) | 70% | 0.0 (0.0 to 0.077) | 0% |

- Changes associated with diabetes or hypertension **[D]**.

Assess brainstem function **[D]**:
- corneal reflex
- oculocephalic reflex (if no cervical spine trauma): rotate head from side to side; if the brainstem is intact, the eyes will move conjugately in the opposite direction from head rotation
- oculovestibular reflex (if unruptured tympanic membrane): inject 200 ml of iced water into one external auditory meatus; a normal response is slow phase of nystagimus towards the irrigated ear.

## INVESTIGATIONS

- Capillary glucose **[D]**.
- Arterial blood gases **[D]**.
- Blood count **[C]**[1].
- Urea and electrolytes **[C]**[1].
- Glucose **[C]**[1].
- Calcium.
- ECG **[D]**.
- Chest X-ray **[D]**.
- CT head **[D]**.

Consider:
- serum and urine drugs screen if overdose suspected **[D]**
- blood culture if evidence of infection **[D]**
- cervical spine X-rays if trauma **[D]**
- lumbar puncture if signs of raised intracranial pressure are absent on CT head, and infection or intracranial haemorrhage are suspected **[D]**.

### Suspected overdose
- Give flumazenil iv **[A]**[19] **[A]**[20].

---

**?** **Why do this?**
- ■ It improves the GCS (by around 2 points) **[B]**[21] and patients are more likely to become fully conscious **[A]**[19] **[A]**[20].
- ■ Watch out for adverse reactions: shivering, agitation, fall in blood pressure, nausea and vomiting – they are relatively common **[A]**[20].

**Flumazenil wakes patients up following an overdose but can causes side-effects**

| Patient [A][20] | Treatment | Comparator | Outcome | CER | RBI | NNT |
|---|---|---|---|---|---|---|
| Coma and suspected overdose | Flumazenil | Placebo | Recovered enough to provide useful information at 15 min | 2% | 2000% (190% to 15000%) | 3 (2 to 4) |
| | | | Adverse reaction | 3% | −342% (−1700% to 0%) | −8 (−57 to −4) |

- Give naloxone **[B]**[2] 400 μg im followed by 400 μg iv **[D]**.

| | | | | |
|---|---|---|---|---|
| **?** **Why?** A complete response to naloxone makes opiate overdose much more likely | | | | |
| *Patient* **[B]**[2] | *Target disorder (reference standard)* | *Diagnostic test* | *LR+(95% CI)* | *Post-test probability* |
| Altered mental state (pre-test probability 10%) | Opiate overdose (physician review of hospital chart) | Complete response to naloxone | 28 (12 to 64) | 76% |
| | | Partial or equivocal response to naloxone | 0.74 (0.18 to 2.9) | 7.7% |
| | | No response to naloxone | 0.19 (0.075 to 0.46) | 2.1% |

## THERAPY

Treat the cause **[A]**.

Remember continuing care of the unconscious patient:
- DVT prophylaxis **[A]**[22] **[A]**[23]
- pressure sore prevention **[D]**
- corneal protection **[D]**
- nutrition **[D]**.

The following chapters provide more information on specific treatments:
- Acute hypoglycaemia
- Diabetic ketoacidosis
- Meningitis
- Hypercalcaemia
- Hypertensive emergency
- Stroke

### Traumatic brain injury
- Cool the patient down **[A]**[24].

**Why?**

■ Patients who have local or systemic cooling to a target temperature of, at most, 34–35°C for at least 12 h are less likely to die or have severe disability **[A]**[24].

**Hypothermia reduces death or severe disability**

| Patient **[A]**[24] | Treatment | Comparator | Outcome | CER | OR | NNT |
|---|---|---|---|---|---|---|
| Moderate or severe closed head injury | Mild hypothermia | Normothermia | Death or severe disability | 62% | 0.40 (0.22 to 0.75) | 4 (3 to 14) |

There is no clear benefit from:
- hyperventilation **[D]**[25]
- CSF drainage **[D]**[25]
- steroids **[D]**[25]
- barbiturates **[D]**[25]
- mannitol **[D]**[25]
- hypertonic saline **[D]**[26].

**Why?**

■ None of these treatments are clearly better than no intervention at reducing mortality. Steroids in particular have no significant effect on death or disability **[D]**[25].

■ Hypertonic saline is not clearly better than Ringer's lactate at reducing neurological problems **[D]**[25].

## PROGNOSIS

### Non-traumatic
- Most patients die. Few make a good recovery **[C]**[1].

**Note**

■ 23% are dead within 1 h (95% CI: 19% to 26%) **[C]**[1].
■ 64% are dead within 1 week (95% CI: 60% to 68%) **[C]**[1].
■ 76% are dead within 1 month (95% CI: 72% to 80%) **[C]**[1].
■ 88% are dead within 1 year (95% CI: 85% to 91%) **[C]**[1].
■ 0.6% make a good recovery (95% CI: 0.0% to 1.3%) **[C]**[1].

Patients are more likely to die or remain in a persistent vegetative state if any of the following are present **[B]**[17]:
- GCS motor score = 1 at day 3
- absent pupillary response at day 3
- burst activity or flat EEG after 1 week
- no cerebral response to somatosensory-evoked potentials after 1 week.

**Why?**
**Poor motor response, no pupil reaction and abnormal EEG and evoked potential predict a bad outcome**

| Patient [B][17] | Prognostic factor | Outcome | Control rate | OR (95% CI) | NNF (95% CI) |
|---|---|---|---|---|---|
| Non-traumatic coma | GCS motor response = 1 on day 3 *independent* | Death or vegetative state | 67% | 1.76 (1.50 to 2.06) | 2 (2 to 3) |
| | Absent pupillary reactions to light on day 3 *independent* | Death or vegetative state | 67% | 1.64 (1.42 to 1.89) | 3 (2 to 4) |
| | Burst-suppression or isoelectric EEG during first week *independent* | Death or vegetative state | 67% | 2.74 (2.31 to 3.25) | 2 (1 to 2) |
| | Somatosensory evoked potential: bilateral absence of N20 (earliest cortical response after median nerve stimulation) during first week *independent* | Death or vegetative state | 67% | 1.78 (1.63 to 1.93) | 2 (2 to 3) |

## Traumatic

A quarter of patients with severe head injury are dead within a year [A][16].

**Note**
■ 23% are dead within 12 months (95% CI: 19% to 28%) [A][16].

Patients are at increased risk of dying if they have [A][16]:
● a haematoma on CT
● neither pupil reacting
● old age
● a low Glasgow Coma Scale
● a high injury severity score.

**Why?**
**Bleeding on CT, no pupil reaction, increasing age and a low GCS predict mortality**

| Patient [A][16] | Prognostic factor | Outcome | Control rate | OR (95% CI) | NNF+(95% CI) |
|---|---|---|---|---|---|
| Severe head injury | Neither pupil reacting *independent* | Death at 12 months | 23.4% | 0.168 (0.06 to 0.50) | 5 (5 to 10) |
| | Age (per 5 years) | Death at 12 months | 23.4% | 0.545 (0.43 to 0.69) | |
| | Injury severity score (per 5 units) | Death at 12 months | 23.4% | 0.737 (0.60 to 0.91) | |
| | No visible haematoma on CT | Death at 12 months | 23.4% | 3.53 (1.43 to 8.73) | −4 (−14 to −2) |
| | GCS total (per unit) | Death at 12 months | 23.4% | 1.31 (1.12 to 1.53) | |

**Guideline writers**: Will Whiteley, Christopher Ball
**CAT writers**: Will Whiteley, Christopher Ball

## REFERENCES

| No | Level | Citation |
| --- | --- | --- |
| 1 | 4 | Levy DE, Bates D, Caronna JJ et al. Prognosis in nontraumatic coma. Ann Intern Med 1981; 94: 293–301 |
| 2 | 2b | Hoffman JR, Schriger DL, Luo JS et al. The empiric use of naloxone in patients with altered mental status: a reappraisal. Ann Emerg Med 1991; 20: 246–52 |
| 3 | 4 | Hoffman JR, Schriger DL, Votey SR et al. The empiric use of hypertonic dextrose in patients with altered mental status: a reappraisal. Ann Emerg Med 1992; 21: 20–4 |
| 4 | 1b | Lavery RF, Allegra JR, Cody RP et al. A prospective evaluation of glucose reagent teststrips in the prehospital setting. Am J Emerg Med 1991; 9: 304–8 |
| 5 | 2b | Scott PA, Wolf LR, Spadafora MP. Accuracy of reagent strips in detecting hypoglycemia in the emergency department. Ann Emerg Med 1998; 32: 305–9 |
| 6 | 1b | Degroote NE, Pieper B. Blood glucose monitoring at triage. J Emerg Nurs 1993; 19: 131–3 |
| 7 | 1b | Jones JL, Ray VG, Gough JE et al. Determination of prehospital blood glucose: a prospective, controlled study. J Emerg Med 1992; 10: 679–82 |
| 8 | 5 | Boyle PJ, Schwartz NS, Shah SD et al. Plasma glucose concentrations at the onset of hypoglycemic symptoms in patients with poorly controlled diabetes and nondiabetics. N Engl J Med 1988; 318: 1487–92 |
| 9 | 4 | Wrenn KD, Murphy F, Slovis CM. A toxicity study of parenteral thiamine hydrochloride. Ann Emerg Med 1989; 18: 867–70 |
| 10 | 4 | Dunne JW, Summers QA, Stewart-Wynne EG. Non-convulsive status epilepticus: a prospective study in an adult general hospital. Q J Med 1987; 62: 117–26 |
| 11 | 1b | Lowenstein DH, Aminoff MJ. Clinical and EEG feature of status epilepticus in comatose patients. Neurology 1992; 42: 100–4 |
| 12 | 1b | Treiman DM et al. A comparison of four treatments for generalised convulsive status epilepticus. N Engl J Med 1998; 339: 792–8 |
| 13 | 1b | Treiman DM et al. A comparison of four treatments for generalised convulsive status epilepticus: NEJM (1998): 339: 792–8 |
| 14 | 1b – | Leppik IE et al. A double-blind study of lorazepam and diazepam in status epilepticus. JAMA 1983; 249: 1452–4 |
| 15 | 1a | Teasdale G, Knill-Jones R, van der Sande J. Observer variability in assessing impaired consciousness and coma. J Neurol Neurosurg Psychiatry 1978; 41: 603–10 |
| 16 | 1a | Signorini DF, Andrews PJ, Jones PA et al. Predicting survival using simple clinical variable: a case study in traumatic brain injury. J Neurol Neurosurg Psychiatry 1999; 66: 20–5 |
| 17 | 2a | Zandbergen EG, de Haan RJ, Stoutenbeek CP et al. Systematic review of early prediction of poor outcome in anoxic-ischaemic coma. Lancet 1998; 352: 1808–12 |
| 18 | 4 | Levin BE. The clinical significance of spontaneous pulsations of the retinal vein. Arch Neurol 1978; 35: 37–40 |

| No | Level | Citation |
|----|-------|----------|
| 19 | 1b | Weinbroum A, Rudick V, Sorkine P et al. Use of flumazenil in the treatment of drug overdose: a double-blind and open clinical study in 110 patients. Crit Care Med 1996; 24: 199–206 |
| 20 | 1b | Hojer J, Baehrendtz S, Matell G et al. Diagnostic utility of flumazenil in coma with suspected poisoning: a double-blind randomised controlled study. BMJ 1990; 301: 1308–11 |
| 21 | 2b | Ritz R, Zuber M, Elsasser S. Use of flumazenil in intoxicated patients with coma: a double-blind placebo-controlled study in ICU. Intensive Care Med 1990; 16: 242–7 |
| 22 | 1b | Geerts WH et al. A comparison of low-dose heparin and LMWH as prophylaxis against venous thromboembolism after major trauma. N Engl J Med 1996; 335: 701–7 |
| 23 | 1a | Antiplatelet Trialists' Collaboration. Collaborative overview of randomised trials of antiplatelet therapy. III: Reduction of venous thromboembolism and pulmonary embolism by antiplatelet prophylaxis amongst surgical and medical patients. BMJ 1994; 308: 235–45 |
| 24 | 1a | Signorini DF, Alderson P. Therapeutic hypothermia for head injury (Cochrane Review). In: The Cochrane Library, Issue 3, 1999. Oxford: Update Software |
| 25 | 1a – | Roberts I, Schierhout G, Alderson P et al. Absence of the evidence for the effectiveness of five interventions routinely used in the intensive care management of severe head injury: a systematic review. J Neurol Neurosurg Psychiatry 1998; 65: 729–33 |
| 26 | 1b – | Shackford SR, Bourguignon PR, Wald SL et al. Hypertonic saline resuscitation of patients with head injury: a prospective, randomized clinical trial. J Trauma 1998; 44: 50–7 |

## PREVALENCE

Heart failure is common, particularly in:

- breathless patients [B][1]
- patients with a recent myocardial infarction [B][1]
- older patients [B][2].

| Note | |
|---|---|
| Heart failure increases with age | |
| *Prevalence of heart failure* [B][2] | (%) |
| Aged 25–54 years | 1.1% |
| Aged 55–64 years | 3.7% |
| Aged 65–74 years | 4.5% |

- Prevalence of left ventricular preload with a recent MI. 24% to 75% [B][1].
- Prevalence of left ventricular preload with dyspnoea: 26% to 31% [B][1].

## CAUSES

Think about a cause. These include [D]:

- fluid overload
  - excess iv fluids
  - renal failure
- pump failure
  - MI
  - valvular heart disease
  - arrhythmias
  - PE
  - myocarditis, constrictive pericarditis
  - atrial myoxoma
  - hypertensive crisis
- drugs and toxins
  - failure to take medication: digitalis, diuretics
  - NSAIDs, beta-blockers, tricyclics
  - alcohol
  - thiamine deficiency
- increased metabolic demands
  - pregnancy
  - fever
  - hyperthyroidism
  - anaemia.

## CLINICAL FEATURES

Ask about:

- a previous MI [B][3-5]

> **? Why?**
> A previous MI increases the risk of left ventricular systolic failure
>
> | Patient [B][3] | Target disorder (reference standard) | Diagnostic test | LR+ (95% CI) | Post-test probability | LR– (95% CI) | Post-test probability |
> |---|---|---|---|---|---|---|
> | Suspected heart failure (pre-test probability 17%) | Left ventricular systolic failure (echocardiogram) | MI | 4.1 (2.7 to 6.2) | 44% | 0.48 (0.33 to 0.70) | 8% |

- previous episodes of congestive heart failure [A][6]

> **? Why?**
> A history of congestive heart disease increases the risk for further episodes
>
> | Patient [A][6] | Prognostic factor | Outcome | Control rate | OR (95% CI) | NNF+ (95% CI) |
> |---|---|---|---|---|---|
> | Frail elderly | History of congestive heart disease *independent* | Congestive heart disease at 12 months | 15% | 7.0 (2.9 to 17) | 2 (2 to 5) |

- orthopnoea [B][5]
- dyspnoea on exertion [B][3]

> **? Why?**
> No dyspnoea on exertion makes left ventricular failure very unlikely
>
> | Patient [B][3] | Target disorder (reference standard) | Diagnostic test | LR+ (95% CI) | Post-test probability | LR– (95% CI) | Post-test probability |
> |---|---|---|---|---|---|---|
> | Suspected heart failure (pre-test probability 17%) | Left ventricular systolic failure (echocardiogram) | Dyspnoea on exertion | 1.2 (1.1 to 1.3) | 18% | 0.0 (0.0 to 0.084) | 0% |

- current medication and alcohol use [D].

Look for:

- tachycardia [B][5]
- hypotension or hypertension [B][5]
- dyspnoea [B][5]
- crackles on chest examination [B][5]
- oedema [B][5]

---

**Note**
**Number of findings relates to probability of heart failure**

| No. of features | Prevalence of reduced ejection fraction (%) |
| --- | --- |
| 3 or more | >83% |
| 1–2 | 23% to 41% |
| None | <10% |

---

**Why?**
**Clinical features can help diagnose increased filling pressure, a low ejection fraction and diastolic dysfunction**

| Findings [B][5] | Increased filling pressure | Ejection fraction < 40% | Diastolic dysfunction |
| --- | --- | --- | --- |
| Very helpful | ■ Radiographic distribution<br>■ Raised JVP | ■ Radiographic cardiomegaly or redistribution<br>■ anterior q waves<br>■ LBBB<br>■ Abnormal apical impulse | ■ Current hypertension (systolic > 160, diastolic > 100 mm Hg) |
| Somewhat helpful | ■ Dyspnoea<br>■ Orthopnoea<br>■ Tachycardia<br>■ Decreased systolic blood pressure<br>■ Proportional pulse pressure (systolic – diastolic/systolic) <25%<br>■ Third heart sound<br>■ Abnormal abdominojugular reflex<br>■ Radiographic cardiomegaly | ■ Pulse >90 beats/min<br>■ Systolic BP < 90 mmHg<br>■ Proportional pulse pressure <33%<br>■ Third heart sound<br>■ Crackles<br>■ Dyspnoea<br>■ Prior MI<br>■ CK >200 in post-infarct patient | ■ Obesity<br>■ No tachycardia<br>■ Elderly<br>■ Non-smoker<br>■ No coronary artery disease |
| Helpful when positive | ■ Oedema | ■ Raised JVP<br>■ Oedema | ■ Normal radiographic heart size |

---

- an elevated JVP [B][3] [B][5] [B][7]

*Remember:*
Use a well-lit room; lay the patient at 30–45° to horizontal; turn the patient's head and look for the right internal jugular vein. Raise or lower the patient as required (normal patients may need to be laid almost flat). The JVP is the vertical height from the highest point of the pulsation to the angle of Louis.

**Why?**
**A raised JVP makes an elevated CVP more likely**

| Patient [B][7] | Target disorder (reference standard) | Diagnostic test | LR+ (95% CI) | Post-test probability |
|---|---|---|---|---|
| Suspected heart failure (pre-test probability 31%) | Elevated CVP (> 5 cm) | JVP high | 4.1 (1.3 to 13) | 65% |
| | | JVP normal | 0.8 (0.5 to 1.3) | 26% |
| | | JVP low | 0.2 (0.02 to 1.3) | 8% |

**A raised JVP makes left ventricular failure more likely**

| Patient [B][3] | Target disorder (reference standard) | Diagnostic test | LR+ (95% CI) | Post-test probability | LR– (95% CI) | Post-test probability |
|---|---|---|---|---|---|---|
| Suspected heart failure (pre-test probability 17%) | Left ventricular systolic failure (echocardiogram) | Jugular venous distension | 9.3 (2.9 to 30) | 64% | 0.84 (0.73 to 0.97) | 14% |

**Note**
■ Physicians agree only moderately about the position of the JVP.

● an abnormal abdominojugular reflex [B][5] [B][7]

*Remember:*
Ask the patient to relax and breathe through an open mouth. Place the palm of your hand on the mid-abdomen and push at pressure 20–35 mmHg for 15–30 s:

- – positive if sustained increase in JVP ≥ 4 cm
- – negative if sustained increase ≤ 3 cm, or transient increase ≥ 4 cm.

Repeat the test if there is pain or if the patient holds the breath or bears down.

**Why?**
**An abnormal abdominojugular reflex makes congestive heart failure more likely**

| Patient [B][7] | Target disorder (reference standard) | Diagnostic test | LR+ (95% CI) | Post-test probability | LR– (95% CI) | Post-test probability |
|---|---|---|---|---|---|---|
| Suspected congestive heart failure (pre-test probability 25%) | Congestive heart failure (clinicoradiographic score) | Abnormal abdominojugular reflex | 6.0 (1.3 to 29) | 67% | 0.7 (0.5 to 1.1) | 19% |

- an abnormal apical pulse **[A]**[8] **[B]**[5]

*Remember:*
Detect this using simultaneous auscultation and palpation: the impulse must be at least two-thirds of systole to be called sustained. Use a tongue blade pressed over the apex to produce a visual demonstration of the impulse (or S3) **[D].** Any increase in size can be detected by percussion **[A]**[9].

---

**? Why?**

**A displaced apex makes left ventricular failure more likely**

| Patient **[B]**[3] | Target disorder (reference standard) | Diagnostic test | LR+ (95% CI) | Post-test probability | LR− (95% CI) | Post-test probability |
|---|---|---|---|---|---|---|
| Suspected heart failure (pre-test probability 17% | Left ventricular systolic failure (echocardiogram) | Apex displaced | 16 (8.1 to 31) | 75% | 0.36 (0.23 to 0.55) | 6% |

**A displaced apex or enlarged heart on percussion makes radiographic cardiomegaly slightly more likely**

| Patient | Target disorder (reference standard) | Diagnostic test | LR+ (95% CI) | Post-test probability | LR− (95% CI) | Post-test probability |
|---|---|---|---|---|---|---|
| Suspected cardiomegaly (pre-test probability 25%) | Cardiomegaly (PA chest X-ray) | Apex palpable beyond mid-clavicular line **[A]**[8] | 2.5 (1.5 to 4.2) | 45% | 0.53 (0.32 to 0.86) | 15% |
| Suspected cardiomegaly (pre-test probability 36%) | Cardiomegaly (PA chest X-ray) | Dull to percussion at >10.5 cm from mid-sternal line **[A]**[9] | 2.9 (2.0 to 4.1) | 62% | 0.083 (0.021 to 0.32) | 4% |
| | | Dull to percussion at >11 cm from mid-sternal line **[A]**[9] | 8.1 (4.0 to 17) | 82% | 0.12 (0.049 to 0.32) | 7% |

---

**Note**
- 40% to 50% of apices are not palpable **[A]**[8] **[A]**[9].

---

- a third heart sound **[B]**[5]
- a gallop rhythm **[B]**[3].

**? Why?**

**A gallop rhythm makes left ventricular failure much more likely**

| Patient [B][3] | Target disorder (reference standard) | Diagnostic test | LR+ (95% CI) | Post-test probability | LR– (95% CI) | Post-test probability |
|---|---|---|---|---|---|---|
| Suspected heart failure (pre-test probability 17%) | Left ventricular systolic failure (echocardiogram) | Gallop rhythm | 27 (6.1 to 120) | 83% | 0.76 (0.64 to 0.91) | 13% |

Listen for heart murmurs:

- evidence of aortic stenosis [B][10]
  - listen for a reduced or absent second heart sound, or a fourth heart sound
  - listen for a murmur loudest in late systole and radiating to the right carotid

**? Why?**

**Heart sounds and a murmur loudest in late systole help diagnose stenosis**

| Patient [B][10] | Target disorder (reference standard) | Diagnostic test | LR+ (95% CI) | Post-test probability | LR– (95% CI) | Post-test probability |
|---|---|---|---|---|---|---|
| Elderly with syncope (pre-test probability 5%) | Aortic stenosis (imaging studies) | Reduced or absent 2nd heart sound | 50 (24 to100) | 72% | 0.45 (0.34 to 0.58) | 2% |
| | | 4th heart sound | 2.5 (2.1 to 3.0) | 12% | 0.26 (0.14 to 0.49) | 1% |
| | | Any murmur | 2.4 (2.2 to 2.7) | 11% | 0.0 (0.0 to 0.13) | 0% |
| | | Murmur loudest in late systole | 101 (25 to 410) | 84% | 0.31 (0.22 to 0.44) | 2% |
| | | Radiation to right carotid | 1.4 (1.3 to 1.5) | 7% | 0.10 (0.13 to 0.40) | 0.5% |

- evidence of mitral regurgitation [B][11]
  - listen for a late or pansystolic murmur in the mitral area
  - listen for any increase on transient arterial occlusion (a blood pressure cuff around both arms simultaneously inflated to 20–40 mmHg > systolic BP; check murmur intensity 20 s later)

**❓ Why?**

**A murmur in the mitral area makes mitral regurgitation more likely**

| Patient [B][11] | Target disorder (reference standard) | Diagnostic test | LR+ (95% CI) | Post-test probability | LR– (95% CI) | Post-test probability |
|---|---|---|---|---|---|---|
| Systolic murmur (pre-test probability 13%) | Any mitral regurgitation (echocardiogram) | Murmur in mitral area | 3.9 (3.0 to 5.1) | 37% | 0.34 (0.23 to 0.47) | 4.8% |
| | | Late/pansystolic murmur | 1.8 (1.2 to 2.5) | 21% | 0.0 (0.0 to 0.8) | 0% |
| | | Transient arterial occlusion causing an increase in murmur intensity | 7.5 (2.5 to 23) | 53% | 0.28 (0.18 to 0.60) | 4.0% |

- evidence of aortic regurgitation
  - a decrescendo early diastolic murmur [A][12]
  - an Austin Flint murmur (low-pitched late diastolic apical murmur) [B][13]
  - listen for any increase on transient arterial occlusion [B][13].

**❓ Why?**

**A typical early diastolic murmur or an Austin Flint murmur makes aortic regurgitation more likely**

| Patient | Target disorder (reference standard) | Diagnostic test | LR+ (95% CI) | Post-test probability | LR– (95% CI) | Post-test probability |
|---|---|---|---|---|---|---|
| Typical early diastolic murmur (pre-test probability 13%) | Any aortic regurgitation (echocardiogram) | Typical early diastolic murmur [A][14] | 32 (16 to 63) | 83% | 0.2 (0.1 to 0.3) | 3% |
| | Moderate or severe aortic regurgitation (echocardiogram) | Typical early diastolic murmur [A][14] | 8.3 (6.2 to 11) | 55% | 0.1 (0.0 to 0.2) | 1% |
| | | Austin Flint murmur (low-pitched late diastolic apical murmur) [B][13] | 25 (2.8 to 240) | 79% | 0.5 (0.2 to 0.7) | 7% |
| | | Popliteal brachial gradient >20 mmHg [B][13] | 8.2 (1.5 to 78) | 55% | 0.2 (0.1 to 0.5) | 3% |
| | | Transient arterial occlusion increases the murmur intensity [B][13] | 8.4 (1.3 to 81) | 56% | 0.3 (0.1 to 0.8) | 4% |

## DIFFERENTIAL DIAGNOSIS

### Dyspnoea

Think about other causes of breathlessness.
Common causes include [B][15]:

- asthma
- COPD
- arrhythmia
- infection
- interstitial lung disease
- anaemia.

**Why?**

**Heart failure is a common cause of dyspnoea**

| Causes of dyspnoea [B][15] | % |
| --- | --- |
| Asthma | 33% |
| Heart failure | 31% |
| COPD | 9% |
| Arrhythmia | 7% |
| Infection | 5% |
| Interstitial lung disease | 4% |
| Anaemia | 2% |
| PE | < 2% |

### Pulmonary oedema on chest X-ray

Think about other causes of pulmonary oedema [B][16].

**Why?**

**Overhydration and ARDS are common causes in intensive care patients**

| Causes of pulmonary oedema in ITU patients [B][16] | % (95% CI) |
| --- | --- |
| Heart failure | 51% (42% to 60%) |
| Overhydration | 25% (17% to 33%) |
| ARDS | 24% (16% to 31%) |

## INVESTIGATIONS

- Blood count [D].
- Urea, electrolytes, creatinine [A].

**Why?**
**A low serum sodium increases the risk of dying**

| Patient | Prognostic factor | Outcome | Control rate | RR (95% CI) | NNF+ (95% CI) |
|---|---|---|---|---|---|
| Severe heart failure | Decrease in serum sodium (by 3 mmol/l) *independent* **[B]**[17] | Death at 15 months | 12% | 1.42 (1.08 to 1.87) | 19 (9 to 100) |

- Cardiac enzymes **[D]**.
- Arterial blood gas if dyspnoeic **[D]**.
- ECG **[B]**[18].
  Look for:
  - anterior q-waves **[B]**[5]
  - LBBB **[B]**[5]

**Why?**
- Anterior q waves and LBBB are very helpful at diagnosing an ejection fraction < 40% **[B]**[5].

**Note**
**A normal ECG makes left ventricular systolic dysfunction less likely**

| Patient **[B]**[18] | Target disorder (reference standard) | Diagnostic test | LR+ (95% CI) | Post-test probability | LR– (95% CI) | Post-test probability |
|---|---|---|---|---|---|---|
| Suspected heart failure (pre-test probability 18%) | Impaired left ventricular systolic dysfunction (echocardiogram) | Abnormal ECG | 2.4 (2.1 to 2.8) | 35% | 0.10 (0.047 to 0.22) | 2% |

- Insert a urinary catheter to monitor urine output **[D]**.
- Chest X-ray.
  Look for **[B]**[1] **[B]**[5]
  - cardiomegaly
  - interstitial oedema
  - inverted pulmonary blood flow distribution.

**Cardiomegaly, interstitial oedema and venous congestion make heart failure slightly more likely**

| Patient | Target disorder (reference standard) | Diagnostic test | LR+ (95% CI) | Post-test probability | LR– (95% CI) | Post-test probability |
|---|---|---|---|---|---|---|
| Dyspnoea and suspected left ventricular dysfunction (pre-test probability 31%) | Increased preload (? echocardiogram) | Cardiomegaly | 4 | 64% | 0.7 | 24% |
| | | Redistribution/ congestion | 2 | 47% | 0.52 | 19% |
| | | Interstitial oedema | 2 | 47% | 0.7 | 22% |
| | Decreased ejection fraction (? echocardiogram) | Cardiomegaly | 2.4 | 52% | 0.62 | 21% |
| | | Redistribution/ congestion | 3 | 57% | 0.6 | 21% |
| | | Interstitial oedema | 4 | 64% | 0.9 | 29% |

In cases of clear pulmonary oedema, look for [B][16]:
- pulmonary blood flow distribution (upper fields predominating make heart failure much more likely)
- pulmonary oedema distribution (even distribution makes heart failure more likely; central or patchy distribution makes it less likely)
- vascular pedicle width (a narrow width makes heart failure less likely).

**Inverted pulmonary blood flow and even pulmonary oedema make heart failure more likely**

| Patient [B][16] | Target disorder (reference standard) | Diagnostic test | LR+ (95% CI) Heart failure | LR+ (95% CI) Overhydration | LR+ (95% CI) ARDS |
|---|---|---|---|---|---|
| On intensive care with radiographic evidence of pulmonary oedema | Heart failure, overhydration or ARDS (physiological evaluation or histology) | Pulmonary blood flow distribution: | | | |
| | | normal | 0.48 (0.23 to 0.97) | 0.57 (0.27 to 1.3) | 2.6 (1.4 to 4.9) |
| | | balanced | 0.58 (0.40 to 0.84) | 1.9 (1.4 to 2.6) | 0.97 (0.64 to 1.5) |
| | | inverted | 14 (3.4 to 55) | 0.0 (0.0 to 0.40) | 0.22 (0.057 to 0.88) |
| | | Distribution of pulmonary oedema: | | | |
| | | patchy | 0.0 (0.0 to 0.24) | 0.0 (0.0 to 0.70) | infinity (13 to inF) |
| | | central | 0.16 (0.066 to 0.38) | 6.5 (3.6 to 12) | 0.67 (0.31 to 1.5) |
| | | even | 3.3 (2.2 to 5.1) | 0.27 (0.13 to 0.56) | 0.52 (0.31 to 0.88) |
| | | Vascular pedicle width: | | | |
| | | narrow | 0.29 (0.083 to 0.98) | 0.0 (0.0 to 0.20) | 11 (3.2 to 37) |
| | | normal | 1.5 (0.85 to 2.5) | 0.45 (0.19 to 1.1) | 1.2 (0.65 to 2.1) |
| | | wide | 1.0 (0.74 to 1.4) | 5.7 (3.4 to 9.7) | 0.43 (0.24 to 0.79) |

**Pulmonary blood-flow distribution:**
- normal: lower lung fields predominate (typical of ARDS)
- balanced: equal in lower and upper lung fields (typical of overhydration and some heart failures)
- inverted: upper lung fields predominate (typical of heart failure, and rules out overhydration)

**Distribution of pulmonary oedema:**
- even: homogeneous from chest wall to heart and obeys gravity (typical of heart failure)
- central: perihilar only (typical of overhydration)
- patchy: spares many areas and often displays air bronchograms (rules out heart and overhydration, and rules in ARDS)

**Vascular pedicle width (just above aortic knob):**
- narrow: <43 mm (virtually rules out overhydration)
- normal: 43–53 mm (seen in all three)
- wide: >53 mm (overhydration)

- Consider an echocardiogram **[D]**.

## THERAPY

- Sit your patient upright **[D]**.
- Give oxygen **[A]**.
- Give salbutamol **[D]** and ipratropium **[B]**[19].

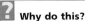

**Why do this?**
- Ipratropium produces small increases in $FEV_1$ **[B]**[19].

- Give morphine in small doses if markedly dyspnoeic **[A]**.
- Give a loop diuretic **[A]** intravenously **[D]**, e.g. frusemide 40–80 mg, and ask patient to remain in bed **[B]**[20].

**Why do this?**
- Patients who lie supine for 6 h compared with walking about have a larger diuresis (on average 500 ml more) and a larger natriuresis (on average 50 mmol more) **[B]**[20].

For large doses, consider using an infusion.

**Why do this?**
- Continuous iv frusemide causes a greater diuresis (on average 600 ml/day) and natriuresis (on average 60 mmol/day) than bolus infusions in patients on high doses **[A]**[21], but has no clear effect on mortality **[D]**[22].

Add a thiazide in resistant cases **[D]**[23].

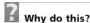
**Why do this?**
- 90% of patients with severe heart failure and fluid retention resistant to loop diuretics who receive thiazide diuretics in addition achieve a diuresis **[D]**[23]
- Bendrofluazide or metolazone are probably equally effective **[D]**[23]

## Pulmonary oedema
- Add high-dose isosorbide dinitrate **[A]**[24] (3 mg bolus iv every 3 min until oxygen saturation is 96% or mean arterial blood pressure decreased by $\geq$ 30% or < 90 mmHg).

**Why do this?**
- It is more effective than low-dose isosorbide dinitrate and high-dose furosemide at reducing MI and the need for mechanical ventilation **[A]**[24].
- There is no clear effect on mortality or adverse events **[A]**[24].
- Patients on high-dose isosorbide dinitrate have a greater rise in oxygen saturation (mean of 5%) and a greater fall in respiratory rate (mean of 6 breaths a minute) **[A]**[24].

- Give an ACE inhibitor **[A]**[23].

**Why do this?**
- It improves symptoms, without clearly preventing the need for ventilation **[A]**[25].

- Give patients with respiratory failure continuous positive airway pressure (CPAP).

**Why do this?**
- It reduces the need for intubation and ventilation, but has no clear effect on mortality **[A]**[26].
- It reduces length of stay on intensive care units (mean of 1.5 days shorter) **[A]**[27].
- Non-invasive positive pressure ventilation (NPPV) is not clearly as effective or safe as CPAP **[A]**[26].

**Severe pulmonary oedema: CPAP reduces endotracheal intubation**

| Patient [A][26] | Treatment | Comparator | Outcome | CER | RRR | NNT |
|---|---|---|---|---|---|---|
| Severe pulmonary oedema | CPAP | No CPAP | Endotracheal intubation at ? admission | 41% | 62% (34% to 78%) | 4 (3 to 8) |

- Consider inotropic support if there is hypotension **[D]**.

There is no clear benefit from:
- balloon counterpulsation **[D]**[28].

**Why?**
- Balloon counterpulsation does not clearly reduce mortality in patients with cardiogenic shock following myocardial infarction **[D]**[28].

## PREVENTION

Give an ACE inhibitor [A][29]

---

### ? Why do this?

■ It reduces death and hospitalisation compared with placebo [A][29].

**ACE inhibitors reduce death and hospitalisation**

| Patient [A][29] | Treatment | Comparator | Outcome | CER | OR | NNT |
|---|---|---|---|---|---|---|
| Severe heart failure | ACE inhibitor | Placebo | Death at 3 months | 22% | 0.77 (0.67 to 0.88) | 24 (16 to 47) |
| | | | Death or hospitalisation from congestive heart failure at 3 months | 33% | 0.65 (0.57 to 0.74) | 12 (9 to 16) |

■ It reduces death compared with isosorbide mononitrate and hydralazine [A][30] and is more cost-effective [A][31].

**Enalapril reduces death and treatment withdrawal better than isosorbide mononitrate and hydralazine**

| Patient [A][30] | Treatment | Comparator | Outcome | CER | RRR | NNT |
|---|---|---|---|---|---|---|
| Men with chronic heart failure | Enalapril mononitrate | Isosorbide at 2 years and hydralazine | Death | 25% | 28% (6% to 45%) | 14 (8 to 70) |
| | | | Medication stopped at 5 years | 29% | 24% (3% to 40%) | 15 (8 to 120) |

---

or losartan [A][32].

---

### ? Why do this?

■ It reduces death and hospital admissions in elderly patients compared with captopril [A][32].
■ Fewer patients discontinue medication, particularly due to coughing [A][32].

**Losartan reduces death and hospital admissions**

| Patient [A][32] | Treatment | Comparator | Outcome | CER | RRR | NNT |
|---|---|---|---|---|---|---|
| Elderly with symptomatic heart failure and an ejection fraction ≤ 40% | Losartan | Captopril | Death at 11 months | 8.7% | 44% (1% to 68%) | 26 (13 to 550) |
| | | | Any hospital admission at 11 months | 30% | 25% (4% to 42%) | 13 (7 to 83) |
| | | | Discontinued medication at 11 months | 21% | 41% (17% to 58%) | 12 (7 to 31) |
| | | | Discontinued medication due to cough at 11 months | 3.8% | 100% | 26 (17 to 54) |

---

Consider monitoring the blood pressure for the first dose.

**Why do this?**
- Falls in systolic blood pressure are usually small (on average 10 mmHg over several hours in elderly patients) on starting ACE inhibitors **[A]**[33], but watch for symptomatic hypotension **[D].**

Consider giving:
- digoxin in patients with a poor left ventricular ejection fraction and normal sinus rhythm **[A]**[34]

**Why do this?**
- It reduces hospital admissions, particularly from worsening heart failure, without reducing mortality **[A]**[34]
- However, more patients are admitted with suspected digoxin toxicity **[A]**[34].
- It is cost-effective **[A]**[35].

**Digoxin reduces hospital admissions**

| Patient **[A]**[34] | Treatment | Comparator | Outcome | CER | RRR | NNT |
|---|---|---|---|---|---|---|
| Symptomatic heart failure LV ejection fraction < 45% Normal sinus rhythm | Digoxin | Placebo | Any hospital admission | 67 | 4% (1% to 7%) | 36 (20 to 200) |
| | | | Hospital admission for worsening heart failure at 3 years | 35 | 23% (17% to 28%) | 13 (10 to 18) |
| | | | Hospital admission with suspected digoxin toxicity at 3 years | 0.91 | −120% (−235% to −44%) | −92 (−190 to −60) |

- spironolactone **[A]**[36]

**Why do this?**
- It reduces mortality and admissions to hospital, and improves symptoms, without clearly increasing the incidence of severe hyperkalaemia **[A]**[36].
- It can cause intolerable side-effects, including gynaecomastia in men **[A]**[36].

**Spironolactone reduces death, hospital admissions and improves symptoms**

| Patient | Treatment | Comparator | Outcome | CER | RRR | NNT |
|---|---|---|---|---|---|---|
| Severe heart failure (LV ejection fraction < 35%) | Digoxin | Placebo | Death at 24 months | 46% | 25% (15% to 33%) | 9 (6 to 15) |
| | | | Hospitalisation due to worsening heart failure at 24 months | 36% | 27% (15% to 37%) | 11 (7 to 20) |
| | | | Improvement in NYHA class at 24 months | 33% | 24% (9% to 41%) | 13 (8 to 30) |
| | | | Discontinuation of medication due to adverse event at 24 months | 4.8% | −59% (−130% to −8%) | −36 (−210 to −20) |
| | | | Gynaecomastia in men at 24 months | 0.95% | −600% (−1370% to −240%) | −17 (−26 to −13) |

● amiodarone in patients with left ventricular dysfunction [A][37][A][38].

> **? Why do this?**
> ■ It reduces mortality [A][37] [A][38].
>
> **Amiodarone reduces the risk of dying suddenly**

| Patient [A][37] [A][38] | Treatment | Comparator | Outcome | CER | OR | NNT |
|---|---|---|---|---|---|---|
| At risk of sudden death | Amiodarone | Placebo, sotalol, propranolol | Death at ? 1 year | 26% | 0.81 (0.69 to 0.94) | 26 (16 to 86) |
| | | | Sudden death at ? 1 year | 13% | 0.70 (0.58 to 0.85) | 28 (20 to 57) |

## Arrange support by a multidisciplinary team [A][39][A][40].

> **? Why?**
> ■ A single visit by a nurse and a pharmacist to assess the need for further intervention and to ensure optimal compliance with medication reduces out-of-hospital deaths [A][37].
>
> **A multidisciplinary team intervention reduces out-of-hospital death**

| Patient [A][39] | Treatment | Comparator | Outcome | CER | RRR | NNT |
|---|---|---|---|---|---|---|
| Discharged following an admission with heart failure | Multidisciplinary team intervention | Usual follow-up | Out-of-hospital death at 18 months | 19% | 78% (4% to 95%) | 7 (4 to 43) |

> **?**
> ■ A nurse-directed multidisciplinary care package (involving patient education, a prescribed diet, social service consultation and planning for an early discharge, medication review and intensive follow-up) reduces readmission in high-risk elderly patients [A][40].
>
> **A multidisciplinary care package reduces hospital readmission in high-risk elderly patients**

| Patient [A][40] | Treatment | Comparator | Outcome | CER | RRR | NNT |
|---|---|---|---|---|---|---|
| Elderly patient with heart failure considered at high-risk for readmission | Nurse-directed multidisciplinary care package | Usual care by primary physician | Readmission at 90 days | 42% | 31% (5% to 50%) | 8 (4 to 45) |
| | | | Readmission for heart failure at 90 days | 39% | 56% (33% to 71%) | 5 (3 to 9) |

Once your patient has been stable for several months, consider:
● beta-blockers for patients with severe heart failure and a poor ejection fraction

**Why?**

■ Beta-blockers improve symptoms **[A]**[41] **[A]**[42] and reduce mortality **[A]**[40] and hospital admissions **[A]**[43] particularly for worsening heart failure.

**Beta-blockers reduce death and improve symptoms**

| Patient **[A]**[40] | Treatment | Comparator | Outcome | CER | RRR | NNT |
|---|---|---|---|---|---|---|
| Stable heart failure | Beta-blockers | Placebo | Death at 8 months | 12% | 32% (22% to 47%) | 26 (18 to 38) |
| | | | Hospitalised for worsening heart failure at 8 months | 17% | 41% (26% to 52%) | 14 (11 to 23) |
| | | | Improvement in NYHA class at 8 months | 21% | –32% (–74% to –1%) | 3 (2 to 4) |

**Beta-blockers reduce hospital admissions**

| Patient **[A]**[43] | Treatment | Comparator | Outcome | CER | RRR | NNH |
|---|---|---|---|---|---|---|
| Stable heart failure | Bisoprolol | Placebo | Admitted to hospital at 1.3 years | 12% | 15% (6% to 23%) | 18 (30–170) |

Avoid D-sotalol **[A]**[44].

 **Why?**

■ It increases mortality **[A]**[44]

**D-sotalol increases mortality**

| Patient | Treatment | Comparator | Outcome | CER | RRR | NNH |
|---|---|---|---|---|---|---|
| Severe heart failure **[A]**[44] | D-sotalol | Placebo | Death at 5 months | 3% | –65% (–135% to –16%) | 50 (30 to 170) |

● long-term exercise training **[A]**[45]

 **Why?**

■ Exercise training (stretching exercises followed by 40 min of exercise cycling twice a week for 14 months) reduces hospital admissions for heart failure and death **[A]**[45]

**Exercise training reduces death and hospitalisation for heart failure**

| Patient **[A]**[45] | Treatment | Comparator | Outcome | CER | RRR | NNT |
|---|---|---|---|---|---|---|
| Stable heart failure | Exercise training | No training | Death at 3.3 years | 41% | 56% (13% to 78%) | 4 (2 to 18) |
| | | | Hospital admission for heart failure at 3.3 years | 29% | 65% (10% to 86%) | 5 (3 to 29) |

● amlodipine for dilated cardiomyopathy **[A]**[46]

**Why?**
- It reduces death and cardiovascular events **[A]**[46].
- There is no clear benefit for patients with heart failure due to ischaemic heart disease **[D]**[47].

**Amlodipine reduces death in dilated cardiomyopathy**

| Patient **[A]**[46] | Treatment | Comparator | Outcome | CER | RRR | NNT |
|---|---|---|---|---|---|---|
| Heart failure due to dilated cardiomyopathy | Amlodipine | Placebo | Death or cardiovascular morbidity at 3 years | 37% | 25% (0% to 43%) | 11 (6 to 650) |
| Death | Amlodipine | Placebo | Death at 3 years | 31% | 43% (19% to 60%) | 7 (5 to 19) |

- coronary artery bypass graft for patients with angina **[B]**[48].

 **Why?**
- CABG reduces mortality in patients with heart failure and angina by 30–50%, and improves functional outcome, assessed as either improvement in ejection fraction or decrease in NYHA class **[B]**[48].
- However, 5% of patients aged < 60 years with mild heart failure die from surgery, and 30% of patients aged > 70 years with severe heart failure and a comorbid condition die from surgery **[B]**[48].
- There is not enough evidence to indicate whether functional status or survival improves in the absence of angina **[B]**[48].

There is no benefit from:
- dofetilide **[A]**[49]

 **Why?**
- It does not reduce mortality **[A]**[49].

- ibopamine **[A]**[50]

**Why?**
- It increase the risk of dying, especially suddenly, without clearly improving symptoms **[A]**[50].

**Ibopamine kills patients**

| Patient **[A]**[50] | Treatment | Comparator | Outcome | CER | RRR | NNH |
|---|---|---|---|---|---|---|
| Severe heart failure | Ibopamine | Placebo | Death at 1 year | 20% | −20% (−42% to −2%) | 24 (13 to 280) |
| | | | Sudden death at 1 year | 4.8% | −50% (−120% to −4%) | 41 (22 to 60) |

- phosphodiesterase inhibitors **[A]**[51]

**Why?**

■ Phosphodiesterase inhibitors increase the risk of dying **[A]**[51].

**Phosphodiesterase inhibitors increase the risk of dying**

| Patient **[A]**[51] | Treatment | Comparator | Outcome | CER | OR | NNH |
|---|---|---|---|---|---|---|
| Overt chronic heart failure | Phosphodiesterase inhibitors (except vesnarinone) | Placebo | Death at 3 months | 17% | 1.42 (1.13 to 1.80) | 18 (10 to 15) |

## PROGNOSIS

Readmission to hospital is common **[B]**[52] **[B]**[53], particularly with heart failure **[B]**[53].

**Note**

■ Two-thirds of patients are readmitted within 18 months (62%; 95% CI: 53% to 72%) **[B]**[52].

Patients are more likely to be readmitted if they have **[B]**[54]:

● symptoms of chronic heart failure
● reduced general health or reduced activities of daily living.

Death is common **[A]**[55] **[B]**[56] **[A]**[57], particularly with acute pulmonary oedema **[A]**[58]. Many patients die suddenly **[A]**[55].

**Note**

■ One in seven patients with heart failure is dead within a year (15%; 95% CI: 13% to 17%) **[A]**[57]. A quarter of patients with heart failure are dead within 3 years (24%; 95% CI: 23% to 25%) **[B]**[56].
■ A third of patients with severe heart failure are dead within a year (38%; 95% CI: 33% to 42%) **[A]**[55]. One in seven die suddenly (14%; 95% CI: 11% to 17%) **[A]**[50].
■ One in seven patients with acute pulmonary oedema dies in hospital (15%; 95% CI 9.6% to 19%) **[A]**[58].

Patients are at increased risk of dying if they have:

- severe heart failure (NYHA class III or IV) **[B]**[56] **[B]**[59]
- had a previous stroke **[B]**[56]
- atrial fibrillation **[B]**[56]
- diabetes mellitus **[B]**[56]
- non-ischaemic heart disease **[A]**[60]
- syncope **[B]**[17]

**Why?**

Severe heart failure and cardiovascular risk factors increase the risk of dying

| Patient | Prognostic factor | Outcome | Control rate | OR (95% CI) | NNF+ (95% CI) |
|---|---|---|---|---|---|
| Heart failure | NYHA class III or IV *independent* | Death at 3 years | 24% | 1.74 (1.53 to 1.97) | 9 (7 to 12) |
| | Ejection fraction per 10% decrease *independent* | | 24% | 1.45 (1.39 to 1.50) | 14 (12 to 16) |
| | Prior stroke *independent* | | 24% | 1.43 (1.20 to 1.71) | 14 (9 to 29) |
| | Atrial fibrillation *independent* | | 24% | 1.34 (1.12 to 1.62) | 18 (10 to 48) |
| | Diabetes mellitus *independent* | | 24% | 1.34 (1.19 to 1.51) | 18 (12 to 30) |

- frequent ventricular tachycardia **[A]**[60]

**Why?**

Ventricular tachycardias increase the risk of dying

| Patient | Prognostic factor | Outcome | Control rate | RR (95% CI) | NNF+ (95% CI) |
|---|---|---|---|---|---|
| Severe heart failure | Non-sustained ventricular tachycardia *independent* **[A]**[55] | Death at 13 months | 24% | 1.62 (1.22 to 2.16) | 5 (3 to 15) |

- an enlarged heart (increased left end-diastolic volume **[A]**[61] or an enlarged cardiothoracic ratio) **[A]**[61]
- reduced heart rate variability **[A]**[61]
- reduced or worsening ejection fraction **[B]**[56] **[B]**[57]

**Why?**
Cardiac enlargement increases the risk of dying

| Patient | Prognostic factor | Outcome | Control rate | RR (95% CI) | NNF+ (95% CI) |
|---|---|---|---|---|---|
| Severe heart failure | Increased left ventricular end-diastolic diameter (by 12 mm) *independent* [B][56] | Death at 15 months | 12% | 1.69 (1.18 to 2.44) | 12 (6 to 45) |
| | Increased cardiothoracic ratio (by 6.5%) *independent* [A][56] | Death at 15 months | 12% | 1.62 (1.23 to 2.14) | 13 (7 to 35) |

A low ejection fraction increases the risk of dying

| Patient [B][51] | Prognostic factor | Outcome | Control rate | OR (95% CI) | NNF+ (95% CI) |
|---|---|---|---|---|---|
| Heart failure | Ejection fraction per 10% decrease *independent* | Death at 12 months | 24% | 1.45 (1.39 to 1.50) | 14 (12 to 16) |

- a reduced serum sodium level [B][17].

 **Why?**
A low serum sodium increases the risk of dying

| Patient | Prognostic factor | Outcome | Control rate | RR (95% CI) | NNF+ (95% CI) |
|---|---|---|---|---|---|
| Severe heart failure | Decrease in serum sodium (by 3 mmol/l) *independent* [B][17] | Death at 15 months | 12% | 1.42 (1.08 to 1.87) | 19 (9 to 100) |

Patients with acute pulmonary oedema are more likely to survive if they [A][58]:

- survived previous attacks
- have a good recovery following emergency treatment
- do not require dopamine support
- have ventricular arrhythmias present.

Arterial thromboembolic events are rare [B][62].

 **Why?**
■ Roughly 2% of patients with chronic heart failure have arterial thromboembolic events per year [B][62].

**Guideline writer**: Christopher Ball
**CAT writers**: Christopher Ball, Clare Wotton, Ati Yates

# REFERENCES

| No | Level | Citation |
|---|---|---|
| 1 | 2a | Badgett RG, Mulrow CD, Otto PM et al. How well can the chest radiograph diagnose left ventricular dysfunction? J Gen Intern Med 1996; 11: 625–34 |
| 2 | 2c | Schocken DD, Arrieta MI, Leaverton PE et al. Prevalence and mortality of congestive heart failure in the United States. J Am Coll Cardiol 1992; 20: 301–6 |
| 3 | 2b | Davie AP, Francis CM, Caruana L et al. Assessing diagnosis in heart failure: which features are any use? Q J Med 1997; 90: 335–9 |
| 4 | 2b | Senni M, Tribouilloy CM, Rodeheffer RJ et al. Congestive heart failure in the community: a study of all incident cases in Olmsted County, Minnesota, in 1991. Circulation 1998; 98: 2282–9 |
| 5 | 2a | Badgett RG et al. Can clinical examination diagnose left-sided heart failure in adults. JAMA 1997; 277: 1712–19 |
| 6 | 1b | Davis KM, Fish LC, Elahi D. Atrial natriuretic peptide levels in the prediction of congestive heart failure risk in frail elderly. JAMA 1992; 267: 2625–9 |
| 7 | 2a | Cook DJ, Simel DL. Does this patient have an abnormal jugular venous pressure? JAMA 1996; 275: 630–4 |
| 8 | 1b | O'Neil TW et al. Diagnostic value of the apex beat. Lancet 1988; i: 410–11 |
| 9 | 1b | Precordial percussion for detecting cardiomegaly. ACP J Club 1992 Jan–Feb; 116: 20. Summary of: Heckerling PS et al. Accuracy of precordial percussion in detecting cardiomegaly. Am J Med. 1991; 91: 328–34 |
| 10 | 3b | Lipsitz LA et al. Syncope in institutionalised elderly: the impact of multiple pathological conditions and situational stress. J Chron Dis 1986; 39: 619–30 |
| 11 | 2a | Etchells E et al. Does this patient have an abnormal systolic murmur? JAMA 1997; 277: 564–71 |
| 12 | 1a | Choudhry NK, Etchells EE. Does this patient have aortic regurgitation? JAMA 1999; 281: 2231–8 |
| 15 | 2a | History and physical examination for dyspnea: a review. ACP J Club 1993 Nov–Dec; 119: 90. Summary of: Mulrow CD et al. Discriminating causes of dyspnea through clinical examination. J Gen Intern Med 1993; 8: 383–92 |
| 16 | 2b | Milne EN, Pistolesi M, Miniati M et al. The radiologic distinction of cardiogenic and noncardiogenic edema. Am J Roentgenol 1985; 144: 879–94 |
| 17 | 2b | Middlekauff HR et al. Syncope in advanced heart failure: high risk of sudden death regardless of origin of syncope. J Am Coll Cardiol 1993; 21: 110–6 |
| 18 | 2b | Davie AP, Francis CM, Love MP et al. Value of the electrocardiogram in identifying heart failure due to left ventricular systolic dysfunction. BMJ 1996; 312: 222 |
| 19 | 2b | Rolla G, Bucca C, Brussino L et al. Bronchodilating effect of ipratropium bromide in heart failure. Eur Respir J 1993; 6: 1492–5 |
| 20 | 2b | Ring-Larsen H, Henriksen JH, Wilken C et al. Diuretic treatment in decompensated cirrhosis and congestive heart failure: effect of posture. BMJ 1986; 292: 1351–3 |

| No | Level | Citation |
|----|-------|----------|
| 21 | 1b | Dormans TPJ et al. Diuretic efficacy of high dose furosemide in severe heart failure: bolus injection versus continuous infusion. J Am Coll Cardiol 1996; 28: 376–82 |
| 22 | 2b- | Schuller D, Lynch JP, Fine D. Protocol-guided diuretic managment: comparison of furosemide by continuous infusion and intermittent bolus. Crit Care Med 1997; 25: 1969–75 |
| 23 | 1b- | Channer KS, McLean KA, Lawson-Matthew P et al. Combination diuretic treatment in severe heart failure: a randomised controlled trial. Br Heart J 1994; 71: 146–50 |
| 24 | 1b | Cotter G et al. Randomised trial of high-dose isosorbide dinitrate plus low-dose furosemide versus high-dose furosemide plus low-dose isosorbide dinitrate in severe pulmonary oedema. Lancet 1998; 351: 389–93 |
| 25 | 1b | Hamilton RJ, Carter WA, Gallagher EJ. Rapid improvement of acute pulmonary edema with sublingual captopril. Academic Emergency Medicine 1996; 3: 205–212 |
| 26 | 1a | Pang D, Keenan SP, Cook DJ et al. The effect of positive pressure airway support on mortality and the need for intubation in cardiogenic pulmonary edema: a systematic review. Chest 1998; 114: 1185–92 |
| 27 | 1b | Bersten AD et al. Treatment of severe cardiogenic pulmonary edema with continuous positive airway pressure delivered by face mask. N Engl J Med 1991; 325: 1825–30 |
| 28 | 2b– | Anderson RD, Ohman EM, Holmes DR et al. Use of intraaortic balloon counterpulsation in patients presenting with cardiogenic shock: observations from GUSTO-1 study. J Am Coll Cardiol 1997; 30: 708–15 |
| 29 | 1a | Garg R, Yusuf S. Overview of randomized trials of angiotensin-converting enzyme inhibitors on mortality and morbidity in patients with heart failure. JAMA 1995; 273: 1450–6 |
| 30 | 1b | Cohn JN et al. A comparison of enalapril with hydralazine-isosorbide dinitrate in the treatment of chronic congestive heart failure. N Engl J Med 1991; 325: 303–10 |
| 31 | 1b | Paul SD, Kuntz KM, Eagle KA et al. Costs and effectiveness of angiotensin converting enzyme inhibition in patients with congestive heart failure. Arch Intern Med 1994; 154: 1143–9 |
| 32 | 1b | Losartan compared with captopril reduced mortality but not renal function in heart failure. ACP J Club 1997 Sep–Oct; 127: 29. Summary of: Pitt B, Segal R, Martinez FA et al. on behalf of ELITE Study Investigators. Randomised trial of losartan versus captopril in patients over 65 with heart failure (Evaluation of Losartan in the Elderly Study, ELITE). Lancet 1997; 349: 747–52 |
| 33 | 1b | MacFadyen RJ, Lees KR, Reid JL. Differences in first dose response to angiotenson converting enzyme inhibition in congestive heart failure: a placebo controlled study. Br Heart J 1991; 66: 206–11 |
| 34 | 1b | Garg R, Gorlin R, Smith T et al. The Digitalis Investigation Group. The effect of digoxin on mortality and morbidity in patients with heart failure. N Engl J Med 1997; 336: 525–33 |
| 35 | 1b | Ward RE, Gheorghiade M, Young JB et al. Economic outcomes of withdrawal of digoxin therapy in adult patients with stable congestive heart failure. J Am Coll Cardiol 1995; 26: 93–101 |
| 36 | 1b | Pitt B, Zannad F, Remme WJ et al. The effect of spironolactone on morbidity and mortality in patients with severe heart failure (RALES). New Engl J Med 1999; 341: 709–17. |
| 37 | 1a | Sim I, McDonald KM, Lavori PW et al. Quantitative overview of randomised trials of amiodarone to prevent sudden cardiac death. Circulation 1997; 96: 2823–9. |

| No | Level | Citation |
|----|-------|----------|
| 38 | 1a | Review: amiodarone reduces mortality after MI and for congestive heart failure. Evidence-Based Med 1998; 3(4): 112. Summary of: Amiodarone Trials Meta-analysis Investigators: effect of prophylactic amiodarone on mortality after acute myocardial infarction and in congestive heart failure: meta-analysis of individual data for 6500 patients in randomised trials. Lancet 1997; 350: 1417–24 |
| 39 | 1b | Stewart S, Pearson S, Horowitz JD. Effects of a home-based intervention among patients with congestive heart failure discharged from acute hospital care. Arch Intern Med 1999; 159: 257–61 |
| 40 | 1b | Rich MW et al. A multidisciplinary intervention to prevent the readmission of elderly patients with congestive heart failure. N Engl J Med 1995; 333: 1190–5 |
| 41 | 1a | Zarembski DG, Nolan PE, Slack MK et al. Meta-analysis of the use of low-dose beta-adrenergic blocking therapy in idiopathic or ischemic dilated cardiomyopathy. Am J Cardiol 1996; 77: 1247–50 |
| 42 | 1a | Lechat P, Packer M, Chalon S et al. Clinical effects of beta-adrenergic blockade in chronic heart failure: a meta-analysis of double-blind, placebo-controlled randomized trials. Circulation 1998; 98: 1184–91 |
| 43 | 1b | CIBIS-II Investigators and Committees et al. The Cardiac Insufficiency Bisoprolol Study II (CIBIS-II): a randomised trial. Lancet 1999; 353: 9–13 |
| 44 | 1b | Waldo AL et al. Effect of d-sotalol on mortality in patients with left ventricular dysfunction after recent and remote myocardial infarction. Lancet 1996; 348: 7–12 |
| 45 | 1b | Belardinelli R, Georgiou D, Cianci G et al. Randomized controlled trial of long-term moderate exercise training in chronic heart failure: effects on functional capacity, quality of life and clinical outcome. Circulation 1999; 99: 1173–82 |
| 46 | 1b | Packer M et al. Effect of amlodipine on morbidity and mortality in severe chronic heart failure. N Engl J Med 1996; 335: 1107–14 |
| 47 | 1b– | Packer M et al. Effect of amlodipine on morbidity and mortality in severe chronic heart failure. N Engl J Med 1996; 335: 1107–14 |
| 48 | 2a | DARE summary of Baker DW et al. Management of heart failure III: the role of revascularization in the treatment of patients with moderate or severe left ventricular systolic dysfunction. JAMA 1994; 272: 1528–34 |
| 49 | 1b | Torp-Pedersen C, Møller M, Bloch-Thomsen PE et al. Dofetilide in patients with congestive heart failure and left ventricular dysfunction. N Engl J Med 1999; 341: 857–65 |
| 50 | 1b | Hampton JR, van Veldhuisen DJ, Kleber FX et al. Randomised study of effect of ibopamine on survival in patients with advanced severe heart failure (PRIME-II). Lancet 1997; 349: 971–7 |
| 51 | 1a | Nony P, Boissel J-P, Lievre M et al. Evaluation of the effect of phosphodiesterase inhibitors on mortality in chronic heart failure patients: a meta-analysis. Eur J Clin Pharmacol 1994; 46: 191–6 |
| 52 | 2b | Stewart S, Pearson S, Horowitz JD. Effects of a home-based intervention among patients with congestive heart failure discharged from acute hospital care. Arch Intern Med 1999; 159: 57–61 |
| 53 | 2b | Rich MW et al. A multidisciplinary intervention to prevent the readmission of elderly patients with congestive heart failure. NEJM 1995; 333: 1190–5 |

| No | Level | Citation |
|---|---|---|
| 54 | 2b | Konstam V, Salem D, Pouleur H et al. Baseline quality of life as a predictor of mortality and hospitalization in 5025 patients with congestive heart failure. Am J Cardiol 1996; 78: 890–5 |
| 55 | 1b | Doval HC, Nul DR, Grancelli HO et al. Nonsustained ventricular tachycardia in severe heart failure: independent marker of increased mortality due to sudden death. Circulation 1996; 94: 3198–203 |
| 56 | 2b | Dries NL, Exner DV, Gersh BJ et al. Atrial fibrillation is associated with an increased risk of mortality and heart failure progression in patients with asymptomatic and symptomatic left ventricular systolic dysfunction: a retrospective analysis of the SOLVD trials. J Am Coll Cardiol 1998; 32: 695–703 |
| 57 | 2b | Cintron G, Johnson G, Francis G et al. Prognostic significance of serial changes in left ventricular ejection fraction in patients with congestive heart failure (suppl VI). Circulation 1993; 87: 17–23 |
| 58 | 1b | Sardella F, Checchini M, Pierini A et al. Prognostic factors in acute cardiogenic pulmonary edema. Eur J Intern Med 1997; 8: 171–6 |
| 59 | 2b | Senni M, Tribouilloy CM, Rodeheffer RJ et al. Congestive heart failure in the community: a study of all incident cases in Olmsted County, Minnesota, in 1991. Circulation 1998; 98: 2282–9 |
| 60 | 1b | Gradman A, Deedwania P, Cody R et al. Predictors of total mortality and sudden death in mild to moderate heart failure. J Am Coll Cardiol 1989; 14: 564–70 |
| 61 | 1b | Nolan J, Batin PD, Andrews R et al. Prospective study of heart rate variability and mortality in chronic heart failure: results of United Kingdom Heart Failure Evaluation and Assessment of Risk Trial (UK-Heart). Circulation 1998; 98: 1510–16 |
| 62 | 2b | Baker DW, and Wright RF. Management of heart failure IV: anticoagulation for patients with heart failure due to left ventricular systolic dysfunction. JAMA 1994; 272: 1614–18 |

# Exacerbation of chronic obstructive pulmonary disease (COPD)

Expiry date 2005

## PREVALENCE

- Exacerbations of chronic obstructive pulmonary disease are a common cause of dyspnoea leading to hospital admission (9%) **[B]**[1].

## CLINICAL FEATURES

Ask about:
- a previous history of COPD **[B]**[1] **[B]**[2]
- smoking **[A]**[3] – and how much for how long **[B]**[2]

---

**Why?**

■ Inhaling cigarettes increases the risk of being admitted to hospital with COPD **[A]**[3].

■ Remember COPD can occur in life-long non-smokers (5.1%; 95% CI: 4.7 to 5.4%) **[B]**[4].

**Heavy smoking makes COPD more likely**

| Patient | Target disorder (reference standard) | Diagnostic test | LR+ (95% CI) | Post-test probability | LR– (95% CI) | Post-test probability |
|---|---|---|---|---|---|---|
| Suspected COPD **[B]**[2] (pre-test probability 9%) | COPD (spirometry) | Smoking history ≥70 pack-years | 8.0 | 44% | 0.63 | 6% |
| Suspected COPD **[A]**[5] (pre-test probability: 9%) | COPD (spirometry) | Ever smoked | 1.2 (1.1 to 1.4) | 11% | 0.23 (0.08 to 0.64) | 2% |

---

- previous exacerbations **[B]**[6]

---

**Why?**

**Frequent exacerbations increase the risk of COPD exacerbations**

| Patient **[B]**[6] | Prognostic factor | Outcome | Control rate | OR (95% CI) | NNF+ (95% CI) |
|---|---|---|---|---|---|
| COPD | Frequent exacerbations in the past *independent* | 3 or more exacerbations of COPD at 1 year | 46% | 1.43 | 11 |

---

- cough **[B]**[1] and any recent increase **[D]**
- wheezing **[B]**[2] and any recent increase **[D]**
- exertional dyspnoea **[B]**[2]
- sputum production **[B]**[2] and any recent increase or purulence **[D]**.

## ❓ Why?

**A history of wheezing, sputum production and severe exertional dyspnoea make COPD more likely**

| Patient | Target disorder (reference standard) | Diagnostic test | LR+ (95% CI) | Post-test probability | LR– (95% CI) | Post-test probability |
|---|---|---|---|---|---|---|
| Suspected COPD **[B]**[2] (pre-test probability 9%) | COPD (spirometry) | Sputum production ≥ 1/4 cup per day | 4.0 | 28% | 0.84 | 8% |
| Suspected COPD **[A]**[5] (pre-test probability 9%) | | Symptoms of chronic bronchitis | 3.8 (2.0 to 7.2) | 27% | 0.66 (0.53 to 0.81) | 6% |
| | | History of wheezing | 3.1 (1.9 to 5.2) | 23% | 0.58 (0.45 to 0.75) | 5% |
| Suspected COPD **[B]**[2] (pre-test probability 9%) | | Severe exertional dyspnoea (grade IV) | 3.0 | 23% | 0.98 | 9% |
| Suspected COPD **[A]**[5] (pre-test probability 9%) | | Cough | 1.8 (1.2 to 2.6) | 15% | 0.69 (0.52 to 0.90) | 6 |
| | | Any dyspnoea | 1.2 (1.0 to 1.5) | 11% | 0.55 (0.31 to 0.98) | 5% |

**Symptoms of bronchitis and daily wheeze increase the risk of COPD exacerbations**

| Patient **[B]**[6] | Prognostic factor | Outcome | Control rate | OR (95% CI) | NNF+ (95% CI) |
|---|---|---|---|---|---|
| COPD | Daily wheeze *independent* | 3 or more exacerbations of COPD at 1 year | 46% | 1.34 | 14 |
| | Symptoms of bronchitis *independent* | | | 1.56 | 9 |

Look for **[A]**[5] **[B]**[2]:

- a barrel chest
- subxyphoid cardiac apical pulse
- decreased cardiac dullness on percussion
- decreased breath sounds
- wheezing
- crackles
- hyperresonance

## ? Why?

**Wheezing, a barrel chest and decreased cardiac dullness make COPD more likely**

| Patient | Target disorder (reference standard) | Diagnostic test | LR+ (95% CI) | Post-test probability | LR– (95% CI) | Post-test probability |
|---|---|---|---|---|---|---|
| Suspected COPD **[A]**[5] (pre-test probability 9%) | COPD (spirometry) | Wheezing on examination | 12 (1.7 to 98) | 54% | 0.87 (0.79 to 0.96) | 8% |
| Suspected COPD **[B]**[2] (pre-test probability 9%) | | Barrel chest | 10 | 50% | 0.90 | 8% |
| | | Decreased cardiac dullness | 10 | 50% | 0.88 | 8% |
| | | Crackles | 5.9 | 37% | 0.95 | 9% |
| | | Hyperresonance | 4.8 | 32% | 0.73 | 7% |
| | | Subxyphoid cardiac apical impulse | 4.6 | 31% | 0.94 | 7% |
| | | Decreased breath sounds | 3.7 | 27% | 0.70 | 9% |

- a prolonged expiratory time **[B]**[2]; measure the time that expiratory sounds are audible over the sternum during forced expiration.

## ? How?

**A prolonged expiratory time makes COPD more likely**

| Patient | Target disorder (reference standard) | Diagnostic test | LR+ (95% CI) | Post-test probability |
|---|---|---|---|---|
| Suspected COPD **[B]**[2] (pre-test probability 9%) | COPD (spirometry) | Forced expiratory time | | |
| | | >9 s | 4.8 | 32% |
| | | 6–9 s | 2.7 | 21% |
| | | <6 s | 0.45 | 4% |

## Note

- Clinical examination cannot safely diagnose or exclude COPD **[A]**[5].

**Clinical impression of moderate or severe COPD makes it more likely**

| Patient | Target disorder (reference standard) | Diagnostic test | LR+ (95% CI) | Post-test probability |
|---|---|---|---|---|
| Suspected COPD **[A]**[5] (pre-test probability 9%) | COPD (spirometry) | Clinical impression: moderate-severe | 4.2 (2.2 to 8.0) | 29% |
| | | Clinical impression: mild | 0.82 (0.55 to 1.2) | 8% |
| | | Clinical impression: no disease | 0.42 (0.25 to 0.70) | 4% |

## DIFFERENTIAL DIAGNOSIS

Think about other common causes of dyspnoea leading to hospital admission **[B]**[1]:

- asthma
- heart failure
- arrhythmias
- infection.

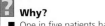
**Why?**
**Asthma and heart failure are common causes of dyspnoea**

| Hospital admissions **[B]**[1] | Cause of dyspnoea |
|---|---|
| Asthma | 33% |
| Heart failure | 31% |
| COPD | 9% |
| Arrhythmia | 7% |
| Infection | 5% |
| Interstitial lung disease | 4% |
| Anaemia | 2% |
| PE | <2% |

Remember other causes of COPD exacerbations:

- pneumothorax **[D]**
- ischaemic heart disease **[D]**.

## INVESTIGATIONS

- Blood count **[D]**.
- Urea and electrolytes, creatinine **[D]**.
- Cardiac enzymes **[D]**.
- Blood culture if strong clinical suspicion of infection **[D]**.
- Sputum culture if strong clinical suspicion of infection **[D]**.
- Arterial blood gases **[B]**[7].

**Why?**
■ One in five patients has carbon dioxide retention: (19%; 95% CI: 14% to 23%) **[B]**[7]

- ECG – look for evidence of right heart failure or ischaemic heart disease **[A]**[8].

**Why?**
**Right heart failure or ischaemic heart disease on ECG increases the risk of dying**

| Patient | Prognostic factor | Outcome | Control rate | OR (95% CI) | NNF+ (95% CI) |
|---|---|---|---|---|---|
| Severe COPD [A][8] | ECG signs of RVH or overload | Death at 3.4 years | 84% | 1.76 (1.30 to 2.38) | 16 (12 to 32) |
| | ECG signs of ischaemic heart disease | Death at 3.4 years | 84% | 1.79 (1.05 to 3.02) | 16 (10 to 160) |

- Chest X-ray [C][9] in all patients [A][10].

**Why?**
- Abnormal chest radiographs are common (40%; 95% CI: 37% to 49%) and clinical features do not usefully predict normal films [A][10].
- A fifth of patients have a chest X-ray that alters management (21%; 95% CI: 14% to 28%) [C][9].

- Peak expiratory flow rate [A][5] [B][11].
- Spirometry when recovered [A].

**Why?**
- This is the reference standard.

## THERAPY

- Give oxygen if hypoxic ($Pao_2 < 8.0$ kPa) [A][12] via mask or nasal cannula [D].

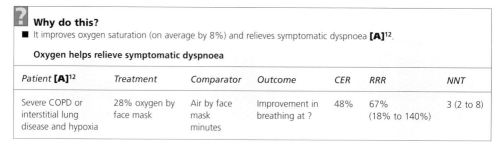
**Why do this?**
- It improves oxygen saturation (on average by 8%) and relieves symptomatic dyspnoea [A][12].

**Oxygen helps relieve symptomatic dyspnoea**

| Patient [A][12] | Treatment | Comparator | Outcome | CER | RRR | NNT |
|---|---|---|---|---|---|---|
| Severe COPD or interstitial lung disease and hypoxia | 28% oxygen by face mask | Air by face mask | Improvement in breathing at ? minutes | 48% | 67% (18% to 140%) | 3 (2 to 8) |

Use low concentrations to prevent $CO_2$ narcosis and monitor $Pco_2$ levels [D].
- Give salbutamol nebulisers [D].
- Give antibiotics [A][13] [A][14].

**❓ Why do this?**
- More patients recover and patients spend less time in hospital (on average 1.5 days less) **[A]**[14].
- Antibiotics increase peak flows slightly (on average 11 l/min) **[A]**[13].

**Antibiotics increase recovery rate and shorten hospital stay**

| Patient **[A]**[14] | Treatment | Comparator | Outcome | CER | RRR | NNT |
|---|---|---|---|---|---|---|
| Outpatient acute exacerbation of COPD | Antibiotics | Placebo | No resolution or worsening symptoms at 21 days | 45% | 29% (8% to 46%) | 8 (4 to 31) |

- Consider any of:

    - a second-generation cephalosporin (e.g. ceftibuten) **[A]**[15] **[A]**[16]
    - co-amoxiclav **[A]**[17]
    - a quinolone **[A]**[18]
    - a macrolide **[A]**[18] **[A]**[19]

**❓ Why?**
- These antibiotics are all equally effective at curing COPD exacerbations **[A]**[15–19], although cephalosporins may cause fewer adverse effects than macrolides **[A]**[16].

**Ceftibuten causes fewer adverse effects than clarithromycin**

| Patient **[A]**[16] | Treatment | Comparator | Outcome | CER | RRR | NNT |
|---|---|---|---|---|---|---|
| Acute exacerbation of COPD | Ceftibuten | Clarithromycin | Adverse effects at 7 days | 22% | 76% (50% to 88%) | 6 (4 to 11) |

**⓵ Note**
- Fewer patients are cured on trimethoprim-sulfamethoxazole than ofloxacin **[A]**[20].

**Trimethoprim-sulfamethoxazole cures fewer patients than ofloxacin**

| Patient **[A]**[16] | Treatment | Comparator | Outcome | CER | RRR | NNT |
|---|---|---|---|---|---|---|
| Acute exacerbation of COPD | Ofloxacin | Trimethoprim-sulfamethoxazole | Cure at 14 days | 52% | 55% (22% to 96%) | 4 (2 to 7) |

- Consider systemic steroids **[A]**[21].

**Why?**

■ Steroids help reduce length of hospital stay (on average by a day) **[A]**[21] and improve respiratory function (increasing $FEV_1$ on average by 70 l/min) **[A]**[22], although there is no clear reduction in treatment failure or deaths **[A]**[21].

■ However, steroids commonly cause adverse effects, particularly diabetes **[A]**[21].

**Steroids cause hyperglycaemia and other adverse effects**

| Patient **[A]**[21] | Treatment | Comparator | Outcome | CER | RRR | NNH |
|---|---|---|---|---|---|---|
| Acute exacerbation of COPD | Steroids for 2 or 8 weeks | Placebo | Hyperglycaemia at 6 months | 4% | −316% (−1066% to −49%) | 9 (21 to 6) |
| | | | Other adverse events at 6 months | 14% | −69% (−187% to 0%) | 10 (157 to 5) |

● Consider aminophylline **[A]**[23] in severe cases **[D]**.

**Why?**

■ It reduces hospital admissions in patients with acute exacerbations of COPD or asthma attending the emergency department, without clearly improving symptoms or respiratory function **[A]**[23].

■ Side-effects (nausea and vomiting) are common. **[A]**[24].

**Note**

■ Be wary of blood levels in patients on oral theophylline.

**Aminophylline reduces hospital admissions, but causes side effects**

| Patient | Treatment | Comparator | Outcome | CER | RRR | NNT |
|---|---|---|---|---|---|---|
| Asthma or COPD exacerbation **[A]**[23] | iv aminophylline | Placebo | Hospital admission at 2 h | 21% | 70% (14% to 90%) | 7 (4 to 31) |
| COPD exacerbation **[A]**[24] | iv aminophylline | Placebo | Adverse effects | 7.7% | −510% (−4200% to 14%) | −3 (−10 to −1) |

For patients with respiratory failure, consider:
● non-invasive ventilation **[B]**[25]

**Why?**

■ It reduces the need for endotracheal intubation and death **[B]**[25], and helps reduce days on mechanical ventilation if used as an adjunct to weaning (on average 6 days) **[A]**[26].

**Non-invasive ventilation reduces intubation and death in severe cases**

| Patient | Treatment | Comparator | Outcome | CER | RRR (%) | NNT |
|---|---|---|---|---|---|---|
| Acute exacerbation of COPD **[B]**[25] | Non-invasive ventilation | No ventilation | Required endotracheal intubation | 74% | 65% (40% to 80%) | 2 (1 to 3) |
| | | | Death at discharge | 26% | 67% (7% to 89%) | 5 (3 to 32) |
| COPD on mechanical ventilation **[A]**[26] | Non-invasive ventilation weaning | Standard weaning | Failure to wean | 52% | 69% (19% to 88%) | 3 (2 to 9) |

There is no clear benefit from:
- doxapram **[D]**[27]

**Why?**
- It does not clearly prevent deterioration in blood gas values nor reduce the rate of intubation and ventilation **[A]**[27].

- ipratropium **[D]**[28–30]

**Why?**
- Adding ipratropium to beta-agonists does not clearly improve respiratory function **[D]**[28] **[D]**[29] nor reduce days on nebulisers or in hospital **[D]**[30].

- magnesium sulphate **[D]**[31].

**Why?**
- It does not clearly improve respiratory function or prevent hospital admissions **[D]**[31].

## PREVENTION

- Advise patients to stop smoking **[A]**[32].

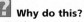

**Why do this?**
- It improves respiratory function (FEV$_1$ increases on average by 73 1/min after 1 year in mild cases); however, respiratory function continues to decline at the same rate as in patients who fail to stop after this **[A]**[32].

- Advise patients to have an influenza vaccination **[B]**[33]

**Why do this?**
- Influenza vaccination reduces pneumonia, hospitalisation and death in elderly patients **[B]**[33].

**Influenza vaccination reduces death and pneumonia**

| Patient **[B]**[33] | Treatment | Comparator | Outcome | CER | OR | NNT |
|---|---|---|---|---|---|---|
| Elderly | Influenza vaccination | No influenza vaccination | Death | 1% | 0.32 (0.24 to 0.44) | 140 (130 to 170) |
| | | | Hospitalisation | 0.8% | 0.50 (0.35 to 0.72) | 260 (200 to 460) |
| | | | Pneumonia | 1% | 0.47 (0.34 to 0.65) | 150 (120 to 220) |

and a pneumococcal vaccination **[A]**[34].

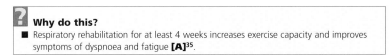

**Why do this?**
■ Pneumococcal vaccination reduces pneumococcal pneumonia, although it has no clear effect on mortality or the overall rate of pneumonia **[A]**[34].

**Pneumococcal vaccination reduces pneumococcal pneumonia**

| Patient **[A]**[34] | Treatment | Comparator | Outcome | CER | OR | NNT |
|---|---|---|---|---|---|---|
| Elderly | Influenza vaccination | No influenza vaccination | Pneumococcal pneumonia | 1% | 0.34 (0.24 to 0.48) | 150 (130 to 190) |

Consider:

● respiratory rehabilitation **[A]**[35]

**Why do this?**
■ Respiratory rehabilitation for at least 4 weeks increases exercise capacity and improves symptoms of dyspnoea and fatigue **[A]**[35].

● home oxygen in patients with severe hypoxia ($Po_2 < 7.5$ kPa or < 8.0 kPa with oedema) **[A]**[36] **[A]**[37] given continuously **[A]**[37]

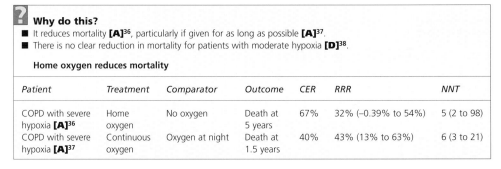

**Why do this?**
■ It reduces mortality **[A]**[36], particularly if given for as long as possible **[A]**[37].
■ There is no clear reduction in mortality for patients with moderate hypoxia **[D]**[38].

**Home oxygen reduces mortality**

| Patient | Treatment | Comparator | Outcome | CER | RRR | NNT |
|---|---|---|---|---|---|---|
| COPD with severe hypoxia **[A]**[36] | Home oxygen | No oxygen | Death at 5 years | 67% | 32% (−0.39% to 54%) | 5 (2 to 98) |
| COPD with severe hypoxia **[A]**[37] | Continuous oxygen | Oxygen at night | Death at 1.5 years | 40% | 43% (13% to 63%) | 6 (3 to 21) |

● mucolytics **[A]**[39].

**Why do this?**
■ Oral mucolytics may reduce exacerbations (on average one fewer a year) and days of sickness (on average 6 a year) **[A]**[39].

There is no clear benefit from:

● immunostimulating agents **[D]**[40].

## PROGNOSIS

Further exacerbations **[B]**[6] and readmissions are common **[B]**[7].

> **Note**
>
> ■ 54% will have three or more exacerbations in the next year (95% CI: 43% to 66%) **[B]**[6].
> ■ 70% are readmitted within a year (95% CI: 62% to 78%) **[B]**[7].

The risk is increased with **[B]**[6]:

- symptoms of bronchitis
- daily wheeze
- frequent exacerbations in the past.

> **Note**
>
> **Symptoms of bronchitis, frequent exacerbations and daily wheeze increase the risk of COPD exacerbations**
>
> | Patient **[B]**[6] | Prognostic factor | Outcome | Control rate | OR (95% CI) | NNF+ (95% CI) |
> |---|---|---|---|---|---|
> | COPD | Symptoms of bronchitis *independent* | 3 or more exacerbations of COPD at 1 year | 46% | 1.56 | 9 |
> | | Frequent exacerbations in the past *independent* | 3 or more exacerbations of COPD at 1 year | 46% | 1.43 | 11 |
> | | Daily wheeze *independent* | 3 or more exacerbations of COPD at 1 year | 46% | 1.34 | 14 |

Death is common **[B]**[7] **[B]**[41], particularly with worsening disease **[A]**[8] **[A]**[42] **[A]**[43].

> **Note**
> ■ One in 12 die in hospital (8.6%; 95% CI: 3.7% to 13%) **[B]**[7].
> ■ A quarter are dead within 3 years (23%; 95% CI: 21% to 26%) **[B]**[41].
> ■ A fifth of patients on home oxygen are dead at 2 years (22%; 95% CI: 15% to 28%) **[A]**[43].
> ■ A third with severe COPD and hypercapnia are dead at 6 months (33%: 95% CI: 30% to 36%) **[A]**[42]; 84% are dead at 3.5 years (95% CI: 80% to 89%) **[A]**[8].
> ■ Half of elderly patients are dead within 7 years (48%; 95% CI: 46% to 50%) **[B]**[44].

The risk of dying is increased with:

- increasing age **[A]**[8] **[A]**[43] **[B]**[41]
- worsening respiratory function **[A]**[43]
- worsening physical disability **[A]**[42] **[B]**[41]
- heart failure **[A]**[42] **[A]**[43]
- ischaemic heart disease **[A]**[8]
- chronic renal failure **[A]**[8].

## ❓Why?
### Heart failure, ischaemic heart disease and renal failure increase the risk of dying

| Patient | Prognostic factor | Outcome | Control rate | OR (95% CI) | NNF+ (95% CI) |
|---|---|---|---|---|---|
| Severe COPD [A][42] | Acute exacerbation due to congestive heart failure | Survival at 6 months | 67% | 0.66 (0.45 to 0.97) | 4 (3 to 49) |
| | Cor pulmonale | Survival at 6 months | 67% | 0.67 (0.45 to 0.99) | 4 (3 to 150) |
| Severe COPD [A][8] | Chronic renal failure | Death at 3.4 years | 84% | 1.42 (1.02 to 1.96) | 25 (14 to 390) |
| | ECG signs of RVH or overload | Death at 3.4 years | 84% | 1.76 (1.30 to 2.38) | 16 (12 to 32) |
| | ECG signs of ischaemic heart disease | Death at 3.4 years | 84% | 1.79 (1.05 to 3.02) | 16 (10 to 160) |

**Guideline writer**: Christopher Ball
**CAT writers**: Robert Philips, Clare Wotton, Christopher Ball

## REFERENCES

| No | Level | Citation |
|---|---|---|
| 1 | 2a | History and physical examination for dyspnoea: a review. ACP J Club 1993 Nov- Dec; 119:90. Summary of:Mulrow CD et al. Discriminating causes of dyspnoea through clinical examination. J Gen Intern Med 1993; 8: 383–92 |
| 2 | 2a | Holleman DR, Simel DL. Does the clinical examination predict airflow limitation? JAMA 1995; 275: 313–9 |
| 3 | 1b | Prescott E, Bjerg AM, Andersen PK et al. Gender difference in smoking effects on lung function and risk of hospitalization for COPD: results from a Danish longitudinal population study. Eur Respir J 1997; 10: 822–7 |
| 4 | 2c | Whittemore AS, Perlin SA, DiCiccio Y. Chronic obstructive pulmonary disease in lifelong nonsmokers: results from NHANES. Am J Public Health 1995; 85: 702–6 |
| 5 | 1b | Holleman DL, Simel DL, Goldberg JS et al. Diagnosis of obstructive airways disease from the clinical examination. J Gen Intern Med 1993; 8: 63–8 |
| 6 | 2b | Seemungal TAR, Donaldson GC, Paul EA et al. Effect of exacerbation on quality of life in patients with chronic obstructive pulmonary disease. Am J Respir Crit Care Med 1998; 157: 1418–22 |
| 7 | 2c | Gibson PG, Wlodarczyk JH, Wilson AJ et al. Severe exacerbations of chronic obstructive airways disease: health resource use in general practice and hospital. J Qual Clin Pract 1998; 18: 125–33 |
| 8 | 1b | Incalzi RA, Fuso L, De Rosa M et al. Co-morbidity contributes to predict mortality of patients with chronic obstructive pulmonary disease. Eur Respir J 1997; 10: 2794–800 |
| 9 | 4c | Tsai TW, Gallagher EJ, Lombardi G et al. Guidelines for the selective ordering of admission chest radiography in adult obstructive airway disease. Ann Emerg Med 1993; 22: 1854–8 |
| 10 | 1a | Emerman CL, Cydulka RK. Evaluation of high-yield criteria for chest radiography in acute exacerbation of chronic obstructive pulmonary disease. Ann Emerg Med 1993; 22: 680–4 |

| No | Level | Citation |
|----|-------|----------|
| 11 | 2a | Badgett RG, Tanaka DJ, Hunt DK et al. The clinical evaluation for diagnosing obstructive airways disease in high-risk patients. Chest 1994; 106: 1427–31 |
| 12 | 1b | Swinburn CR, Mould H, Stone TN et al. Symptomatic benefit of supplemental oxygen in hypoxemic patients with chronic lung disease. Am Rev Respir Dis 1991; 143: 913–15 |
| 13 | 1a | Saint S, Bent S, Vittinghoff E et al. Antibiotics in chronic obstructive pulmonary disease exacerbations. JAMA 1995; 273: 957–60 |
| 14 | 1b | Anthonisen NR, Manfreda J, Warren CP et al. Antibiotic therapy in exacerbations of chronic obstructive pulmonary disease. Ann Intern Med 1987; 106: 196–204 |
| 15 | 1b | McAdoo MA, Rice K, Gordon GR et al. Comparison of ceftibuten once daily and amoxicillin-clavulanate three times daily in the treatment of acute exacerbations of chronic bronchitis. Clin Ther 1998; 20: 88–100 |
| 16 | 1b | Ziering W, McElvaine P. Randomized comparison of once-daily ceftibuten and twice-daily clarithromycin in the treatment of acute exacerbation of chronic bronchitis. Infection 1998; 26: 72–9 |
| 17 | 1b | Allegra L, Konietzko N, Leophonte P et al. Comparative safety and efficacy of sparfloxacin in the treatment of acute exacerbations of chronic obstructive pulmonary disease: a double-blind, randomised, parallel, multicentre study. J Antimicrob Chemother 1996; 37: 93–104 |
| 18 | 1b | Chodosh S, Laksminarayan S, Swarz H et al. Efficacy and safety of a 10-day course of 400 or 600 milligrams of grepafloxacin once daily for treatment of acute bacterial exacerbations of chronic bronchitis: comparison with a 10-day course of 500 milligrams of ciprofloxacin twice daily. Antimicrob Agents Chemother 1998; 42: 114–20 |
| 19 | 1b | Anzueto A, Niederman MS, Haverstock DC et al. Efficacy of ciprofloxacin and clarithromycin in acute bacterial exacerbation of complicated chronic bronchitis: interim analysis. Clin Ther 1997; 19: 989–1001 |
| 20 | 1b | Perez-Gonzalvo ME, Mosquera-Pestana JA, Ramos D et al. Ofloxacin versus trimethoprim-sulfamethoxazole in the treatment of patients with acute exacerbation of chronic bronchitis. Clin Ther 1996; 18: 440–7 |
| 21 | 1b | Niewoehner DE et al. Effect of systemic glucocorticoids on exacerbations of chronic obstructive pulmonary disease. N Engl J Med 1999; 340: 1941–7 |
| 22 | 1b | Thompson WH, Nielson CP, Carvalho P et al. Controlled trial of oral prednisone in outpatients with acute COPD exacerbation. Am J Respir Crit Care Med 1996; 154: 407–12 |
| 23 | 1b | Wrenn K et al. Aminophylline therapy for acute bronchospastic disease in the emergency room. Ann Intern Med 1991; 115: 241–7 |
| 24 | 1b | Rice KL, Leatherman JW, Duane PG et al. Aminophylline for acute exacerbations of chronic obstructive pulmonary disease: a controlled trial. Ann Intern Med 1987; 107: 305–9 |
| 25 | 2b | Brochard L, Mancebo J, Wysocki M et al. Noninvasive ventilation for acute exacerbations of chronic obstructive pulmonary disease. N Engl J Med 1995; 333: 817–22 |
| 26 | 1b | Nava S, Ambrosino N, Clini E et al. Noninvasive mechanical ventilation in the weaning of patients with respiratory failure due to chronic obstructive pulmonary disease: a randomized, controlled trial. Ann Intern Med 1998; 128: 721–8 |
| 27 | 1a – | Greenstone M et al. Doxapram for ventilatory failure due to exacerbations of chronic obstructive pulmonary disease (Cochrane Review). In: The Cochrane Library, Issue 3, 1999. Oxford: Update Software. |

| No | Level | Citation |
| --- | --- | --- |
| 28 | 1b – | O'Driscoll BR et al. Nebulised salbutamol with and without ipratropium bromide in acute airflow obstruction. Lancet 1989; 1: 1418–20 |
| 29 | 1b – | Rebuck AS et al. Nebulised anticholinergic and sympathomimetic treatment of asthma and chronic obstructive airways disease in the emergency room. Am J Med 1987; 82: 59–64 |
| 30 | 1b | Moayyedi P, Congleton J, Page RL et al. Comparison of nebulised salbutamol and ipratropium bromide with salbutamol alone in the treatment of chronic obstructive pulmonary disease. Thorax 1995; 50: 834–7 |
| 31 | 1b | Skorodin MS, Tenholder MF, Yetter B et al. Magnesium sulphate in exacerbations of chronic obstructive pulmonary disease. Arch Intern Med 1995; 155: 496–500 |
| 32 | 1b | Anthonisen NR, Connett JE, Kiley JP et al. Effects of smoking intervention and the use of an inhaled anticholinergic bronchodilator on the rate of decline of $FEV_1$: the Lung Health Study. JAMA 1994; 272: 1497–505 |
| 33 | 2a | Gross PA, Hermogenes AW, Sacks HS et al. The efficacy of influenza vaccine in elderly persons: a meta-analysis and review of the literature. Ann Intern Med 1995; 123: 518–27 |
| 34 | 1a | Fine MJ, Smith MA, Carson CA et al. Efficacy of pneumococcal vaccination in adults: a meta-analysis of randomized controlled trials. Arch Intern Med 1994; 154: 2666–77 |
| 35 | 1a | Lacasse Y, Wong E, Guyatt GH et al. Meta-analysis of respiratory rehabiliation in chronic obstructive pulmonary disease. Lancet 1996; 348: 1115–19 |
| 36 | 1b | Medical Research Council Working Party et al. Long term domiciliary oxygen therapy in chronic hypoxic cor pulmonale complicating chronic bronchitis and emphysema. Lancet 1981; i: 681–5 |
| 37 | 1b | Nocturnal Oxygen Therapy Trial Group et al. Continuous trial of nocturnal oxygen therapy in hypoxemic chronic obstructive disease: a clinical trial. Ann Intern Med 1980; 92: 391–8 |
| 38 | 1b– | Gorecka D, Gorzela K, Sliwinski P et al. Effect of long term oxygen therapy on survival in patients with chronic obstructive pulmonary disease with moderate hypoxia. Thorax 1997; 52: 674–9 |
| 39 | 1a | Poole PJ and Black PN. Mucolytic agents for chronic bronchitis (Cochrane Review). In: The Cochrane Library, Issue 3, 1999. Oxford: Update Software |
| 40 | 1b– | Collet JP, Shapiro S, Ernst P et al. Effects of an immunostimulating agent on acute exacerbations and hospitalisations in patients with chronic obstructive pulmonary disease. Am J Respir Crit Care Med 1997; 156: 1719–24 |
| 41 | 2b | Anthonisen NR, Wright EC, Hodgkin JE et al. Prognosis in chronic obstructive pulmonary disease. Am Rev Respir Dis 1986; 133: 14–20 |
| 42 | 1b | Connors AF, Dawson NV, Thomas C et al. Outcomes following acute exacerbations of severe chronic obstructive lung disease. Am J Respir Crit Care Med 1996; 154: 959–67 |
| 43 | 1b | Dallari R, Barozzi G, Pinelli G et al. Predictors of survival in subjects with chronic obstructive pulmonary disease treated with long-term oxygen therapy. Respiration 1994; 61: 8–13 |
| 44 | 2c | Vilkman S et al. Survival and cause of death among elderly chronic obstructive pulmonary disease patients after first admission to hospital. Respiration 1997; 64: 281–4 |

## PREVALENCE

● Around a quarter of patients attending hospital with a suspected DVT have one **[A]**[1]; however, it is rare in the community (<0.02%) **[B]**[2], especially in young people (<0.003%) **[B]**[3].

 **Note**
- 0.02% of women in the community develop a DVT **[B]**[2]; the risk is even lower in healthy women aged under 40 years (0.003%) **[B]**[3].
- 15–40% of patients with a suspected DVT attending hospital have one **[A]**[4] **[A]**[5].

## CLINICAL FEATURES

● Use the clinical prediction rule (Box 1) to rank patients for their risk of having a DVT **[A]**[1]. For patients with symptoms in both legs, use the most symptomatic leg.
● Remember DVT cannot be safely diagnosed or excluded on history and physical examination alone. Imaging studies are necessary **[A]**[6].

| Box 1 Clinical prediction rule to rank DVT risk | Score |
|---|---|
| Ask about: | |
| ■ Active cancer (on-going treatment, diagnosed within the last 6 months or having palliative care) | +1 |
| ■ Paralysis, paresis or plaster immobilisation of a leg | +1 |
| ■ Recently bedridden >3 days or major surgery within past 4 weeks | +1 |
| Look for: | |
| ■ Localised tenderness over distribution of the deep veins **[A]** | +1 |
| ■ Entire leg swollen | +1 |
| ■ Calf circumference 10 cm below tibial tuberosity >3 cm greater than other calf | +1 |
| ■ Pitting oedema only in the symptomatic leg **[A]** | +1 |
| ■ Collateral dilated (but not varicose) veins | +1 |
| ■ An alternative diagnosis as or more likely than DVT | −2 |

■ Match the patient's score to the risk

| Score **[A]**[1] | Risk of DVT |
|---|---|
| 3 or more | High |
| 1–2 | Moderate |
| 0 or less | Low |

**Why do this?**

When combined with ultrasonography (see below):

■ Few cases of DVT are missed (0.6%) **[A]**[1]. If all suspected cases have ultrasound scanning only, then 5% of DVT are missed **[A]**[7]. If all suspected cases have venography only, then 2% of DVT are missed **[C]**[8].

■ Few patients require a venogram (5.6%); however, one in three will have an extra hospital visit for additional testing **[A]**[1].

■ It helps clinicians agree about the risk of DVT. $K_{interobservor}$ for prediction rule =0.75 (two nurses and two doctors) **[A]**[1].

| Patient **[A]**[1] | Target disorder (reference standard) | Diagnostic test | LR (95% CI) | Post-test probability |
|---|---|---|---|---|
| Suspected DVT (pre-test probability 16%) | DVT (ultrasound, venogram, follow-up) | Score: 3 or more | 15 (9.5 to 25) | 75% |
| | | Score: 1 to 2 | 1.0 (0.76 to 1.4) | 17% |
| | | Score: 0 or less | 0.16 (0.091 to 0.30) | 3% |

In addition, ask about features that might affect your management:

● recurrent venous thromboemblism **[A]**[9]

● a known clotting disorder **[B]**[10]

● a history of clotting disorders in first-degree relatives **[C]**[11]

**Why?**

■ Thrombophilia is quite common, especially in patients who develop a DVT under 25 years of age **[C]**[11].

■ Factor $V_{Leiden}$ is the commonest disorder **[B]**[10].

**A family history and early or recurrent venous thromboemoblism makes thrombophilia more likely**

| Patient **[C]**[11] | Target disorder (reference standard) | Diagnostic test | LR+ (95% CI) | Post-test probability | LR– (95% CI) | Post-test probability |
|---|---|---|---|---|---|---|
| Suspected thrombophilia (pre-test probability 8%) | Thrombophilia (thrombophilia blood tests) | Family history (first-degree relative) | 2.2 (1.3 to 3.5) | 16% | 0.67 (0.45 to 1.0) | 6% |
| | | Family history + first episode aged <41 years | 3.2 (1.4 to 7.0) | 22% | 0.81 (0.63 to 1.0) | 7% |
| | | Family history, first episode aged <41 years and previous PE, DVT | 4.7 (1.3 to 17) | 30% | 0.89 (0.76 to 1.1) | 7% |

**Why?**

Factor $V_{Leiden}$ is the commonest thrombophilia

| Thrombophilia [B][10] [C][11] | Prevalence (95% CI) |
|---|---|
| Factor $V_{Leiden}$ | 21% (17% to 26%) |
|    aged <45 years | 23% |
|    aged <25 years | 42% |
| Protein C deficiency | 3% (1% to 5%) |
| Protein S deficiency | 2% (0% to 4%) |
| Plasminogen deficiency | 1% (0% to 2%) |
| Antithrombin III deficiency | 1% (0% to 2%) |

**Thrombophilia increases the risk of venous thromboembolism**

| Outcome | Risk factor | PEER | OR (95% CI) | NNH (95% CI) |
|---|---|---|---|---|
| Venous thromboembolism [B][2] | Factor $V_{Reiden}$ independent | 0.021% | 9.3 (3.6 to 24.1) | 570 (200 to 1800) |
| Venous thromboembolism [B][12] | homocysteinaemia not independent | 0.021% | 2.95 (2.08 to 4.17) | 2400 (1500 to 4400) |

- oral contraceptive pill use [B][13] (especially with a known thrombophilia) [B][2]

**Why?**

- It increases the risk of developing venous thromboembolism [A][13].
- Third-generation oral contraceptives are slightly more dangerous than second-generation [B][2] [B][3].
- There is no clear evidence to suggest that women on HRT are at increased risk of venous thromboembolism [A][13].

**Oral contraceptive pill increases the risk of venous thromboembolism very slightly**

| Patient [A][33] | Prognostic factor | Outcome | Control rate | OR (95% CI) | NNF+ (95% CI) |
|---|---|---|---|---|---|
| Healthy | Oral contraceptive pill independent | Venous thromboembolism | 0.003% | 2.4 (1.6 to 3.5) | 6000 (3400 to 14 000) |

**Third-generation contraceptives increase the risk of venous thromboembolism slightly more than second-generation**

| Outcome [B][2] [B][3] | Risk factor | PEER | OR (95% CI) | NNH (95% CI) |
|---|---|---|---|---|
| Venous thromboembolism | Nesogestrel or gestodene compared to levnogestrel independent | 0.012% | 2.2 (1.0 to 4.7) | 7000 (2300 to infinity) |

**Patients with factor $V_{Leides}$ who take an oral contraceptive are at greatly increased risk of venous thromboembolism**

| Outcome [B][2] | Risk factor | PEER | OR (95% CI) | NNH (95% CI) |
|---|---|---|---|---|
| Venous thromboembolism | Oral contraceptive and factor $V_{Leiden}$ not independent | 18% | 34.7 (7.8 to 154) | 140 (32 to 700) |

**Note**

The following are not particularly helpful in diagnosing DVT:

■ Asking about age, sex, symptom duration, recent trauma, a family history of venous thromboembolism, erythema or recent hospital admission **[A]**[1].

■ Looking for Homan's sign: it does not help diagnose or exclude DVT in hospital patients **[A]**[14] **[A]**[15].

● current or recent pregnancy **[B]**[16] (especially if known thrombophilia) **[C]**[17].

**Why?**

During pregnancy and the puerperium women are at increased risk for venous thromboembolism **[C]**[18], but it is rare (0.01% of pregnancies) **[B]**[16].

**Pregnancy especially with thrombophilia increases the risk of venous thromboembolism**

| Outcome | Risk factor | PEER | OR (95% CI) | NNH (95% CI) |
|---|---|---|---|---|
| Venous thromboembolism **[C]**[18] | Pregnant or puerperal *not independent* | 0.021% | 9.3 (3.6 to 24.1) | 570 (200 to 1800) |
| Venous thromboembolism **[C]**[17] | Thrombophilia and pregnant *not independent* | 0.078% | 9.0 (1.07 to 75) | 160 (18 to 18 000) |

In pregnant women:

● ask which leg is affected: a DVT is less likely if the right leg is affected clinically **[A]**[19].

**Why?**

**In pregnancy a DVT is less likely if the right leg is clinically affected**

| Patient **[A]**[19] | Target disorder (reference standard) | Diagnostic test | LR (95% CI) | Post-test probability |
|---|---|---|---|---|
| Suspected DVT in pregnancy (pre-test probability 42%) | DVT (serial impedance plethysmography) | Left leg affected clinically | 1.4 (1.0 to 1.8) | 49% |
| | | Right leg affected clinically | 0.23 (0.075 to 0.73) | 14% |
| | | Both legs affected clinically | Infinity (0.15 to infinity) | 100% |

Don't bother asking how long she has been pregnant: the trimester does not help predict DVT **[B]**[20].

**? Why?**

■ DVTs are equally likely to occur in all three trimesters **[B]**[20].

**DVT can occur in any trimester**

| Trimester **[B]**[20] | DVT occurrence (95% CI) |
|---|---|
| First (0 to 91 days) | 22% (13% to 35%) |
| Second (92 to 182 days) | 47% (33% to 60%) |
| Third (183 days to term) | 32% (19% to 44%) |

## DIFFERENTIAL DIAGNOSIS

Think about other causes of unilateral leg swelling. Common causes include **[A]**[4] **[A]**[5]:

● cellulitis
● muscle injury
● superficial thrombosis.

**? Why?**

| Differential diagnosis **[A]**[4] **[A]**[5] | Prevalence in emergency departments |
|---|---|
| DVT | 16%–30% |
| Cellulitis | 6%–9% |
| Muscular injury | 6%–7% |
| Superficial thrombosis | 5%–7% |
| Ruptured Baker's cyst | 2%–6% |
| Chronic oedema | 3% |
| Chronic venous insufficiency | 3% |
| Post-operative swelling | 3% |
| Arthritis | 2% |
| Pelvic tumour | 1% |

*Remember* **[A]**[4] **[A]**[5]

● Chronic oedema or venous insufficiency
● Pelvic tumours compressing lymphatic or venous drainage
● A ruptured Baker's cyst.

Look for **[A]**[21]:
– crepitus on flexing the knee
– a history of arthritis
– a positive ultrasound scan.

## Why?
**Arthritis, knee crepitus or a positive ultrasound scan make a Baker's cyst more likely**

| Patient [A][21] | Target disorder (reference standard) | Diagnostic test | LR+ (95% CI) | Post-test probability | LR– (95% CI) | Post-test probability |
|---|---|---|---|---|---|---|
| Suspected Baker's cyst (pre-test probability 37%) | Baker's cyst (arthrogram) | Crepitus on flexing knee | 3.0 (1.2 to 7.5) | 64% | 0.54 (0.30 to 0.96) | 24% |
| | | History of arthritis | 3.4 (1.2 to 9.4) | 67% | 0.59 (0.35 to 0.98) | 26% |
| | | Ultrasound scan | Infinity (0.16 to infinity) | 100% | 0.88 (0.73 to 1.1) | 34% |

## Note
- Baker's cysts are common: a third of patients with a suspected DVT have a Baker's cyst (ruptured or not) [A][21].
- Remember that the presence of a Baker's cyst does not exclude a DVT [A][21].

**A Baker's cyst (ruptured or not) does not exclude a DVT**

| Patient [A][21] | Target disorder (reference standard) | Diagnostic test | LR+ (95% CI) | Post-test probability | LR– (95% CI) | Post-test probability |
|---|---|---|---|---|---|---|
| Suspected DVT (pre-test probability 33%) | DVT (venogram) | Presence of Baker's cyst | 0.77 (0.33 to 1.8) | 31% | 1.16 (0.74 to 1.8) | 41% |
| | | Presence of ruptured Baker's cyst | 1.1 (0.21 to 6.0) | 40% | 0.98 (0.78 to 1.2) | 37% |

## INVESTIGATIONS

- Blood count: check platelets [D].
- Clotting: to provide baseline measurements and to exclude problems pre-anticoagulation [D].
- Consider thrombophilia screen if:
  - episode confirmed [D]
  - indicated; a family history of thrombophilia and a first thromboemoblic event aged <41 years [A][11].

## Note
Send factor $V_{Leiden}$, protein C, S, antithrombin, plasminogen, antiphospholipid antibodies.

- Consider D-dimer [A][22] [A][23] in clinically low-risk patients [A][24].

**Why?**
A negative D-dimer rules out DVT in clinically low-risk patients

| Patient [A]24 | Target disorder (reference standard) | Diagnostic test | LR+ (95% CI) | Post-test probability | LR– (95% CI) | Post-test probability |
|---|---|---|---|---|---|---|
| Suspected DVT and clinical low-risk (pre-test probability 3%) | DVT (venogram and follow-up) | Positive whole blood assay D-dimer | 5.2 (4.0 to 6.7) | 14% | 0.14 (0.072 to 0.30) | 0.43% |

**Note**
- D-dimer test characteristics vary greatly [A]25.
- ELISA studies are best at excluding DVT but take several hours [A]25.
- Whole blood agglutination studies can be done at the bedside and are simple and quick to perform and read, but are less good at excluding DVT [A]25.

- Ultrasonography [A]1 of the common femoral vein and popliteal vein to the trification. (Positive if any vein not fully compressible).

**Why?**
- DVT isolated in the femoral or illiac veins is rare (<0.5% of patients) [B]26.

Using the clinical prediction rule ranking [A]1, read the ultrasound result as follows:

*High risk for DVT*
Positive scan: DVT.
Negative scan: Venous thromboembolism remains so likely that venography is needed.

- If the venogram is positive: DVT.
- If the venogram is negative: no DVT.

*Moderate risk for DVT*
Positive scan: DVT.
Negative scan: Repeat the scan in 1 week [A] and withhold anticoagulation [C].

- If it is positive: DVT.
- If it is negative: no DVT.

**Why do this?**
- Few patients have a positive second scan. In a study that rescanned all patients with a first negative scan, only 0.9% had a positive second scan and 0.06% developed further symptoms in the intervening week [A]27.
- DVT is very rare if two scans are negative: 0.6% of patients with two negative ultrasounds one week apart develop a DVT in the next 3 months [A]28.

*Low risk for DVT*
Positive scan: Venous thromboembolism remains so unlikely that
venography is needed.
● If the venogram is positive: DVT.
● If the venogram is negative: no DVT.
Negative scan: no DVT.

**?  Why?**
An ultrasound scan can help diagnose and exclude a DVT

| Patient | Target disorder (reference standard) | Diagnostic test | LR+ (95% CI) | Post-test probability | LR– (95% CI) | Post-test probability |
|---|---|---|---|---|---|---|
| Suspected DVT **[A]**[7] (pre-test probability 16%) | DVT (venogram) | Ultrasound | 23 (18 to 28) | 81% | 0.08 (0.06 to 0.10) | 1.5% |
| Clinical high risk for a DVT (pre-test probability 75%) **[A]**[1] **[A]**[29] | | Ultrasound | Infinity | 100% | 0.09 | 21% |
| Clinical moderate risk for a DVT (pre-test probability 17%) **[A]**[1] **[A]**[29] | | Ultrasound | 53 | 92% | 0.39 | 7% |
| Clinical low risk for a DVT (pre-test probability 3%) **[A]**[1] **[A]**[29] | | Ultrasound | 24 | 43% | 0.34 | 1% |

*Remember*
● Ultrasound scans can diagnose recurrent DVT in patients with a
recent DVT **[A]**[30]. (Positive if veins non-compressible or ≥2 mm
increase in clot diameter from last measurement.)

**?  Why?**
An ultrasound scan can help diagnose and exclude a recurrent DVT

| Patient **[A]**[30] | Target disorder (reference standard) | Diagnostic test | LR+ (95% CI) | Post-test probability | LR– (95% CI) | Post-test probability |
|---|---|---|---|---|---|---|
| Suspected recurrent DVT (pre-test probability 38%) | DVT (venogram) | Ultrasound | >100 (3.5 to infinity) | 100% | 0.091 (0.014 to 0.59) | 5% |

**‖  Note**
■ Around a half of patients with DVT have normal ultrasound scans after 1 year **[A]**[30].

● There is little benefit in scanning asymptomatic high-risk patients (e.g. following orthopaedic surgery) **[A]**[31] **[A]**[32].

---

**?** **Why?**
**An ultrasound scan cannot safely diagnose and exclude an asymptomatic DVT**

| Patient **[A]**[7] | Target disorder (reference standard) | Diagnostic test | LR+ (95% CI) | Post-test probability | LR– (95% CI) | Post-test probability |
|---|---|---|---|---|---|---|
| Suspected asymptomatic first DVT (pre-test probability 15%) | DVT (venogram) | Ultrasound | 9.8 (7.6 to 13) | 78% | 0.60 (0.56 to 0.65) | 18% |

---

Alternatives include:

● Impedance plethysmography **[A]**[33]. This is less good than ultrasonography **[A]**[7] **[A]**[34].

---

**?** **Why?**
■ Ultrasound scanning is better than IPG at diagnosing and excluding DVT in patients with symptoms **[A]**[7] **[A]**[34].
■ There are fewer uninterpretable scans using ultrasound **[A]**[33], although the study used has no clear effect on recurrent venous thromboembolism or death **[A]**[33].

**More ultrasound scans are interpretable than IPG**

| Patient | Treatment | Comparator | Outcome | CER | RRR | NNT |
|---|---|---|---|---|---|---|
| Suspected DVT **[A]**[33] | IPG | Ultrasound | Uninterpretable non-invasive test or venogram at 8 days | 4.5% | 55% (5% to 78%) | 41 (21 to 440) |

---

Using the clinical prediction rule ranking **[A]**[4] **[A]**[5], read the IPG result as follows:

*High risk for DVT*
Positive scan: DVT.
Negative scan: Venous thromboembolism remains so likely that venography is needed.

● If the venogram is positive: DVT.
● If the venogram is negative: no DVT.

*Moderate risk for DVT*
Positive scan: DVT.
Negative scan: Repeat the scan in 1 week **[A]** and withhold anticoagulation **[C]**.

● If it is positive: DVT.
● If it is negative: no DVT.

> **? Why do this?**
> ■ Few DVTs are missed: 1.1% **[A]**[4].
> ■ DVT is very rare if two scans are negative **[A]**[5].

*Low risk for DVT*

Positive scan: venous thromboembolism remains so unlikely that venography is needed.

● If the venogram is positive: DVT.
● If the venogram is negative: no DVT.

Negative scan: no DVT.

> **? Why?**
> **IPG can help diagnose and exclude a DVT**
>
> | Patient **[A]**[7] | Target disorder (reference standard) | Diagnostic test | LR+ (95% CI) | Post-test probability | LR− (95% CI) | Post-test probability |
> |---|---|---|---|---|---|---|
> | Suspected first DVT (pre-test probability 18%) | DVT (venogram) | IPG | 11 (8.8 to 150) | 70% | 0.20 (0.16 to 0.25) | 4% |

Combination with a whole blood agglutination D-dimer test makes IPG better at diagnosing and excluding DVT **[A]**[24].

> **? Why?**
> **D-dimer and IPG can diagnose and exclude DVT**
>
> | Patient **[A]**[24] | Target disorder (reference standard) | Diagnostic test | LR (95% CI) | Post-test probability |
> |---|---|---|---|---|
> | Suspected DVT (pre-test probability 18%) | DVT (venogram, follow-up) | IPG+, D-dimer+ | 61 (19 to 190) | 93% |
> | | | IPG+,D-dimer− | 6.3 (1.4 to 27) | 57% |
> | | | IPG−,D-dimer+ | 2.0 (1.3 to 3.0) | 30% |
> | | | Either test positive | 2.3 (1.5 to 3.3) | 33% |
> | | | IPG−,D-dimer− | 0.070 (0.027 to 0.18) | 1.5% |

*Remember*

● IPG can diagnose recurrent DVT in patients with a recent DVT **[C]**[35].

> **? Why?**
> ■ In patients with a DVT, IPG returns to normal within a year in 95% of cases (most within 9 months) **[C]**[35].

- There is little benefit in scanning asymptomatic high-risk patients (e.g. following orthopaedic surgery) **[A]**[7].

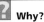

**Why?**

**An ultrasound scan cannot safely diagnose and exclude an asymptomatic DVT**

| Patient **[A]**[7] | Target disorder (reference standard) | Diagnostic test | LR+(95% CI) | Post-test probability | LR–(95% CI) | Post-test probability |
|---|---|---|---|---|---|---|
| Suspected asymptomatic first DVT (pre-test probability 7%) | DVT (venogram) | IPG | 3.8 (2.6 to 5.6) | 53% | 0.88 (0.84 to 0.92) | 21% |

- Venography **[A]**: the reference standard.

**Why?**

It is the current reference standard, but it is not perfect.
- Some DVTs are missed: 2% of patients with a negative venogram develop DVT **[C]**[8].
- It may not be technically possible (5%) **[C]**[36].
- Pain is a common side-effect (20%). Serious side-effects are rare **[C]**[36].
- It may cause DVT **[C]**[36].

It can be safely performed in pregnant women if necessary **[B]**[37].

**Why?**

- Babies exposed to low-dose radiation *in utero* are probably slightly more likely to develop cancer (in 11 retrospective case-control and cohort studies, the relative risk ranged from 1.2 to 1.7. Assuming a cancer rate of 0.1% in neonates, NNH = 5000. The teratogenic risks are probably even smaller **[B]**[37].

- MRI **[B]**[38] from inferior vena cava to popliteal veins. (Positive if central signal void with hyperintense signal or no flow in vessel (with or without intraluminal thrombus).)

**Why?**

**MRI can help diagnose and exclude DVT**

| Patient **[B]**[38] | Target disorder (reference standard) | Diagnostic test | LR+(95% CI) | Post-test probability | LR–(95% CI) | Post-test probability |
|---|---|---|---|---|---|---|
| Suspected DVT (pre-test probability 28%) | DVT (venography) | MRI | 25 (8.1 to 75) | 90% | 0.0 (0.0 to 0.11) | 0% |

Avoid:
- [125I] fibrinogen leg scanning: it cannot safely diagnose or exclude DVT **[C]**[39].

**Why?**

**Fibrinogen leg scanning cannot diagnose or exclude DVT**

| Patient [C][39] | Target disorder (reference standard) | Diagnostic test | LR+(95% CI) | Post-test probability | LR–(95% CI) | Post-test probability |
|---|---|---|---|---|---|---|
| Suspected DVT (pre-test probability 30%) | DVT (venography) | [$^{125}$I] fibrinogen leg scanning | 3.2 (1.8 to 5.5) | 57% | 0.63 (0.48 to 0.84) | 21% |

## THERAPY

- Give pain relief if necessary **[D]**.
- Anticoagulate all patients with suspected venous thromboembolism, **[A]**[40].

**Why do this?**

- Recurrent venous thromboembolism and death are common without anticoagulation. Anticoagulation reduces both **[A]**[40].

**Anticoagulation reduces death and recurrent PE**

| Patient | Treatment | Comparator | Outcome | CER | RRR | NNT |
|---|---|---|---|---|---|---|
| PE **[A]**[40] | Anticoagulation | No anticoagulation | Death at 3 months | 26% | 100% | 4 (2 to 15) |
| | | | Recurrent PE at 3 months | 32% | 100% | 3 (2 to 9) |

including patients with calf DVT.

**Why do this?**

- Complications are common. Calf DVTs can propogate (6% to 23%), and lead to recurrent DVT (4% to 9%) or chronic venous insufficiency (21% to 79%) **[C]**[41].
- Anticoagulation reduces recurrent venous thromboembolism. Patients with calf DVT who are anticoagulated with heparin followed by warfarin for 3 months are less likely to have recurrences than patients just given heparin for 5 days **[A]**[40].

**Anticoagulation reduces recurrent venous thromboembolism in patients with a calf DVT**

| Patient [A][40] | Treatment | Comparator | Outcome | CER | RRR | NNT |
|---|---|---|---|---|---|---|
| Calf DVT | Heparin for 5 days and warfarin for 3 months | Heparin for 5 days | Recurrence of venous thromboembolism at 1 year | 32% | 87% (27% to 100%) | 4 (2 to 12) |

Give low molecular weight heparin (LMWH) **[A]**[42] (e.g. tinzaparin 175 units/kg sc) while waiting for the results of investigations. No monitoring is necessary for LMWH **[D]**.

**Why do this?**
- It is more effective than unfractionated heparin **[A]**[42].
- It causes fewer bleeds than unfractionated heparin **[A]**[42].
- It may be more cost-effective than intravenous unfractionated heparin **[A]**[43].

**LMWH and warfarin reduce death and causes less bleeding than heparin and warfarin**

| Patient | Treatment | Comparator | Outcome | CER | OR | NNT |
|---|---|---|---|---|---|---|
| Venous thromboembolism **[A]**[42] | LMWH and warfarin | Heparin and warfarin | Death at 3–6 months | 5.7% | 0.78 (0.62 to 0.99) | 84 (48 to 1860) |
| | | | Major bleed at 3–6 months | 2.0% | 0.60 (0.39 to 0.93) | 127 (83 to 730) |
| Cancer and venous thromboembolism **[A]**[42] | LMWH and warfarin | Heparin and warfarin | Death at 3–6 months | 24% | 0.53 (0.33 to 0.85) | 10 (7 to 35) |

In addition **[A]**[44] give warfarin **[A]**[40] **[A]**[45]**[A]**[46] (e.g. 5 mg **[A]**[47] at 1800 hours **[C]**[48]), as soon as DVT has been demonstrated **[A]**[49].

**Why do this?**
- Heparin and warfarin together is safer than warfarin alone. Patients who remain on heparin while awaiting satisfactory oral anticoagulation with warfarin have fewer recurrent symptomatic DVTs **[A]**[44].
- The effect on major bleeding is unclear **[A]**[44].

**Starting anticoagulation with heparin and warfarin reduces symptomatic recurrent DVT**

| Patient | Treatment | Comparator | Outcome | CER | RRR | NNT |
|---|---|---|---|---|---|---|
| Proximal DVT **[A]**[44] | Heparin and warfarin | Warfarin alone | Symptomatic recurrent DVT at 6 months | 20% | 13% (1.4% to 25%) | 8 (4 to 71) |

- A loading dose of 5 mg of warfarin leads to more successful anticoagulation than a loading dose of 10 mg **[A]**[47].

**More patients given a loading dose of 5 mg of warfarin are therapeutically stable after 5 days**

| Patient **[A]**[47] | Treatment | Comparator | Outcome | CER | RRR | NNT |
|---|---|---|---|---|---|---|
| Starting anticoagulation | 5 mg loading dose of warfarin | 10 mg loading dose of warfarin | INR 2.0–3.0 on 2 consecutive days, and never > 3.0 at 5 days | 68% | 190% (27% to 540%) | 2 (1 to 5) |

Give warfarin:

- for 6 weeks for transient risk factors (e.g. surgery, recently bed-ridden) **[D]**[50]
- for 6 months **[A]**[45] or longer **[D]** for permanent risk factors (e.g. cancer, leg paralysis)
- indefinitely for idiopathic cases **[A]**[51] or recurrent venous thromboembolism **[A]**[46].

**Why do this?**

- Six months of anticoagulation is not clearly better than 6 weeks for patients with temporary risk factors (e.g. surgery, trauma, plaster casts) **[D]**[50].
- Patients with permanent risk factors are at increased risk for recurrent venous thromboembolism compared with patients with transient risk factors **[C]**[57]. Six months of anticoagulation leads to fewer recurrent episodes of venous thromboembolism in patients with permanent risk factors (e.g. cancer, thrombophilia, paresis) than 6 weeks. The effect on mortality and major haemorrhage is unclear **[A]**[45].
- Indefinite oral anticoagulant therapy for a first idiopathic episode of a DVT or PE leads to fewer recurrences of venous thromboembolism than 3 months of therapy without clearly increasing bleeding or mortality **[A]**[51].
- Indefinite oral anticoagulant therapy for a second episode of a DVT or PE leads to fewer recurrences of venous thromboembolism than 6 months of therapy without clearly increasing bleeding or mortality **[A]**[46].

**Indefinite anticoagulation reduces recurrent venous thromboembolism for idiopathic or recurrent episodes**

| Patient | Treatment | Comparator | Outcome | CER | RRR | NNT |
|---------|-----------|------------|---------|-----|-----|-----|
| First PE or DVT **[A]**[45] | Anticoagulation for 6 months | Anticoagulation for 6 weeks | Recurrent venous thromboembolism at 2 years | 18% | 48% (26% to 63%) | 12 (8 to 24) |
| First idiopathic PE or DVT **[A]**[51] | Indefinite anticoagulation | Anticoagulation for 3 months | Recurrent venous thromboembolism at 10 months | 21% | 94% (55% to 99%) | 5 (4 to 10) |
| Second PE or DVT **[A]**[46] | Indefinite anticoagulation | Anticoagulation for 6 months | Recurrent venous thromboembolism at 4 years | 21% | 88% (60% to 96%) | 6 (4 to 10) |

*Remember*
- Anticoagulation can be done on an outpatient basis in uncomplicated cases **[D]**[53] **[D]**[54]. Avoid in patients with **[D]**:
  - active bleeding
  - problems being followed-up.

 **Why do this?**

- Outpatient anticoagulation is not clearly less effective or safer than inpatient anticoagulation **[D]**[53] **[D]**[54].
- LMWH and warfarin given to outpatients is cheaper than heparin and warfarin given to inpatients **[A]**[54].

- Monitor the response using daily INR **[C]**[48], and aim for a therapeutic range of 2.0–3.0 **[C]**[54] **[C]**[57]. Use a set protocol (preferably computerised **[A]**[58]) to prescribe the amount of warfarin.
- Continue the LMWH for at least 5 days, and until the INR is in range for 2 days **[D]**. Seek expert advice if there are problems **[A]**[59] **[A]**[56].

 **Why do this?**

- A therapeutic and stable INR is achieved sooner by using a computer program to predict dosing. Patients are also more likely to have a therapeutic INR after 2 weeks **[A]**[55] **[A]**[58].
- Hospital stays are shorter: patients spend on average a week less in hospital **[A]**[55] **[A]**[58].
- Fewer patients have anticoagulant-related bleeding if guideline-based consultation is used **[A]**[56] **[A]**[59].
- Fewer patients have new or recurrent PE or DVT if guideline-based consultation is used **[A]**[56] **[A]**[59].

> **? Why do this?**
> Guideline-based anticoagulation reduces bleeding and recurrent PE or DVT
>
> | Patient | Treatment | Comparator | Outcome | CER | RRR | NNT |
> |---|---|---|---|---|---|---|
> | Requiring anticoagulation **[A]**⁵⁹ | Guideline-based anticoagulation with expert advice | Standard care | Major or minor bleeding at 3 months | 31% | 58% (2% to 82%) | 6 (3 to 45) |
> | | | | New or recurrent PE or DVT at 3 months | 16% | 73% (−17% to 94%) | 8 (4 to 160) |

- Check platelets after 5 days to exclude heparin-induced thrombocytopenia **[B]**⁶⁰ **[B]**⁴¹.

> **? Why do this?**
> ■ Heparin-induced thrombocytopenia is uncommon (3% of patients on heparin, <1% on LMWH) **[B]**⁶⁰ **[B]**⁶¹ but may increase the risk of venous thromboembolism **[C]**⁶².
>
> **Heparin-induced thrombocytopenia increases the risk of venous thromboembolism**
>
> | Patient **[C]**⁶² | Prognostic factor | Outcome | Control rate | OR (95% CI) | NNF+ (95% CI) |
> |---|---|---|---|---|---|
> | On heparin or LMWH | Heparin-induced thrombocytopenia *not independent* | Venous thromboembolism | 18% | 4.98 (3.75 to 6.62) | 1 (1 to 2) |

(See **Anticoagulation** chapter for further details.)

- Ask patients to wear knee-length sized-to-fit elasticated stockings during the day **[A]**⁶³.

> **? Why do this?**
> ■ Patients with proximal DVT are less likely to develop post-thrombotic leg syndrome (leg pain, swelling and ulcers) if they wear knee-length sized-to-fit elasticated stockings daily for at least 2 years; however, stockings do not clearly prevent recurrent DVT or ulcers **[A]**⁶³.
> ■ Patient compliance is good: 93% wear stockings all or most of the time **[A]**⁶³.
>
> **Sized-to-fit elasticated stockings worn daily reduce thrombotic leg syndrome**
>
> | Patient | Treatment | Comparator | Outcome | CER | RRR | NNT |
> |---|---|---|---|---|---|---|
> | Proximal DVT **[A]**⁶³ | Sized-to-fit elasticated stockings daily for at least 2 years | No stockings | Mild-to-moderate post-thrombotic leg syndrome at 5 years | 47% | 58% (34% to 73%) | 4 (3 to 7) |
> | | | | Severe post-thrombotic leg syndrome at 5 years | 23% | 51% (5% to 75%) | 8 (4 to 68) |

There is no clear benefit from:

- thrombolysis **[A]**[64] **[A]**[65]

 **Why?**

- Patients given streptokinase or tPA have better clot lysis, **[A]**[64] **[A]**[65], but are more likely to have a major bleed **[A]**[65].
- The route of administration (systemic or local) has no clear effect on the incidence of bleeding **[A]**[66].

**Streptokinase lyses clots but increases the risk of major bleeding**

| Patient | Treatment | Comparator | Outcome | CER | OR | NNT |
|---|---|---|---|---|---|---|
| DVT **[A]**[65] | Streptokinase | Heparin | Clot lysis at 1 week | 18% | 3.7 (2.5 to 5.7) | 4 (3 to 6) |
| | | | Major bleed at 1 week | 23% | 2.9 (1.1 to 8.1) | 17 (5 to 310) |

- vena caval filters combined with anticoagulation for preventing PE in high-risk patients **[A]**[67].

**Why?**

- There is an increased risk of recurrent DVT, with no clear reduction in subsequent PE. Patients with a proximal DVT who are at high-risk for PE have fewer PE in the first 12 days, but not clearly over the next 2 years. Furthermore, patients are more likely to have recurrent DVT **[A]**[67].

**Vena caval filters in addition to anticoagulation increase recurrent DVT with clearly reducing PE**

| Patient | Treatment | Comparator | Outcome | CER | RRR | NNT |
|---|---|---|---|---|---|---|
| Proximal DVT considered at high risk for PE **[A]**[67] | Inferior vena caval filter anticoagulation | Anticoagulation | PE | 4.5% | 78% (–2% to 95%) | 29 (15 to 320) |
| | | | Symptomatic PE | 6.0% | 50% (–31% to 81%) | 33 (NNT = 14 to infinity; NNH = 95 to infinity) |
| | | | Recurrent DVT | 11% | –71% (–183% to –4%) | –13 (–145 to –7) |

Vena caval filters may be useful in patients at high risk for further venous thromboembolism who have a contraindication to anticoagulation **[D]**.

## PREVENTION

All patients who are:

- having major surgery (especially orthopaedic) **[A]**[69] **[A]**[70] **[A]**[71] **[A]**[72]
- likely to have poor mobility **[A]**[73]
  - major trauma **[A]**[74]
  - leg plaster cast **[A]**[73]

- spinal cord injury **[A]**[75]
- stroke **[A]**[75]
- decompensated heart failure **[A]**[75]
- myocardial infarction or unstable angina **[A]**[75]

- at increased risk for DVT
  - old **[A]**[76]
  - active cancer having chemotherapy **[A]**[77]
  - recurrent venous thromboembolism **[A]**[77]
  - pregnant with thrombophilia **[C]**[78] **[D]**[79]

should have venous thromboembolism prophylaxis **[A]**[80]

---

**? Why do this?**

■ Venous thromboembolism prophylaxis reduces DVT in all these groups.
■ Heparin prophylaxis reduces DVT and PE but increases the risk of having an episode of excessive bleeding or requiring a blood transfusion **[A]**[80].
■ It reduces fatal PE without clearly increasing death from haemorrhage **[A]**[80].

**Heparin prophylaxis reduces venous thromboembolism and fatal PE but increases excessive bleeding**

| Patient **[A]**[80] | Treatment | Comparator | Outcome | CER | OR | NNT |
|---|---|---|---|---|---|---|
| Undergoing general, orthopaedic or urological surgery | Subcutaneous heparin | Placebo | DVT at? | 27% | 0.68 (0.65 to 0.71) | 15 (13 to 16) |
| | | | Non-fatal PE at? | 2.0% | 0.40 (0.29 to 0.51) | 83 (70 to 100) |
| | | | Fatal PE at ? | 0.83% | 0.64 (0.49 to 0.80) | 340 (240 to 610) |
| | | | Episodes of excessive bleeding or need for transfusion at? | 3.8% | 1.66 (1.55 to 1.77) | −43 (−51 to −37) |

**Heparin reduces venous thromboembolism in elderly patients with infection**

| Patient **[A]**[81] | Treatment | Comparator | Outcome | CER | RRR | NNT |
|---|---|---|---|---|---|---|
| Elderly patients with infection | Heparin | Nothing | Non-fatal venous thromboembolism at 60 days | 2.0% | 38% (17% to 54%) | 130 (83 to 340) |

**LMWH reduces venous thromboembolism in patients wearing leg plaster casts**

| Patient **[A]**[73] | Treatment | Comparator | Outcome | CER | RRR | NNT |
|---|---|---|---|---|---|---|
| Below knee or cylindrical leg plaster cast | LMWH | Nothing | DVT at 19 days | 4.3% | 100% | 23 (14 to 85) |

using
- thigh-length graduated compression stockings [A][70] [A][82]

 **Why do this?**
- It reduces DVT and PE in patients having major abdominal or gynaecological surgery if worn until discharge [A][70].
- It saves money: using compression stockings is more cost-effective than doing nothing [B][83].

**Graduated compression stockings reduce symptomatic venous thromboembolism**

| Patient | Treatment | Comparator | Outcome | CER | OR | NNT |
|---|---|---|---|---|---|---|
| Major abdominal or gynaecological surgery [A][70] | Compression stockings until discharge | No stockings | Symptomatic venous thromboembolism at 60 days | 18% | 0.28 (0.23 to 0.42) | 8 (8 to 11) |

- Mechanical devices (compression stockings, calf or foot pumps) reduce DVT in elderly patients after surgery for proximal hip fractures [A][84]

**Mechanical devices reduce DVT in elderly patients having surgery for a hip fracture**

| Patient | Treatment | Comparator | Outcome | CER | OR | NNT |
|---|---|---|---|---|---|---|
| Elderly with a hip fracture [A][84] | Mechanical devices | Nothing | DVT at ? discharge | 20% | 0.24 (0.13 to 0.44) | 7 (6 to 10) |

with heparin [A][69] or an LMWH [A][71]

 **Why do this?**
- Adding heparin [A][69] or an LMWH [A][68] [A][71] to compression stockings or pneumatic compression [A][72] reduces symptomatic venous thromboembolism in neurosurgery, major abdominal surgery or orthopaedic surgery. There is no clear effect on the rate of bleeding [A][68].

| Patient | Treatment | Comparator | Outcome | CER | RRR | NNT |
|---|---|---|---|---|---|---|
| Elective cranial or spinal surgery [A][68] | Compression stockings and enoxaparin until discharge | Compression stockings until discharge | Symptomatic venous thromboembolism at 60 days | 6.9% | 89% (14% to 99%) | 16 (9 to 65) |
| Elective major abdominal surgery [A][69] | Compression stockings and heparin for 5 days | Heparin for 5 days | Venous thromboembolism at 7 days | 12% | 84% (23% to 100%) | 10 (6 to 35) |
| Total knee replacement or tibial osteotomy [A][91] | Compression stockings and ardeparin | Compression stockings | DVT at 14 days | 58% | 50% (29% to 65%) | 3 (2 to 6) |
| Open heart surgery | Pneumatic compression and heparin for 14 days | Heparin for 14 days | Symptomatic PE at 30 days | 4.0% | 50% (17% to 83%) | 50 (30 to 150) |

*in moderate-risk cases*
- low-dose heparin **[A]**[84] 5000 units every 12 h (adjusted so aPTT is at the upper limit of normal) **[A]**[86]

 **Why do this?**
- ■ Both heparin and LMWH reduce DVT in elderly patients after surgery for proximal hip fractures **[A]**[84].
- ■ Adjusted low-dose heparin prevents more DVT than fixed dose heparin **[A]**[85].
- ■ Heparin is more cost-effective than LMWH in lower risk patients **[A]**[86].

**Heparin and LMWH reduce DVT in elderly patients with a hip fracture**

| Patient | Treatment | Comparator | Outcome | CER | OR | NNT |
|---|---|---|---|---|---|---|
| Elderly with a hip fracture **[A]**[84] | Heparin or LMWH | Placebo or nothing | DVT at ? discharge | 24% | 0.41 (0.31 to 0.55) | 5 (4 to 8) |

**Adjusted dose heparin prevents more DVT than fixed dose**

| Patient | Treatment | Comparator | Outcome | CER | RRR (%) | NNT |
|---|---|---|---|---|---|---|
| Elective total hip replacement **[A]**[85] | Adjusted dose heparin | Fixed dose heparin | DVT at 9 days | 39% | 67 (20 to 100) | 4 (2 to 13) |

*in high-risk cases* (major abdominal, gynaecological, neurosurgical, cardiovascular or orthopaedic surgery) any of:

- LMWH **[A]**[74] **[A]**[82]**[A]**[87], e.g. 40 mg enoxaparin daily **[A]**[88]

**Why do this?**
- ■ Both heparin and LMWH reduce DVT in elderly patients after surgery for proximal hip fractures **[A]**[84].
- ■ LMWH is better than unfractionated heparin for preventing venous thromboembolism in general surgery, orthopaedic and trauma patients **[A]**[74] **[A]**[87]. It reduces wound haematomas but has no clear effect on major bleeding **[A]**[89]. Around 2% of patients on LMWH have a major bleed **[A]**[82].
- ■ LMWH is more cost-effective than heparin in high-risk cases **[B]**[86].
- ■ 40 mg of enoxaparin daily reduces more DVT than lower doses but increases the risk of bleeding. Higher doses are not clearly more effective **[A]**[88].

**LMWH prevents more DVT and PE than heparin in patients having orthopaedic or general surgery**

| Patient **[A]**[87] | Treatment | Comparator | Outcome | CER | OR | NNT |
|---|---|---|---|---|---|---|
| General surgery | LMWH | Heparin | DVT at ? discharge | 6.7% | 0.79 (0.65 to 0.95) | 33 (23 to 87) |
| | LMWH | Heparin | PE at ? discharge | 0.44% | 0.44 (0.21 to 0.95) | 260 (180 to 2800) |
| Orthopaedic surgery | LMWH | Heparin | DVT at ? discharge | 21% | 0.68 (0.54 to 0.86) | 15 (10 to 34) |
| | LMWH | Heparin | PE at ? discharge | 4.1% | 0.43 (0.22 to 0.82) | 43 (31 to 140) |

**Why do this?**
LMWH prevents more DVT than heparin in trauma patients

| Patient [A][87] | Treatment | Comparator | Outcome | CER | RRR | NNT |
|---|---|---|---|---|---|---|
| Major trauma [A][74] | Enoxaparin for 14 days | Heparin for 14 days | DVT | 35% | 33% (5% to 52%) | 9 (5 to 56) |

**40 mg of enoxaparin prevents more DVT but causes more major bleeding than 10 mg**

| Patient | Treatment | Comparator | Outcome | CER | RRR | NNT |
|---|---|---|---|---|---|---|
| Major trauma [A][88] | Enoxaparin 40 mg daily | Enoxaparin 10 mg daily | DVT at 7 days | 25% | 44% (10% to 77%) | 9 (5 to 39) |
| | | | Major bleed at 7 days | 5% | −120% (−100% to −10%) | −17 (−200 to −9) |

- thigh-length intermittent pneumatic compression [A][84]

**Why do this?**
- It reduces venous thromboembolism [A][90] and, when combined with heparin, it reduces PE better than heparin alone [A][72].
- It is cost-effective [B][83].
- Calf pneumatic compression is not clearly as safe as thigh pneumatic compression during major urological surgery [D][91].

**Pneumatic compression reduces venous thromboembolism**

| Patient | Treatment | Comparator | Outcome | CER | RRR | NNT |
|---|---|---|---|---|---|---|
| Elective total hip replacement [A][90] | Thigh-length intermittent pneumatic compression | Nothing | Venous thromboembolism at 3 months | 49% | 51 (30% to 72%) | 4 (3 to 7) |
| Open heart surgery [A][72] | Pneumatic compression and heparin | Heparin | Symptomatic PE at 30 days | 4.0% | 50 (17% to 83%) | 50 (30 to 150) |

- warfarin [A][88].

**Why do this?**
- Warfarin reduces venous thromboembolism in patients having elective total hip replacement [A][82] or with metastatic breast carcinoma receiving chemotherapy [A][24].
- LMWH and warfarin are equally cost-effective in preventing DVT in patients undergoing total hip or knee replacement. The final decision depends on local drug costs and the costs of monitoring warfarin therapy and treating bleeds [A][92].

**Warfarin reduces venous thromboembolism in patients having elective total hip replacement**

| Patient | Treatment | Comparator | Outcome | CER | OR | NNT |
|---|---|---|---|---|---|---|
| Elective total hip replacement [A][82] | Warfarin | Placebo or nothing | Venous thromboembolism at ? discharge | ? | 0.24 (0.13 to 0.34) | 4 (3 to 8) |
| Cancer patients having chemotherapy [A][77] | Warfarin | Nothing | DVT at 19 days | 4.3% | 100 | 23 (14 to 85) |

Alternatives include:

● hirudin [A][93]

**Why do this?**

■ Hirudin is more effective than heparin at preventing venous thromboembolism in patients undergoing first total hip replacement [A][13].

**Hirudin is more effective than heparin at preventing venous thromboembolism**

| Patient | Treatment | Comparator | Outcome | CER | RRR | NNT |
|---------|-----------|------------|---------|-----|-----|-----|
| Elective total hip replacement [A][93] | Hirudin | Heparin | DVT at 1.5 months | 18% | 67% (41% to 81%) | 8 (5 to 16) |
| | | | PE at 1.5 months | 1.8% | 100% | 55 (28 to 1900) |

● antiplatelet drugs [A][75] (aspirin, dipyridamole, hydroxychloroquine, ticlodipine).

**Why do this?**

■ It reduces venous thromboembolism in high-risk medical and surgical patients. The benefits are greater the more risky the surgery (traumatic orthopaedic > elective orthopaedic > general surgery) [A][75].
■ However, bleeds requiring transfusion or reoperation are more common. Wound haematoma and associated infection are also more common [A][75].
■ There is no clear benefit from combining antiplatelet drugs with heparin or LMWH [D][94].

**Antiplatelet drugs reduce venous thromboembolism but increase bleeding**

| Patient | Treatment | Comparator | Outcome | CER | OR | NNT |
|---------|-----------|------------|---------|-----|-----|-----|
| High-risk surgery | Antiplatelet drug | Placebo | DVT at 2 weeks | 35% | 0.39 (0.33 to 0.45) | 11 (9 to 16) |
| High-risk surgery | | | PE at 2 weeks | 2.7% | 0.64 (0.48 to 0.80) | 58 (44 to 86) |
| High-risk medical | | | DVT at 2 weeks | 23% | 0.42 (0.25 to 0.59) | 13 (7 to 75) |
| High-risk medical or surgical | | | Non-fatal bleed requiring transfusion at 2 weeks | 0.39% | 87 (0 to 250) | 290 (150 to 16000) |
| High-risk medical or surgical | | | Bleed requiring reoperation, wound haematoma, infection due to bleed at 2 weeks | 5.6% | 39 (12 to 74) | 45 (27 to 130) |

Continue prophylaxis for as long as the patient is at risk [A][95].

**Why do this?**

■ A fifth of patients have a DVT within 21 days of leaving hospital after a total hip replacement **[A]**[95].
■ Enoxaparin given for 35 days post-operation reduces DVT occurrence, clearly affecting mortality **[A]**[95].

**Extended LMWH prophylaxis reduces DVT following total hip replacement**

| Patient **[A]**[95] | Treatment | Comparator | Outcome | CER | RRR | NNT |
|---|---|---|---|---|---|---|
| Total hip replacement | LMWH for 50 days following surgery | LMWH for 15 days following surgery | DVT at 3 months | 19% | 63% (12% to 85%) | 8 (5 to 42) |

## PROGNOSIS

Silent PE is common **[B]**[96] **[B]**[97], although few patients develop serious problems if anticoagulated **[A]**[98]

**Note**

■ 40-50% of patients with a symptomatic DVT have a silent PE **[B]**[96] **[B]**[97].
■ Fatal PE in patients with treated venous thromboembolism is rare (2% during anticoagulation; 0.3% per 100 patient-years after).
■ More recurrent events are fatal in patients who initially present with PE (26%) compared with DVT (< 10%) **[A]**[98].

Patients are at increased risk of:

● recurrent venous thromboembolism (a quarter within 5 years) **[A]**[99]
● Post-thrombotic leg (a quarter within 5 years)**[A]**[99]
  – symtoms: pain, cramps, heaviness, pruritus, paraesthesia
  – signs: pretibial oedema, skin induration, hyperpigmentation, redness, pain on calf compression
● dying (a quarter within 5 years) **[A]**[99].

**Note**
**Recurrent venous thromboembolism, death and post-thrombotic leg are all common**

| Time after DVT **[A]**[99] | Recurrent VTE | Death | Post-thrombotic leg | Severe post-thrombotic leg |
|---|---|---|---|---|
| 3 months | 4.9% | | | |
| 1 year | 8.6% | 17% | 17% | 2.6% |
| 2 years | 18% | 20% | 23% | 9.3% |
| 5 years | 25% | 25% | 28% | |
| 8 years | 30% | 30% | | |

The risk of recurrent venous thromboembolism is increased with **[A]**[99]:

● cancer
● impaired coagulation inhibition

and reduced with [A][99]

- recent surgery
- recent trauma or fracture.

---

**? Why?**
**Cancer and clotting disorders increase the risk of venous thromboembolism**

| Patient [A][99] | Prognostic factor | Outcome | Control rate | OR (95% CI) | NNF+ (95% CI) |
|---|---|---|---|---|---|
| First DVT | Cancer *independent* | Recurrent venous thromboembolism at 2 years | 18% | 1.72 (1.31 to 2.25) | 8 (5 to 19) |
| | Impaired coagulation inhibition *independent* | Recurrent venous thromboembolism at 2 years | 18% | 1.44 (1.02 to 2.01) | 14 (7 to 270) |
| | Recent surgery *independent* | Recurrent venous thromboembolism at 2 years | 18% | 0.36 (0.21 to 0.62) | −7 (−13 to −5) |
| | Recent trauma or fracture *independent* | Recurrent venous thromboembolism at 2 years | 18% | 0.51 (0.32 to 0.87) | −10 (−40 to −7) |

---

The risk of dying is increased with [A][99]:

- cancer.

---

**? Why?**
**Cancer increases the risk of dying**

| Patient [A][99] | Prognostic factor | Outcome | Control rate | OR (95% CI) | NNF+ (95% CI) |
|---|---|---|---|---|---|
| First DVT | Cancer *independent* | Death at 2 years | 20% | 8.1 (3.6 to 18.1) | 2 (2 to 3) |

---

Patients are at a slightly greater risk of having cancer diagnosed in the next year [C][100] [C][101].

---

**Note**
- Roughly 1% of patients with a DVT have a cancer diagnosed in the next year [C][100] [C][101].
- After 1 year the risk is little different from the general population [C][100] [C][101].

---

## UPPER-LIMB DVT

Treat in a similar way to lower limb DVT [C][102].
Common causes include [C][102]:

- central venous line or pacemaker

- malignancy
- history of venous thromboembolism
- current leg DVT.

**Why?**
**Central lines and malignancy are the commonest causes of upper limb DVT**

| Causes [C]102 | % |
|---|---|
| Central venous line or pacemaker | 65% |
| Malignancy | 37% |
| History of venous thromboembolism | 11% |
| Current leg DVT | 11% |

Death is common. PE and arm swelling are rarer [C]102.

**Note**
- 7% of patients develop symptomatic PE (95% CI: 3.2% to 11%) and 6% develop arm swelling (95% CI: 2.4% to 9.6%) [C]102
- 16% are dead within a month (95% CI: 11% to 22%), and 34% within 3 months (95% CI: 27% to 41%) [C]102

**Guideline writers**: Christopher Ball
**CAT writers**: Christopher Ball, Robert Phillips

## REFERENCES

| No | Level | Citation |
|---|---|---|
| 1 | 1a | Wells PS et al. Value of assessment of pre-test probability of deep-vein thrombosis in clinical management. Lancet 1997; 350: 1795–8 |
| 2 | 3b | Vanderbroucke JP et al. Increased risk of venous thromboembolism in oral-contraceptive users who are carriers of factor V Leiden mutation. Lancet 1994; 344: 1453–7 |
| 3 | 3b | Nonfatal venous thromboembolism was associated with oral contraceptives that contain desogestrel and gestodene. ACP J Club 1996 May-June; 124:79. Evidence-Based Med 1996 May-June; 1:126. Summary of: Jick H et al. Risk of idiopathic cardiovascular death and nonfatal venous thromboembolism in women using oral contraceptives with differing progestogen components. Lancet 1995; 346: 1589–93 |
| 4 | 1b | Wells PS et al. A simple clinical model for the diagnosis of DVT combined with impedance plethysmography: potential for an improvement in the diagnostic process. J Intern Med 1998; 243: 15–23 |
| 5 | 1b | Huisman MV et al. Serial impedance plethysmogram for suspected deep venous thrombosis in outpatients: Amsterdam General Practitioner Study. N Engl J Med 1986; 314: 823–8 |
| 6 | 1a | Anand SS et al. The rational clinical exam: does this patient have deep vein thrombosis? JAMA 1998; 279: 1094–9 |
| 7 | 1a | Kearon C et al. Non-invasive diagnosis of deep vein thrombosis. Ann Intern Med 1998; 128: 663–77 |

| No | Level | Citation |
|----|-------|----------|
| 8 | 4 | Hull RD et al. Clinical validity of a negative venogram in patients with clinically suspected venous thrombosis. Circulation 1981; 64: 622–4 |
| 9 | 1b | Schulman S et al. The duration of oral anticoagulation after a second episode of venous thromboembolism. N Engl J Med 1997; 336: 393–8 |
| 10 | 2c | Koster V et al. Venous thromboembolism due to poor anticoagulation response to APC. Lancet 1993; 342: 1503–6 |
| 11 | 4 | Heijboer H et al. Deficiencies of coagulation-inhibiting and fibrinolytic proteins in out-patients with deep vein thrombosis. N Engl J Med 1990; 323: 1512–6 |
| 12 | 3a | Ray JG et al. Meta-analysis of hyperhomocysteinemia as a risk factor for venous thromboembolic disease. Arch Intern Med 1998; 158: 2101–6 |
| 13 | 2a | Doukatis JD et al. A re-evaulation of the risk of venous thromboembolism with the use of oral contraceptives or hormone replacement therapy. Arch Intern Med 1997; 157: 1522–30 |
| 14 | 1b | Sandler DR et al. Homans' sign and medical education. Lancet 1985; ii: 1130–1 |
| 15 | 1b | Cranley JJ et al. The diagnosis of deep venous thrombosis: fallibility of clinical symptoms and signs. Arch Surg 1976; 111: 34–6 |
| 16 | 2c | McColl MD et al. Risk factors for pregnancy associated venous thromboembolism. Thromb Haemost 1997; 78: 1183–8 |
| 17 | 4 | Friederich PW et al. Frequency of pregnancy-related venous thromboembolism in anticoagulant factor deficient women: implications for prophylaxis. Ann Intern Med 1996; 125: 955–60 |
| 18 | 4 | Kirkegaard A. Incidence and diagnosis of DVT associated with pregnancy. Arch Obst Gynecol Scand 1983; 62: 239–43 |
| 19 | 1b | de Boer K et al. Deep vein thrombosis in obstetric patients: diagnosis and risk factors. Thromb Haemost 1992; 61: 4–7 |
| 20 | 2c | Ginsberg JS et al. Venous thrombosis during pregnancy: leg and trimester of presentation. Thromb Haemost 1992; 67(S): 519–20 |
| 21 | 1b | Simpson FW et al. A prospective study of thrombophlebitis and 'pseudothrombophlebitis'. Lancet 1980; i: 331–3 |
| 22 | 1b | Freyburger G et al. D-dimer strategy in thrombus exclusion: a gold standard study in 100 patients suspected of deep venous thrombosis or pulmonary embolism: 8 d-dimer methods compared. Thromb Haemost 1998; 79: 32–7 |
| 23 | 1b | Dale S et al. Comparison of 3 d-dimer assays for the diagnosis of DVT: ELISA, latex and an immunofiltration assay Nycocard D-Dimer. Thromb Haemost 1994; 71: 270–4 |
| 24 | 1b | D-dimer testing and impedance plethysmography were effective for the exclusion of deep venous thrombosis. Evidence – Based Med 1997; 2; 186. Summary of: Ginsberg JS et al. The use of d-dimer testing and impedance plethysmographic examination in patients with clinical indications of deep venous thrombosis. Arch Intern Med 1997; 157: 1077–81 |
| 25 | 1a | Becher DM et al. D-dimer testing and acute venous thromboembolism: a shortcut to accurate diagnosis? Arch Intern Med 1996; 156: 939–46 |
| 26 | 2c | Cogo A et al. Distribution of thrombosis in patients with symptomatic deep vein thrombosis: implications for simplifying the diagnostic process with compression ultrasound. Arch Intern Med 1993; 153: 2777–80 |

| No | Level | Citation |
|----|-------|----------|
| 27 | 1b | Cogo A et al. Compression ultrasonography for diagnostic management of patients with clinically suspected deep vein thrombosis: prospective cohort study. BMJ 1998; 316: 17–20 |
| 28 | 1b | Birdwell BG et al. Clinical validity of normal compression ultrasound in outpatients suspected of having deep venous thrombosis. Ann Intern Med 1998; 128: 1–7 |
| 29 | 1a | Wells PS, Hirsch J, Anderson DR et al. Accuracy of clinical assessment of deep-vein thrombosis. Lancet 1995; 345: 1326–30 |
| 30 | 1b | Prandoni P et al. A simple ultrasound approach for the detection of recurrent proximal vein thrombosis. Circulation 1993; 88: 1730–5 |
| 31 | 1a | Wells PS et al. Accuracy of ultrasound for the diagnosis of deep vein thrombosis in asymptomatic patients after orthopedic surgery. Ann Intern Med 1995; 122: 47–51 |
| 32 | 1b | Ginsberg JS et al. Venous thromboembolism in patients who have undergone major hip or knee surgery: detection with compression ultrasound and impedance plethysmography. Radiology 1991; 181: 651–4 |
| 33 | 1b | Heijboer H et al. Comparison of real-time compression ultrasound with impedance plethysmography for the diagnosis of DVT in symptomatic outpatients. N Engl J Med 1993; 329: 1365–9 |
| 34 | 1b | Wells PS et al. Comparison of accuracy of impedance plethysmography and compression ultrasound in outpatients with clinically suspected DVT: a 2 centre paired-design trial. Thromb Haemost 1995; 74: 1423–7 |
| 35 | 4 | Huisman MV et al. Impedance plethysmography in the diagnosis of recurrent deep vein thrombosis. Arch Intern Med 1988; 148: 681–3 |
| 36 | 4 | Lensing AW et al. Lower extremity venography with iohexol; results and complications. Radiology 1990; 177: 503–5 |
| 37 | 2a | Ginsberg JS et al. Risks to the fetus of radiologic procedures used in the diagnosis of maternal venous thromboembolic disease. Thromb Haemost 1989; 61: 189–96 |
| 38 | 2b | Carpenter JP et al. Magnetic resonance venography for the detection of deep vein thrombosis: comparison with contrast venography and duplex doppler ultrasound. J Vasc Surg 1993; 18: 734–41 |
| 39 | 4 | Browse NL et al. Diagnosis of established deep venous thrombosis with I 125 fibrinogen uptake scan. BMJ 1971; iv: 325–8 |
| 40 | 1b | Lagerstedt CL et al. Need for long-term anticoagulation treatment in symptomatic calf-vein thrombosis. Lancet 1985; ii: 515–8 |
| 41 | 4 | Fulbrick and Becker DL. Calf DVT: a wolf in sheep's clothing? Arch Intern Med 1988; 148: 2131–8 |
| 42 | 1a | van den Belt AGM et al. Fixed dose subcutaneous low molecular weight heparins versus adjusted dose unfractionated heparin for venous thromboembolism (Cochrane Review). In: The Cochrane Library, Issue 2, 1999. Oxford: Update Software |
| 43 | 1b | Hull RD et al. Treatment of proximal vein thrombosis with subcutaneous LMWH versus intravenous heparin: an economic perspective. Arch Intern Med 1997; 157: 289–94 |
| 44 | 1b | Brandjes DP et al. Acencoumarol and heparin compared with acencoumarol alone in the initial treatment of proximal vein thrombosis. N Engl J Med 1992; 327: 1485 |

| No | Level | Citation |
|----|-------|----------|
| 45 | 1b | Fewer venous thromboembolism recurrences occurred with 6 months than with 6 weeks of anticoagulant therapy. ACP J Club 1996 Jan-Feb; 124:9. Evidence-Based Med 1996 Jan-Feb; 1:42. Summary of: Schulman S, Rhedin AS, Lindmarker P et al. and the Duration of Anticoagulation Trial Study Group. A comparison of six weeks with six months of oral anticoagulant therapy after a first episode of venous thromboembolism. N Engl J Med 1995; 332: 1661–5 |
| 46 | 1b | Schulman S et al. and the Duration of Anticoagulation Trial Study Group. The duration of oral anticoagulation after a second episode of venous thromboembolism. N Engl J Med 1997; 336: 393–8 |
| 47 | 1b | Crowther MA, Ginsberg JB, Kearon C et al. A randomized trial comparing 5-mg and 10-mg warfarin loading doses. Arch Intern Med 1999; 159: 46–8 |
| 48 | 4 | Fennerty A et al. Flexible induction dose regimen for warfarin and prediction of maintenance dose. BMJ 1984; 288: 1268–70 |
| 49 | 1b | Mohiuddin SM et al. Efficacy and safety of early versus late initiation of warfarin during heparin therapy in acute thromboembolism. Am Heart J 1992; 123: 729–32 |
| 50 | 1b – | Fewer venous thromboembolism recurrences occurred with 6 months than with 6 weeks of anticoagulant therapy: ACP Journal Club. 1996 Jan-Feb; 124:9. Evidence-Based Medicine 1996 Jan-Feb; 1:42. Summary of: Schulman S, Rhedin AS, Lindmarker P, et al. and the Duration of Anticoagulation Trial Study Group. A comparison of six weeks with six months of oral anticoagulant therapy after a first episode of venous thromboembolism. N Engl J Med. 1995 Jun 22; 332: 1661–5. |
| 51 | 1b | Kearon C, Gent M, Hirsch J et al. A comparison of three months of anticoagulation with extended anticoagulation for a first episode of idiopathic venous thromboembolism. N Engl J Med 1999; 340: 901–7 |
| 52 | 4 | Levine MN et al. Optimal duration of oral anticoagulation treatment: a randomised trial comparing 4 weeks with 3 months of warfarin in patients with proximal deep vein thrombosis. Thromb Haemost 1995; 74: 606–11 |
| 53 | 1b – | Low-molecular-weight heparin at home was as effective as unfractionated heparin in the hospital in proximal DVT. ACP J Club 1996 July-Aug; 125:3. Evidence-Based Med 1996 July-Aug; 1:141. Summary of: Levine M, Gent M, Hirsh J et al. A comparison of low-molecular-weight heparin administered primarily at home with unfractionated heparin administered in the hospital for proximal deep-vein thrombosis. N Engl J Med 1996; 334: 677–81 |
| 54 | 1b – | Low-molecular-weight heparin at home was as effective as unfractionated heparin in the hospital in proximal DVT. ACP J Club. 1996 July-Aug; 125:2. Evidence-Based Med 1996 July-Aug; 1:140. Summary of: Koopman MM et al. Treatment of venous thrombosis with intravenous unfractionated heparin administered in the hospital as compared with subcutaneous low-molecular-weight heparin administered at home. N Engl J Med 1996; 334: 682–7 |
| 55 | 1b | van den Belt AG et al. Replacing inpatient care by outpatient care in the treatment of DVT: an economic evaluation. Thromb Haemost 1998; 79: 259–63 |
| 56 | 1b | Schulman S et al. and the Duration of Anticoagulation Trial Study Group. The duration of oral anticoagulation after a second episode of venous thromboembolism. N Engl J Med. 1997; 336: 393–8 |

| No | Level | Citation |
|----|-------|----------|
| 57 | 4b | Fewer venous thromboembolism recurrences occurred with 6 months than with 6 weeks of anticoagulant therapy: ACP Journal Club. 1996 Jan-Feb; 124:9. Evidence-Based Medicine 1996 Jan-Feb; 1:42. Summary of: Schulman S, Rhedin AS, Lindmarker P, et al. and the Duration of Anticoagulation Trial Study Group. A comparison of six weeks with six months of oral anticoagulant therapy after a first episode of venous thromboembolism. N Engl J Med. 1995 Jun 22; 332: 1661–5 |
| 58 | 1b | White RH et al. Initiation of warfarin therapy: comparison of physician dosing with computer-assisted dosing. J Gen Intern Med 1987; 2: 141–8 |
| 59 | 1b | Consultation and guidelines to reduce anticoagulant-related bleeding. ACP J Club. 1992 Sept-Oct; 117:61. Summary of: Landefeld CS, Anderson PA. Guideline-based consultation to prevent anticoagulant-related bleeding. A randomized, controlled trial in a teaching hospital. Ann Intern Med 1992; 16: 829–37 |
| 60 | 2b | Cohen M et al. A comparison of low-molecular weight heparin with unfractionated heparin for unstable coronary disease. N Engl J Med 1997; 337: 447–52 |
| 61 | 2b | Warkentin TE et al. Heparin-induced thrombocytopenia in patients treated with LWMH or unfractionated heparin. N Engl J Med 1995; 332: 1330–5 |
| 62 | 4 | Warkentin TE et al. heparin-induced thrombocytopenia in patients treated with LWMH or unfractionated heparin: NEJM 1995; 332: 1330–5 |
| 63 | 1b | Brandjes DP et al. Randomised trial of compression stockings in patients with symptomatic proximal-vein thrombosis: Lancet 1997; 349: 759–62 |
| 64 | 1b | Goldhaber SZ et al. A randomised controlled trial in proximal deep vein thrombosis. Am J Med 1990; 88: 235–40 |
| 65 | 1a | Goldhaber SZ et al. Pooled analysis of randomised trials of streptokinase and heparin in phlebographically documented acute deep vein thrombosis. Am J Med 1984; 76: 393–7 |
| 66 | 1b – | Schweider G et al. Intermittent regional treatment with rt-PA is not superior to systemic thrombolysis in deep vein thrombosis: a German multicenter trial. Thromb Haemost 1995; 74: 1240–3 |
| 67 | 1b | Decousus H et al. A clinical trial of vena caval filters in the prevention of pulmonary embolism in patients with proximal deep venous thrombosis. N Engl J Med 1998; 338: 409–15 |
| 68 | 1b | Agnelli G et al. Enoxaparin plus compression stockings compared with compression stockings alone in the prevention of venous thromboembolism after elective neurosurgery. N Engl J Med 1998; 339: 80–5 |
| 69 | 1b | Wille-Jorgensen P et al. Heparin with and without graded compression stockings in the prevention of thromboembolic complications of major abdominal surgery: a randomised trial. Br J Surg 1985; 72: 579–81 |
| 70 | 1a | Graduated compression stockings prevent postoperative deep venous thrombosis. ACP J Club 1994 July-Aug; 121:8. Wells PS, Lensing AW, Hirsh J. Graduated compression stockings in the prevention of postoperative venous thromboembolism. A meta-analysis. Arch Intern Med 1994; 154: 67–72 |
| 71 | 1b | Ardeparin plus graduated compression stockings prevented DVT after knee surgery. ACP J Club 1996 Nov-Dec; 125:63. Evidence-Based Med 1996 Nov-Dec; 1: 213. Summary of: Levine MN et al. Ardeparin (low-molecular-weight heparin) vs graduated compression stockings for the prevention of venous thromboembolism. A randomized trial in patients undergoing knee surgery. Arch Intern Med 1996; 156: 851–6 |

| No | Level | Citation |
|----|-------|----------|
| 72 | 1b | Ramos R et al. The efficacy of pneumatic compression stockings in the prevention of pulmonary embolism after cardiac surgery. Chest 1996; 109: 82–5 |
| 73 | 1b | Kock HJ et al. Thromboprophylaxis with low-molecular weight heparin in outpatients with plaster-cast immobilisation of the leg. Lancet 1995; 346: 459–61 |
| 74 | 1b | Geerts WH et al. A comparison of low-dose heparin and LMWH as prophylaxis against venous thromboembolism after major trauma. N Engl J Med 1996; 335: 701–7 |
| 75 | 1a | Antiplatelet Trialists' Collaboration. Collaborative overview of randomised trials of antiplatelet therapy: III: Reduction of venous thromboembolism and pulmonary embolism by antiplatelet prophylaxis amongst surgical and medical patients. BMJ 1994; 308: 235–45 |
| 76 | 1b | Gardlund B. Randomised controlled trial of low-dose heparin for the prevention of fatal pulmonary embolism in patients with infectious disease. Lancet 1996; 347: 1357–61 |
| 77 | 1b | Very-low-dose warfarin reduces thromboembolism in patients with metastatic breast cancer receiving chemotherapy. ACP J Club 1994 Sept-Oct; 121:34. Summary of: Levine M et al. Double-blind randomised trial of very-low-dose warfarin for prevention of thromboembolism in stage IV breast cancer. Lancet 1994; 343: 886–9 |
| 78 | 4 | Melissari E et al. Use of low-molecular weight heparin in pregnancy: Thromb Haemost 1992; 68: 652–6 |
| 79 | 1b – | Howell R et al. The risks of antenatal subcutaneous heparin prophylaxis: a controlled trial. Br J Obstet Gynaecol 1983; 90: 1124–8 |
| 80 | 1a | Collins R, Scrimgeour A, Yusuf S et al. Reduction in fatal pulmonary embolism and venous thrombosis in perioperative admininstration of subcutaneous heparin: overview of results of randomized trials in general, orthopedic and urologic surgery. N Engl J Med 1988; 318: 1162–73 |
| 81 | 1b | Gardlund B. Randomised controlled trial of low-dose heparin for the prevention of fatal pulmonary embolism in patients with infectious disease. Lancet 1996; 347: 1357–61 |
| 82 | 1a | Low-molecular-weight heparin and compression stockings are most effective for preventing venous thromboembolism in hip replacement. ACP J Club 1994 Nov-Dec; 121:61. Summary of: Imperiale TF, Speroff T. A meta-analysis of methods to prevent venous thromboembolism following total hip replacement. JAMA 1994; 271: 1780–5 |
| 83 | 2b | Oster G et al. Prevention of venous thromboembolism after general surgery: cost-effectiveness analysis of alternative approaches to prophylaxis. Am J Med 1987; 82: 889–99 |
| 84 | 1a | Handoll HH et al. Prophylaxis using heparin, low molecular weight heparin and physical methods against deep vein thrombosis and pulmonary embolism in hip fracture surgery. In: Gillespie WJ et al (eds) Musculoskeletal injuries module of Cochrane Database of systematic reviews (updated 1/12/97). Available in the Cochrane Library Database on disk or CD-ROM. The Cochrane Collection, Issue 1, 1998. Oxford: Udate Software |
| 85 | 1b | Leyvroz PF et al. Adjusted versus fixed dose subcutaneous heparin in the prevention of deep vein thrombosis after total hip replacement. N Engl J Med 1983; 309: 954–8 |
| 86 | 2b | Bergqvist D et al. Comparison of cost of preventing post-operative DVT with either unfractionated or LMWH. Br J Surg 1996; 83: 1548–52 |
| 87 | 1a | Nurmohamed MT et al. Low molecular weight heparin versus standard heparin in general and orthopaedic surgery: a meta-analysis. Lancet 1992; 340: 152–6 |
| 88 | 1b | Spiro TE et al. Efficacy and safety of enoxaparin to prevent DVT after hip replacement surgery. Ann Intern Med 1994; 121: 81–9 |

| No | Level | Citation |
|----|-------|----------|
| 89 | 1b | Kakkar VV et al. Low molecular weight versus standard heparin for prevention of venous thromboembolism after major abdominal surgery. Lancet 1993; 341: 259–65 |
| 90 | 1b | Hull RD et al. Effectiveness of intermittent pneumatic leg compression for preventing deep vein thrombosis after total hip replacement. JAMA 1990; 263: 2313–17 |
| 91 | 1b – | Soderdahl DW et al. A comparison of intermittent pneumatic compression of the calf and whole leg in preventing DVT in urological surgery. J Urol 1997; 157: 1774–6 |
| 92 | 1b | Hull RD et al. Subcutaneous LMWH versus warfarin for the prophylaxis of DVT after hip or knee implantation: an economic perspective. Arch Intern Med 1997; 157: 298–303 |
| 93 | 1b | Eriksson BI et al. Prevention of thromboembolism with use of recombinant hirudin. J Bone Joint Surg 1997; 79A: 326–33 |
| 94 | 1b – | Monreal M et al. Platelet count, antiplatelet therapy and pulmonary embolism: a prospective study in patients with hip surgery. Thromb Haemost 1995; 73: 380–5 |
| 95 | 1b | Planes A et al. Risk of deep venous thrombosis after hospital discharge in patients having undergone total hip replacement: a double-blind randomised comparison of enoxaparin versus placebo: Lancet 1996; 348: 224–28 |
| 96 | 2c | Moser KM et al. Frequent asymptomatic pulmonary embolism in patients with DVT. JAMA 1994; 271: 223–5 |
| 97 | 2c | Nielsen HK et al. Silent pulmonary embolism in patients with deep venous thrombosis: incidence and fate in a randomised trial of anticoagulation versus no anticoagulation. J Intern Med 1994; 235: 457–61 |
| 98 | 1a | Doukatis JD et al. Risk of fatal pulmonary embolism in patients with treated venous thromboembolism. JAMA 1998; 279: 458–62 |
| 99 | 1b | Prandoni P et al. The long-term clinical course of acute deep venous thrombosis. Ann Intern Med 1996; 125: 1–7 |
| 100 | 4 | Sorensen HT et al. The risk of a diagnosis of cancer after primary deep venous thrombosis or pulmonary thrombosis. N Engl J Med 1998; 338: 1169–73 |
| 101 | 4 | Baron JA et al. Venous thromboembolism and cancer. Lancet 1998; 351: 1077–80 |
| 102 | 4 | Hingorani A et al. Upper extremity deep vein thrombosis and its impact on morbidity and mortality rates in a hospital-based population. J Vasc Surg 1997; 26: 853–60 |

## PREVALENCE

Diabetic ketoacidosis is defined as [D][1]:
- hyperglycaemia (> 14 mmol/l)
- metabolic acidosis (pH < 7.35 or bicarbonate < 15 mmol/l)
- high anion gap (anion gap = $Na + K - HCO_3$) [C][2]
- ketonaemia.

Hyperglycaemic hyperosmolar non-ketosis [D][1] is different:
- blood glucose is higher (often > 33 mmol/l)
- no acidosis
- one plus ketonuria at the most on urine dipstick
- higher $Na^+$ (often > 150 mmol/l).

DKA is relatively common [B][3] in patients with diabetes and is often recurrent [B][4]. Roughly one in seven patients with hyperglycaemia who feel unwell have DKA [C][2].

**Note**
- 8.9% of patients with diabetes have an episode of DKA in 1 year (95% CI: 7.7% to 10%) [B][3].
- 42% of patients with DKA have another episode (95% CI: 32% to 52%) [B][4].
- 14% of patients with a blood glucose > 11 mmol/l and any complaint have DKA (95% CI: 12% to 17%) [C][2].

Up to a quarter of cases are patients with new-onset diabetes [C][8].

**Note**
- 27% of patients with DKA have new-onset diabetes (95% CI: 22% to 33%).

## CAUSES

Common causes of DKA include [B][3] [B][4] [C][5] [C][6]:
- infection
- treatment error
- new-onset diabetes
- other medical illness

but it is often of unknown aetiology.

**❓ Why?**

**The cause of many cases of DKA is unknown**

| [B]3 [B]4 [C]5 [C]6 | Prevalence |
|---|---|
| Unknown | 19%–38% |
| Infection | 27%–38% |
| Treatment error | 12%–28% |
| Other medical illness | 11% |
| ■ pancreatitis | 2%–3% |
| ■ myocardial infarction | 1%–7% |
| ■ GI bleed | 1% |
| ■ heart failure | 2% |
| Affected by drugs or alcohol | 9% |
| Newly diagnosed diabetes | 10%–27% |

## CLINICAL FEATURES

Ask about:
- known diabetes mellitus [B]3 [B]4:
- previous episodes of DKA [B]3 [B]4
- current medication [A]7, and any recent changes or mistakes [B]3 [B]4
- recent illness [B]3 [B]4
- polyuria, polydipsia and weakness [D].

**❓ Why do this?**

■ Patients who have intensive insulin therapy are at increased risk of ketoacidosis; however, there is no clear effect on mortality [A]7.

■ In particular, patients on continuous insulin infusions are at increased risk of ketoacidosis. There is no clear increase in ketoacidosis for patients on multiple daily injections [A]7.

**Intensive insulin regimens, particularly insulin pumps, increase the risk of DKA**

| Patient [A]7 | Treatment | Comparator | Outcome | CER | OR | NNH |
|---|---|---|---|---|---|---|
| Insulin-dependent diabetes | Intensified insulin regimen | Standard insulin regimen | DKA at 2–6 years | 6.4% | 2.88 (2.38 to 3.48) | 4 (3 to 5) |
| Insulin-dependent diabetes | Insulin pump | Standard insulin regimen | DKA at 2–6 years | 0.86% | 5.76 (2.88 to 11.50) | 26 (12 to 64) |

Look for evidence of [B]3 [B]4:
- dehydration
- infection (e.g. lobar pneumonia, urinary tract infection)
- associated disease (e.g. MI, pancreatitis).

Think about acidosis in any hyperventilating patient [D]8.

## INVESTIGATIONS

Take a capillary blood glucose **[A]**.

Take a urine sample and test for:
- ketones **[C]**[2]
- leucocytes or nitrites: if abnormal send for culture **[D]**.

**Why?**

**No ketones on urine dipstick make DKA very unlikely**

| Patient [C][2] | Target disorder (reference standard) | Diagnostic test | LR+(95% CI) | Post-test probability | LR−(95% CI) | Post-test probability |
|---|---|---|---|---|---|---|
| Suspected DKA (pre-test probability 14%) | DKA (elevated glucose, metabolic acidosis and ketonaemia) | Positive urine ketone dipstick | 3.2 (2.9 to 3.7) | 35% | 0.015 (0.0021 to 0.10) | 0.24% |

Take the following blood tests:
- blood glucose
- urea and electrolytes, creatinine **[C]**[9]

**Why?**
- 40% of patients with DKA have abnormal potassium levels: 28% hyperkalemia; 12% hypokalaemia **[C]**[9].

- ketones **[A]**
- pH **[A]** from venous blood **[C]**[10]

**Why?**
- Venous blood pH and bicarbonate levels correlate closely in patients with DKA **[C]**[10].

- bicarbonate **[C]**[2].

Calculate the anion gap (Na + K − $HCO_3$) **[C]**[2].

**Why?**

**A normal anion gap makes DKA unlikely, and a low bicarbonate makes it very likely**

| Patient [C][2] | Target disorder (reference standard) | Diagnostic test | LR+ (95% CI) | Post-test probability | LR−(95% CI) | Post-test probability |
|---|---|---|---|---|---|---|
| Suspected DKA (pre-test probability 14%) | DKA (elevated glucose, metabolic acidosis and ketonaemia) | Anion gap > 16 mmol/l | 6.3 (5.1 to 7.6) | 51% | 0.096 (0.049 to 0.19) | 1.5% |
| | | Serum bicarbonate < 15 mmol/l | 100 (42 to 240) | 94% | 0.16 (0.11 to 0.26) | 2.6% |

The following tests may help identify the cause:
- blood count [D]
- cardiac enzymes [B][3] [B][4]
- amylase [B][3] [B][4]
- blood cultures
- chest X-ray [B][3] [B][4]
- 12-lead and continuous ECG [B][3] [B][4].

Repeat electrolytes and glucose levels [C][9] [C][11] at least hourly [D] until biochemical normality is achieved. A chart for vital signs, laboratory results and fluid balance is helpful [D].

## THERAPY

- Resuscitate and seek help if required [D].
- Give intravenous fluids: initially 0.9% saline [C][11] (e.g. 1 litre over 30 min, 1 litre over 1 h, 1 litre over 2 h, 1 litre over 4 h).

If none of the following are present, fluids can safely be given more slowly if necessary [D][12]:
- circulatory shock
- oliguria (< 30 ml/h) during the first 4 h of admission
- renal insufficiency (urea > 21 mmol/l or creatinine > 350 μmol/l).

 **Why do this?**
- If there is no evidence of severe dehydration, normal saline given at 500 ml/h for 4 h followed by 250 ml/h for 4 h does not clearly affect time to normalised biochemistry compared with normal saline 1 litre/h for 4 h followed by 500 ml/h for 4 h [D][12].

In dehydrated or comatose patients, consider [D]:
- a urinary catheter
- a central venous line.

- Monitor electrolytes [C][9] [C][11] and capillary glucose [D] frequently. Give potassium supplementation [A] after insulin therapy has begun if K+ < 5.5 mmol/l [D]. Provide 10–30 mmol/h [C][9].

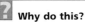 **Why do this?**

■ Potassium abnormalities are common: 28% of patients have hyperkalaemia on admission (95% CI: 10% to 46%) and 12% have hypokalaemia (95% CI: 0% to 25%) **[C]**[9].
■ Patients require on average 30–40 mmol of potassium per litre of fluid to keep serum potassium normal during rehydration **[C]**[9].
■ A patient whose serum sodium concentration falls or fails to rise during rehydration is at increased risk of developing cerebral oedema. A failure to rise suggests rehydration with excess free water **[C]**[11].

**A failure of sodium to rise on rehydration increases the risk of cerebral oedema**

| Patient [C][11] | Prognostic factor | Outcome | Control rate | RR (95% CI) | NNF+ (95% CI) |
|---|---|---|---|---|---|
| DKA | No rise in serum sodium on rehydration *not independent* | Cerebral oedema | 2.3% (0.0% to 5.5%) | 6.56 (1.56 to 27.53) | 8 (2 to 76) |

● Give broad-spectrum antibiotics if there is evidence of infection **[A]**.
● Give soluble insulin **[A]** in low doses (e.g. 5–10 units/h) **[A]**[13] intravenously **[D]** at regular intervals or continuously **[D]**.

**Why do this?**

■ A low-dose insulin regimen is less likely to cause hypoglycaemia or hypokalaemia than a high-dose regimen **[A]**[13].
■ There is no clear difference in the time taken to return to biochemical normality **[A]**[13].

**A low-dose insulin regimen reduces the risk of hypoglycaemia or hypokalaemia**

| Patient | Treatment | Comparator | Outcome | CER | RRR | NNT |
|---|---|---|---|---|---|---|
| DKA | Low-dose insulin | High-dose insulin | Hypoglycaemia (< 2.8 mmol/l) at 12 h | 25% | 100% | 4 (2 to 13) |
| | | | Hypokalaemia (< 3.4 mmol/l) at 12 h | 29% | 86% (–7% to 98%) | 4 (2 to 19) |

■ The route used to administer insulin in patients has no clear effect on the time taken to return to biochemical normality or the amount of insulin required **[D]**[14] **[D]**[15].
■ A continuous insulin infusion is not clearly more likely to cause a faster fall in glucose levels nor shorten the time to reach a glucose < 14 mmol/l than a bolus followed by regular injections **[D]**[16].

● Continue giving insulin by this route until **[A]**[17]:
  – glucose < 10 mmol/l, and
  – ketones are cleared (3-hydroxybutyrate < 0.5 mmol/l).

If glucose < 10 mmol/l but ketones are still raised, continue insulin infusion with 20% glucose iv to maintain glucose 5–10 mmol/l.

**Why do this?**
■ Patients with DKA who receive an extended insulin regimen have a more rapid fall in ketones than those on a conventional regimen (~16 h difference) **[A]**[17].

● Once patients have stabilised, swap to subcutaneous insulin.
Give 5% glucose and insulin infusion (at 8 units/h), with subcutaneous insulin as necessary to maintain blood glucose < 10 mmol/l until patients are eating **[C]**[17].
Give the first subcutaneous dose before stopping the infusion **[D]**.

There is no clear benefit from:
● sodium bicarbonate **[D]**[18] **[D]**[19]

**Why?**
■ Patients with severe DKA who receive bicarbonate do not clearly return more quickly to biochemical stability **[D]**[18] **[D]**[19].
■ The effect on hypokalaemic or hypoglycaemic episodes is unclear **[D]**[18] **[D]**[19].

● routine phosphate supplementation **[A]**[20]

**Why?**
■ It reduces the risk of hypophosphataemia but increases the risk of infection, and has no clear effect on mortality **[A]**[20].
■ Patients do not recover consciousness more quickly nor leave hospital sooner **[A]**[20].
■ It has no clear effect on pH, phosphate, calcium or glucose levels at 24 h **[D]**[21] **[D]**[22].

● hypertonic glucose **[D]**[23].

**Why?**
■ Patients with a glucose < 14 mmol/l do not clearly have a faster improvement in biochemical markers following 10% glucose and insulin rather than 5% glucose and insulin **[D]**[23].

## PREVENTION

● Refer your patient to the diabetes team and educate the patient about diabetes **[A]**[24].

**Why do this?**
■ It improves glycaemic control and reduces readmissions **[A]**[24].
■ There is no clear effect on length of hospital stay **[A]**[24].

**Why do this?**
A diabetic team improves glycaemic control and reduces hospital readmissions

| Patient [A][24] | Treatment | Comparator | Outcome | CER | RRR | NNT |
|---|---|---|---|---|---|---|
| Inpatient with diabetes | Diabetic team intervention | No intervention | Good glycaemic control at 1 month | 46% | 65 % (28% to 112%) | 3 (2 to 6) |
| | | | Readmission at 3 months | 32% | 52 % (14% to 73%) | 6 (3 to 22) |

## PROGNOSIS

Watch for cerebral oedema during resuscitation of patients aged < 30 years, particularly in patients whose serum sodium concentration fails to rise during rehydration [C][11].

**Note**

■ Around 10% of patients with DKA suffer complications of brain swelling (mostly minor); 3% die [C][11].

Few patients die: death is mainly from associated disease [B][3] [B][25].

**Note**

■ 3–5% with DKA die during admission; 15% of patients with hyperosmolar coma die [B][3] [B][25].
■ The commonest causes of death are pneumonia, MI and bowel or limb ischaemia [B][25].

Recurrent episodes are common [B][4].
Patients with recurrent episodes are at increased risk of dying or having diabetic complications [C][26] [C][27].

**Note**
Half of patients have another episode

| Number of subsequent episodes of DKA [B][4] | % of patients |
|---|---|
| 0 | 58% |
| 1 | 23% |
| 2 | 10% |
| ≥3 | 9% |

■ 20% of women with recurrent DKA are dead within 10 years [C][26] [C][27].
■ Two-thirds have a diabetic complication and ~75% have a pregnancy complication in this time [C][26] [C][27].
■ Only 10% still have recurrent DKA after 10 years [C][26] [C][27].

**Guideline writers**: Richard Hardern, Christopher Ball
**CAT writers**: Richard Hardern, Chris Ball

## REFERENCES

| No | Level | Citation |
|---|---|---|
| 1 | 5 | Kitabchi AE, Wal BM. Diabetic ketoacidosis (narrative review). Med Clin North Am 1995; 79: 9–37 |
| 2 | 4 | Schwab TM, Hendey GW, Soliz TC et al. Screening for ketonemia in patients with diabetes. Ann Emerg Med 1999; 34: 342–6 |
| 3 | 2c | Snorgaard O et al. Diabetic ketoacidosis in Denmark: epidemiology, incidence rates, precipitating factors and mortality rates. J Intern Med 1989; 226: 223–8 |
| 4 | 2c | Johnson DD et al. Diabetic ketoacidosis in a community-based population. Mayo Clin Proc 1980; 55: 83–8 |
| 5 | 4 | Westphal SA: The occurrence of diabetic ketoacidosis in non-insulin-dependent diabetes and newly diagnosed diabetic adults: Am J Med 1996; 101: 19–24 |
| 6 | 4 | Basu A, Close CF, Jenkins D et al. Persisting mortality in diabetic ketoacidosis. Diabet Med 1993; 10: 282–4 |
| 7 | 1a | Egger M, Davey Smith G, Stettler C et al. Risk of adverse effects of intensified treatment in insulin dependent diabetes mellitus: a meta-analysis. Diabet Med 1997; 14: 919–28 |
| 8 | 5 | Treasure RA et al. Misdiagnosis of diabetic ketoacidosis as hyperventilation syndrome (case report). BMJ 1987; 294: 630 |
| 9 | 4 | Soler NG et al. Potassium balance during the treatment of diabetic ketoacidosis. Lancet 1972; ii: 665–7 |
| 10 | 4 | Brandenburg MA, Dire DJ. Comparison of arterial and venous blood gas values in the initial emergency department evaluation of patients with diabetic ketoacidosis. Ann Emerg Med 1998; 31: 459–65 |
| 11 | 4 | Harris GD et al. Minimizing the risk of brain herniation during treatment of diabetic ketoacidosis: a retrospective and prospective study. J Pediatr 1990; 117: 22–31 |
| 12 | 1b – | Adrogue HJ, Barrero J, Eknoyan G. Salutary effects of modest fluid replacement in the treatment of adults with diabetic ketoacidosis. Use in patients without extreme volume deficit. JAMA 1989; 262: 2108–13 |
| 13 | 1b | Kitabchi AE, Ayyagari V, Guerra SM. The efficacy of low dose versus conventional therapy of insulin for treatment of diabetic ketoacidosis. Ann Intern Med 1976; 84: 633–8 |
| 14 | 1b – | Fisher JN et al. Diabetic ketoacidosis: low-dose insulin therapy by various routes. N Engl J Med 1977; 297: 238–41 |
| 15 | 1b – | Sacks HS et al. Similar responsiveness of diabetic ketoacidosis to low-dose insulin by intramuscular injection and albumin-free solution. Ann Intern Med 1979; 90: 36–42 |
| 16 | 1b – | Heber D, Molitch ME, Sperling MA. Low-dose continuous insulin therapy for diabetic ketoacidosis: prospective comparison with 'conventional' insulin therapy. Arch Intern Med 1977; 137: 1377–80 |

| No | Level | Citation |
|----|-------|----------|
| 17 | 1b | Wiggam MI et al. Treatment of diabetic ketoacidosis using normalization of blood 3-hydroxybutyrate concentration as the endpoint of emergency management. Diabetes Care 1997; 20: 1347–51 |
| 18 | 4 | Morris LR, Murphy MB, Kitabchi AE. Bicarbonate therapy in severe diabetic ketoacidosis. Ann Intern Med 1986; 105: 836–40 |
| 19 | 4 | Hale PJ, Crase J, Nattrass M. Metabolic effects of bicarbonate in the treatment of diabetic ketoacidosis. BMJ 1984; 289: 1035–8 |
| 20 | 1b | Keller U, Berger W. Prevention of hypophosphatemia by phosphate infusion during treatment of diabetic ketoacidosis and hyperosmolar coma. Diabetes 1980; 29: 87–95 |
| 21 | 1b – | Wilson HK, Keuer SP, Lea AS et al. Phosphate therapy in diabetic ketoacidosis. Arch Intern Med 1982; 142: 517–20 |
| 22 | 1b – | Fisher JN, Kitabchi AE. A randomized study of phosphate therapy in the treatment of diabetic ketoacidosis. J Clin Endocrinol Metab 1983; 57: 177–80 |
| 23 | 1b – | Krentz AJ, Hale PJ, Singh BM et al. The effect of glucose and insulin infusion on the fall of ketone bodies during treatment of diabetic ketoacidosis. Diabet Med 1989; 6: 31–6 |
| 24 | 1b | Koproski J et al. Effects of an intervention by a diabetes team in hospitalized patients with diabetes. Diabetes Care 1997; 20: 1553–5 |
| 25 | 2c | Hamblin PS et al. Deaths associated with diabetic ketoacidosis and hyperosmolar coma 1973–1988. Med J Aust 1989; 151: 439–44 |
| 26 | 4 | Kent LA, Gill GV, Williams G. Mortality and outcome of patients with brittle diabetes and recurrent ketoacidosis. Lancet 1994; 344: 778–81 |
| 27 | 4 | Tattersall R et al. Course of brittle diabetes: 12 year follow-up. BMJ 1991; 302: 1240–3 |

Resuscitate your patient before doing anything else **[A]**:
- airway (head down if bleeding)
- breathing–give oxygen **[D]**
- circulation – two large-bore iv catheters in the antecubital veins **[D]**.

## PREVALENCE

Upper gastrointestinal (GI) bleeding is relatively common in:
- patients on non-steroidal anti-inflammatory drugs (NSAIDs) **[A]**
- patients on intensive care units **[B]**[2]
- elderly patients **[B]**[3].

**Note**
- Around 1 in 1000 patients recently started on NSAIDs have a GI haemorrhage or perforation (0.11%; 95% CI: 0.094% to 0.13%) **[A]**[1].
- One in 12 patients on intensive care units for longer than 2 days have an upper GI bleed (8.7%; 95% CI: 6.8% to 11%) **[B]**[2].

**Old age increases the risk for a bleeding peptic ulcer**

| Patient [B][3] | Prognostic factor | Outcome | Control rate | OR (95% CI) | NNF+ (95% CI) |
|---|---|---|---|---|---|
| Well | Aged > 75 years | Bleeding peptic ulcer at 19 months | 0.13% | 5.1 (3.3 to 7.8) | 190 (110 to 330) |

- Suspicion of an upper GI bleed is proved correct in a third of inpatients (39%; 95% CI: 27% to 51% **[C]**[4].

## CAUSES

Common causes include **[B]**[5]:
- gastric or duodenal ulcers
- gastric erosions
- varices
- Mallory–Weiss tear
- oesophagitis.

Rarer causes include:
- tumours **[B]**[5]
- angiodysplasia.

**Note**
**Upper GI bleeding: differential diagnoses**

| Differential diagnosis [B]⁵ [C]⁶ | Prevalence (95% CI) |
|---|---|
| Duodenal ulcer | 24% (23% to 26%) |
| Gastric erosions | 24% (22% to 25%) |
| Gastric ulcer | 21% (20% to 23%) |
| Varices | 10% (9.0% to 12%) |
| Mallory–Weiss tear | 7.2% (6.1% to 8.3%) |
| Oesophagitis | 6.3% (5.3% to 7.3%) |
| Erosive duodenitis | 5.8% (4.8% to 6.7%) |
| Neoplasm | 2.9% (2.2% to 3.6%) |
| Stomal ulcer | 1.8% (1.3% to 2.4%) |
| Oesophageal ulcer | 1.7% (1.1% to 2.2%) |
| Osler–Rendu–Weber telangiectasia | 0.49% (0.20% to 0.79%) |
| Other | 6.3% (5.2% to 7.3%) |

## CLINICAL FEATURES

Ask about:
- any haematemesis or melaena before admission, and its colour [C]⁷ and amount [D]

**Why?**
**Haematemesis and melaena make a peptic ulcer slightly more likely**

| Patient [C]⁷ | Target disorder (reference standard) | Diagnostic test | LR+ (95% CI) | Post-test probability |
|---|---|---|---|---|
| History of haematemesis or melaena (pre-test probability 51%) | Peptic ulcer (endoscopy) | Black haematemesis with melaena | 2.4 (1.5 to 3.9) | 71% |
| | | Red haematemesis with melaena | 1.5 (1.1 to 2.0) | 61% |
| | | Melaena only | 1.3 (0.88 to 1.8) | 57% |
| | | Red haematemesis only | 0.66 (0.48 to 0.91) | 41% |
| | | Black haematemesis only | 0.43 (0.30 to 0.62) | 31% |

**Red haematemesis makes varices slightly more likely**

| Patient [C]⁷ | Target disorder (reference standard) | Diagnostic test | LR+ (95% CI) | Post-test probability |
|---|---|---|---|---|
| History of haematemesis or melaena (pre-test probability 11%) | Varices (endoscopy) | Red haematemesis +/– melaena | 1.7 (1.4 to 2.0) | 17% |
| | | Black haematemesis or melaena | 0.43 (0.27 to 0.69) | 5% |

> **❓ Why?**
> **Black haematemesis or melaena makes a Mallory–Weiss tear unlikely**
>
> | Patient [C][7] | Target disorder (reference standard) | Diagnostic test | LR+ (95% CI) | Post-test probability |
> |---|---|---|---|---|
> | History of haematemesis or melaena (pre-test probability 3.5%) | Mallory–Weiss tear (endoscopy) | Red haematemesis +/– melaena | 2.1 (2.0 to 2.3) | 7% |
> |  |  | Black haematemesis or melaena | 0.0 (0.0 to 0.29) | 0% |

- other illnesses [A][8] [B][9]
  - previous peptic ulcers [B][3] and any previous peptic ulcer surgery [B][10]
  - *Helicobacter pylori* infection [B][10]
  - alcohol-related disorders [B][2] [B][3]
  - liver cirrhosis, oesophageal varices or portal vein thrombosis [A][8] [A][9] [B][2] [B][3]
  - renal failure [A][8] [A][9]
  - disseminated malignancy [A][8] [A][9]
  - heart disease and heart failure [A][8] [A][9]

> **❓ Why?**
> - Comorbidity (particularly liver failure, renal failure or disseminated malignancy) increases the risk of rebleeding or dying (see prognosis for Rockall score) [A][8] [A][9].
> - *H. pylori* infection is common in patients who have had peptic ulcer surgery: 50% of patients with a partial gastrectomy (95% CI: 46% to 54%) and 83% of patients with a vagotomy (95% CI: 80% to 86%) are infected [B][10].
>
> **Peptic ulcer disease, alcohol abuse, liver disease and *H. pylori* infection increase the risk of upper GI bleeding**
>
> | Patient | Prognostic factor | Outcome | Control rate | OR (95% CI) | NNF + (95% CI) |
> |---|---|---|---|---|---|
> | Well [B][3] | History of a peptic ulcer | Bleeding peptic ulcer at 19 months | 0.13% | 6.5 (4.4 to 9.7) | 140 (88 to 220) |
> |  | Alcohol-related diagnosis | As above | 0.13% | 4.1 (2.3 to 7.5) | 250 (120 to 590) |
> |  | Liver cirrhosis, oesophageal varices or portal vein thrombosis | As above | 0.13% | 4.1 (2.2 to 7.6) | 250 (120 to 630) |
> | On ITU for 2 or more days [B][2] | *H. pylori* infection | Upper GI bleed | 8.7% | 1.92 | 15 |

- how long a nasogastric tube has been *in situ* [B][2]

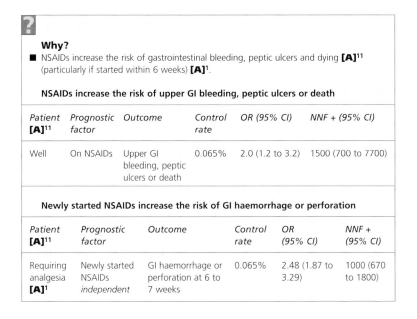

| Patient | Prognostic factor | Outcome | Control rate | OR (95% CI) | NNF + (95% CI) |
|---|---|---|---|---|---|
| On ITU for 2 or more days **[B]**[2] | Nasogastric tube *in situ* for 6 days | Upper GI bleed | 8.7% | 2.59 | 9 |

**Why?**
A nasogastric tube *in situ* for 6 or more days increases the risk of upper GI bleeding

- current medication, particularly:
  - anticoagulants **[A]**
  - NSAIDs **[A]**[1] **[A]**[11].

**Why?**
■ NSAIDs increase the risk of gastrointestinal bleeding, peptic ulcers and dying **[A]**[11] (particularly if started within 6 weeks) **[A]**[1].

NSAIDs increase the risk of upper GI bleeding, peptic ulcers or death

| Patient [A][11] | Prognostic factor | Outcome | Control rate | OR (95% CI) | NNF + (95% CI) |
|---|---|---|---|---|---|
| Well | On NSAIDs | Upper GI bleeding, peptic ulcers or death | 0.065% | 2.0 (1.2 to 3.2) | 1500 (700 to 7700) |

Newly started NSAIDs increase the risk of GI haemorrhage or perforation

| Patient [A][11] | Prognostic factor | Outcome | Control rate | OR (95% CI) | NNF + (95% CI) |
|---|---|---|---|---|---|
| Requiring analgesia [A][1] | Newly started NSAIDs *independent* | GI haemorrhage or perforation at 6 to 7 weeks | 0.065% | 2.48 (1.87 to 3.29) | 1000 (670 to 1800) |

Look for:
- evidence of acute bleeding **[B]**[12]
  - supine tachycardia (pulse >100 beats/min)
  - supine hypotension (systolic blood pressure >95 mmHg)
  - postural pulse increase of ≥30 beats/min or severe dizziness on sitting upright, then on standing.

**? Why?**

Severe dizziness and a pulse increase >30 beats/min on standing make a significant acute bleed more likely

| Patient [B][12] | Target disorder (reference standard) | Diagnostic test | LR+ | Post-test probability | LR– | Post-test probability |
|---|---|---|---|---|---|---|
| Suspected acute blood loss (pre-test probability 7.3%) | Acute severe blood loss (venesection of 630–1150 ml) | Postural pulse increase >30 beats/min or severe postural dizziness on sitting from supine | 39 | 75% | 0.22 | 1.7% |
| | Acute severe blood loss (venesection of 630–1150 ml) | Postural pulse increase >30 beats/min or severe postural dizziness on standing from supine | 49 | 79% | 0.030 | 0.24% |
| | Acute moderate blood loss (venesection of 350–600 ml) | Postural pulse increase > 30 beats/min or severe postural dizziness on standing from supine | 44 | 78% | 0.80 | 5.9% |
| | Acute severe blood loss (venesection of 630–1150 ml) | Supine tachycardia | 4.0 | 24% | 0.92 | 6.8% |
| | Acute severe blood loss (venesection of 630–1150 ml) | Supine hypotension | 11 | 46% | 0.68 | 5.1% |
| | Acute moderate blood loss (venesection of 350–600 ml) | Supine hypotension | 4.3 | 24% | 0.90 | 6.8% |

**Note**

- Evidence of shock increases the risk of rebleeding or dying [A][8] [A][9].
- Postural hypotension (fall in systolic > 20 mmHg on standing) does not usefully diagnose acute blood loss [B][12].
- Absence of supine tachycardia does not exclude moderate acute blood loss [B][12].

In uncertain cases, look for:
- evidence of anaemia
- conjunctival pallor [A][13]

> **❓ Why?**
> Conjunctival pallor makes anaemia more likely, but a normal colour cannot rule it out
>
> | Patient [A][13] | Target disorder (reference standard) | Diagnostic test | LR+ (95% CI) | Post-test probability |
> |---|---|---|---|---|
> | Inpatient (pre-test probability 18%) | Severe anaemia (haemoglobin < 9.0 g/dl) | Pale conjunctivae<br>Borderline conjunctivae<br>Normal conjunctivae | 4.5 (1.8 to 11)<br>1.8 (1.2 to 2.7)<br>0.61 (0.45 to 0.82) | 50%<br>29%<br>12% |
>
> - Pale: little or no evidence of red colour on anterior rim which matched the fleshy part of the posterior aspect of the palpebral conjunctiva.
> - Borderline: neither clearly red nor clearly pale or those with one conjunctiva red and the other pale.
> - Normal: full or nearly full redness of the anterior rim.

– facial pallor [B][14]
– palmar pallor [B][14]

The more that are present, the greater the chance of anaemia [B][14].

> **❓ Why?**
> Conjunctival pallor, facial or palmar pallor make anaemia more likely
>
> | Patient [B][14] | Target disorder (reference standard) | Diagnostic test | LR + (95% CI) | Post-test probability | LR – (95% CI) | Post-test probability |
> |---|---|---|---|---|---|---|
> | Suspected anaemia (pre-test probability 19%) | Anaemia (haematocrit <0.41 men or < 0.31 women) | Conjunctival pallor | 3.1 (1.4 to 6.8) | 42% | 0.65 (0.50 to 0.84) | 13% |
> | | | Facial pallor | 3.6 (1.3 to 9.8) | 46% | 0.72 (0.59 to 0.89) | 14% |
> | | | Palmar pallor | 2.2 (1.2 to 4.0) | 34% | 0.62 (0.46 to 0.85) | 13% |
> | | | Any present | 2.3 (1.4 to 3.8) | 35% | 0.48 (0.32 to 0.72) | 10% |
> | | | Two present | 3.0 (1.4 to 6.6) | 41% | 0.67 (0.52 to 0.86) | 14% |
> | | | All present | 5.5 (1.3 to 23) | 56% | 0.77 (0.66 to 0.91) | 15% |

– dyspnoea [C][15]

> **❓ Why?**
> Dyspnoea makes anaemia slightly more likely
>
> | Patient | Target disorder (reference standard) | Diagnostic test | LR + (95% CI) | Post-test probability | LR – (95% CI) | Post-test probability |
> |---|---|---|---|---|---|---|
> | Suspected anaemia (pre-test probability 19%) | Anaemia (haemoglobin <8.0 g/dl) | Upper GI symptoms [C][15] | 1.4 (1.0 to 1.8) | 25% | 0.67 (0.44 to 1.0) | 14% |

Do not bother looking for the following – they are little help at diagnosing or excluding anaemia:
- nail bed pallor **[B]**[14]
- palmar crease pallor **[B]**[14]
- koilonychia **[C]**[15]

**Note**
- No clinician agreed with another when identifying palmar crease pallor **[B]**[14].

- evidence of cirrhosis, specifically **[A]**[16]
  - facial telangiectasia
  - vascular spiders
  - abdominal wall veins
  - white nails
  - fatness
  - peripheral oedema.

**Why?**
**Facial telangiectasia, vascular spiders, white nails and abdominal wall veins help diagnose cirrhosis**

| Patient [A][16] | Target disorder (reference standard) | Diagnostic test | LR + (95% CI) | Post-test probability | LR − (95% CI) | Post-test probability |
|---|---|---|---|---|---|---|
| Suspected cirrhosis (pre-test probability 27%) | Cirrhosis (liver biopsy) | Facial telangiectasia | 20 (7.0 to 59) | 88% | 0.20 (0.11 to 0.36) | 7% |
| | | Vascular spiders | 6.1 (2.1 to 18) | 69% | 0.37 (0.34 to 0.65) | 12% |
| | | White nails | 5.8 (1.5 to 22) | 68% | 0.78 (0.46 to 0.74) | 22% |
| | | Abdominal wall veins | 4.4 (0.9 to 21) | 62% | 0.77 (0.66 to 0.90) | 18% |
| | | Fatness | 2.9 (1.1 to 7.8) | 52% | 0.61 (0.42 to 0.90) | 18% |

Perform a rectal examination **[D]** and a faecal occult blood test **[A]**[17].

**Why?**
**A positive faecal occult blood test makes a GI bleed more likely**

| Patient | Target disorder (reference standard) | Diagnostic test | LR + (95% CI) | Post-test probability | LR − (95% CI) | Post-test probability |
|---|---|---|---|---|---|---|
| Iron-deficiency anaemia (pre-test probability 19%) | Probable GI bleed (gastroscopy, colonoscopy) | Guaiac occult blood test **[A]**[17] | 2.6 (1.8 to 3.6) | 37% | 0.39 (0.22 to 0.69) | 8% |

**Note**
- Epigastric tenderness does not help diagnose peptic ulcer disease **[B]**[18].

Look at the appearance of any vomit or nasogastric aspirate, and test it using a gastro-occult dipstick [C][19].

**Why?**

**Whitish or yellow-green aspirate makes upper GI bleeding less likely**

| Patient [C][19] | Target disorder (reference standard) | Diagnostic test | LR+ (95% CI) | Post-test probability |
|---|---|---|---|---|
| Suspected acute upper GI bleeding (pre-test probability 39%) | Upper GI bleeding (endoscopy) | Grossly bloody aspirate | 2.5 (1.4 to 4.6) | 62% |
| | | Slightly bloody aspirate | 1.1 (0.33 to 3.4) | 40% |
| | | Coffee grounds aspirate | 0.95 (0.25 to 3.6) | 38% |
| | | Whitish or yellow-green aspirate | 0.093 (0.013 to 0.66) | 6% |

**A negative gastro-occult test makes upper GI bleeding much less likely**

| Patient [C][19] | Target disorder (reference standard) | Diagnostic test | LR + (95% CI) | Post-test probability | LR – (95% CI) | Post-test probability |
|---|---|---|---|---|---|---|
| Suspected acute upper GI bleeding (pre-test probability 39%) | Upper GI bleeding (endoscopy) | Gastro-occult positive | 5.2 (2.7 to 10) | 77% | 0.051 (0.0075 to 0.35) | 3% |

**Note**

■ Looking for bile is little use at diagnosing or excluding upper GI bleeding [C][19].

## INVESTIGATIONS

● Blood count [A].
● Clotting screen [D].
● Group and save serum, or cross-match 2–6 units depending on blood loss [D].
● Urea, electrolytes and creatinine [A][20].

**Note**

**A urea:creatinine ratio ≥ 100 can help diagnose an upper GI bleed**

| Patient [A][20] | Target disorder (reference standard) | Diagnostic test | LR + (95% CI) | Post-test probability | LR – (95% CI) | Post-test probability |
|---|---|---|---|---|---|---|
| Suspected upper GI bleed (pre-test probability 74%) | Upper GI bleed (endoscopy or barium studies) | Urea:creatinine ratio ≥ 100 (SI units) | 4.4 (1.5 to 13) | 93% | 0.41 (0.27 to 0.61) | 54% |

■ The greater the ratio, the greater the bleed [A][20].

- Liver function tests **[D]**.

Consider inserting:
- a central venous catheter to monitor fluid resuscitation **[D]**.
- a urinary catheter to monitor urine output **[D]**.

In patients found to have peptic ulcer disease, test for *H. pylori*.

 **Why?**
- *H. pylori* infection is common: 48%–62% of patients with peptic ulcer disease have it **[A]**[21] **[C]**[22].

The most helpful tests are:
- CLO test **[C]**[22]
- histology looking for antral inflammation **[C]**[22] and *H. pylori* bacteria **[A]**[21]
- urease breath test **[C]**[22].

**Why?**
**The CLO test and histology are most helpful at diagnosing *H. pylori* infection**

| Patient | Target disorder (reference standard) | Diagnostic test | LR + (95% CI) | Post-test probability | LR – (95% CI) | Post-test probability |
|---|---|---|---|---|---|---|
| Suspected *H. pylori* infection **[C]**[22] (pre-test probability 65%) | *H. pylori* infection (4 concordant tests) | CLO test | Infinity (29 to infinity) | 100% | 0.10 (0.067 to 0.16) | 16% |
| | | Acute antral inflammation | 0.14 (6.2 to 30) | 96% | 14 (0.097 to 0.21) | 21% |
| | | Chronic antral inflammation | 3.0 (2.2 to 3.9) | 84% | 0.0 (0.0 to 0.026) | 0% |
| | | Warthin–Starry stain | 88 (13 to 620) | 99% | 0.070 (0.041 to 0.12) | 11% |
| Suspected *H. pylori* infection **[A]**[21] (pre-test probability 48%) | *H. pylori* infection (histology) | Giemsa stain | 25 (3.6 to 170) | 96% | 0.043 (0.0064 to 0.30) | 4% |
| | | Urease breath test | 25 (3.6 to 170) | 96% | 0.043 (0.0064 to 0.30) | 4% |
| Suspected *H. pylori* infection **[C]**[22] (pre-test probability 65%) | *H. pylori* infection (4 concordant tests) | Serum IgG | 11 (5.6 to 21) | 95% | 0.095 (0.058 to 0.15) | 15% |
| | | Serum IgA | 4.8 (3.0 to 7.9) | 90% | 0.34 (0.26 to 0.43) | 38% |
| Undergoing upper GI endoscopy **[C]**[23] (pre-test probability 62%) | *H. pylori* infection (2 positive from histology, culture, rapid urease breath test) | Stool immunoassay | 12 (4.9 to 32) | 92% | 0.043 (0.011 to 0.17) | 4% |

## THERAPY

Order an endoscopy **[A]**:

- urgently **[A]**[24] to control bleeding **[A]**[25-27]

**Why do this?**
- Patients with acute non-variceal upper GI bleeding who have endoscopic therapy are less likely to rebleed, require surgery or diex **[A]**[24], **[A]**[25].
- Endoscopic ligation **[A]**[26] or sclerotherapy **[A]**[27] reduces rebleeding and death in patients with bleeding oesophageal varices.

**Endoscopic therapy reduces rebleeding, surgery and death**

| Patient [A][24] [A][25] | Treatment | Comparator | Outcome | CER | OR | NNT |
|---|---|---|---|---|---|---|
| Non-variceal upper GI bleed | Endoscopic therapy | No endoscopic therapy | Further bleeding at unknown | 39% | 0.38 (0.32 to 0.45) | 5 (5 to 6) |
| | | | Surgery at unknown | 26% | 0.36 (0.28 to 0.45) | 7 (6 to 8) |
| | | | Death at unknown | 9.9% | 0.55 (0.40 to 0.76) | 24 (18 to 46) |

- to make a diagnosis and determine future risk of bleeding or death (using the Rockall score, see Prognosis) **[A]**[8] **[A]**[9].

  Look for endoscopic stigmata of recent haemorrhage **[A]**[8] **[A]**[9]:
  - blood in upper GI tract
  - an adherent clot
  - a visible or spurting vessel.

**Why?**
- Malignancy increases the risk of dying or rebleeding; a Mallory–Weiss tear or a normal examination make both less likely **[A]**[8] **[A]**[9].
- Endoscopic stigmata increase the risk of dying or rebleeding **[A]**[8] **[A]**[9]:
  - blood in upper GI tract
  - adherent clot
  - visible or spurting vessel.

*Remember*
- Endoscopy is not necessary for all patients **[D]**[28].
- Endoscopy is safe **[B]**[29].

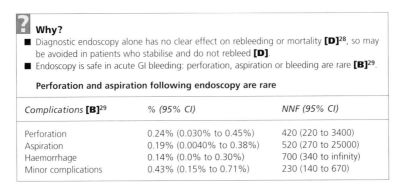

**Why?**

■ Diagnostic endoscopy alone has no clear effect on rebleeding or mortality **[D]**[28], so may be avoided in patients who stabilise and do not rebleed **[D]**.

■ Endoscopy is safe in acute GI bleeding: perforation, aspiration or bleeding are rare **[B]**[29].

**Perforation and aspiration following endoscopy are rare**

| Complications **[B]**[29] | % (95% CI) | NNF (95% CI) |
|---|---|---|
| Perforation | 0.24% (0.030% to 0.45%) | 420 (220 to 3400) |
| Aspiration | 0.19% (0.0040% to 0.38%) | 520 (270 to 25000) |
| Haemorrhage | 0.14% (0.0% to 0.30%) | 700 (340 to infinity) |
| Minor complications | 0.43% (0.15% to 0.71%) | 230 (140 to 670) |

● Patients with a Mallory–Weiss tear or an ulcer (with a clean base, a flat pigmented spot or an adherent clot) can start eating immediately on recovery from endoscopy **[D]**[30].

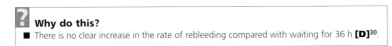

**Why do this?**

■ There is no clear increase in the rate of rebleeding compared with waiting for 36 h **[D]**[30].

If your patient's prothrombin time is prolonged (or INR raised):
● give a concentrate of factors II, VII, IX and X at a dose of 50 units of factor IX/kg body weight **[C]**[31]

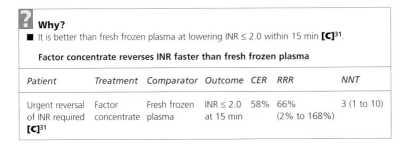

**Why?**

■ It is better than fresh frozen plasma at lowering INR ≤ 2.0 within 15 min **[C]**[31].

**Factor concentrate reverses INR faster than fresh frozen plasma**

| Patient | Treatment | Comparator | Outcome | CER | RRR | NNT |
|---|---|---|---|---|---|---|
| Urgent reversal of INR required **[C]**[31] | Factor concentrate | Fresh frozen plasma | INR ≤ 2.0 at 15 min | 58% | 66% (2% to 168%) | 3 (1 to 10) |

● if no concentrate is available give fresh frozen plasma (~ 1 litre for an adult) **[D]**
● stop warfarin if your patient is on it and it is safe to do so **[C]**[32]
● consider giving 5 mg vitamin K by slow (5 min) iv infusion **[A]**.

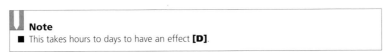

**Note**

■ This takes hours to days to have an effect **[D]**.

While waiting for endoscopy, consider giving:
● somatostatin or octreotide **[A]**[33]

**Why do this?**

■ Somatostatin or octreotide reduces rebleeding and the need for surgery in non-variceal bleeding **[A]**[33].

■ Somatostatin or octreotide reduces the need for transfusion (on average two fewer) and reduces the number of units of blood required (on average one fewer) in variceal bleeding **[A]**[34].

■ There is no clear effect on control of initial haemostasis, rebleeding, need for balloon tamponade or mortality in variceal bleeding **[A]**[34].

**Non-variceal bleeding: somatostatin or octreotide reduces rebleeding and the need for surgery**

| Patient [A][33] | Treatment | Comparator | Outcome | CER | OR | NNT |
|---|---|---|---|---|---|---|
| Non-variceal bleeding | Somatostatin or octreotide for 2–5 days | Placebo or H₂ antagonists | Continued bleeding or rebleeding at unknown | 38% | 0.53 (0.43 to 0.63) | 6 (5 to 7) |
| | | | Continued bleeding at unknown | 36% | 0.44 (0.33 to 0.55) | 5 (4 to 6) |
| | | | Surgery at unknown | 28% | 0.71 (0.61 to 0.81) | 12 (9 to 19) |

● thiamine 100 mg **[D]** iv **[C]**[35] to alcoholics or malnourished patients **[D]**.

**Note**

■ Few patients develop adverse effects when given thiamine iv (0.1%; 95% CI: 0.0% to 0.3%) **[C]**[35].

There is no clear benefit from:
● immediate surgery for all patients with non-variceal bleeding **[C]**[36]

**Why?**

■ Patients who have surgery within 6 h of admission are not clearly less likely to die than patients who only have surgery in an emergency (massive bleed or continued to bleed despite endoscopy) **[C]**[36].

● giving proton-pump inhibitors **[D]**[37] or H₂ antagonists **[D]**[38] to all patients.

**Why?**

■ There is no clear reduction in recurrent bleeding, need for surgery or death **[D]**[37] **[D]**[38].

## Ulcers

Perform endoscopic haemostasis **[A]**[24] using adrenaline **[A]**[39].

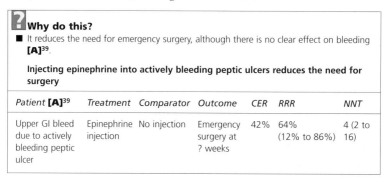

**? Why do this?**

■ It reduces the need for emergency surgery, although there is no clear effect on bleeding **[A]**[39].

**Injecting epinephrine into actively bleeding peptic ulcers reduces the need for surgery**

| Patient **[A]**[39] | Treatment | Comparator | Outcome | CER | RRR | NNT |
|---|---|---|---|---|---|---|
| Upper GI bleed due to actively bleeding peptic ulcer | Epinephrine injection | No injection | Emergency surgery at ? weeks | 42% | 64% (12% to 86%) | 4 (2 to 16) |

There is no clear reduction in bleeding or mortality from adding:

● alcohol **[D]**[40]
● ethanolamine **[D]**[41]
● polidocanol **[D]**[42]
● laser photocoagulation **[D]**[43]
● heat probe coagulation **[D]**[44].

There is no clear benefit from a routine repeat endoscopy **[D]**[45].

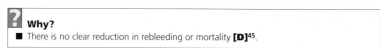

**? Why?**

■ There is no clear reduction in rebleeding or mortality **[D]**[45].

Give patients with a bleeding peptic ulcer a proton-pump inhibitor (e.g. omeprazole) **[A]**[46–48].

**? Why do this?**

■ Omeprazole reduces rebleeding and the need for surgery, although there is no clear effect on mortality **[A]**[46–48].
■ Omeprazole is more effective than cimetidine **[A]**[49] at preventing rebleeding.

**Bleeding peptic ulcer: omeprazole reduces rebleeding and emergency surgery**

| Patient **[A]**[47] | Treatment | Comparator | Outcome | CER | RRR | NNT |
|---|---|---|---|---|---|---|
| Bleeding peptic ulcer | Omeprazole | Placebo | Continued or further bleeding at ? weeks **[A]**[47] | 36% | 70% (46% to 83%) | 4 (3 to 7) |
| | | | Surgery needed at 30 days **[A]**[47] | 28% | 69% (35% to 85%) | 6 (4 to 14) |
| Bleeding peptic ulcer or visible vessel on endoscopy | Omeprazole | Cimetidine | Rebleeding at 14 days **[A]**[49] | 24% | 83% (29% to 96%) | 5 (3 to 14) |

Give antacids **[A]**[50].

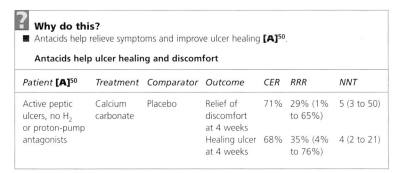

**?** **Why do this?**
- Antacids help relieve symptoms and improve ulcer healing **[A]**[50].

**Antacids help ulcer healing and discomfort**

| Patient **[A]**[50] | Treatment | Comparator | Outcome | CER | RRR | NNT |
|---|---|---|---|---|---|---|
| Active peptic ulcers, no H₂ or proton-pump antagonists | Calcium carbonate | Placebo | Relief of discomfort at 4 weeks | 71% | 29% (1% to 65%) | 5 (3 to 50) |
| | | | Healing ulcer at 4 weeks | 68% | 35% (4% to 76%) | 4 (2 to 21) |

Advise patients to stop smoking **[B]**[51].

**?** **Why do this?**
- Ulcers are more likely to heal **[B]**[51].

Discuss any patient likely to rebleed (see Rockall score) with surgeons and anaesthetists to determine criteria for operation **[D]**.

Patients who rebleed (defined as vomiting of fresh blood, hypotension and melaena or a requirement for 4 units of blood in the 72 h after endoscopic treatment) should be re-endoscoped **[A]**[52].

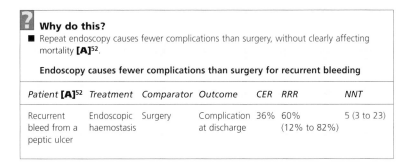

**?** **Why do this?**
- Repeat endoscopy causes fewer complications than surgery, without clearly affecting mortality **[A]**[52].

**Endoscopy causes fewer complications than surgery for recurrent bleeding**

| Patient **[A]**[52] | Treatment | Comparator | Outcome | CER | RRR | NNT |
|---|---|---|---|---|---|---|
| Recurrent bleed from a peptic ulcer | Endoscopic haemostasis | Surgery | Complication at discharge | 36% | 60% (12% to 82%) | 5 (3 to 23) |

Consider surgery for patients who have evidence of **[D]**[53] **[D]**[54]:
- persistent haemorrhage despite endoscopic therapy
- recurrent haemorrahge despite endoscopic therapy.

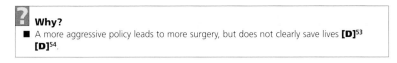

**?** **Why?**
- A more aggressive policy leads to more surgery, but does not clearly save lives **[D]**[53] **[D]**[54].

**Note**
- A partial gastrectomy prevents rebleeding and reoperation more effectively than oversewing and a vagotomy for patients with bleeding duodenal ulcers, but leads to more duodenal leaks **[B]**[55].
- There is no clear effect on mortality **[B]**[55].

**A partial gastrectomy reduces rebleeding and reoperations better than oversewing and vagotomy**

| Patient [B][55] | Treatment | Comparator | Outcome | CER | RRR | NNT |
|---|---|---|---|---|---|---|
| Bleeding duodenal ulcer | Partial gastrectomy | Oversewing and vagotomy | Rebleeding at 4 weeks | 17% | 81% (16% to 96%) | 7 (4 to 31) |
| | | | Reoperations at 4 weeks | 14% | 88% (6% to 98%) | 8 (5 to 37) |
| | | | Duodenal leaks at 4 weeks | 3.5% | −290% (−1600% to 14%) | −10 (−1200 to −5) |

Consider tranexamic acid **[A]**[56] for patients likely to rebleed **[D]**. (3.6 g iv daily for 3 days, followed by 3.6 g orally daily for 3.5 days).

**Why do this?**
- It reduces death, without clearly affecting rebleeding or need for emergency surgery **[A]**[56].
- Thromboembolic events are rare: 0.04% have an event (mainly superficial thrombophlebitis) **[A]**[56].

**Tranexamic acid reduces mortality**

| Patient [A][56] | Treatment | Comparator | Outcome | CER | OR | NNT |
|---|---|---|---|---|---|---|
| Upper GI bleed | Tranexamic acid | Placebo | Death at unknown | 10% | 0.60 (0.40 to 0.89) | 26 (17 to 97) |

Consider iron supplements **[B]**[57] **[B]**[58] for patients with anaemia, e.g. oral ferrous sulphate 200 mg three times a day **[D]**.

**Why do this?**
- Iron supplementation increases haemoglobin levels (on average 70 g/l within 70 days) and improves exercise capacity **[B]**[57] **[B]**[58].
- Watch for constipation **[B]**[57].

| Patient [B][57] | Treatment | Comparator | Outcome | CER | RRR (%) | NNT |
|---|---|---|---|---|---|---|
| Iron-deficiency anaemia | Ferrous succinate | Placebo | Constipation | 14% | −150% (−470% to −4%) | −5 (−39 to −3) |

## Varices

Perform:

- endoscopic ligation **[A]**[59]

**Why do this?**
- It is more effective than sclerotherapy at reducing rebleeding, death (particularly from bleeding) **[A]**[59].
- It causes fewer oesophageal strictures **[A]**[59].
- Fewer sessions are required to achieve variceal obliteration (on average two fewer) **[A]**[59].

**Bleeding varices: endoscopic ligation reduces rebleeding and death better than sclerotherapy**

| Patient **[A]**[59] | Treatment | Comparator | Outcome | CER | OR | NNT |
|---|---|---|---|---|---|---|
| Bleeding oesophageal varices | Endoscopic ligation | Sclerotherapy | Rebleeding at unknown | 47% | 0.52 (0.37 to 0.74) | 7 (5 to 14) |
| | | | Death at unknown | 32% | 0.67 (0.46 to 0.98) | 12 (7 to 230) |
| | | | Death from rebleeding at unknown | 14% | 0.49 (0.24 to 0.996) | 15 (10 to 2100) |
| | | | Oesophageal strictures at unknown | 11% | 0.10 (0.03 to 0.29) | 10 (9 to 13) |

- or sclerotherapy **[A]**[27] within 6 h **[B]**[60]

**Why do this?**
- It reduces rebleeding and death **[A]**[27] particularly if performed within 6 h **[B]**[60].
- It is more effective than balloon tamponade, though not clearly more effective than somatostatin **[A]**[27].
- However, complications are common: 18% of patients have severe complications from emergency sclerotherapy (bleeding from post-sclerosis ulcers, stenosis, oesophageal perforation) and of these 15% die **[A]**[27].

**Sclerotherapy controls bleeding and reduces mortality**

| Patient **[A]**[27] | Treatment | Comparator | Outcome | CER | OR | NNT |
|---|---|---|---|---|---|---|
| Bleeding oesophageal varices | Sclerotherapy | Sham procedure | Failure to control bleeding at ? | 40% | 0.13 (0.05 to 0.36) | 3 (3 to 5) |
| | | | Death at ? | 48% | 0.39 (0.17 to 0.95) | 5 (3 to 78) |
| | Sclerotherapy | Balloon tamponade | Failure to control bleeding at ? | 38% | 0.15 (0.04 to 0.53) | 3 (4 to 10) |

**Early sclerotherapy reduces rebleeding**

| Patient **[B]**[60] | Treatment | Comparator | Outcome | CER | RRR | NNT |
|---|---|---|---|---|---|---|
| Large bleeding oesophageal varices | Sclerotherapy within 6 h | Sclerotherapy after 24 h | Bleeding at 1 year | 34% | 66% (14% to 87%) | 4 (3 to 20) |

- and give octreotide or somatostatin in addition (e.g. somatostatin 6 mg in 500 ml saline iv over 24 h for 5 days).

 **Why do this?**

- Octreotide and band ligation reduces rebleeding and need for a balloon tamponade compared with band ligation alone **[A]**[61].
- Somatostatin and sclerotherapy reduce treatment failure (extra transfusions, additional sclerotherapy, balloon tamponade or TIPS, or death) more than sclerotherapy alone **[A]**[62].
- Endoscopists find sclerotherapy easier to perform **[A]**[62].
- Octreotide and sclerotherapy reduce rebleeding more than sclerotherapy alone. There is no clear effect on mortality **[A]**[63].

**Somatostatin or octreotide added to sclerotherapy reduces treatment failure**

| Patient | Treatment | Comparator | Outcome | CER | RRR | NNT |
|---|---|---|---|---|---|---|
| Bleeding oesophageal varices | Band ligation and octreotide | Band ligation | Rebleeding at 30 days **[A]**[61] | 38% | 78% (39% to 92%) | 3 (2 to 7) |
| | | | Balloon tamponade required at 30 days **[A]**[61] | 21% | 90% (25% to 99%) | 5 (3 to 15) |
| Cirrhosis and upper GI bleeding | Sclerotherapy and somatostatin | Sclerotherapy | Treatment failure at 5 days **[A]**[62] | 35% | 37% (13% to 54%) | 5 (3 to 15) |
| Acute variceal bleeding | Sclerotherapy and octreotide | Octreotide | Rebleeding at 15 days **[A]**[64] | 29% | 50% (12% to 72%) | 7 (4 to 31) |

Consider balloon tamponade **[A]**[65] for patients who do not stop bleeding **[D]**.

 **Why do this?**

- It is more likely to control bleeding than terlipressin at 24 h, although there is no clear effect on mortality **[A]**[65].
- However, the risk of rebleeding and complications (gastro-oesophageal ulcers, arterial hypertension, thoracic pain) is greater **[A]**[65].

**Balloon tamponade controls bleeding faster than terlipressin, but causes more complications**

| Patient **[A]**[65] | Treatment | Comparator | Outcome | CER | RRR | NNT |
|---|---|---|---|---|---|---|
| Bleeding oesophageal varices | Balloon tamponade | Terlipressin | Failure to control bleeding at 24 h | 30% | 83% (−26% to 98%) | 4 (2 to 36) |
| | | | Rebleeding at 7 days | 10% | −250% (−1400% to 98%) | −4 (−330 to −2) |
| | | | Complications at 7 days | 15% | −330% (−1200% to −45%) | −2 (−4 to −1) |

Consider performing a portocaval shunt [A][27] for patients who do not stop bleeding [D]:

- transjugular intrahepatic portosystemic shunts (TIPS) [A][66–70].

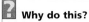
**Why do this?**

- TIPS is more effective than banding [A][66] or sclerotherapy [A][67–70] at preventing rebleeding, but causes more encephalopathy [A][67] [A][69] and increases readmissions to hospital [A][71].
- There is no clear effect on mortality [A][66–70].

**Varices: TIPS reduces rebleeding but increases hepatic encephalopathy compared with banding or sclerotherapy**

| Patient | Treatment | Comparator | Outcome | CER | RRR | NNT |
|---|---|---|---|---|---|---|
| Cirrhosis and bleeding varices [A][66] | TIPS | Endoscopic banding | Rebleeding at 16 months | 52% | 81% (42% to 94%) | 2 (2 to 5) |
| Cirrhosis and bleeding varices [A][67] | TIPS | Sclerotherapy | Rebleeding at 19 months | 51% | 54% (12% to 76%) | 4 (2 to 14) |
| | | | Moderate or severe hepatic encephalopathy at 19 months | 23% | –140% (–340% to –29%) | –3 (–8 to –2) |
| Cirrhosis and recent bleeding varices | TIPS | Sclerotherapy | Readmission to hospital at 2.7 years | 23% | –200% (–450% to –61%) | –2 (–4 to –2) |

Alternatives include:

- distal splenorenal shunts [A][72].

**Why do this?**

- Distal splenorenal shunts reduce rebleeding, but have no clear effect on mortality [A][72].

Avoid:

- staple transection of the oesophagus.

**Why?**

- It leads to fewer rebleeds than sclerotherapy [A][73], but increases early mortality [A][74].

**Oesophageal staple transection reduces rebleeding but increases mortality**

| Patient | Treatment | Comparator | Outcome | CER | RRR | NNT |
|---|---|---|---|---|---|---|
| Bleeding varices not controlled by medication or transfusion [A][73] | Staple transection of the oesophagus | Sclerotherapy | Rebleeding at 5 days | 38% | 69% (29% to 87%) | 4 (2 to 10) |
| Recent bleeding oesophageal varices [A][74] | Oesophagogastric devascularisation with oesophageal transection | Sclerotherapy | Death at 3 months | 2.0% | –900% (–7500% to –31%) | –6 (–18 to –3) |

## PREVENTION

### Ulcers and erosions

● Stop NSAIDs **[A]**.

If patients need to continue, consider:
- topical NSAIDs **[B]**[75]

**Why do this?**
■ Topical NSAIDs do not clearly increase the risk of GI bleeding or perforation, unlike oral NSAIDs **[B]**[75].

- ibuprofen **[B]**[76] at the lowest possible dose **[B]**[77]

**Why do this?**
■ It is least likely to cause serious GI complications **[B]**[76] **[B]**[77].
■ The risk of GI complications increases with higher daily doses **[B]**[77].

**Ibuprofen is the safest NSAID**

| Outcome | Risk factor | PEER | OR (95% CI) | NNH (95% CI) |
|---|---|---|---|---|
| Bleeding peptic ulcer | Ibuprofen independent | 0.05% | 2.0 (1.4 to 2.8) | 2000 (1100 to 5000) |

- a COX-2 inhibitor such as rofecoxib **[A]**[78] or celecoxib **[B]**[79]

**Why do this?**
■ Celecoxib is as effective as naproxen **[B]**[79].
■ Fewer patients develop gastroduodenal ulcers **[A]**[78] **[B]**[79] and fewer discontinue medication or have GI complications compared with NSAIDs **[A]**[78].

**Rofecoxib causes fewer GI complications or withdrawals than NSAIDs**

| Patient | Treatment | Comparator | Outcome | CER | RRR | NNT |
|---|---|---|---|---|---|---|
| Osteoarthritis **[A]**[78] | Rofecoxib | NSAIDs | Discontinued medication 4 months | 37% | 17% (10% to 23%) | 16 (11 to 29) |
| | | | Discontinuation due to adverse GI symptoms 4 months | 4.8% | 27% (3% to 45%) | 78 (40 to 1930) |
| | | | Gastroduodenal ulcer on endoscopy 4 months | 8.1% | 77% (68% to 83%) | 16 (13 to 21) |
| | | | GI perforation, symptomatic gastroduodenal ulcer or upper GI bleeding 4 months | 1.5% | 63% (33% to 80%) | 100 (61 to 320) |

- adding in regular omeprazole 40 mg daily **[A]**[80] or misoprostol **[A]**[80] **[A]**[81]

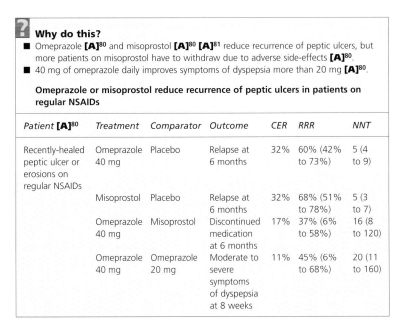

**? Why do this?**

■ Omeprazole **[A]**[80] and misoprostol **[A]**[80] **[A]**[81] reduce recurrence of peptic ulcers, but more patients on misoprostol have to withdraw due to adverse side-effects **[A]**[80].

■ 40 mg of omeprazole daily improves symptoms of dyspepsia more than 20 mg **[A]**[80].

**Omeprazole or misoprostol reduce recurrence of peptic ulcers in patients on regular NSAIDs**

| Patient **[A]**[80] | Treatment | Comparator | Outcome | CER | RRR | NNT |
|---|---|---|---|---|---|---|
| Recently-healed peptic ulcer or erosions on regular NSAIDs | Omeprazole 40 mg | Placebo | Relapse at 6 months | 32% | 60% (42% to 73%) | 5 (4 to 9) |
| | Misoprostol | Placebo | Relapse at 6 months | 32% | 68% (51% to 78%) | 5 (3 to 7) |
| | Omeprazole 40 mg | Misoprostol | Discontinued medication at 6 months | 17% | 37% (6% to 58%) | 16 (8 to 120) |
| | Omeprazole 40 mg | Omeprazole 20 mg | Moderate to severe symptoms of dyspepsia at 8 weeks | 11% | 45% (6% to 68%) | 20 (11 to 160) |

- *H. pylori* eradication therapy for infected patients without ulcers **[A]**[82]

**? Why do this?**

■ Eradication therapy reduces development of peptic ulcers **[A]**[82].

**Eradication therapy reduces peptic ulcers in patients starting long-term NSAIDs**

| Patient **[A]**[80] | Treatment | Comparator | Outcome | CER | RRR | NNT |
|---|---|---|---|---|---|---|
| *H. pylori* infection starting NSAIDs | *H. pylori* eradication therapy | Placebo | Peptic ulcer on endoscopy at 8 weeks | 26% | 74% (14% to 92%) | 5 (3 to 23) |

For patients with peptic ulcers:
- give *H. pylori* eradication therapy to infected patients **[A]**[83]

**❓ Why do this?**
- More ulcers heal **[A]**[83] **[A]**[84] and fewer patients rebleed **[A]**[85].
- Eradication therapy is more effective than long-term ranitidine at healing ulcers **[A]**[86].

***H. pylori* eradication therapy helps heal ulcers and reduces rebleeding**

| Patient | Treatment | Comparator | Outcome | CER | OR | NNT |
|---------|-----------|------------|---------|-----|-----|-----|
| Peptic ulcer **[A]**[83] | *H. pylori* eradication therapy | No therapy | Healing of peptic ulcer at ? | 91% | 6.60 (4.10 to 10.6) | 13 (12 to 14) |

| Patient | Treatment | Comparator | Outcome | CER | RRR | NNT |
|---------|-----------|------------|---------|-----|-----|-----|
| Bleeding peptic ulcer **[A]**[85] | *H. pylori* eradication therapy | No therapy | Rebleeding at 10 months | 29% | 100% | 4 (2 to 20) |
| Bleeding peptic ulcer **[A]**[86] | *H. pylori* eradication therapy | Long-term ranitidine | Recurrent ulcer at 12 months | 9% | 89% (17% to 99%) | 15 (9 to 58) |

using triple therapy **[B]**[87] **[B]**[88]:
- a proton-pump inhibitor plus any two of amoxicillin, clarithromycin or nitroimidazole **[B]**[89]
- a bismuth compound plus nitroimidazole plus tetracycline **[B]**[88]

**❓ Why do this?**
- Triple therapy is more effective than dual therapy **[B]**[88] **[B]**[89].
- Eradication rates are highest using a proton-pump triple therapy (87%; 95% CI: 86% to 87%) **[B]**[89], followed by a bismuth compound plus nitroimidazole plus tetracycline (82%; 95% CI: 80% to 84%) **[B]**[88].

- continue giving proton-pump inhibitors long-term **[A]**[90].

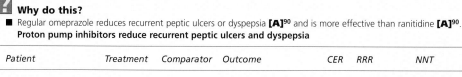

**❓ Why do this?**
- Regular omeprazole reduces recurrent peptic ulcers or dyspepsia **[A]**[90] and is more effective than ranitidine **[A]**[90].
**Proton pump inhibitors reduce recurrent peptic ulcers and dyspepsia**

| Patient | Treatment | Comparator | Outcome | CER | RRR | NNT |
|---------|-----------|------------|---------|-----|-----|-----|
| Recently-healed peptic ulcer remaining on NSAIDs | Omeprazole | Placebo | Recurrent peptic ulcers, dyspepsia or stopped treatment at 8 weeks **[A]**[90] | 41% | 31% (10% to 48%) | 8 (5 to 26) |
| | Omeprazole | Ranitidine | Recurrent peptic ulcers, dyspepsia or stopped treatment at 8 weeks **[A]**[90] | 37% | 47% (24% to 63%) | 6 (4 to 13) |

## Varices

Continue endoscopic ligation **[A]**[59] or sclerotherapy **[A]**[27] until varices are obliterated.

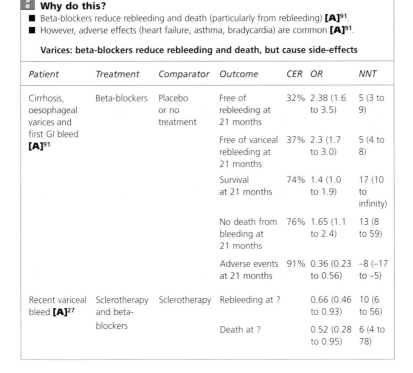

> **?** **Why do this?**
> ■ Sclerotherapy reduces rebleeding and death, and is more effective than beta-blockers alone **[A]**[27].
>
> **Sclerotherapy to obliterate varices reduces rebleeding and death**
>
> | Patient **[A]**[27] | Treatment | Comparator | Outcome | CER | OR | NNT |
> |---|---|---|---|---|---|---|
> | Recent variceal bleed | Sclerotherapy | Non-active treatment | Rebleeding at ? | 65% | 0.63 (0.49 to 0.79) | 9 (6 to 18) |
> |  |  |  | Death at ? | 44% | 0.77 (0.61 to 0.98) | 16 (9 to 200) |
> |  | Sclerotherapy | Beta-blockers | Rebleeding at ? | 58% | 0.66 (0.50 to 0.88) | 12 (6 to 410) |

In addition give:
- beta-blockers **[A]**[27] **[A]**[91]

> **?** **Why do this?**
> ■ Beta-blockers reduce rebleeding and death (particularly from rebleeding) **[A]**[91].
> ■ However, adverse effects (heart failure, asthma, bradycardia) are common **[A]**[91].
>
> **Varices: beta-blockers reduce rebleeding and death, but cause side-effects**
>
> | Patient | Treatment | Comparator | Outcome | CER | OR | NNT |
> |---|---|---|---|---|---|---|
> | Cirrhosis, oesophageal varices and first GI bleed **[A]**[91] | Beta-blockers | Placebo or no treatment | Free of rebleeding at 21 months | 32% | 2.38 (1.6 to 3.5) | 5 (3 to 9) |
> |  |  |  | Free of variceal rebleeding at 21 months | 37% | 2.3 (1.7 to 3.0) | 5 (4 to 8) |
> |  |  |  | Survival at 21 months | 74% | 1.4 (1.0 to 1.9) | 17 (10 to infinity) |
> |  |  |  | No death from bleeding at 21 months | 76% | 1.65 (1.1 to 2.4) | 13 (8 to 59) |
> |  |  |  | Adverse events at 21 months | 91% | 0.36 (0.23 to 0.56) | −8 (−17 to −5) |
> | Recent variceal bleed **[A]**[27] | Sclerotherapy and beta-blockers | Sclerotherapy | Rebleeding at ? |  | 0.66 (0.46 to 0.93) | 10 (6 to 56) |
> |  |  |  | Death at ? |  | 0.52 (0.28 to 0.95) | 6 (4 to 78) |

- or isosorbide mononitrate slow-release 50 mg po daily [A][92]

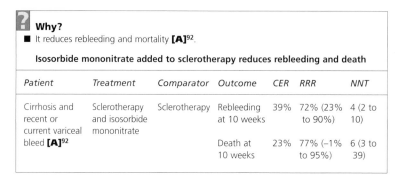

**Why?**
- It reduces rebleeding and mortality [A][92].

**Isosorbide mononitrate added to sclerotherapy reduces rebleeding and death**

| Patient | Treatment | Comparator | Outcome | CER | RRR | NNT |
|---|---|---|---|---|---|---|
| Cirrhosis and recent or current variceal bleed [A][92] | Sclerotherapy and isosorbide mononitrate | Sclerotherapy | Rebleeding at 10 weeks | 39% | 72% (23% to 90%) | 4 (2 to 10) |
| | | | Death at 10 weeks | 23% | 77% (−1% to 95%) | 6 (3 to 39) |

There is no clear benefit from combining beta-blockers and isosorbide mononitrate [D][93].

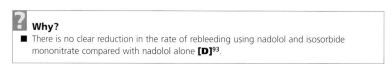

**Why?**
- There is no clear reduction in the rate of rebleeding using nadolol and isosorbide mononitrate compared with nadolol alone [D][93].

- or octreotide (50 mg twice daily for 6 months).

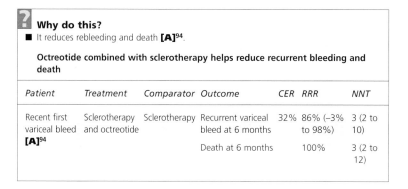

**Why do this?**
- It reduces rebleeding and death [A][94].

**Octreotide combined with sclerotherapy helps reduce recurrent bleeding and death**

| Patient | Treatment | Comparator | Outcome | CER | RRR | NNT |
|---|---|---|---|---|---|---|
| Recent first variceal bleed [A][94] | Sclerotherapy and octreotide | Sclerotherapy | Recurrent variceal bleed at 6 months | 32% | 86% (−3% to 98%) | 3 (2 to 10) |
| | | | Death at 6 months | | 100% | 3 (2 to 12) |

## PROGNOSIS

Death and further rebleeding are common, particularly for:
- inpatients [A][9]
- patients with varices [A][95].

> **Note**
> - One in seven die in hospital (14%; 95% CI: 13% to 15%) and one in six rebleed (18%; 95% CI: 17% to 19%) **[A]**[9] **[A]**[96].
> - One in 15 die from further bleeding (6.6%; 95% CI: 5.8% to 7.3%) **[A]**[9].
> - One in three inpatients who have a GI bleed die in hospital (33%; 95% CI: 29% to 37%) **[A]**[9].
> - A third of patients with bleeding varices fail to stop bleeding **[B]**[97], half rebleed in the next year **[B]**[98] **[B]**[99] and a third are dead within 2 months (37%; 95% CI: 30 to 45%) **[A]**[95].

Rank your patient for risk of rebleeding or dying **[A]**[8] **[A]**[9] (Box 1).

### Box 1 The Rockall score can help rank your patient for risk of rebleeding and mortality

| **[A]**[8] **[A]**[9] | Score 0 | Score 1 | Score 2 | Score 3 |
|---|---|---|---|---|
| Age (years) | ➤ <60 | ➤ 60–79 | ➤ >80 | |
| Shock | ➤ Pulse < 100 beats/min<br>➤ Systolic BP > 100 mmHg | ➤ Pulse > 100 beats/min<br>➤ Systolic BP > 100 mmHg | ➤ Pulse > 100 beats/min<br>➤ Systolic BP < 100 mmHg | |
| Comorbidity | ➤ No major comorbidity | | ➤ Cardiac failure<br>➤ Ischaemic heart disease<br>➤ Any other comorbidity | ➤ Renal failure<br>➤ Liver failure<br>➤ Disseminated malignancy |
| Endoscopic stigmata | ➤ None<br>➤ Dark spot seen | | ➤ Blood in upper GI tract<br>➤ Adherent clot<br>➤ Visible or spurting vessel | |
| Diagnosis | ➤ Mallory Weiss tear<br>➤ No lesion seen and No stigmata of recent haemorrhage | ➤ All other diagnoses | ➤ Malignancy of upper GI tract | |

| Pre-endoscopy score **[A]**[8] **[A]**[9] | Death | Post-endoscopy score | Death **[A]**[8] **[A]**[9] | Rebleeding |
|---|---|---|---|---|
| 7 | 75% (45% to 100%) | 8+ | 405% (30% to 51%) | 37% (27% to 47%) |
| 6 | 62% (50% to 73%) | 7 | 23% (15% to 31%) | 37% (28% to 46%) |
| 5 | 35% (27% to 43%) | 6 | 12% (6.3% to 17%) | 27% (20% to 34%) |
| 4 | 21% (17% to 25%) | 5 | 11% (6.3% to 15%) | 25% (19% to 31%) |
| 3 | 12% (8.6% to 16%) | 4 | 8.0% (4.0% to 12%) | 15% (10% to 21%) |
| 2 | 5.6% (2.8% to 8.5%) | 3 | 1.9% (0.0% to 3.9%) | 125 (6.8% to 17%) |
| 1 | 3.0% (0.63% to 5.35) | 0 to 2 | 0.0% (0.0% to 0.93%) | 5.9% (3.3% to 8.5%) |
| 0 | 0.0% (0.0% to 1.2%) | | | |

## Varices

The risk of dying from varices is increased with **[A]**[95]:
- worsening Pugh score
- alcoholism
- increasing age
- hepatocellular carcinoma.

## Peptic ulcers

Peptic ulcers heal slowly and relapses are common **[C]**[100].

**Note**
- 24%–43% of ulcers are not healed at 8 weeks. **[B]**[101] **[B]**[51].
- A third of patients with a healed peptic ulcer relapse within 12 months (36%; 95% CI: 30% to 43%) **[C]**[100].

Ulcers are less likely to heal **[B]**[51]:
- with increasing age
- with cigarette smoking
- in men
- with persisting ulcer symptoms **[B]**[101]
- with a duodenal ulcer diameter larger than 20 mm **[B]**[101].

Relapse is more likely with **[C]**[100]
- duodenal ulcer
- psychological stress
- endoscopic findings of scars at ulcer sites on healing
- no acute therapy.

**Guideline writers**: Alain Townsend, Christopher Ball
**CAT writers**: Alain Townsend, Christopher Ball, Clare Wotton

## REFERENCES

| No | Level | Citation |
|---|---|---|
| 1 | 1b | McMahon AD, Evans JM, White G et al. A cohort study (with re-sampled comparator groups) to measure the association between new NSAID prescribing and upper gastrointestinal hemorrhage and perforation. J Clin Epidemiol 1997; 50: 351–6 |
| 2 | 2b | Ellison RT, Perez-Perez G, Welsh CH et al. Risk factors for upper gastrointestinal bleeding in intensive care patients: role of *Helicobacter pylori*. Crit Care Med 1996; 24: 1974–81 |
| 3 | 2b | Hallas J, Lauritsen J, Dalsgard Villadsen H et al. Non-steroidal anti-inflammatory drugs and upper gastrointestinal bleeding: identifying high-risk groups by excess risk estimates. Scand J Gastroenterol 1995; 30: 438–44 |
| 4 | 4 | Cuellar R. Gastrointestinal tract hemorrhage: the value of a nasogastric hemorrhage. Arch Intern Med 1990; 150: 1381–4 |

| No | Level | Citation |
| --- | --- | --- |
| 5 | 2c | Silverstein FE, Gilbert DA, Tedesco FJ et al. The National ASGE survey on upper gastrointestinal bleeding. Gastrointest Endosc 1981; 27: 73–103 |
| 6 | 4 | Masson J, Bramley PN, Herd K et al. Upper gastrointestinal bleeding in an open-access dedicated unit. J R Coll Physicians Lond 1996; 30: 436–442 |
| 7 | 4 | Wara P, Stodkilde H. Bleeding pattern before admission as guideline for emergency endoscopy. Scand J Gastroenterol 1985; 20: 72–8 |
| 8 | 1a | Rockall TA, Logan RF, Devlin HB et al. Risk assessment after acute upper gastrointestinal haemorrhage. Gut 1996; 38: 316–21 |
| 9 | 1a | Rockall TA, Logan RF, Devlin HB. Incidence of and mortality from acute upper gastrointestinal haemorrhage in the United Kingdom. BMJ 1995; 311: 222–6 |
| 10 | 2a | Danesh J, Appleby P, Peto R et al. How often does surgery for peptic ulceration erradicate H. pylori: Systematic review of 36 studies. BMJ 1998; 316: 746–7 |
| 11 | 1a | Bollini P, Garcia Rodriguez LA, Perez Gutthann SP et al. The impact of research quality and study design on epidemiologic estimates of the effect of non-steroidal anti-inflammatory drugs on upper gastrointestinal tract disease. Arch Intern Med 1992; 152: 1289–95 |
| 12 | 2a | McGee S et al. Is this patient hypovolemic? JAMA 1999; 281: 1022–9 |
| 13 | 1b | Sheth TN et al. The relation of conjunctival pallor to the presence of anemia. J Gen Intern Med 1997; 12: 102–6 |
| 14 | 2b | Nardone DA et al. Usefulness of physical examination in detecting the presence or absence of anemia: Arch Intern Med 1990; 150: 201–4 |
| 15 | 4 | Dawson AA et al. Evaluation of diagnostic significance of certain symptoms and physical signs in anaemic patients. BMJ 1969; 3: 436–9 |
| 16 | 1b | Hamberg KJ et al. Accuracy of clinical diagnosis of cirrhosis among alcohol-abusing men. J Clin Epidemiol 1996; 49: 1295–1301 |
| 17 | 1b | Moran A et al. Diagnostic value of a guaiac occult blood test and faecal alpha 1-antitrypsin. Gut 1995; 36: 87–9 |
| 18 | 3b | Priebe WM, DaCosta LR, Beck IT. Is epigastric tenderness a sign of peptic ulcer disease? Gastroenterology 1982; 82: 16–19 |
| 19 | 4 | Cuellar R. Gastrointestinal tract hemorrhage. The value of a nasogastric hemorrhage. Arch Intern Med 1990; 150: 1381–4 |
| 20 | 1b | Mortensen PB et al. The diagnostic value of serum urea/creatinine ratio in distinguishing between upper and lower gastrointestinal bleeding. A prospective study. Dan Med Bull 1994; 41: 237–40 |
| 21 | 1b | Fallone CA, Mitchell A, Paterson WG. Determination of the test performance of less costly methods of Helicobacter pylori detection. Clin Invest Med 1995; 18: 177–85 |
| 22 | 4 | Cutler AF, Havstad S, MaC CK, et al. Accuracy of invasive and noninvasive tests to diagnose Helicobacter pylori infection. Gastroenterology 1995; 109: 136–41 |
| 23 | 4 | Lehmann F, Drewe J, Terracciano L et al. Comparison of stool immunoassay with standard methods for detecting Helicobacter pylori infection. BMJ 1999; 319: 1409 |
| 24 | 1a | Sacks HS, Chalmers TC, Blum AL et al. Endoscopic haemostasis: an effective therapy for bleeding peptic ulcers. JAMA 1990; 264: 494–9 |
| 25 | 1a | Cook DJ et al. Endoscopic therapy for acute nonvariceal upper gastrointestinal hemorrhage: a meta-analysis. Gastroenterology 1993; 102: 139–48 |

| No | Level | Citation |
|---|---|---|
| 26 | 1a | Laine L, Cook D. Endoscopic ligation compared with sclerotherapy for treatment of esophageal variceal bleeding: a meta-analysis. Ann Intern Med 1995; 123: 280–7 |
| 27 | 1a | D'Amico G, Pagliaro L, Bosch J. The treatment of portal hypertension: a meta-analytic review. Hepatology 1995; 22: 332–54 |
| 28 | 1b – | Peterson WL, Barnett CC, Smith HJ et al. Routine endoscopy in upper-gastrointestinal-tract bleeding. N Eng J Med 1981; 304: 925–9 |
| 29 | 2c | Gilbert DA, Silverstein FE, Tedesco FJ et al. National ASGE survey on upper gastrointestinal bleeding: complications of endoscopy supplement. Dig Dis Sci 1981; 26: 55–9 |
| 30 | 1b – | Laine L, Cohen H, Brodhead J et al. Prospective evaluation of immediate versus delayed refeeding and prognostic value of endoscopy in patients with upper gastrointestinal hemorrhage. Gastroenterology 1992; 102: 314–16 |
| 31 | 4 | Makris M et al. Emergency oral anticoagulant reversal; the relative efficacy of infusions of fresh frozen plasma and clotting factor concentrate on correction of the coagulopathy. Thromb Haemost 1997; 77: 477–80 |
| 32 | 4 | White RH et al. Temporary discontinuation of warfarin therapy: changes in international normalised ratio. Ann Intern Med 1995; 122: 40–2 |
| 33 | 1a | Imperiale TF, Birgisson S. Somatostatin or octreotide compared with $H_2$ antagonists and placebo in the management of acute non-variceal upper gastrointestinal haemorrhage: a meta-analysis. Ann Intern Med 1997; 127: 1062–71 |
| 34 | 1a | Gotzsche PC. Somatostatin or octreotide versus placebo or no treatment in acute bleeding oesophageal varices (Cochrane Review). In: The Cochrane Library, Issue 3, 1999. Oxford: Update Software |
| 35 | 4 | Wrenn KD, Murphy F, Slovis CM. A toxicity study of parenteral thiamine hydrochloride. Ann Emerg Med 1998; 18: 867–70 |
| 36 | 4 | Wong J, Lam SK, Lee NW. Immediate operation for acute non-variceal gastrointestinal haemorrhage in patients aged 50 years and over. Aust N Z J Surg 1980; 50(2): 150–4 |
| 37 | 1b – | Daneshmend TK, Hawkey CJ, Langman MJ. Omeprazole versus placebo for acute gastrointestinal bleeding: randomised double-blind controlled trial. BMJ 1992; 304: 143–7 |
| 38 | 1b – | La Brooy SJ, Misiewicz JJ, Edwards J et al. Controlled trial of cimetidine in upper gastrointestinal haemorrhage. Gut 1979; 20: 892–5 |
| 39 | 1b | Chung SC, Leung JW, Steele RJ et al. Endoscopic injection of adrenaline for actively bleeding ulcers: a randomised trial. BMJ 1988; 296: 1631–3 |
| 40 | 1b – | Chung SCS, Leong H-T, Chan ACW et al. Epinephrine or epinephrine plus alcohol for injection of bleeding ulcers: a prospective randomized trial. Gastrointest Endosc 1996; 43: 591–5 |
| 41 | 1b – | Choudari CP, Palmer KR. Endoscopic injection therapy for bleeding peptic ulcer: a comparison of adrenaline alone with adrenaline plus ethanolamine oleate. Gut 1994; 35: 608–10 |
| 42 | 1b – | Villanueva C, Balanzo J, Equinos JC et al. Endoscopic injection therapy of bleeding ulcer: a prospective and randomized comparison of adrenaline alone or with polidocanol. J Clin Gastroenterol 1993; 17: 195–200 |
| 43 | 1b – | Loizou LA, and Bown SG. Endoscopic treatment for bleeding peptic ulcers: randomised comparison of adrenaline injection and adrenaline injection + Nd:YAG laser photocoagulation. Gut 1991; 32: 1100–1103 |

| No | Level | Citation |
|----|-------|----------|
| 44 | 1b – | Chung SS, Lau JY, Sung JJ et al. Randomised comparison between adrenaline injection alone and adrenaline injection plus heat probe treatment for actively bleeding ulcers. BMJ 1997; 314: 1307–11 |
| 45 | 1b – | Villanueva C, Balanzo J, Torras X, et al. Value of second-look endoscopy after injection therapy for bleeding peptic ulcer: a prospective and randomized trial. Gastrointestinal Endoscopy 1994; 40: 34–39 |
| 46 | 1b | Hasselgren G, Lind T, Lundell L et al. Continuous intravenous infusion of omeprazole in elderly patients with peptic ulcer bleeding: results of a placebo-controlled multicenter study. Scand J Gastroenterol 1997; 32: 328–33 |
| 47 | 1b | Khuroo MS, Yattoo GN, Javid G et al. A comparison of omeprazole and placebo for bleeding peptic ulcer. N Engl J Med 1997; 336: 1054–8 |
| 48 | 1b | Schaffalitzky de Muckadell OB, Havelund T, Harling T et al. Effect of omeprazole on the outcome of endoscopically treated bleeding peptic ulcers: randomized double-blind placebo-controlled multicentre study. Scand J Gastroenterol 1997; 32: 320–7 |
| 49 | 1b | Lin HJ, Lo WC, Lee FY. A prospective randomized comparative trial showing that omeprazole prevents rebleeding in patients with bleeding peptic ulcer after successful endoscopic therapy. Arch Intern Med 1998; 158: 54–8 |
| 50 | 1b | Hollander D, Harlan J. Antacids versus placebos in peptic ulcer therapy: a controlled double-blind investigation. JAMA 1973; 226: 1181–5 |
| 51 | 2b | Sonnenberg A, Muller-Lissner SA, Vogel E et al. Predictors of duodenal ulcer healing and relapse. Gastroenterology 1981; 81: 1061–7 |
| 52 | 1b | Lau JY, Sung JJ, Lam Y-H et al. Endoscopic retreatment compared with surgery in patients with recurrent bleeding after initial endoscopic control of bleeding ulcers. N Engl J Med 1999; 340: 751–6 |
| 53 | 1b | Morris DL, Hawker PC, Brearley S et al. Optimal timing of operation for bleeding peptic ulcer: prospective randomised trial. BMJ 1984; 288: 1277–80 |
| 54 | 1b | Saperas E, Pique JM, Perez Ayuso R et al. Conservative management of bleeding duodenal ulcer without a visible vessel: prospective randomized trial. Br J Surg 1987; 74: 784–6 |
| 55 | 2b | Millat B, Hay J-M, Valleur P et al. Emergency surgical treatment for bleeding duodenal ulcer: oversewing plus vagotomy versus gastric resection, a controlled randomized trial. World J Surg 1993; 17: 568–4 |
| 56 | 1a | Henry DA, O'Connell DL. Effects of fibrinolytic inhibitors on mortality from upper gastrointestinal haemorrhage. BMJ 1989; 298: 1142–6 |
| 57 | 2b | Rybo E et al. Effect of iron supplementation to women with iron deficiency. Scand J Haematol 1986; 35: 103–13 |
| 58 | 2b | Gardner GW et al. Cardiorespiratory, hematological and physical performance responses of anemic subjects to iron treatment. Am J Clin Nutr 1975; 28: 982–88 |
| 59 | 1a | Laine L, Cook D. Endoscopic ligation compared with sclerotherapy for treatment of esophageal variceal bleeding: a meta-analysis. Ann Intern Med 1995; 123: 280–7 |
| 60 | 2b | Shemesh E, Czerniak A, Klein E et al. A comparison between emergency and delayed endoscopic injection sclerotherapy of bleeding esophageal varices in nonalcoholic portal hypertension. J Clin Gastroenterol 1990; 12: 5–9 |

| No | Level | Citation |
|----|-------|----------|
| 61 | 1b | Sung JJ, Chung SC, Yung MY et al. Prospective randomised study of effect of octreotide in rebleeding from oesophageal varices after endoscopic ligation. Lancet 1995; 346: 1666–9 |
| 62 | 1b | Avgerinos A, Nevens F, Raptis S et al. Early administration of somatostatin and efficacy of sclerotherapy in acute oesophageal variceal bleeds: the European Acute Bleeding Oesophageal Variceal Episodes (ABOVE) randomised trial. Lancet 1997; 350: 1495–9 |
| 63 | 1b | Besson I et al. Sclerotherapy with or without octreotide for acute variceal bleeding. N Engl J Med 1995; 333: 555–60 |
| 64 | 1b | Besson I et al. Sclerotherapy with or without octreotide for acute variceal bleeding N Engl J Med 1995; 333: 555–60 |
| 65 | 1b | Garcia-Compean D, Blanc P, Bories J-M, et al. Treatment of active gastroesophageal variceal bleeding with terlipressin or hemostatic balloon in patients with cirrhosis. A randomized controlled trial. Archives of Medical Research 1997; 28: 241–245 |
| 66 | 1b | Jalan R, Forrest E, Stanley AJ et al. A randomized trial comparing transjugular intrahepatic portosystemic stent-shunt with variceal band ligation in the prevention of rebleeding from esophageal varices. Hepatology 1997; 26: 1115–22 |
| 67 | 1b | Merli M, Salerno F, Riggio O et al. Transjugular intrahepatic portosystemic shunt versus endoscopic sclerotherapy for the prevention of variceal bleeding in cirrhosis: a randomized multicenter trial. Hepatology 1998; 27: 40–5 |
| 68 | 1b | Garcia-Villareal L, Martinez-Lagares F, Sierra A et al. Transjugular intrahepatic portosystemic shunt versus endoscopic sclerotherapy for the prevention of variceal rebleeding after recent variceal hemorrhage. Hepatology 1999; 29: 27–32 |
| 69 | 1b | Carbrera J, Maynar M, Granados R et al. Transjugular intrahepatic portosystemic shunt versus sclerotherapy in the elective treatment of variceal hemorrhage. Gastroenterology 1996; 110: 832–9 |
| 70 | 1b | Cello JP et al. Endoscopic sclerotherapy compared with percutaneous transjugular intrahepatic portosystemic shunt after initial sclerotherapy in patients with acute variceal hemorrhage. A randomized, controlled trial. Ann Intern Med 1997; 126: 858–65 |
| 71 | 1b | Sanyal AJ, Freedman AM, Luketic VA et al. Transjugular intrahepatic portosystemic shunts compared with endoscopic sclerotherapy for the prevention of recurrent variceal hemorrhage: a randomized, controlled trial. Ann Intern Med 1997; 126: 849–57 |
| 72 | 1a | Spina GP, Henderson JM, Rikkers LF et al. Distal spleno-renal shunt versus endoscopic sclerotherapy in the prevention of variceal rebleeding: a meta-analysis of 4 randomized clinical trials. J Hepatol 1992; 16: 338–45 |
| 73 | 1b | Burroughs AK, Hamilton G, Phillips A et al. Comparison of sclerotherapy with staple transection of the esophagus for the emergency control of bleeding from esophageal varices. N Engl J Med 1989; 321: 857–62 |
| 74 | 1b | Triger DR, Johnson AG, Brazier JE et al. A prospective trial of endoscopic sclerotherapy versus oesophageal transection and gastric devascularisation in the long term management of bleeding oesophageal varices. Gut 1992; 33: 1553–8 |
| 75 | 3b | Evans JM, McMahon AD, McGilchrist MM et al. Topical non-steroidal anti-inflammatory drugs and admission to hospital for upper gastrointestinal bleeding and perforation: a record linkage case-control study. British Medical Journal 1995; 311: 22–26 |
| 76 | 3a | Henry D, Lim L, Rodriguez G et al. Variability in risk of gastrointestinal complications with individual non-steroidal anti-inflammatory drugs: results of a collaborative meta-analysis. BMJ 1996; 312: 1563–6 |

| No | Level | Citation |
|----|-------|----------|
| 77 | 3b | Langman MJ, Weil J, Wainwright P, et al. Risks of bleeding peptic ulcer associated with individual non-steroidal anti-inflammatory drugs. Lancet 1994; 343: 1075–1078 |
| 78 | 1b | Langman MJ, Jensen DM, Watson DJ et al. Adverse upper gastrointestinal effects of rofecoxib compared with NSAIDs. JAMA 1999; 282: 1929–33 |
| 79 | 2b | Simon LS, Weaver AL, Graham DY et al. Anti-inflammatory and upper gastrointestinal effects of celecoxib in rheumatoid arthritis: a randomized controlled trial. JAMA 1999; 282: 1921–8 |
| 80 | 1b | Hawkey CJ, Karrasch JA, Szczepanski L et al. Omeprazole compared with misoprostol for ulcers associated with nonsteroidal anti-inflammatory drugs. N Engl J Med 1998; 338: 727–34 |
| 81 | 1a | Koch M, Dezi A, Ferrario F et al. Prevention of nonsteroidal anti-inflammatory drug-induced gastrointestinal mucosal injury: a meta-analysis of randomized controlled clinical trials. Arch Intern Med 1996; 156: 2321–32 |
| 82 | 1b | Chan FK, Sung JJ, Chung SC et al. Randomised trial of eradication of *Helicobacter pylori* before non-steroidal anti-inflammatory drug therapy to prevent peptic ulcers. Lancet 1997; 350: 975–9 |
| 83 | 1a | Treiber G, Lambert JR. The impact of *Helicobacter pylori* eradication on peptic ulcer healing. Am J Gastroenterol 1998; 93: 1080–4 |
| 84 | 1b | Hawkey CJ, Tulassay Z, Szczepanski L et al. Randomised controlled trial of *Helicobacter pylori* eradication in patients on non-steroidal anti-inflammatory drugs: HELP NSAIDs study. Lancet 1998; 352: 1016–21 |
| 85 | 1b | Graham DY, Hepps KS, Ramirez FC, et al. Scand J Gastroenterol 1993; 28: 939–942 |
| 86 | 1b | Sung JJ, Leung WK, Suen R, et al. One-week antibiotics versus maintenance acid suppression therapy for *Helicobacter pylori*-associated peptic ulcer bleeding. Digestive Diseases and Sciences 1997; 42 (12): 2524–2528 |
| 87 | 2a | Penston JG, McColl KE. Eradication of *Helicobacter pylori*: an objective assessment of current therapies. Br J Clin Pharmacol 1997; 43: 223–43 |
| 88 | 2a | Unge P, Berstad A. Pooled analysis of anti-*Helicobacter pylori* treatment regimens (supplement). Scand J Gastroenterol 1996; 31: 27–40 |
| 89 | 2a | Penston JG, McColl KE. Eradication of *Helicobacter pylori*: an objective assessment of current therapies. Br J Clin Pharmacol 1997; 43: 223–43 |
| 90 | 1b | Yeomans ND, Tulassay Z, Juhasz L et al. A comparison of omeprazole with ranitidine for ulcers associated with nonsteroidal anti-inflammatory drugs. N Engl J Med 1998; 338: 719–26 |
| 91 | 1a | Bernard B et al. Beta-adrenergic antagonists in the prevention of gastrointestinal rebleeding in patients with cirrhosis: a meta-analysis: Hepatology 1997; 25: 63–70 |
| 92 | 1b | Bertoni G, Sassatelli R, Fornaciari G et al. Oral isosorbide-5 mononitrate reduces the rebleeding rate during the course of injection sclerotherapy for esophageal varices. Scand J Gastroenterol 1994; 29(4): 363–70 |
| 93 | 2b – | Merkel C, Marin R, Enzo E et al. Randomised trial of nadolol alone or with isosorbide mononitrate for primary prophylaxis of variceal bleeding in cirrhosis. Lancet 1996; 348: 1677–81 |
| 94 | 1b | Jenkins SA, Baxter JN, Critchley M et al. Randomised trial of octreotide for long term management of cirrhosis after variceal haemorrhage. BMJ 1997; 315: 1338–41 |

| No | Level | Citation |
|----|-------|----------|
| 95 | 1b | Merkel C, Gatta A, Bellumat A et al. Optimizing the time-frame for the definition of bleeding-related death after acute variceal bleeding in cirrhosis. Eur J Gastroenterol Hepatol 1996; 8: 75–9 |
| 96 | 1b | Villanueva C, Balanzo J, Espinos JC et al. Prediction of therapeutic failure in patients with bleeding peptic ulcer treated with endoscopic injection. Dig Dis Sci 1993; 38: 2062–70 |
| 97 | 2b | Garcia-Compean D, Blanc P, Bories J-M et al. Treatment of active gastroesophageal variceal bleeding with terlipressin or hemostatic balloon in patients with cirrhosis. A randomized controlled trial. Archives of Medical Research 1997; 28: 241–245 |
| 98 | 2b | Jalan R, Forrest E, Stanley AJ, et al. A randomized trial comparing transjugular intrahepatic portosystemic stent-shunt with variceal band ligation in the prevention of rebleeding from esophageal varices. Hepatology 1997; 26: 1115–1122 |
| 99 | 2b | Merli M, Salerno F, Riggio O et al. Transjugular intrahepatic portosystemic shunt versus endoscopic sclerotherapy for the prevention of variceal bleeding in cirrhosis: a randomized multicenter trial. Hepatology 1998; 27: 40–45 |
| 100 | 4 | Ishimori A, Kawakami K, Inoue S et al. Predictors of relapse in peptic ulcer. Hepatogastroenterology 1992; 39: 396–9 |
| 101 | 2b | Battaglia G, di Mario F, Dotto P et al. Markers of slow-healing peptic ulcer in the elderly: a study of 1052 ranitidine-treated patients. Dig Dis Sci 1993; 38: 1414–21 |

## PREVALENCE

Classically, giant cell or temporal arteritis occurs in patients aged > 50 presenting with a headache, malaise, weight loss, jaw claudication, scalp tenderness and visual disturbance.

**Note**

- Giant cell arteritis is common in strongly suspected cases (~30% to 50%) **[B]**[1] **[C]**[2].

## CLINICAL FEATURES

Ask about:

- recent onset headache **[B]**[1]
- jaw claudication **[B]**[1]
- anorexia **[C]**[3]
- tongue claudication **[C]**[4]

**? Why do this?**

**A recent headache and jaw claudication make giant cell or arteritis more likely**

| Patient | Target disorder (reference standard) | Diagnostic test | LR+ (95% CI) | Post-test probability | LR− (95% CI) | Post-test probability |
|---|---|---|---|---|---|---|
| Suspected giant cell arteritis having a temporal artery biopsy **[B]**[1] (pre-test probability 53%) | Giant cell arteritis (positive temporal artery biopsy) | Recent onset headache | 1.7 (1.3 to 2.3) | 57% | 0.37 (0.20 to 0.70) | 23% |
| Suspected giant cell arteritis having a temporal artery biopsy **[B]**[1] (pre-test probability 53%) | Giant cell arteritis (positive temporal artery biopsy) | Jaw claudication | 3.5 (1.6 to 7.6) | 73% | 0.66 (0.50 to 0.86) | 34% |
| Suspected giant cell arteritis having a temporal artery biopsy **[C]**[4] (pre-test probability 40%) | Giant cell arteritis (clinical features or temporal artery biopsy) | Tongue claudication | 0.11 (0.027 to 0.44) | 7% | 1.5 (1.2 to 1.7) | 50% |
| Suspected giant cell arteritis having a temporal artery biopsy **[C]**[3] (pre-test probability 36%) | Giant cell arteritis (positive temporal artery biopsy) | Anorexia | 3.8 (1.4 to 10) | 69% | 0.77 (0.63 to 0.95) | 31% |

- visual disturbances **[D]**.

Look for:

- an abnormal temporal artery (hot, red, tender) **[B]**[1]

? **Why do this?**
A red, hot, tender temporal artery makes giant cell arteritis more likely

| Patient | Target disorder (reference standard) | Diagnostic test | LR+ (95% CI) | Post-test probability | LR– (95% CI) | Post-test probability |
|---|---|---|---|---|---|---|
| Suspected giant cell arteritis having a temporal artery biopsy [B][1] (pre-test probability 53%) | Giant cell arteritis (positive temporal artery biopsy) | Red, hot, tender temporal artery | 2.3 (1.6 to 3.4) | 64% | 0.24 (0.12 to 0.49) | 16% |

- complications, e.g. vision loss, stroke, neuropathy [D]
- other causes of a headache [D].

**Note**
- Patients without a recent onset headache, jaw claudication or an abnormal temporal artery are unlikely to have giant cell arteritis [B][1].

**Why do this?**
No recent headache, jaw claudication or abnormal temporal artery make giant cell arteritis unlikely

| Patient | Target disorder (reference standard) | Diagnostic test | LR+ (95% CI) | Post-test probability | LR– (95% CI) | Post-test probability |
|---|---|---|---|---|---|---|
| Suspected giant cell arteritis having a temporal artery biopsy [B][1] (pre-test probability 53%) | Giant cell arteritis (positive temporal artery biopsy) | Any of recent onset headache, jaw claudication, abnormal temporal artery | 2.9 (2.0 to 4.1) | 69% | 0.0 (0.0 to 0.098) | 0% |

No other clinical findings have been shown to be particularly useful for diagnosing giant cell arteritis [B][1].

## DIFFERENTIAL DIAGNOSIS

Think about other causes of these symptoms.
Common causes include [C][4]:

- non-specific headache
- infection.

<table>
<tr><td colspan="2">Note</td></tr>
</table>

| Differential diagnosis of giant cell arteritis [C]⁴ | % (95% CI) |
|---|---|
| Non-specific headache | 16% (10% to 23%) |
| Infection | 9.0% (4.1% to 14%) |
| Cardiac emboli or atherosclerosis | 9.0% (4.1% to 14%) |
| Connective tissue disease | 9.0% (4.1% to 14%) |
| Other causes | 10% (5.3% to 16%) |

## INVESTIGATIONS

● ESR or plasma viscosity.

**Note**
■ A normal ESR or plasma viscosity does not rule out giant cell arteritis.

**Why do this?**
An elevated ESR or plasma viscosity helps diagnose giant cell artertis

| Patient | Target disorder (reference standard) | Diagnostic test | LR+ (95% CI) | Post-test probability | LR– (95% CI) | Post-test probability |
|---|---|---|---|---|---|---|
| Suspected giant cell arteritis (pre-test probability 48%) | Giant cell arteritis (posiive temporal artery biopsy) | ESR ≥ 60 mm/h | 6.9 (1.9 to 26) | 87% | 0.16 (0.041 to 0.56) | 13% |
| Suspected giant cell arteritis (pre-test probability 48%) | Giant cell arteritis (positive temporal artery biopsy | Plasma viscosity ≥ 1.8 units | 5.3 (1.3 to 13) | 81% | 0.16 (0.044 to 0.61) | 13% |

Around 20% of patients with giant cell arteritis have a normal ESR
when first seen [A]⁵.

● Blood count.

**Why do this?**
Anaemia makes giant cell arteritis more likely

| Patient | Target disorder (reference standard) | Diagnostic test | LR+ (95% CI) | Post-test probability | LR– (95% CI) | Post-test probability |
|---|---|---|---|---|---|---|
| Suspected giant cell arteritis having a temporal artery biopsy [C]³ (pre-test probability 36%) | Giant cell arteritis (positive temporal artery biopsy) | Anaemia | 2.0 (1.3 to 3.2) | 53% | 0.58 (0.39 to 0.87) | 25% |

- Bilateral **[C]**[6] temporal artery biopsy **[A]** in areas of pain or inflammation (this increases the chance of a positive biopsy) **[C]**[6].

---

**? Why do this?**

■ Temporal artery biopsy is the reference standard.

**A normal temporal artery biopsy does not rule out giant cell arteritis**

| Patient | Target disorder (reference standard) | Diagnostic test | LR+ (95% CI) | Post-test probability | LR– (95% CI) | Post-test probability |
|---|---|---|---|---|---|---|
| Suspected giant cell arteritis having a temporal artery biopsy **[C]**[3] (pre-test probability 36%) | Giant cell arteritis (diagnostic criteria and follow-up) | Temporal artery biopsy | Infinity (14 to infinity) | 100% | 0.18 (0.10 to 0.32) | 17% |
| Suspected giant cell arteritis having a temporal artery biopsy **[C]**[3] (pre-test probability 21%) | Giant cell arteritis (temporal artery biopsy and follow-up) | Temporal artery biopsy at sites of pain or inflammation | 6.0 (3.5 to 10) | 61% | 0.47 (0.33 to 0.67) | 11% |

---

Patients with negative biopsies who meet all the following criteria should be diagnosed with giant cell arteritis **[D]**[7]:

1. aged > 55
2. a positive response to steroids within 48 h
3. a history lasting > 2 weeks
4. at least three of the following:

   - proximal and symmetrical girdle or upper arm muscle pain, stiffness or tenderness
   - jaw claudication
   - clinically abnormal temporal artery (tender, thickened, red)
   - systemic symptoms or sign (malaise, anorexia, weight loss, anaemia, pyrexia)
   - recent onset headache
   - visual disturbance (loss, dip, blurring).

---

## THERAPY

- Give corticosteroids **[A]**[8] **[A]**[9] immediately in all suspected cases **[D]**[1].

---

**? Why do this?**

- Vision loss is common without steroids (40% – and 10% lose vision in both eyes). This is less common (~20%) on steroids **[A]**[8] **[A]**[9].
- Symptoms resolve rapidly on steroids. A response within 48 h supports the diagnosis **[D]**[1].

---

Start with 40 mg prednisolone **[D]** daily **[A]**[8,9] with vitamin D and calcium supplements **[A]**[14].

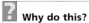

**Why do this?**

- Patients on lower doses are more likely to require increases to control symptoms, although there is no clear difference in the rate of ocular complications **[C]**[10] **[D]**[11].
- There are fewer side-effects. Patients with greater doses of steroid have more side-effects **[B]**[12].
- Alternate day regimens cause fewer steroid side-effects, but are worse at controlling symptoms **[A]**[13].
- Patients on long-term steroids who take vitamin D and calcium have less bone loss in the lumbar spine and forearm, although the effect on non-traumatic fractures is unclear **[A]**[14].

**High-dose steroids help control symptoms in giant cell arteritis**

| Patient | Treatment | Comparator | Outcome | CER | RRR | NNT |
|---|---|---|---|---|---|---|
| Giant cell arteritis **[C]**[10] | Prednisolone ≥ 20 mg daily | Prednisolone < 20 mg daily | Dose increase required to control symptoms or lower ESR up to 40 weeks | 46% | 89% (51% to 100%) | 2 (2 to 4) |
| Giant cell arteritis **[A]**[13] | Prednisolone alternate days | Prednisolone daily | Symptom resolution by 4 weeks | 85% | −65% (−92% to −38%) | −2 (−3 to −1) |
| Giant cell arteritis **[A]**[13] | Prednisolone alternate days | Prednisolone daily | Adverse effects due to steroids by 8 weeks | 65% | 100% | 2 (1 to 2) |

Warn patients that they may be on steroids for a long time, and that side-effects are common with long-term use **[A]**.
Common problems include weight gain and vertebral fracture **[D]**.
Watch out for iatrogenic Cushing's syndrome, bacterial sepsis and hypertension **[A]**.

**Note**

- Around a third of patients with giant cell arteritis who are on steroids have side-effects, the most common being weight gain (~50%) and vertebral fractures (~15%) **[C]**[15].
- Dyspepsia symptoms are more common with steroids, but there is no clear increase in the occurrence of peptic ulcers **[A]**[16].

**Cushing's syndrome is common in patients on long-term steroids**

| Patient **[A]**[16] | Treatment | Comparator | Outcome | CER | OR (95% CI) | NNF (95% CI) |
|---|---|---|---|---|---|---|
| Giant cell arteritis | Steroid use | Placebo | Cushing's syndrome/ acne/hirsutism at 2 months | 2.6% | 4.5 (3.5 to 5.7) | 12 (9 to 17) |
| Giant cell arteritis | Steroid use | Placebo | Bacterial sepsis at 2 months | 4.8% | 1.2 (1.0 to 1.6) | 110 (38 to infinity) |
| Giant cell arteritis | Steroid use | Placebo | Hypertension at 2 months | 0.24% | 2.2 (1.4 to 3.8) | 350 (150 to 1100) |
| Giant cell arteritis | Steroid use (mean of 35 mg prednisolone for 2 months) | Placebo | Ulcer symptoms at 2 months | 0.25% | 1.9 (1.1 to 3.0) | 440 (200 to 4000) |
| Giant cell arteritis | Steroid use• | Placebo | Diabetes mellitus at 2 months | 0.32% | 1.7 (1.1 to 2.6) | 450 (200 to 3100) |

Consider starting:

- antacid medication if patients complain of dyspepsia **[D]**
- bisphosphonates **[A]**[17].

 **Why do this?**
- Patients on long-term corticosteroids who take bisphosphonates maintain lumbar bone density better than controls **[A]**[17].
- There is no clear effect on new vertebral fractures.

There is no clear benefit from combining steroids with methotrexate **[D]** or azathioprine **[A]**.

**Why?**
- Methotrexate does not reduce the dose or duration of steroids required to control polymyalgia rheumatica or giant cell arteritis **[D]**[18].
- Azathioprine does not produce a clinically significant decrease in the steroid dose required to control polymyalgia rheumatica or giant cell arteritis **[D]**[19].

## PROGNOSIS

Relapses are common but decrease over time (60% within 2 years). Half are triggered by attempting to reduce the steroid dose **[B]**[11]. The ESR or CRP alone do not usefully predict which patients relapse or develop complications **[C]**[5], so adjustments in steroid dose should be based on patient's symptoms **[D]**. Long-term steroid use is common: mean duration of steroid use is about 2 years **[B]**[11] **[B]**[20]. Complications are common despite steroids (Table 1) **[C]**[21]; However, there is no effect on mortality **[C]**[22].

Table 1 Complications in patients with giant cell arteritis are common

| Complications **[C]**[21] | % (95% CI) |
| --- | --- |
| Large artery disease | 31% (24% to 38%) |
| ■ upper limb | 18% (12% to 23%) |
| ■ lower limb | 9.0% (4.7% to 13%) |
| Ophthalmic | 21% (15% to 27%) |
| ■ amaurosis fugax | 10% (5.6% to 15%) |
| ■ permanent vision loss | 8.4% (4.2% to 13%) |
| Carotid arteries affected | 19% (13% to 25%) |
| Neuropathy | 14% (8.6% to 19%) |
| Stroke or TLA | 7.2% (3.3% to 11%) |

**Guideline writer**: Chris Ball
**CAT writer**: Chris Ball

# REFERENCES

| No. | Level | Citation |
|-----|-------|----------|
| 1 | 2b | Vilaseca J et al. Clinical usefulness of temporal artery biopsy. Ann Rheum Dis 1987; 46: 262–85 |
| 2 | 4 | Brittain GP et al. Plasma viscosity or erythrocyte sedimentation rate in the diagnosis of giant cell arteritis? Br J Ophthalmol 1991; 75: 656–9 |
| 3 | 4 | Fernandez-Herlihy L. Temporal arteritis: clinical aids to diagnosis. J Rheumatol 1988; 15: 1797–801 |
| 4 | 4 | Hall S et al. Therapeutic impact of temporal artery biopsy. Lancet 1983; ii: 1217–20 |
| 5 | 1b | Ellis ME, Ralston S. The erthyrocyte sedimentation rate in the diagnosis and management of polymyalgia rheumatica and giant cell arteritis syndrome. Ann Rheum Dis 1983; 42: 168–70 |
| 6 | 4 | Ponge T et al. The efficacy of selective unilateral temporal artery biopsy versus bilateral biopsies for diagnosing giant cell arteritis. J Rheumatol 1988; 15: 997–1000 |
| 7 | 5 | Vilaseca J et al. Clinical usefulness of temporal artery biopsy. Ann Rheum Dis 1987; 46: 262–285 |
| 8 | 1c | Huston KA et al. Temporal arteritis: a twenty-five year epidemiological, clinical and pathological study. Ann Intern Med 1978; 88: 162–7 |
| 9 | 1c | Caselli RJ et al. Neurologic disease in biopsy-proven giant cell (temporal arteritis). Neurology 1988; 38: 352–9 |
| 10 | 4 | Myles AB et al. Prevention of blindness in giant cell arteritis by corticosteroid treatment. Br J Rheumatol 1992; 31: 103–5 |
| 11 | 1b– | Kyle V, Hazleman BL. Treatment of polymyalgia rheumatica and giant cell arteritis. I Steroid regimens in the first two months. Ann Rheum Dis 1989; 48: 658–61 |
| 12 | 2c | Kyle V, Hazleman BL. Treatment of polymyalgia rheumatica and giant cell arteritis. II Relation between steroid dose and steroid associated side effects. Ann Rheum Dis 1989; 48: 662–6 |
| 13 | 1b | Hunder GG et al. Alternate day corticosteroid regimens in the treatment of giant cell arteritis: comparison in a prospective study. Ann Intern Med 1975; 82: 613–18 |
| 14 | 1a | Homik J et al. Osteoporosis (OP): Calcium (Ca) and vitamin D for the treatment of corticosteroid-induced osteoporosis (Cochrane Review). In: The Cochrane Library, Issue 2, 1998. Oxford: Update Software. |
| 15 | 4 | Kyle V, Hazleman BL. Clinical and laboratory course of polymyalgia rheumatica and giant cell arteritis after the first 2 months of therapy. Ann Rheum Dis 1993; 52: 847–50 |
| 16 | 1a | Conn HO, Poynard T. Corticosteroids and peptic ulcer: a meta-analysis of adverse events during steroid therapy. J Intern Med 1994; 236: 619–32 |
| 17 | 1a | Homik J et al. Bisphosphonates for steroid induced osteoporosis (Cochrane Review). In: The Cochrane Library, Issue 3, 1999. Oxford: Update Software. |
| 18 | 1b– | van der Veen MJ et al. Can methotrexate be used as a steroid sparing agent in the treatment of polymyalgia rheumatica and giant cell arteritis? Ann Rheum Dis 1996; 55: 218–23 |

| No. | Level | Citation |
|-----|-------|----------|
| 19 | 1b– | de Silva M, Hazleman BL. Azathioprine in giant cell arteritis/polymyalgia rheumatica. Ann Rheum Dis 1986; 45: 136–8 |
| 20 | 2c | Delecoeuillerie G, Joly P, Cohen de Lara A et al. PMR and TA: a retrospective analysis of prognostic features and different corticosteroid regimes. Ann Rheum Dis 1998; 47: 733–9 |
| 21 | 4 | Caselli RJ et al. Neurologic disease in biopsy-proven giant cell (temporal arteritis). Neurol 1988; 38: 352–9 |
| 22 | 4 | Huston KA et al. Temporal arteritis: a twenty-five year epidemiological, clinical and pathological study. Ann Intern Med 1978; 88: 162–7 |

## PREVALENCE

Hypercalcaemia is uncommon in patients in hospital.

> **Note**
> ■ The prevalence of hypercalcaemia ranges from 0.17% to 2.9% among hospitalised patients **[A]**[1].

## CAUSES

Common causes include **[C]**[2] **[C]**[3]:

- primary hyperparathyroidism
- malignancy
- renal failure.

Rarer causes include **[C]**[2] **[C]**[3]

- sarcoidosis
- thyrotoxicosis
- excessive vitamin D therapy.

> **Note**
> **Primary hyperparathyroidism is the commonest cause in outpatients**
>
> | Hospital outpatients | **[C]**[2] % |
> | --- | --- |
> | Primary hyperparathyroidism | 54% (47% to 60%) |
> | Malignancy | 35% (28% to 41%) |
> | Unknown | 9.2% (5.2% to 13%) |
> | Sarcoidosis | 1.0% (0.0% to 2.3%) |
> | Thyrotoxicosis | 0.5% (0.0% to 1.4%) |
> | Immobilisation | 0.5% (0.0% to 1.4%) |
> | Vitamin D intoxication | 0.5% (0.0% to 1.4%) |
>
> **Malignancy is the commonest cause in inpatients**
>
> | Hospital inpatients **[C]**[3] | % (95% CI) |
> | --- | --- |
> | Malignancy | 47% (42% to 51%) |
> | No cause found | 22% (18% to 26%) |
> | On renal dialysis | 15% (11% to 18%) |
> | Primary hyperparathyroidism | 13% (9.6% to 16%) |
> | Excessive vitamin D therapy | 2.1% (0.8% to 3.4%) |
> | Other causes | 1.3% (0.3% to 2.3%) |
> | Thyrotoxicosis | 0.9% (0.0% to 1.7%) |
> | Sarcoidosis | 0.2% (0.0% to 0.6%) |

## CLINICAL FEATURES

Many patients with hypercalcaemia are asymptomatic.
Clinical features can be non-specific.

Ask about:
- known malignancy [C][2] [C][3].
- medication [D]
  - which may exacerbate hypercalcaemia (e.g. thiazides, vitamin D)
  - which may be more toxic (e.g. digoxin [D][4]).

Look for [C][2] [C][5] [C][6]:
- dehydration
- polyuria
- gastrointestinal symptoms (nausea, vomiting, constipation)
- confusion and psychiatric symptoms.

| Why?<br>Many cases of hypercalcaemia are asymptomatic | |
| --- | --- |
| Clinical feature [C][2] [C][5] | % (95% CI) |
| Asymptomatic | 51%–57% |
| Confusion and dehydration | 14% |
| Symptoms of hypercalcaemia (lethargy, polyuria) | 8% |
| Renal (stones or decreased function) | 7%–18% |
| Hypertension | 5% |
| Psychiatric disorder | 5%–20% |
| Gastrointestinal symptoms | 4%–8% |
| Bone disease | 0%–20% |

## INVESTIGATIONS

- Calcium [A].
- Albumin [A].

Calculate the corrected calcium:

$$\text{corrected calcium (mmol/l)} = \text{uncorrected calcium (mmol/l)} + 0.02 \times (40\text{-albumin}) \text{ (g/L)} \textbf{ [A]}$$

| Why?<br>A calcium level $\geq$ 3.50 mmol/l makes malignancy more likely | | | | |
| --- | --- | --- | --- | --- |
| Patient [C][3] [C][7] | Target disorder (reference standard) | Diagnostic test | LR (95% CI) | Post-test probability |
| Hypercalcaemia (pre-test probability 47%) | Malignancy (hospital records) | Calcium<br>≥3.50 mmol/l<br>3.00–3.49 mmol/l<br>< 3.00 mmol/l | 5.7 (2.9 to 11)<br>1.7 (1.2 to 2.5)<br>0.63 (0.54 to 0.73) | 84%<br>60%<br>36 % |

- Alkaline phosphatase [D] and liver function tests [D].
- Urea and electrolytes (including phosphate, magnesium and creatinine) [C][3].
- Parathyroid hormone [C][7] [C][8] – positive if > 4.0 pmol/l or within reference range (0.9–4.0 pmol/l) that is high in relation to calcium.

**Why?**
**PTH can diagnose and exclude primary hyperparathyroidism**

| Patient [C][7] [C][8] | Target disorder (reference standard) | Diagnostic test | LR+ (95% CI) | Post-test probability | LR– (95% CI) | Post-test probability |
|---|---|---|---|---|---|---|
| Hypercalcaemia (pre-test probability 13%) | Primary hyperparathyroidism (investigations) | PTH | 58 (8.3 to 400) | 90% | 0.0 (0.0 to 0.048) | 0% |

- PTH-related protein [C][7] [C][8].

**Why?**
**PTH-related protein can help diagnose malignancy but absence cannot safely exclude it**

| Patient [C][7] [C][8] | Target disorder (reference standard) | Diagnostic test | LR+ (95% CI) | Post-test probability | LR– (95% CI) | Post-test probability |
|---|---|---|---|---|---|---|
| Hypercalcaemia (pre-test probability 47%) | Malignancy (investigations) | PTH-related protein detected | 8.7 (4.0 to 19) | 89% | 0.22 (0.13 to 0.37) | 25% |

- Thyroid function tests [C][3].

Look for a cause [A], e.g. evidence of malignancy.
Consider electrocardiogram (especially in those with pre-existing cardiac conditions or on digoxin).

## THERAPY

### Malignancy
- Give fluid: 0.9% saline iv – at once [A].
- Consider use of additional monitoring (such as central venous pressure and urinary catheter) in patients with critical fluid balance (e.g. severe cardiac failure or renal insufficiency).
- Give furosemide.

**Why?**
■ High-dose furosemide reduces the calcium and magnesium levels – and potassium (measure and replace appropriately) **[C]**[9].

● Give pamidronate **[A]**[10] 90 mg over 1 h iv **[A]**[10].

 **Why?**
■ It speeds return to normocalcaemia and reduces relapse **[A]**[10].
■ Fever is a common side-effect **[A]**[10].
■ 90 mg of pamidronate is more effective than 30 or 60 mg **[A]**[10].
■ It is more effective than etidronate **[A]**[11], clodronate and mithramycin **[A]**[12] and the effects lasts longer (on average 2 weeks) **[A]**[12].

**90 mg of pamidronate helps correct hypercalcaemia and prevents relapse**

| Patient | Treatment | Comparator | Outcome | CER | RRR | NNT |
|---|---|---|---|---|---|---|
| Hypercalcaemia **[A]**[10] | Pamidronate | Placebo | Normocalcaemia at 7 days | 22% | –220% (–611% to –44%) | 2 (1 to 4) |
| | | | Fever due to medication at 7 days | 0.0% | | –5 (–10 to –3) |
| | | | Relapse at 7 days following normocalcaemia | 91% | 43% (23% to 585%) | 3 (12 to 5) |
| Hypercalcaemia **[A]**[13] | Pamidronate 90 mg iv | Pamidronate 60 mg iv | Normocalcaemia | 100% | –64% (–137% to –13%) | 3 (2 to 6) |
| Hypercalcaemia **[A]**[12] | Pamidronate | Etidronate | Normocalcaemia at 7 days | 40% | –75 % (–180% to –10%) | 3 (2 to 14) |
| Hypercalcaemia **[A]**[12] | Pamidronate | Clodronate | Normocalcaemia at 7 days | 80% | –25 (–56% to 0%) | 5 (3 to 40) |
| Hypercalcaemia **[A]**[14] | Pamidronate | Mithramycin | Normocalcaemia at 9 days | 86% | –270% (–860% to –40%) | 1 (1 to 2) |

Alternatives include:

● gallium nitrate (200 mg/m$^2$ per day iv for 5 days) **[A]**[15].

 **Why?**
■ It is more effective than etidronate **[A]**[15] or calcitonin **[A]**[16] at lowering calcium levels.
■ It reduces the need for further treatment **[A]**[15].
■ It increases the risk of hypophosphataemia **[A]**[15].

**Gallium nitrate helps correct hypercalcaemia and reduces the need for further treatment**

| Patient | Treatment | Comparator | Outcome | CER | RRR | NNT |
|---|---|---|---|---|---|---|
| Hypercalcaemia **[A]**[15] | Gallium nitrate | Etidronate | Normocalcaemia at 7 days | 43% | –90% (–184% to –28%) | 3 (2 to 5) |
| | | | Additional treatment required at 7 days | 27% | 67% (9% to 90%) | 5 (3 to 99) |
| | | | Hypophosphataemia at 7 days | 41% | –118% (–228% to –45%) | –2 (–4 to –1) |

Consider dialysis for patients with severe renal insufficiency **[D]**.
There is no clear role for:
- steroids **[C]**[17] except in steroid-responsive malignancy (breast cancer **[A]**[18], myeloma
- calcitonin **[D]**[19].

 **Why?**
- Women with breast cancer and hypercalcaemia who take prednisobne are more likely to become normocalcaemic **[A]**[18].
- Adding calcitonin to prednisolone has no clear effect on calcium levels **[D]**[19].

**Prednisolone helps achieve normocalcaemia in breast cancer**

| Patient **[A]**[18] | Treatment | Comparator | Outcome | CER | RRR | NNT |
|---|---|---|---|---|---|---|
| Breast cancer and hypercalcaemia | Prednisolone, frusemide, rehydration | Frusemide, rehydration | Normocalcaemic at 8 days | 0% | 47% (14% to 67%) | 2 (1 to 5) |

## Primary hyperparathyroidism
- Treat asymptomatic and mild cases conservatively.

 **Why?**
- Patients with mild asymptomatic primary hyperparathyroidism who are treated conservatively do not develop worsening disease **[A]**[20].

- Hormone replacement therapy may be beneficial in post-menopausal women. **[C]**[20]

 **Why?**
- Ethinyl oestradiol and norethisterone reduce calcium levels slightly in post-menopausal women with primary hyperparathyroidism (on average by 0.18 mmol/l **[C]**[21].

- Refer for parathyroidectomy in symptomatic cases **[A]**[19].

 **Why?**
- Surgery for primary hyperparathyroidism reduces renal stones, osteitis, constipation and neuropsychiatric symptoms in symptomatic patients. It has little effect on hypertension or renal function **[A]**[20].
- Around 10% of patients develop hypoparathyroidism, 5% have a permanently hoarse voice, and surgery fails to lower calcium levels in 2% **[C]**[22].

**The commonest long-term complications of parathyroidectomy are hypoparathyroidism and vocal cord paralysis**

| Complications **[C]**[22] | % (95% CI) |
|---|---|
| Transient hypocalcaemia at first post-operative week | 51% (41% to 61%) |
| Any complication at 5 years | 18% (8.6% to 27%) |
| Persistent hypoparathyroidism at 5 years | 8.8% (2.1% to 16%) |
| Persistent vocal cord paresis at 5 years | 4.4% (0.0% to 9.3%) |
| Transient vocal cord paralysis at 5 years | 2.9% (0.0% to 7.0%) |
| Persistent hypercalcaemia at 5 years | 1.5% (0.0% to 4.3%) |

## PREVENTION

Repeat the pamidronate infusion (60 mg) every 2 weeks [A][23].

---

**Why?**

- Regular doses every 2 weeks compared with every 3 weeks reduce recurrent symptomatic hypercalcaemia [A][23].
- It increases survival (by roughly 2 weeks) [A][23].

**Pamidronate given every 2 weeks reduces symptomatic hypercalcaemia**

| Patient | Treatment | Comparator | Outcome | CER | RRR | NNT |
|---|---|---|---|---|---|---|
| Malignancy and hypercalcaemia [A][23] | Pamidronate every 2 weeks | Pamidronate every 3 weeks | Symptomatic hypercalcaemia at 16 weeks | 53% | 78% (12% to 94%) | 2 (1 to 8) |

---

Give bisphophonates to patients with:

- breast cancer and bony metastases [A][24] [A][25]

---

**Why?**

- Regular pamidronate reduces skeletal complications, non-vertebral pathological fractures [A][24].
- Fewer patients require surgery or radiation to bone [A][24].
- Fewer patients develop hypercalcaemia [A][24].
- Patients require less analgesia [A][25].

**Breast cancer and bony metastases: pamidronate reduces hypercalcaemia and skeletal complications**

| Patient | Treatment | Comparator | Outcome | CER | RRR | NNT |
|---|---|---|---|---|---|---|
| Breast cancer and bony metastases [A][24] | Pamidronate every 2 weeks | Placebo | Any skeletal complication at 12 months | 56% | 13% (3.2% to 23%) | 8 (4 to 31) |
| | | | Non-vertebral pathological fracture at 12 months | 30% | 10% (1.3% to 19%) | 10 (5 to 75) |
| | | | Radiation to bone at 12 months | 33% | 14% (4.8% to 22%) | 7 (4 to 21) |
| | | | Surgery on bone at 12 months | 61% | 5.9% (0.91% to 11%) | 17 (9 to 110) |
| | | | Hypercalcaemia at 12 months | 51% | 6.2% (0.54% to 12%) | 16 (8 to 190) |

---

- multiple myeloma [A][25].

**Why?**

■ It reduces skeletal complications and pathological fractures without clearly affecting hypercalcaemia **[A]**[26].
■ Fewer patients require radiation to bone **[A]**[26].

**Multiple myeloma: regular pamidronate reduces skeletal complications**

| Patient | Treatment | Comparator | Outcome | CER | RRR | NNT |
|---|---|---|---|---|---|---|
| Multiple myeloma and ≥1 osteolytic lesion **[A]**[26] | Pamidronate 90 mg every 4 weeks | Placebo | Any skeletal complication at 9 months | 41% | 41% (20% to 57%) | 6 (4 to 13) |
| | | | Pathological fracture at 9 months | 30% | 42% (15% to 60%) | 8 (5 to 25) |
| | | | Radiation treatment to bone at 9 months | 22% | 35% (0% to 58%) | 13 (6 to 3000) |

## PROGNOSIS

● Recurrent hypercalcaemia is common **[A]**[23].
● Survival is poor in patients with bony metastases **[A]**[27] **[A]**[23].

**Note**

■ Patients survive on average 10 weeks **[A]**[23].
■ 85% of patients with breast cancer and a first episode of hypercalcaemia are dead within 8 years (95% CI: 80% to 90%) **[A]**[27].

The risk of dying is increased with **[A]**[27]:
● a WHO performance status grade 3 or 4
● visceral metastases
● bony metastases
● a late treatment stage.

**Why?**

**A poor functional status and metastases increase the risk of dying**

| Patient **[A]**[27] | Prognostic factor | Outcome | Control rate | OR (95% CI) | NNF+(95% CI) |
|---|---|---|---|---|---|
| Breast cancer and first episode of hypercalcaemia | WHO performance status grade 3 or 4 | Death at 7.5 years | 85% | 4.12 (2.88 to 5.88) | 9 (8 to 11) |
| | Visceral metastases | Death at 7.5 years | 85% | 4.06 (2.10 to 7.85) | 9 (8 to 14) |
| | Bony metastases | Death at 7.5 years | 85% | 2.42 (1.24 to 4.73) | 12 (9 to 39) |
| | Late treatment stage | Death at 7.5 years | 85% | 1.67 (1.23 to 2.27) | 18 (13 to 41) |

- Patients with asymptomatic hypercalcaemia are at increased risk of dying **[A]**[28].

**Note**
- 41% are dead within 14 years (95% CI: 32% to 49%) **[A]**[28].
- Patients with a raised glucose are at increased risk of dying **[A]**[28].

**Guideline writer**: Christopher Ball
**CAT writers**: Christopher Ball, Clare Wotton

## REFERENCES

| No | Level | Citation |
|----|-------|----------|
| 1 | 1a | Frolich A. Prevalence of hypercalcemia in normal and hospital populations. Dan Med Bull 1998; 45: 436–9 |
| 2 | 4 | Mundy GR et al. Primary hyperparathyroidism: changes in the pattern of clinical presentation. Lancet 1980; 1: 1317–20 |
| 3 | 4 | Fisken RA et al. Hypercalcaemia: a hospital survey. Quart J Med 1980; 196: 405–18 |
| 4 | 4 | Vella A, Gerber TC, Hayes DL et al. Digoxin, hypercalcaemia, and cardiac conduction. Postgrad Med J 1999; 75: 554–6 |
| 5 | 4 | Heath H et al. Primary hyperparathyroidism: incidence, morbidity and potential economic impact in a community. N Engl J Med 1980; (302)4: 189–93 |
| 6 | 4 | Okamoto T, Gerstein HC, Obara T et al. Psychiatric symptoms, bone density and non-specific symptoms in patients with mild hypercalcemia due to primary hyperparathyroidism: a systematic overview of the literature. Endocr J 1997; 44: 367–74 |
| 7 | 4 | Ratcliffe WA et al. Role of assays for parathyroid-hormone-related protein in investigation of hypercalcaemia. Lancet 1992; 339: 164–7 |
| 8 | 4 | Lee J-K, Chuang M-J, Hao L-J et al. Parathyroid hormone and parathyroid hormone related protein assays in the investigation of hypercalcemic patients in hospital in a Chinese population. J Endocrinol Invest 1997; 20: 404–9 |
| 9 | 4 | Suki WN et al. Acute treatment of hypercalcaemia with furosemide. N Engl J Med 1970; 283: 836–40 |
| 10 | 1b | Gucalp R et al. Treatment of calcium-associated hypercalcaemia: a double-blinded comparison of rapid and slow intravenous infusion regimen of pamidronate disodium and saline alone. Arch Intern Med 1994; 154: 1935–44 |
| 11 | 1b | Gucalp R et al. Comparison study of pamidronate disodium and etidronate disodium in the treatment of cancer-related hypercalcaemia. J Clin Oncol 1992; 10: 134–42 |
| 12 | 1b | Purohit OP et al. A randomised double-blind comparison of intravenous pamidronate and clodronate in the hypercalcaemia of malignancy. Br J Cancer 1995; 72: 1289–93 |
| 13 | 1b | Nussbaum SR et al. Single-dose intravenous therapy with pamidronate for the treatment of hypercalcemia of malignancy: comparison of 30-, 60-, and 90-mg dosages. Am J Med 1993; 95: 297–308 |

| No | Level | Citation |
|---|---|---|
| 14 | 1b | Ostenstal B, Andersen OK. Disodium pamidronate versus mithramycin in the management of tumour-associated hypercalcaemia. Acta Oncol 1992; 31: 861–4 |
| 15 | 1b | Warrell RP et al. A randomised double-blinded study of gallium nitrate compared with etidronate for acute control of cancer-related hypercalcaemia. J Clin Oncol 1991; 9: 1467–75 |
| 16 | 1b | Warrell RP et al. Sallium nitrate for acute treatment of cancer-related hypercalcemia: a randomized, double-blind comparison to calcitonin. Ann Intern Med 1988; 108: 669–74 |
| 17 | 4 | Percival RC et al. Role of glucocorticoids in management of malignant hypercalcaemia. BMJ 1984; 289: 287–8 |
| 18 | 1b | Kristensen, Ejlertsen B, Holmegaard S N, et al. Prednisolone in the treatment of severe maligant hypercalcaemia in metastatic breast cancer: a randomized study. J Intern Med 1992; 232: 237–245 |
| 19 | 1b | Ralston SH et al. Comparison of aminohydroxypropylidene phosphonate, mithramycin and corticosteroid/calcitonin in the treatment of calcium associated hypercalcaemia. Lancet 1985; ii: 907–10 |
| 20 | 1b | Sudhaker Rao et al. Lack of biochemical progression or continuation of accelerated bone loss in mild asymptomatic primary hyperparathyroidism: evidence for biphasic disease course. J Clin Endocrinol Metabol 1988; 67: 1294–8 |
| 21 | 4 | Selby P, Peacock M. Ethinyl oestradiol and norethisterone in the treatment of primary hyperparathyroidism in post-menopausal women. N Engl J Med 1986; 314: 1481–5 |
| 22 | 4c | Sudhaker Rao et al: lack of biochemical progression or continuation of accelerated bone loss in mild asymptomatic primary hyperparathyroidism: evidence for biphasic disease course: J Clin Endocrinol Metabol 1988; 67: 1294–8 |
| 23 | 1b | Wimalawansa SJ et al. Optimal frequency of administration of pamidronate in patients with hypercalcaemia of malignancy. Clin Endocrinol 1994; 41: 591–5 |
| 24 | 1b | Hortobagyi GN et al. Efficacy of pamidronate in reducing skeletal complication in patients with breast cancer and lytic bone metastases. N Engl J Med 1996; 335: 1785–91 |
| 25 | 1b | Elomaa I et al. Long-term controlled trial with diphosphonate in patients with osteolytic bone metastases. Lancet 1983; i: 146–8 |
| 26 | 1b | Berenson JR et al. Efficacy of pamidronate in reducing skeletal events in patients with advanced multiple myeloma. N Engl J Med 1996; 334: 488–93 |
| 27 | 1b | Kristensen B, Ejlertsen B, Mouriden HT et al. Survival in breast cancer patients after the first episode of hypercalcaemia. J Intern Med 1998; 244: 189–98 |
| 28 | 1b | Palmer M et al. Survival and renal function in untreated hypercalcaemia: population-based cohort study with 14 years of follow-up. Lancet 1987; 334: 59–62 |

## PREVALENCE

Hyperkalaemia (potassium > 5.5 mmol/l) is uncommon in hospital **[C]**[1], but watch patients on ACE inhibitors **[B]**[2] or with diabetes **[C]**[3].

**Why do this?**
- Around 1% of hospital inpatients have hyperkalaemia (potassium ≥ 5.5 mmol/l) **[C]**[1].
- 0.3% of diabetic outpatients have potassium ≥ 6.0 mmol/l **[C]**[3].
- 10% of patients on ACE inhibitors have raised potassium levels, though few have severe hyperkalaemia (0.2% potassium > 6 mmol/l) in a year **[B]**[2].

## CAUSES

Common causes are **[C]**:
- haemolysis (e.g. poor venepuncture, blood dyscrasias)

**Note**
- Around 20% of samples found on laboratory testing to have high potassium levels are haemolysed **[C]**[1].
- Patients with platelet counts > 500 × 10⁹/l are at increased risk of having a raised potassium (NNH = 29). Potassium levels increase by ~0.3 mmol/l **[C]**[4].

- impaired renal function
- drug treatment (e.g. iv infusion, ACE inhibitors, potassium-sparing diuretics, NSAIDs, trimethoprim)
- redistribution of potassium (e.g. acidosis, mineralocorticoid deficiency).

**Note**

**Impaired renal function, drug treatment and potassium redistribution are the commonest causes of hyperkalaemia**

| Causes of hyperkalaemia **[C]**[1] **[C]**[5] | % (95% CI) |
| --- | --- |
| Impaired renal function | 43% (38% to 47%) |
| Drug treatment | 37% (33% to 42%) |
| Redistribution of potassium | 15% (12% to 19%) |
| Unknown | 4.7% (2.6% to 6.7%) |

## CLINICAL FEATURES

Patients can present with:
- no specific clinical features **[D]**
- non-specific weakness and paraesthesias **[D]**
- sudden cardiac arrest **[D].**

Ask about:
- renal failure, and look at recent electrolytes, urea and creatinine results
- heart failure
- current medication, specifically ACE inhibitors, infusions, diuretics, NSAIDs, trimethoprim
- use of salt substitutes.

---

**Note**

Outpatient's risk of developing hyperkalaemia

| Outcome **[B]**[2] | Risk factor | PEER | Adjusted OR (95% CI) | NNH (95% CI) |
|---|---|---|---|---|
| K > 5.0 mmol/l | Creatinine ≥ 137 μmol/l | 11% | 4.6 (1.8 to 12) | 4 (2 to 14) |
| K > 5.0 mmol/l | Use of long-acting ACE inhibitor (e.g. lisinopril or enalapril) | 11% | 2.8 (1.3 to 6.0) | 7 (3 to 36) |
| K > 5.0 mmol/l | Urea ≥ 6.4 mmol/l | 11% | 2.5 (1.5 to 4.4) | 8 (4 to 22) |
| K > 5.0 mmol/l | Congestive heart failure | 11% | 2.6 (1.4 to 5.1) | 8 (4 to 27) |
| K > 6.0 mmol/l | Aged > 70 years | 0.2% | 5.4 (1.5 to 19) | 140 (35 to 1200) |
| K > 6.0 mmol/l | Urea ≥ 8.9 mmol/l | 0.2% | 4.5 (1.5 to 15) | 170 (44 to 1200) |

---

**Note**

- Patients on loop or thiazide diuretics are at reduced risk of developing hyperkalaemia.

Outpatients' risk of developing hyperkalaemia

| Outcome **[B]**[2] | Risk factor | PEER | Adjusted OR (95% CI) | NNH (95% CI) |
|---|---|---|---|---|
| K > 5.0 mmol/l | Use of loop diuretic | 11% | 0.4 (0.2 to 0.8) | −16 (−51 to −12) |
| K > 5.0 mmol/l | Use of thiazide diuretic | 11% | 0.4 (0.2 to 0.9) | −16 (−100 to −12) |

---

## INVESTIGATIONS

- Repeat the sample if haemolysis is possible **[C].**
- 12-lead ECG **[B].**
- Beware of attributing extreme values to haemolysis alone: obtain ECG while awaiting repeat **[D].**

Look for **[B]**[6]:
- peaked T waves, small P waves

- or worse yet: absent P waves, wide QRS, blurring of ST into T
- or worse yet, sine wave pattern.

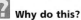

**Note**

ECG diagnosis of hyperkalaemia is poor

| Patient [B][6] | Target disorder (reference standard) | Diagnostic test | LR+ (95% CI) | Post-test probability | LR– (95% CI) | Post-test probability |
|---|---|---|---|---|---|---|
| Suspected hyperkalaemia or renal insufficiency (pre-test probability 37%) | Hyperkalaemia (serum potassium > 5.0 mmol/l) | ECG | 2.8 (1.8 to 4.5) | 65% | 0.68 (0.56 to 0.82) | 31% |

- Consider continuous ECG monitoring [D].

If no obvious cause can be found, do the following investigations [D]:
- blood count
- glucose
- arterial blood gas
- cortisol level
- monitor urine output.

## TREATMENT

### K 6.0–6.5 mmol/L [D]
- No ECG changes: monitor the patient and correct the cause.
- Consider using resins to prevent worsening if no other way to increase potassium output (e.g. oliguric patient).

### K > 6.5 mmol/L [D]
- Give 10 ml of 10% calcium gluconate if urgent correction is required (e.g. haemodynamic instability, significant ECG changes) [D].
- Give 50 ml of 50% glucose iv and short-acting insulin 10 units iv as an iv bolus [C][7].

**Why do this?**
- It lowers potassium by 0.5 mmol/l within 15 min in haemodialysis patients with hyperkalaemia [C][7].
- Onset of action is at 15 min, rather than 30 min for albuterol [C][7].

- Consider adding salbutamol 10 to 20 mg by nebuliser [C][8].

**Note**
- This is 2–4 times the usual dose for severe asthma: watch for adverse effects (tachycardia, hypertension, anxiety).
- About a quarter of patients have very poor responses to nebulised salbutamol **[C]**[8].

**Why do this?**
- It lowers potassium by 0.4–0.9 mmol/l within 1 h in haemodialysis patients with hyperkalaemia **[C]**[8].
- The combination of insulin glucose with salbutamol lowers potassium more than either alone and reduces the hypoglycaemic effect of insulin **[C]**[8].

- Consider combining with hypertonic sodium bicarbonate at 2 mmol/min for one hour. **[B]**[9]

**Why do this?**
- Hypertonic sodium bicarbonate increases the potassium-lowering effect of insulin and glucose by 0.5 mmol/l when given over 1 h in hyperkalaemic patients with end-stage renal disease on maintenance haemodialysis **[B]**[9] **[B]**[10].
- Isotonic bicarbonate infusions have no clear effect when given over 1 h in patients with end-stage renal disease on maintenance haemodialysis **[B]**[11].
- Sodium bicarbonate iv has no clear effect alone **[D]**[12].

- Correct the cause **[D]**.
- Monitor the serum potassium, and repeat therapy if necessary **[D]**.

These agents promote shift within the body and are temporising **[D]**.

If not possible to reverse underlying condition/promote potassium excretion (e.g. acute renal failure, oliguria) or if hyperkalaemia persists, give sodium polystyrene sulphonate or calcium polystyrene sulphonate (calcium resonium) **[A]** 30–60 g by mouth, combined with lactulose **[D]**.
- Avoid using resins combined with sorbitol because of the rare complication of intestinal necrosis **[D]**.
- If unable to give by mouth/by nasogastric tube but lower GI pathology absent, give as retention enema **[D]**.

**Note**
- Procedure is to give cleansing enema, then 30–60 g sodium polystyrene sulphonate in enough tap water to make a slurry, and leave *in situ* for several hours or until evacuated (then tap-water enema to remove residual slurry) **[D]**.
- Rarely, sodium polystyrene sulphonate use may be complicated by volume overload **[D]**.

**Why do this?**
- Calcium resins lower potassium levels in hyperkalaemic patients by ~ 2 mmol/l by 48 h **[A]**[13].

Refer for dialysis if hyperkalaemia persists or renal function is poor [A].

## PROGNOSIS

Hyperkalaemia increases the risk of dying, especially if acute in onset [C].

An increased risk of death [B][2] is associated with:
- potassium $\geq 6.3$ mmol/l
- creatinine $\geq 136$ μol/l
- urea $\geq 10$ mmol/l
- peripheral vascular disease
- pulmonary disease
- use of digoxin.

---

**Note**
**Prognosis with hyperkalaemia**

| Outcome [D][5] | Risk factor | PEER | Unadjusted OR (95 % CI) | NNH (95% CI) |
|---|---|---|---|---|
| Death | Hyperkalaemia | 14% | 2.69 (1.87 to 3.89) | 12 (7 to 22) |

---

**Guideline writers**: Warren Lee, Christopher Ball
**CAT writers**: Warren Lee, Christopher Ball

## REFERENCES

| No | Level | Citation |
|---|---|---|
| 1 | 4 | Moore ML et al. Hyperkalaemia in patients in hospital. N Z Med J 1989; 102: 557–8 |
| 2 | 3b | Reardon LC et al. Hyperkalaemia in outpatients using angiotensin-converting enzyme inhibitors: how much should we worry? Arch Intern Med 1998; 158: 26–32 |
| 3 | 4 | Jarman PR et al. Hyperkalaemia in diabetes: prevalence and associations. Postgrad Med J 1995; 71: 551–2 |
| 4 | 4 | Graber M et al. Thrombocytosis elevates serum potassium. Am J Kidney Dis 1988; 12: 116–20 |
| 5 | 4 | Paice B, Gray JMB et al. Hyperkalaemia in patients in hospital. BMJ 1983; 286: 1189–92 |
| 6 | 2b | Wrenn KD et al. The ability of physicians to predict hyperkalaemia from the ECG. Ann Emerg Med 1991; 20: 1229–32 |
| 7 | 4 | Allon M, Copkney C. Albuterol and insulin for treatment of hyperkalemia in hemodialysis patients. Kidney Int 1990; 38: 869–72 |
| 8 | 4 | Allon M, Dunlay R, Copkney C et al. Nebulized albuterol for acute hyperkalemia in patients on hemodialysis. Ann Intern Med 1989; 110: 426–9 |

| No | Level | Citation |
|---|---|---|
| 9 | 2b | Kim H. Combined effect of bicarbonate and insulin with glucose in acute therapy of hyperkalaemia in end-stage renal disease patients. Nephron 1996; 72: 476–82 |
| 10 | 2b | Gutierrez R, Schlessinger F et al. Effect of hypertonic versus isotonic sodium bicarbonate on plasma potassium concentration in patients with end-stage renal disease. Miner Electrolyte Metab 1991; 17: 297–302 |
| 11 | 3b | Allon M, Shanklin N. Effect of bicarbonate administration on plasma potassium in dialysis patients: interactions with insulin and albuterol. Am J Kidney Dis 1996; 28: 508–14 |
| 12 | 2b – | Kim H. Combined Effect of Bicarbonate and Insulin with Glucose in Acute Therapy of Hyperkalaemia in End-Stage Renal Disease Patients. Nephron 1996; 72: 476–482 |
| 13 | 1c | Berlyne et al. Treatment of hyperkalaemia with a calcium-resin. Lancet 1966; i: 169–72 |

## PREVALENCE

Hypertensive crises are commonly defined as diastolic BP ≥ 120 mmHg.
Hypertensive emergencies involve end-organ damage.
Both are uncommon.

> **Note**
> ■ Roughly 3% of emergency department cases **[B]**[1] or hypertension clinic attenders **[A]**[2] are:
> - emergencies (i.e. evidence of end-organ damage): 0.8% **[B]**[1]
> - urgencies (i.e. no evidence of end-organ damage): 2.4% **[B]**[1].

## CAUSES

Common causes include **[C]**[3] **[C]**[4]:

- essential hypertension
- renovascular disease
- diabetic nephropathy
- neurogenic disease
- phaeochromocytoma.

Other causes include:

- primary hyperaldosteronism
- ingestion of sympathomimetics (e.g. cocaine, amphetamine, LSD, phencyclidine)
- collagen-vascular disease
- pre-eclampsia
- spinal cord syndromes.

> **Why?**
> **The commonest causes of hypertensive urgencies are unknown or due to kidney disease**
>
> | Final diagnosis **[C]**[3] **[C]**[5] | % (95% CI) |
> | --- | --- |
> | Essential | 70.0% (54% to 86%) |
> | Renovascular | 10.0% (0.0% to 21%) |
> | Neurogenic | 6.7% (0.0% to 16%) |
> | Diabetic nephropathy | 10.0% (0.0% to 21%) |
> | Phaeochromocytoma | 3.3% (0.0% to 10%) |
> | Primary hyperaldosteronism | 0.60% (0.46% to 0.75%) |

## CLINICAL FEATURES

Repeat the blood pressure. **[D]**

**Why?**
- Most studies repeat readings over 1 h before initiating therapy.
- But initiate immediate therapy if signs or symptoms of end-organ injury are present (see later).

Ask patients with known hypertension:

- if they have a primary care physician **[B]**[6]
- if they take their antihypertensive medication **[B]**[6].

**Why?**
**Patients who have no primary care physician or who fail to take medication are at increased risk of severe hypertension**

| Outcome **[B]**[6] | Risk factor | PEER | OR (95% CI) | NNH (95% CI) |
|---|---|---|---|---|
| Severe hypertension and grade III or IV hypertensive retinopathy | No primary care physician *not independent* | 2% | 3.5 (1.6 to 7.7) | 15 (6 to 58) |
| | Non-compliance with antihypertensive regimen *not independent* | 2% | 1.9 (1.4 to 2.5) | 39 (24 to 87) |

Ask about:

- headaches, palpitations and sweating attacks **[C]**[7].

**Why?**
**The triad of headaches, palpitations and sweating attacks makes a phaeochromocytoma more likely**

| Patient **[C]**[7] | Target disorder (reference standard) | Diagnostic test | LR+ (95% CI) | Post-test probability | LR– (95% CI) | Post-test probability |
|---|---|---|---|---|---|---|
| Hypertension (pre-test probability 3.3%) | Phaeochromocytoma (surgery or follow-up) | All of headaches, palpitations and sweating attacks | 15 (12 to 19) | 34% | 0.10 (0.15 to 0.63) | 0.34% |

Look for evidence of end-organ damage **[C]**[8]:
- headache
- psychomotor agitation
- epistaxis
- chest pain
- dyspnoea
- arrhythmias.

Particularly concentrate on excluding the following conditions:

- neurological
  - cerebral infarction
  - intracranial haemorrhage or subarachnoid haemorrhage
  - hypertensive encephalopathy
- cardiovascular causes
  - acute pulmonary oedema or acute congestive heart failure
  - acute MI or unstable angina
  - aortic dissection
  - coarctation of the aorta
  - renovascular hypertension (see below)
- eclampsia.

**Why?**
Headache, epistaxis, psychomotor agitation and arrhythmia make end-organ damage much more likely

| Patient [C][8] | Target disorder (reference standard) | Diagnostic test | LR+ (95% CI) | Post-test probability | LR– (95% CI) | Post-test probability |
|---|---|---|---|---|---|---|
| Diastolic blood pressure ≥ 120 mmHg (pre-test probability 24%) | Hyperkalaemia (laboratory and imaging studies) | Headache | 79 (25 to 250) | 96% | 0.31 (0.23 to 0.41) | 9% |
| | | Epistaxis | Infinity (61 to inf) | 100% | 0.46 (0.38 to 0.57) | 13% |
| | | Chest pain | 3.4 (2.1 to 5.3) | 52% | 0.78 (0.69 to 0.88) | 20% |
| | | Dyspnoea | 4.1 (2.5 to 6.6) | 56% | 0.77 (0.68 to 0.87) | 20% |
| | | Psychomotor agitation | Infinity (36 to inf) | 100% | 0.69 (0.60 to 0.78) | 18% |
| | | Arrhythmia | Infinity (21 to inf) | 100% | 0.81 (0.74 to 0.89) | 21% |

**Note**
- No other clinical features are clearly associated with end-organ damage [C][8]

Stroke, heart failure and hypertensive encephalopathy are the commonest examples of end-organ damage

| End-organ damage associated with hypertensive emergencies [C][8] | % (95% CI) |
|---|---|
| Cerebral infarction | 24% (16% to 32%) |
| Acute pulmonary oedema | 22% (14% to 30%) |
| Hypertensive encephalopathy | 17% (9.6% to 24%) |
| Acute congestive heart failure | 14% (7.4% to 20%) |
| Acute MI or unstable angina | 12% (5.9% to 18%) |
| Intracranial haemorrhage or subarachnoid haemorrhage | 4.6% (0.7% to 8.6%) |
| Eclampsia | 4.6% (0.7% to 8.6%) |
| Aortic dissection | 1.9% (0.0% to 4.4%) |

- Fundoscopy (Table 1) [C][9].

| Table 1 Classification of retinal changes | |
|---|---|
| [C][9] | Retinal changes |
| Grade I | Minimal change; No haemorrhages |
| Grade II | Sclerosis of arterioles +/– haemorrhages, no exudates |
| Grade III | Exudates +/– haemorrhages |
| Grade IV | Papilloedema |

- Auscultate for an abdominal bruit [A][10].

**Why?**
Abdominal bruits make renovascular hypertension more likely

| Patient [A][10] | Target disorder (reference standard) | Diagnostic test | LR+ (95% CI) | Post-test probability | LR– (95% CI) | Post-test probability |
|---|---|---|---|---|---|---|
| Diastolic blood pressure ≥120 mmHg (pre-test probability 10%) | Renovascular stenosis (>50% on angiography) | Systolic and diastolic abdominal bruit | 38 (9.5 to 160) | 81% | 0.62 (0.51 to 0.75) | 6.2% |
| | | Any epigastric or flank bruit | 6.4 (3.2 to 12) | 42% | 0.41 (0.25 to 0.68) | 4.4% |
| | | Systolic bruit | 2.1 | 19% | 0.35 | 3.7% |

## INVESTIGATIONS

- Urinalysis and urgent microscopy [B][11].

**Why?**
Absence of blood or protein on urine dipstick makes glomerular disease less likely

| Patient [A][11] | Target disorder (reference standard) | Diagnostic test | LR+ (95% CI) | Post-test probability | LR– (95% CI) | Post-test probability |
|---|---|---|---|---|---|---|
| Undergoing renal biopsy (pre-test probability 3%) | Glomerular disease (renal biopsy) | Blood on dipstick | 2.7 (1.6 to 4.5) | 8% | 0.16 (0.067 to 0.38) | 0.5% |
| | | Protein ≥2+ on dipstick | 1.9 (1.2 to 2.9) | 6% | 0.34 (0.17 to 0.66) | 1% |

Look for, or request examination for:

- dysmorphic red blood cells [B][11]
- pigmented granular casts [B][11].

> **Note**
> ■ 'Pigmented granular' casts are also called 'haem-granular' or 'muddy brown' casts.

> **Why?**
> **Absence of dysmorphic red blood cells or presence of haem-granular casts makes glomerular disease less likely**

| Patient [B][11] | Target disorder (reference standard) | Diagnostic test | LR+ (95% CI) | Post-test probability | LR– (95% CI) | Post-test probability |
|---|---|---|---|---|---|---|
| Undergoing renal biopsy (pre-test probability 3%) | Glomerular disease (renal biopsy) | Dysmorphic red blood cells on microscopy | 4.7 (2.3 to 9.6) | 13% | 0.080 (0.026 to 0.24) | 0.2% |
| | | Haem-granular casts on microscopy | 0.66 (0.48 to 0.92) | 2% | 2.3 (1.1 to 5.1) | 6.6% |
| | | Any features of glomerular disease on microscopy | 4.9 (2.2 to 11) | 13% | 0.23 (0.13 to 0.42) | 0.7% |

– blood count (including MCV and blood smear) **[D]**.
– Urea, electrolytes and glucose **[C][3] [C][4]**.

> **Why?**
> **A low potassium makes primary hyperaldosteronism more likely**

| Patient [C][4] | Target disorder (reference standard) | Diagnostic test | LR + (95% CI) | Post-test probability | LR- (95% CI) | Post-test probability |
|---|---|---|---|---|---|---|
| Suspected primary hyperaldosteronism (pre-test probability 0.6%) | Primary hyperaldosteronism (biochemistry and imaging studies) | Potassium <4.0 mmol/l | 24 (9.2 to 63) | 13% | 0.035 (0.0089 to 0.14) | 0.021% |

> **Note**
> ■ Primary hyperaldosteronism can occur with a normal potassium: 2.7% of cases in one study (95% CI: 0.0% to 6.4%) **[C][12]**

● Electrocardiography **[C][13]**.
● Chest X-ray **[D]**

Consider:

● if cerebral infarction or subarachnoid haemorrhage is suspected [D]
   – CT head
   – lumbar puncture

- if primary hyperaldosteronism is suspected
  - renin and aldosterone levels **[C]**[4]

**Why?**
Aldosterone and renin levels can help diagnose and exclude primary hyperaldosteronism

| Patient **[C]**[4] | Target disorder (reference standard) | Diagnostic test | LR+ (95% CI) | Post-test probability | LR– (95% CI) | Post-test probability |
|---|---|---|---|---|---|---|
| Suspected primary hyperaldosteronism (pre-test probability 0.6%) | Primary hyperaldosteronism (biochemistry and imaging studies) | Supine aldosterone >179 pg/ml | 3.8 (2.7 to 5.4) | 2.2% | 0.11 (0.0047 to 0.26) | 0.066% |
| | | Supine aldosterone: renin ratio >22 | 17 (6.5 to 46) | 9.5% | 0.31 (0.21 to 0.46) | 0.19% |
| | | Erect renin <26 pg/ml | 1.5 (1.2 to 1.8) | 0.90% | 0.38 (0.20 to 0.69) | 0.23% |

- if a phaeochromocytoma is suspected **[C]**[14]
  - plasma catecholamines
  - 24 h urine for catecholamine breakdown products

**Why?**
Raised plasma and urine catecholamines make a phaeochromocytoma more likely

| Patient **[C]**[14] | Target disorder (reference standard) | Diagnostic test | LR+ (95% CI) | Post-test probability | LR– (95% CI) | Post-test probability |
|---|---|---|---|---|---|---|
| Suspected phaeochromocytoma (pre-test probability 6.3%) | Phaeochromocytoma (histology or follow-up) | Plasma catecholamines >950 pg/ml | 13 (8.3 to 20) | 47% | 0.24 (0.12 to 0.50) | 1.6% |
| | | Urinary metanephrines >1.8 mg/24 h | 6.9 (4.7 to 10) | 32% | 0.34 (0.19 to 0.61) | 2.2% |
| | | Urinary vanillylmandelic acid (VMA) >11 mg/24 h | 16 (9.7 to 26) | 51% | 0.24 (0.12 to 0.49) | 1.6% |

- further renal assessment in the presence of suspected renal or renovascular disease **[D]**
  - consider Doppler ultrasound to assess kidney size, symmetry, echogenicity and presence of renal artery stenosis
  - serologic work-up and/or renal biopsy as judged appropriate by renal specialist.

**Note**
- Predictive value of clinical characteristics and diagnostic testing in suspected drug-resistant hypertensives is being assessed by ongoing study [DRASTIC study].

## THERAPY

Give antihypertensive medication **[A]**.

**Why?**
- Symptoms resolve rapidly **[C]**[15].

If there is evidence of end-organ damage, aim to reduce the blood pressure immediately; otherwise aim for a gradual reduction over 24 h **[D]**[16].

Avoid reducing the blood pressure too rapidly **[C]**[17].
Aim for a reduction to < 120 mmHg or a fall > 20 mmHg **[D]**.
Repeat blood pressure readings frequently **[D]**.

**Why?**
- Patients with severe uncontrolled hypertension suffer brain hypoxia if their mean arterial blood pressure falls below 70 mmHg (compared with 40 mmHg in controls) **[C]**[17].
- In patients with severe uncontrolled hypertension, the brain can typically autoregulate cerebral blood supply between 120 and 200 mmHg **[C]**[17].

Try any of:

- nifedipine 5 mg orally chewed then swallowed **[D]**[18] as capsules or sustained-release **[D]**[19]

**Why do this?**
- Patients with severe hypertension who received 10 mg nifedipine rather than 5 mg do not clearly have a larger fall in diastolic blood pressure at 4 h **[D]**[18]
- Sustained-release nifedipine is probably as effective as nifedipine capsules for lowering blood pressure in patients with hypertensive emergencies, and works as quickly **[D]**[19]

- nicardipine 30 mg orally **[A]**[20]

> **? Why do this?**
> - It effectively lowers blood pressure, without clearly causing adverse effects **[A]**[20].
>
> **Nicardipine effectively lowers blood pressure**
>
> | Patient | Treatment | Comparator | Outcome | CER | RRR | NNT |
> |---|---|---|---|---|---|---|
> | Hypertensive crisis | Dicardipine | Placebo | Diastolic BP ≤ 100 mmHg or a fall of ≥ 20 mmHg at 2 h | 22% | 190% (38% to 530%) | 2 (1 to 5) |

- enalapril 0.625 mg orally **[C]**[21] or captopril 25 mg sublingually **[A]**[22]
  - especially in cases of systemic sclerosis **[B]**[23]

> **? Why do this?**
> - Sublingual captopril is probably as effective as sublingual nifedipine in reducing severe hypertension, but with fewer side-effects (headache, facial flushing) **[A]**[22].
> - Around two-thirds of patients with hypertensive crises have a significant fall in their blood pressure when given iv enaprilat. 0.625 mg is probably as effective as higher doses **[C]**[21].
> - In scleroderma crises, ACE-inhibitors are effective at reducing mortality **[B]**[23].
>
> | Patient | Treatment | Comparator | Outcome | CER | RRR | NNT |
> |---|---|---|---|---|---|---|
> | Hypertensive crisis **[A]**[22] | Captopril | Nifedipine | Side-effects at 1 h | 30% | 100% | 3 (2 to 63) |
> | Scleroderma crisis **[B]**[23] | ACE inhibitor | Other agent | Mortality at 1 year | 85% | 80% | 2 (1 to 2) |

- labetalol orally **[D]**[24]
  - especially in phaeochromocytoma crises

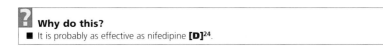

> **? Why do this?**
> - It is probably as effective as nifedipine **[D]**[24].

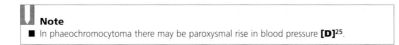

> **! Note**
> - In phaeochromocytoma there may be paroxysmal rise in blood pressure **[D]**[25].

- oral clonidine **[A]**[26].

**Why do this?**
- It causes a slower fall in blood pressure than nifedipine but lasts longer.
- Side-effects (particularly sedation) are more common.

**Clonidine prevents recurrence of hypertension more effectively than nifedipine but causes sedation**

| Patient [A]²² | Treatment | Comparator | Outcome | CER | RRR | NNT |
|---|---|---|---|---|---|---|
| Hypertensive crisis | Clonidine | Nifedipine | Diastolic blood pressure < 120 mmHg at 45 min | 21% | 290% (%85 to 700%) | 2 (1 to 3) |
| | | | Recurrence of diastolic > 120 mmHg at 6 h | 3.6% | 750% (13% to 6300%) | −4 (−15 to −2) |
| | | | Side-effects at 6 h | 61% | 50% (0% to 75%) | 3 (2 to 24) |

- The indications for parenteral therapy (usually with short-acting and titratable agents) are unclear. It is commonly used for patients with severe end-organ damage [D]. Seek assistance if you think this is indicated [D].

## PROGNOSIS

Mortality is high [A]²⁷ [B]²⁸.

**Note**
- 25–40% of patients with hypertensive emergencies are dead within 3 years, mainly from renal failure or stroke [A]²⁷ [B]²⁸.

The risk increases with:

- increasing age [A]²⁷
- essential hypertension [A]²⁷
- increasing creatinine levels [A]²⁷ [A]²⁹
- serum urea ≥ 10 mmol/l [B]²⁶
- increasing duration of known hypertension [B]²⁶
- grade II, IV hypertensive retinopathy [C]⁹.

**Note**
**Worsening hypertensive retinopathy increases the risk of death**

| [C]⁹ Retinopathy | Survival at 20 years |
|---|---|
| Grade I | 46% |
| Grade II | 21% |
| Grade III | 5% |
| Grade IV | 4% |

Few patients require haemodialysis **[B]**[28] unless there is glomerulonephritis **[A]**[29].

**Note**
- 3.2% develop renal failure requiring haemodialysis (95% CI: 1.2% to 5.1%) **[B]**[28].
- Patients with malignant hypertension secondary to chronic glomerulonephritis are more likely to require renal dialysis, and far sooner than patients with essential hypertension (3.5 years sooner) **[A]**[29].
- Most patients are on haemodialysis within 18 months (>90%) **[A]**.

**Guideline writers**: Nick Shenker, Christopher Ball
**CAT writers**: Nick Shenker, Christopher Ball

## REFERENCES

| No | Level | Citation |
|---|---|---|
| 1 | 2c | Zampaglione B et al. Hypertensive urgencies and emergencies: prevalence and clinical presentation. Hypertension 1996; 27: 144–7 |
| 2 | 1b | Webster J et al. Accelerated hypertension: Patterns of mortality and clinical factors affecting outcome in treated patients. Quart J Med 1993; 86: 485–93 |
| 3 | 4 | Bertel et al. Nifedipine in hypertensive emergencies. BMJ 1983; 286: 19–21 |
| 4 | 4 | Davis BA et al. Prevalence of renovascular hypertension in patients with grade III or IV hypertensive retinopathy. N Engl J Med 1979; 301: 1273–6 |
| 5 | 4 | Massien-Simon C, Battaglia C, Chatellier G et al. Adenome de Conn: valeur diagnostique et pronostique de la mesure du potassium, de la renine, de l'aldosterone et du rapport aldosterone/renine. Presse Med 1995; 24: 1238–42 |
| 6 | 3b | Shea S et al. Predisposing factors for severe uncontrolled hypertension in an inner-city minority population. N Engl J Med 1992; 327: 776–81 |
| 7 | 4 | Plouin P-F, Degoulet P, Tugaye A et al. Le depistage du pheochromocytome: chez quels hypertendus? Etude semiologique chez 2585 hypertendus dont 11 ayant un pheochromocytome. Nouv Presse Med 1981; 10: 869–72 |
| 8 | 4 | Zampaglione B et al. Hypertensive urgencies and emergencies: prevalence and clinical presentation: Hypertension 1996; 27: 144–147 |
| 9 | 4 | Breslin DJ et al. Prognostic importance of ophthalmoscopic findings in essential hypertension. JAMA 1966; 195: 335–8 |
| 10 | 1c | Turnbull JM. Is listening for abdominal bruits useful in the evaluation of hypertension? JAMA 1995; 274: 1299–301 |
| 11 | 2b | Marcussen N et al. Analysis of cytodiagnostic urinalysis findings in 77 patients with concurrent renal biopsies. Am J Kidney Dis 1992; 20: 618–28 |
| 12 | 4 | Brown MA, Zammit VC, Cramp HA et al. Primary hyperaldosteronism: a missed diagnosis in 'essential hypertensives'? Aust N Z J Med 1996; 26: 533–8 |
| 13 | 4 | Zampaglione B et al. Hypertensive urgencies and emergencies: prevalence and clinical presentation: Hypertension 1996; 27: 144–147 |

| No | Level | Citation |
|----|-------|----------|
| 14 | 4 | Young MY, Dmuchowski C, Wallis JW et al. Biochemical tests for pheochromocytoma: strategies in hypertensive patients. J Gen Intern Med 1989; 4: 273–6 |
| 15 | 4 | Krogsgaard AR, McNair A, Hilden T et al. Reversibility of cerebral symptoms in severe hypertension in relation to acute antihypertensive therapy: a Danish multicenter study. Acta Med Scand 1986; 220: 25–31 |
| 16 | 5 | The sixth report of the Joint National Committee on prevention, detection, evaluation and treatment of high blood pressure. Arch Intern Med 1997; 157: 2413 (consensus statement) |
| 17 | 4 | Strandgaard S et al. Autoregulation of brain circulation in severe arterial hypertension. BMJ 1973; i: 507–10 |
| 18 | 1b– | Maharaj B et al. A comparison of the acute hypotensive effects of two different doses of nifedipine. Am Heart J 1992; 124: 720–5 |
| 19 | 1b– | Damasceno A et al. Nifedipine-retard versus nifedipine-capsules for the therapy of hypertensive crisis in black patients. J Cardiovasc Pharmacol 1998; 31: 165–9 |
| 20 | 1b | Habib GB et al. Evaluation of the efficacy and safety of oral nicardipine in treatment of urgent hypertension: a multicenter, randomised double-blind parallel placebo-controlled clinical trial. Am Heart J 1995; 129: 917–23 |
| 21 | 1b– | Hirschl MM et al. Clinical evaluation of different doses of intravenous enalaprilat in patients with hypertensive crises. Arch Intern Med 1995; 155: 2217–23 |
| 22 | 1b | Angeli P et al. Comparison of sublingual captopril and nifedipine in immediate treatment of hypertensive emergencies: a randomised, single-blind clinical trial. Arch Intern Med 1991; 151: 678–82 |
| 23 | 2b | Steen VD et al. Outcome of renal crisis in systemic sclerosis: relation to availability of angiotensin converting enzyme (ACE) inhibitors. Ann Intern Med 1990; 113: 352–7 |
| 24 | 1b– | McDonald AJ, Yealy DM, Jacobson S. Oral labetolol versus oral nifedipine in hypertensive urgencies in the ED. Am J Emerg Med 1993; 11: 460–3 |
| 25 | 4 | Briggs RS et al. Hypertensive response to labetalol in pheochromocytoma. Lancet 1978; i: 1045–6 |
| 26 | 1b | Jaker M et al. Oral nifedipine versus oral clonidine in the treatment of urgent hypertension. Arch Intern Med 1989; 149: 260–5 |
| 27 | 1b | Webster J et al. Accelerated hypertension: patterns of mortality and clinical factors affecting outcome in treated patients. Quart J Med 1993; 86: 485–93 |
| 28 | 2b | Lip GY et al. Complications and survival of 315 patients with malignant-phase hypertension. J Hypertens 1995; 13: 915–24 |
| 29 | 1b | Kawazoe N et al. Long term prognosis of malignant hypertension: difference between underlying diseases such as essential hypertension and chronic glomerulonephritis. Clin Nephrol 1988; 29: 53–7 |

## PREVALENCE

Think about hypoglycaemia in patients with:
- a reduced level of consciousness **[C]**[1]
- hemiparesis **[C]**[2]
- seizures **[C]**[2].

**Why?**
- 7% of patients with altered consciousness have hypoglycaemia (95% CI: 3.2% to 11%) **[A]**[3].
- Seizures and hemiparesis are uncommon presentations of hypoglycaemia (7% and 2% of cases) **[C]**[2].

Hypoglycaemia is common in patients with diabetes mellitus.

**Why?**
- 37% of patients with type 1 diabetes have symptoms of hypoglycaemia once a week (33% to 40%) **[B]**[4].
- 32% of patients with type 1 diabetes on intensive therapy have severe hypoglycaemia over 6 years (28% to 35%) **[B]**[5].

## CAUSES

Most patients with hypoglycaemia have diabetes **[C]**[6].

**Note**
**Diabetes and alcohol consumption are the commonest causes of hypoglycaemia**

| Patient **[C]**[6] | % (95% CI) |
|---|---|
| Type 1 diabetes mellitus (insulin-dependent diabetes mellitus) | 59% (45% to 72%) |
| Type 2 diabetes mellitus (non-insulin-dependent diabetes mellitus) | 16% (6% to 26%) |
| Insulin-treated diabetes secondary to chronic pancreatitis | 6% (0% to 12%) |
| Alcohol-induced hypoglycaemia without underlying diabetes | 18% (7% to 28%) |
| Parasuicide without diabetes | 2% (0% to 6%) |

Common causes in diabetics include **[B]**[7] **[C]**[2] **[C]**[6] **[C]**[8]:
- a missed meal
- alcohol consumption
- insulin overdose (accidental or intentional)
- exercise.

Common causes in non-diabetics include **[B]**[7] **[C]**[2] **[C]**[6] **[C]**[8]:
- alcohol consumption
- drug overdose.

**Note**
Missed meals, alcohol and insulin overdose cause hypoglycaemia

| Cause of hypoglycaemia **[B]**[7] **[C]**[2] **[C]**[6] **[C]**[8] | Prevalence (95% CI) |
|---|---|
| Missed meal | 25%–52% |
| Alcohol | 22%–48% |
| Unidentified causes | 19%–24% |
| Insulin overdosage (deliberate or accidental) | 15%–20% |
| Exercise | 6%–14% |
| Multiple causes | 25% |
| Drugs (propranolol, glibenclamide and metoprolol) | 4% |
| Renal failure | 1% |

## CLINICAL FEATURES

Ask about:

- current insulin regimen **[A]**[9]

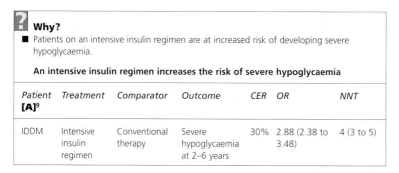
**Why?**
■ Patients on an intensive insulin regimen are at increased risk of developing severe hypoglycaemia.

**An intensive insulin regimen increases the risk of severe hypoglycaemia**

| Patient **[A]**[9] | Treatment | Comparator | Outcome | CER | OR | NNT |
|---|---|---|---|---|---|---|
| IDDM | Intensive insulin regimen | Conventional therapy | Severe hypoglycaemia at 2–6 years | 30% | 2.88 (2.38 to 3.48) | 4 (3 to 5) |

**Note**
■ Human insulin use does not increase the risk of developing hypoglycaemia **[B]**[4].

- duration of diabetes **[B]**[10]

**Why?**
**Longstanding diabetes increases the risk of severe hypoglycaemia**

| Outcome **[B]**[10] | Risk factor | PEER | OR (95% CI) | NNH (95% CI) |
|---|---|---|---|---|
| Severe hypoglycaemia | Duration of diabetes *independent* | 30% | 3.6 (1.2 to 11) | 3 (2 to 25) |

- glycaemic control **[A]**[11] **[B]**[10] and HbA$_{1c}$ levels **[B]**[12]
- any previous episodes of hypoglycaemia **[B]**[12]

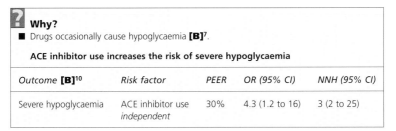

**Why?**

■ Frequently low blood glucose levels **[A]**[11] or HbA$_{1c}$ **[B]**[12] help predict patients at increased risk for hypoglycaemia.

**Diabetes: history of hypoglycaemia or a low HbA$_{1c}$ increase the risk of hypoglycaemia**

| Patient **[B]**[12] | Prognostic factor | Outcome | Control rate | OR (95% CI) | NNF (95% CI) |
|---|---|---|---|---|---|
| Type 1 diabetes | History of hypoglycaemia at 6.5 years *independent* | Hypoglycaemia requiring assistance at 6.5 years | 41% (38% to 45%) | 1.33 (1.17 to 1.52) | 14 (10 to 26) |
| | Fall in HbA$_{1c}$ by 10% (at baseline of 9%) *independent* | Hypoglycaemia requiring assistance at 6.5 years | 41% | 1.53 (1.43 to 1.64) | 9 (8 to 11) |

**Diabetes: poor glycaemic control may increase the risk of severe hypoglycaemia**

| Outcome **[B]**[10] | Risk factor | PEER | OR (95% CI) | NNH (95% CI) |
|---|---|---|---|---|
| Severe hypoglycaemia | Poor glycaemic control *independent* | 30% | 3.0 (1.0 to 9.0) | 4 (2 to infinity) |

- current medication, particularly ACE inhibitor **[B]**[10], oral hypoglycaemic **[B]**[7] and beta-blocker use

**Why?**

■ Drugs occasionally cause hypoglycaemia **[B]**[7].

**ACE inhibitor use increases the risk of severe hypoglycaemia**

| Outcome **[B]**[10] | Risk factor | PEER | OR (95% CI) | NNH (95% CI) |
|---|---|---|---|---|
| Severe hypoglycaemia | ACE inhibitor use *independent* | 30% | 4.3 (1.2 to 16) | 3 (2 to 25) |

- any cardiac problems **[B]**[10].

**Why?**

**Diabetes: cardiac disease increases the risk of hypoglycaemia**

| Outcome **[B]**[10] | Risk factor | PEER | OR (95% CI) | NNH (95% CI) |
|---|---|---|---|---|
| Severe hypoglycaemia | Cardiovascular comorbidity *independent* | 30% | 3.2 (1.2 to 5.3) | 4 (3 to 25) |

Look for:
- symptoms of hypoglycaemia (sweating, tachycardia, altered consciousness, aggression, confusion) **[C]**[1] **[C]**[13] but do not assume patients who are asymptomatic are normoglycaemic **[C]**[1] **[C]**[13]**[C]**[14].

---

**?** **Why?**

■ Patients with insulin-dependent diabetes are not good at judging whether they are hypoglycaemic: sensitivity 55% (95% CI: 45% to 65%) **[C]**[14].

**Altered mental state: absence of hypoglycaemic symptoms does not exclude hypoglycaemia**

| Patient [C][1] | Target disorder (reference standard) | Diagnostic test | LR + (95% CI) | Post-test probability | LR – (95% CI) | Post-test probability |
|---|---|---|---|---|---|---|
| Altered mental state (pre-test probability 9%) | Hypoglycaemia (blood glucose or clinical diagnosis) | Any of tachycardia, sweating or available history of diabetes mellitus | 1.7 (1.3 to 2.1) | 14% | 0.45 (0.23 to 0.86) | 4% |

**Diabetes: absence of hypoglycaemic symptoms does not exclude hypoglycaemia**

| Patient [C][13] | Target disorder (reference standard) | Diagnostic test | LR + (95% CI) | Post-test probability | LR – (95% CI) | Post-test probability |
|---|---|---|---|---|---|---|
| IDDM (pre-test probability 6%) | Hypoglycaemia (blood glucose < 3 mmol/l) | Symptoms of hypoglycaemia | 8.3 (6.5 to 10.5) | 35% | 0.56 (0.48 to 0.66) | 3% |

---

## INVESTIGATIONS

- Measure glucose rapidly using reagent strips **[A]**[15] **[B]**[16] or a capillary blood glucose in triage **[A]**[17].

---

**?** **Why?**

**Normoglycaemia on a reagent strip makes hypoglycaemia unlikely**

| Patient [A][3] | Target disorder (reference standard) | Diagnostic test | LR + (95% CI) | Post-test probability | LR – (95% CI) | Post-test probability |
|---|---|---|---|---|---|---|
| Altered mental state (pre-test probability 7%) | Hypoglycaemia (blood glucose) | Reagent strip | 12.1 (6.8 to 21) | 48% | 0.090 (0.014 to 0.6) | 0.68% |

**Why?**
- Immediate blood glucose measurement reduces time to definitive care (mean 2 h to nursing care, 1 h to medical care) **[A]**[17].

- Send a specimen for formal laboratory blood glucose measurement **[A]**.

*Remember*
Patients with diabetes may experience symptoms of hypoglycaemia at 'normoglycaemic' levels.

**Why?**
- Patients with poorly controlled diabetes experience symptoms of hypoglycaemia at higher blood glucose levels than patients without diabetes (on average 1.4 mmol/l higher) **[D]**[18].

- If you believe hypoglycaemia is present, try a test dose of 50% glucose iv (20–50 ml).

**Why?**
**A full recovery following 50% glucose diagnosing hypoglycaemia**

| Patient **[C]**[1] | Target disorder (reference standard) | Diagnostic test | LR+ (95% CI) | Post-test probability |
|---|---|---|---|---|
| Altered mental consciousness (pre-test probability 9%) | Hypoglycaemia (blood glucose or clinical diagnosis) | Complete response to 50% glucose | 43 (18 to 110) | 80% |
| | | Partial response to 50% glucose | 1.2 (0.47 to 3.2) | 10% |
| | | No response to 50% glucose | 0.20 (0.089 to 0.44) | 1.8% |

## THERAPY

- Encourage ambulance crews to give a high-sugar drink and glucagon **[C]**[19].

**Why?**
- Few patients given a sugar drink and glucagon require iv glucose or admission **[C]**[19].

**Few patients given sugar drinks and glucagon require iv glucose or admission**

| Outcome if received sugar drink and glucagon | % (95% CI) |
|---|---|
| Recovery without hospitalisation | 23% (15% to 32%) |
| Attended emergency department but required no more than oral treatment | 60% (51% to 70%) |
| Attended emergency department and required glucose but no admission | 10% (4% to 15%) |
| Admission to hospital | 7% (2% to 12%) |

- If semiconscious **[D]** give glucose iv **[A]**[20] **[A]**[21], e.g. 50% **[C]**[1].

>  **Why?**
> - Recovery from coma is faster than on glucagon (on average 2 min) **[A]**[20] **[A]**[21].

or glucagon **[A]**[19] **[A]**[20] iv or im **[D]**[22].
- If conscious **[D]** give a sugar drink **[C]**[19].
- Follow any urgent measure with long-acting carbohydrate **[D]**.

## PREVENTION

- Refer your patient to the diabetes team and educate about diabetes **[A]**[23].

>  **Why do this?**
> - It improves glycaemic control and reduces readmissions **[A]**[23].
> - There is no clear effect on length of hospital stay **[A]**[23].
>
> **A diabetic team improves glycaemic control and reduces hospital readmissions**
>
> | Patient [A][23] | Treatment | Comparator | Outcome | CER | RRR | NNT |
> |---|---|---|---|---|---|---|
> | Inpatient with diabetes | Diabetic team intervention | No intervention | Good glycaemic control at 1 month | 46% | 65% (28% to 112%) | 3 (2 to 6) |
> | | | | Readmission at 3 months | 32% | 52% (14% to 73%) | 6 (3 to 22) |

- Consider giving patients with type 1 diabetes on an intensive regimen insulin lispro **[A]**[23].

>  **Why?**
> - It reduces episodes of severe hypoglycaemia and hypoglycaemic coma **[A]**[24].
>
> **Insulin lispro causes fewer episodes of severe hypoglycaemia than soluble insulin**
>
> | Patient [A][24] | Treatment | Comparator | Outcome | CER | RRR | NNT |
> |---|---|---|---|---|---|---|
> | Type 1 diabetes mellitus | Insulin lispro | Short-acting insulin (soluble) | Severe hypoglycaemia at 12 weeks | 29% | 38% (10% to 57%) | 9 (5 to 36) |
> | | | | Hypoglycaemic coma at 12 weeks | 8% | 81% (37% to 94%) | 15 (5 to 52) |

## PROGNOSIS

Headache is common on recovery **[B]**[25].
Few patients require admission **[C]**[6].

> **Note**
> ■ 51% of patients with severe hypoglycaemia have a headache on recovery (95% CI:
> 37% to 65%) **[B]**[25].
> ■ 0.4% of patients require admission to hospital (95% CI: 0.3% to 0.5%) **[C]**[6].

Recurrence is common **[B]**[4]. The risk is increased with:
● an intensive insulin regimen **[A]**[5]
● a history of hypoglycaemia **[B]**[12]
● a low HbA$_{1c}$ **[B]**[12].

> **Why?**
> **An intensive insulin regimen increases the risk of severe hypoglycaemia**
>
> | Patient **[A]**[5] | Treatment | Comparator | Outcome | CER | OR | NNT |
> |---|---|---|---|---|---|---|
> | Type 1 diabetes mellitus | Intensive insulin regimen | Conventional therapy | Severe hypoglycaemia at 2 to 6 years | 30% | 2.88 (2.38 to 3.48) | 4 (3 to 5) |
>
> **A history of hypoglycaemia or a low HbA$_{1c}$ increases the risk of hypoglycaemia**
>
> | Patient **[B]**[12] | Prognostic factor | Outcome | Control rate | OR (95% CI) | NNF (95% CI) |
> |---|---|---|---|---|---|
> | Type 1 diabetes | History of hypoglycaemia at 6.5 years *independent* | Hypoglycaemia requiring assistance at 6.5 years | 41% (38% to 45%) | 1.33 (1.17 to 1.52) | 14 (10 to 26) |
> | | Fall in HbA$_{1c}$ by 10% (at baseline of 9%) *independent* | Hypoglycaemia requiring assistance at 6.5 years | 41% | 1.53 (1.43 to 1.64) | 9 (8 to 11) |

A single episode of hypoglycaemic coma does not clearly cause brain
damage **[B]**[26], but recurrent attacks do **[C]**[27].

> **Why?**
> ■ No patients with hypoglycaemic coma in the last 4 weeks develop neuropsychological
> problems (95% CI: 0% to 5%) **[B]**[26].
> ■ More than five attacks of hypoglycaemia lead to a fall in IQ **[C]**[27].

Hypoglycaemia in inpatients often heralds a poor prognosis **[C]**[28].

> **Why?**
> ■ 27% of patients found to have a low blood glucose are dead within 6 months (95%
> CI: 18% to 36%) **[C]**[28].
> ■ All deaths were felt to be related to severe underlying disease (e.g. sepsis, hepatic failure).

**Guideline writer**: Christopher Ball
**CAT writers**: Matthew Taylor, Christopher Ball, Richard Hardern

## REFERENCES

| No | Level | Citation |
|----|-------|----------|
| 1 | 4 | Hoffman JR, Schriger DL, Votey SR et al. The empiric use of hypertonic dextrose in patients with altered mental status: a reappraisal. Ann Emerg Med 1992; 21: 20–4 |
| 2 | 4 | Malouf R, Brust JCM. Hypoglycaemia: causes, neurological manifestations, and outcome. Ann Neurol 1985; 17: 421–30 |
| 3 | 1b | Jones JL, Ray VG. Determination of prehospital blood glucose: a prospective, controlled study. J Emerg Med 1992; 10: 679–82 |
| 4 | 2b | Klein BEK, Klein R, Moss SE. Risk of hypoglycaemia in users of human insulin. Diabetes Care 1997; 20: 336–9 |
| 5 | 2a | Egger M, Davey Smith G, Stettler C et al. Risk of adverse effects of intensified treatment in insulin dependent diabetes mellitus: a meta-analysis. Diabetic Medicine 1997; 14: 919–28 |
| 6 | 4 | Hart SP, Frier BM. Causes, management and morbidity of acute hypoglycaemia in adults requiring hospital admission. Q J Med 1998; 51: 505–10 |
| 7 | 2c | Feher MD, Grout P, Kennedy A et al. Hypoglycaemia in an inner-city accident and emergency department: a 12-month survey. Arch Emerg Med 1989; 6: 183–8 |
| 8 | 4 | Collier A, Steedman DJ. Comparison of intravenous glucagon and dextrose in treatment of severe hypoglycaemia in an accident and emergency department. Diabetes Care 1989; 10: 712–15 |
| 9 | 1a | Egger M, Davey Smith G, Stettler C, Diem P. Risk of adverse effects of intensified treatment in insulin dependent diabetes mellitus: a meta-analysis. Diabetic Medicine 1997; 14: 919–28 |
| 10 | 3b | Morris AD, Boyle DIR, McMahon AD et al. ACE inhibitor use is associated with hospitalization for severe hypoglycaemia in patients with diabetes. Diabetes Care 1997; 20: 1363–7 |
| 11 | 1a | Kovatchev BP, Cox DJ. Assessment of risk for severe hypoglycaemia among adults with IDDM. Diabetes Care 1998; 21: 1870–5 |
| 12 | 2b | DCCT Research Group et al. Hypoglycaemia in the Diabetes Control and Complications Trial. Diabetes 1997; 46: 271–86 |
| 13 | 4 | Pramming S, Thorsteinsson B, Bendtson I. The relationship between symptomatic and biochemical hypoglycaemia in insulin-dependant diabetic patients. J Intern Med 1990; 228: 641–6 |
| 14 | 4 | Fritsche A, Stumvoll M. Diabetes teaching program improves glycaemic control and preserves perception of hypoglycaemia. Diabetes Res Clin Pract 1998; 40: 129–35 |
| 15 | 1b | Lavery RF, Allegra JR. A prospective evaluation of glucose reagent test strips in the prehospital setting. Am J Emerg Med 1991; 9: 304–8 |
| 16 | 2b | Scott PA, Wolf LR, Spadafora MP. Accuracy of reagent strips in detecting hypoglycaemia in the emergency department. Ann Emerg Med 1998; 32: 305–9 |
| 17 | 1b | Degroote NE, Pieper B. Blood glucose monitoring at triage. J Emerg Nurs 1993; 19: 131–3 |

| No | Level | Citation |
|----|-------|----------|
| 18 | 5 | Boyle PJ, Schwartz NS, Shah SD et al. Plasma glucoseconcentrations at the onset of hypoglycaemic symptoms inpatients with poorly controlled diabetes and nondiabetics. N Engl J Med 1988; 318: 1487–92 |
| 19 | 4 | Steele JM, Allwinkle J. Use of Lucozade and glucagon byambulance staff for treating hypoglycaemia. BMJ 1992;394: 1283–4 |
| 20 | 1b | Collier A, Steedman DJ. Comparison of intravenous glucagonand dextrose in treatment of severe hypoglycaemia in anaccident and emergency department. Diabetes Care 1989;10: 712–15 |
| 21 | 1b | Patrick AW, Collier A. Comparison of intramuscular glucagonand intravenous glucose in the treatment of hypoglycaemiccoma in an A+E department. Arch Emerg Med 1990; 7: 72–7 |
| 22 | 1b – | MacCuish A, Munro JF, Duncan LJP. Treatment of hypoglycaemic coma with glucagon, intavenous dextrose andmannitol in 100 diabetics. Lancet 1970; ii: 946–9 |
| 23 | 1b | Koproski J et al. Effects of an intervention by a diabetesteam in hospitalized patients with diabetes. Diabetes Care1997; 20: 1553–5 |
| 24 | 1b | Holleman F, Schmitt H. Reduced frequency of severehypoglycaemia and coma in well-controlled IDDM patientstreated with insulin lispro. Diabetes Care 1997; 20: 1827–32 |
| 25 | 2b | Collier A, and Steedman DJ. Comparison of intravenousglucagon and dextrose in treatment of severe hypoglycaemiain an accident and emergency department. Diabetes Care 1989; 10(6): 712–15 |
| 26 | 3b | Kramer L, and Fasching P. Previous episodes ofhypoglycaemic coma are not associated with permanentcognitive brain dysfunction in IDDM patients on intensiveinsulin treatment. Diabetes 1998; 47: 1909–14 |
| 27 | 4 | Langan SJ, and Deary IJ. Cumulative cognitive impairmentfollowing recurrent severe hypoglycaemia in adult patientswith insulin-treated diabetes mellitus. Diabetologia 1991;34: 337–44 |
| 28 | 4 | Fischer KF, Lees JA, Newman JH. Hypoglycaemia inhospitalized patients: causes and outcomes. N Engl J Med1986; 315: 1245–50 |

## PREVALENCE

- Hyponatraemia: Na < 130 mmol/l [D][1].
- Hyponatraemia is a rare cause of admission to hospital [C][1].
- However, it often develops in elderly patients in hospital, but is usually mild [C][1].

> **Note**
> - 0.9% of elderly patients are admitted to hospital with hyponatraemia (95% CI: 0.3 to 1.6%), but 20% develop it during their stay (95% CI: 18% to 23%) [C][1].
> - Only 3% of these have a sodium level below 121 mmol/l (95% CI: 0.4% to 5%); three-quarters only fall to 130–134 mmol/l [C][1].

## CAUSES (Box 1)

| Box 1   Causes of hyponatraemia | | |
|---|---|---|
| **Dehydration [C][2] [C][3]** | **No dehydration or oedema** | **Oedema** |
| Renal losses | Artefact | Congestive heart failure |
| ➤ diuretics | ➤ sample taken iv from arm | Nephrotic syndrome |
| ➤ adrenal insufficiency | | Cirrhosis |
| ➤ osmotic diuresis (glucose, | Pseudohyponatraemia | Renal failure |
| urea, mannitol) | ➤ hyperglycaemia, | |
| ➤ renal tubular acidosis | hypertriglyceridaemia, | |
| | hyperproteinaemia | |
| Fluid loss | | |
| ➤ vomiting, diarrhoea | Acute onset | |
| ➤ sweating | ➤ excess intravenous intake | |
| | post-operatively | |
| | ➤ psychogenic polydipsia | |
| | Chronic onset | |
| | ➤ syndrome of inappropriate | |
| | ADH secretion (SIADH) | |
| | ➤ hypothyroidism | |
| | ➤ glucocorticoid deficiency | |
| | ➤ pain, emotion or drugs | |

### Syndrome of inappropriate ADH secretion

SIADH is diagnosed when all of the following are present [D]:
- a low serum sodium
- a concentrated urine and dilute plasma (urine osmolality > 100 mOsmol/kg plasma osmolality < 270 mOsmol/kg)
- a normal circulating volume (no postural hypotension, normal CVP, no pre-renal failure)
- a normal renal, adrenal and thyroid function.

Causes include **[D]**:
- cancers: small cell of lung, duodenum, pancreas, thymus, brain, lymphoma
- infections: pneumonia, CNS, tuberculosis, Guillain–Barré syndrome
- brain injury: stroke, tumour, haemorrhage, hydrocephalus
- drugs: commonly diuretics, carbamazepine, psychotropics, nicotine.

> **Note**
> Common causes of severe hyponatraemia are diuretics and SIADH

| Causes of severe hyponatraemia Na < 110 mol/l **[C]**[3] | % (95% CI) |
|---|---|
| Chronic causes | 84% (76% to 93%) |
| ■ diuretic agents only | 36% (24% to 48%) |
| ■ SIADH | 28% (17% to 39%) |
| ■ oedematous disorders | 14% (5.5% to 23%) |
| ■ Addison's disease | 4.7% (0.0% to 9.9%) |
| ■ chronic renal failure | 1.6% (0.0% to 4.6%) |
| Acute causes | 16% (6.7% to 25%) |
| ■ parenteral fluids and SIADH | 7.8% (1.2% to 14%) |
| ■ psychotic polydipsia | 6.3% (0.3% to 12%) |
| ■ Addison's disease | 1.6% (0.0% to 4.6%) |

## CLINICAL FEATURES

Ask about:
- recent illness
  - diarrhoea and vomiting **[C]**[1]
  - sweating **[C]**[1]
- fluid intake **[D]**
- current medical problems
  - heart failure **[C]**[2] **[C]**[3]
  - renal disease **[C]**[2] **[C]**[3]
  - liver failure and ascites **[C]**[1]
  - diabetes mellitus **[C]**[1]
  - any psychiatric problems **[C]**[3]
- current medication (particularly diuretics, NSAIDs, antibiotics) **[C]**[1].

**? Why?**

Hepatic failure, gastrointestinal losses increase the risk of hyponatraemia

| Outcome [C][1] | Risk factor | PEER | OR (95% CI) | NNH (95% CI) |
|---|---|---|---|---|
| Hyponatraemia (Na < 135 mmol/l) | Hepatic failure *not independent* | 4.6% | 2.91 (1.63 to 5.21) | 6 (3 to 17) |
| | GI losses *not independent* | 11.1% | 1.99 (1.27 to 3.11) | 11 (6 to 39) |
| | Diabetes mellitus *not independent* | 17.6% | 1.62 (1.09 to 2.41) | 12 (6 to 78) |
| | Ascites *not independent* | 2.1% | 2.63 (1.12 to 6.17) | 31 (10 to 410) |
| | Sweating *not independent* | 1.6% | 5.39 (2.40 to 12.10) | 15 (7 to 46) |
| | NSAIDs *not independent* | 7.7% | 1.86 (1.10 to 3.14) | 17 (8 to 140) |
| | Potassium-sparing diuretics *not independent* | 7.1% | 1.93 (1.13 to 3.30) | 17 (8 to 120) |
| | Trimethoprim/ sulfamethoxazole *not independent* | 1.9% | 3.51 (1.54 to 7.97) | 22 (9 to 100) |

Patients may have nausea, cramps, confusions or seizures [D]; However, unless the serum sodium is falling rapidly, levels in the range 125–135 mmol/l are usually asymptomatic [D].

Look for:
- evidence of oedema or dehydration [C][2] [C][3].

When assessing dehydration, look for [B][4]:
- sunken eyes
- dry axillae
- dry nasal or oral mucous membranes
- longitudinal furrows on the tongue.

**? Why?**

Sunken eyes, dry axillae, dry mucous membranes and tongue furrows make dehydration more likely

| Patient [B][4] | Target disorder (reference standard) | Diagnostic test | LR+ (95% CI) | Post-test probability | LR– (95% CI) | Post-test probability |
|---|---|---|---|---|---|---|
| Suspected hypovolaemia not due to blood loss (pre-test probability 15%) | Hypovolaemia not due to blood loss (biochemistry) | Sunken eyes | 3.4 (1.0 to 12.2) | 38% | 0.5 (0.3 to 0.7) | 8% |
| | | Dry axilla | 2.8 (1.4 to 5.4) | 33% | 0.6 (0.4 to 1.0) | 10% |
| | | Dry oral and nasal mucous membranes | 2.0 (1.0 to 4.0) | 26% | 0.3 (0.1 to 0.6) | 5% |
| | | Longitudinal furrows on tongue | 2.0 (1.0 to 4.0) | 26% | 0.3 (0.1 to 0.6) | 5% |

**Note**

The following are not very helpful at diagnosing dehydration **[B]**[4]:
■ postural changes in pulse or blood pressure
■ neurological signs or symptoms (including confusion and slurred speech).

## INVESTIGATIONS

● Urea and electrolytes, creatinine **[A]**.
● Glucose **[D]**.
● Serum osmolality **[A]**.

If indicated **[D]**:
● cortisol
● thyroid function tests.

Send a urine sample for biochemistry:
● urine sodium **[C]**[5] **[C]**[7]
● urine chloride **[C]**[6]
● urine creatinine
● urine osmolality **[C]**[5] **[C]**[7].

**?** **Why?**

**A low urine sodium makes pre-renal failure more likely**

| Patient **[C]**[5] | Target disorder (reference standard) | Diagnostic test | LR (95% CI) | Post-test probability |
|---|---|---|---|---|
| Acute renal failure (pre-test probability 24%) | Pre-renal failure (response to pre-renal therapy) | Urine sodium: < 10 mmol/l 10–20 mmol/l > 20 mmol/l | 3.5 (1.6 to 7.4) 1.4 (0.56 to 3.6) 0.41 (0.20 to 0.82) | 53% 21% 12% |

**A low urine chloride makes pre-renal failure more likely**

| Patient **[C]**[6] | Target disorder (reference standard) | Diagnostic test | LR (95% CI) | Post-test probability |
|---|---|---|---|---|
| Acute renal failure (pre-test probability 31%) | Pre-renal failure (response to pre-renal therapy) | Urine chloride: < 10 mmol/l 10–20 mmol/l > 20 mmol/l | infinity (6.9 to infinity) 3.6 (1.3 to 9.7) 0.21 (0.088 to 0.52) | 100% 62% 9% |

Calculate:
● the fractional excretion of sodium **[C]**[5] **[C]**[7]:

$$\frac{[\text{Urine Na} \times \text{plasma creatinine}]}{[\text{plasma Na} \times \text{urine creatinine}]} \times 100$$

- the fractional excretion of chloride [C][6]

$$\frac{[\text{Urine Cl} \times \text{plasma creatinine}]}{[\text{plasma Cl} \times \text{urine creatinine}]} \times 100$$

### Why?
**A low fractional excretion of sodium or chloride makes pre-renal failure more likely**

| Patient [C][6] | Target disorder (reference standard) | Diagnostic test | LR+ (95% CI) | Post-test probability | LR− (95% CI) | Post-test probability |
|---|---|---|---|---|---|---|
| Acute renal failure (pre-test probability 31%) | Pre-renal failure (possible cause and response to pre-renal therapy) | Fractional excretion of sodium ≤ 1% | 10 (3.9 to 26) | 82% | 0.16 (0.055 to 0.45) | 7% |
| | | Fractional excretion of chloride ≤ 1% | 22 (5.8 to 87) | 91% | 0.050 (0.0073 to 0.34) | 2% |

**A high urine osmolality makes pre-renal failure more likely**

| Patient [C][5] | Target disorder (reference standard) | Diagnostic test | LR+ (95% CI) | Post-test probability | LR− (95% CI) | Post-test probability |
|---|---|---|---|---|---|---|
| Acute renal failure (pre-test probability 24%) | Pre-renal failure (response to pre-renal therapy) | Urine osmolality > 500 mosmol/kg | 7.9 (1.6 to 38) | 71% | 0.79 (0.62 to 1.0) | 20% |

## THERAPY

Treat the underlying cause [A]. Ask for specialist advice if hyponatraemia fails to correct or recurs [D].

### Dehydration
- Give 0.9% saline – avoid giving fluid too rapidly [C][8].
  Aim to correct sodium levels at 0.5 mmol/l per hour with a maximum rise of 12 mmol in 24 hours [D].

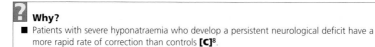

### Why?
- Patients with severe hyponatraemia who develop a persistent neurological deficit have a more rapid rate of correction than controls [C][8].

- Monitor urea and electrolytes regularly [D].

## No dehydration or oedema

- Restrict water intake to 1.5 l/day **[D]** followed by 1 l/day if no response **[D]**.
  Aim to correct sodium levels at 0.5 mmol/l per hour with a maximum rise of 12 mmol in 24 hours **[D]**.
- Consider demeclocycline 300 mg 8-hourly if no response **[D]**.

## Oedema

- Give frusemide **[C]**[9] and monitor fluid balance carefully.

**Why?**

- It is more effective than chlorthiazide at correcting urine/plasma osmolality abnormalities. **[C]**[9]

## PROGNOSIS

- Most patients with severe hyponatraemia recover well **[C]**[3] **[C]**[10].
- Patients with acute hyponatraemia or rapid correction are more likely to die **[C]**[2] **[C]**[8].
- Neurological complications (including encephalopathy) are uncommon **[C]**[3] **[C]**[11].

**Note**

- 8% of patients with severe hyponatraemia die (95% CI: 1.3% to 15%) **[C]**[3]; 50% of patients with acute hyponatraemia (onset < 12 h die (95% CI: 24% to 76%) **[C]**[2].
- 11% suffer neurological complications (95% CI: 3.4% to 19%) **[C]**[3] **[C]**[11].
- The risk of developing encephalopathy is not clearly related to the speed of onset or the magnitude of hyponatraemia **[C]**[2].

**Guideline writers**: Tim Ringrose, Christopher Ball
**CAT writers**: Tim Ringrose, Christopher Ball

## REFERENCES

| No | Level | Citation |
|---|---|---|
| 1 | 4 | Rosenblatt DE et al. Incidence of hyponatremia in elderly patients on hospital admission. J Geriatr Drug Ther 1996; 11: 71–84 |
| 2 | 4 | Arieff AI et al. Neurological manifestations and morbidity or hyponatremia: correlation with brain water and electrolytes. Medicine 1976; 55: 121–9 |
| 3 | 4 | Sterns RH. Severe symptomatic hyponatremia: treatment and outcome. A study of 64 cases. Ann Intern Med 1987; 107: 656–64 |
| 4 | 2a | McGee S, Abernethy WB, Simel DL. Is this patient hypovolemic? JAMA 1999; 281: 1022–29 |
| 5 | 4 | Espinel CH, Gregory AW. Differential diagnosis of acute renal failure. Clin Nephrol 1980; 13: 73–7 |

| No | Level | Citation |
|----|-------|----------|
| 6 | 4 | Anderson RJ et al. Urinary chloride concentration in acute renal failure. Miner Electrolyte Metab 1984; 10: 92–7 |
| 7 | 4 | Miller TR et al. Urinary diagnostic indices in acute renal failure. Ann Intern Med 1978; 89: 47–50 |
| 8 | 4 | Brunner JE et al. Central pontine myelinolysis and pontine lesions after rapid correction of hyponatremia: a prospective magnetic resonance imaging study. Ann Neurol 1990; 27: 61–6 |
| 9 | 4 | Szatalowicz VL, Miller PD, Lacher JW et al. Comparative effect of diuretics on renal water excretion in hyponatraemic oedematous disorders. Clin Sci 1982; 62: 235–8 |
| 10 | 4 | Ayus JC et al. Treatment of symptomatic hyponatremia and its relation to brain damage: a prospective study. N Engl J Med 1987; 317: 1190–5 |
| 11 | 4 | Ayus JC, Wheeler JM, Arieff AI. Post-operative hyponatraemic encephalopathy in menstruant women. Ann Intern Med 1992; 117: 891–7 |

## PREVALENCE

Infective endocarditis is uncommon **[B]**[1], even in patients with bacteraemia **[C]**[2] or prosthetic valves **[A]**[3]; however, it can easily be missed **[C]**[2].

> **Note**
> - Infective endocarditis occurs in 3% of patients with *Staphylococcus aureus* bacteraemia **[C]**[2].
> - 6% of patients with newly inserted prosthetic valves develop infective endocarditis over 7 years **[A]**[3].
> - 55% of cases of *Staph. aureus* infective endocarditis are diagnosed at autopsy or surgery **[C]**[2].

In clinically suspicious cases, infective endocarditis is common **[C]**[4], as are vegetations **[A]**[5].

> **Note**
> - Pre-test probability of infective endocarditis in suspected cases: 48% **[C]**[4].
> - Pre-test probability of echocardiography-detectable vegetation or abscess cavity in suspected cases: 45% **[A]**[5].

## CLINICAL FEATURES

Ask about:

- valvular heart disease **[B]**[6] (including mitral valve prolapse) **[B]**[6]
  - which valves are affected **[B]**[6]
  - severity of disease **[B]**[6]
  - any recent valvular surgery in the last 2 months **[A]**[3]
  - any prosthetic valves **[B]**[1]
- previous rheumatic fever **[B]**[6]
- previous endocarditis **[B]**[6]
- intravenous drug use **[B]**[1]
- any infectious episode in the last 3 months **[B]**[7], particularly superficial wound infections **[A]**[3]
- any skin wounds in the last 3 months **[B]**[7].

**Note**
- Recent dental, surgical or medical procedures do not clearly predict an increased risk of developing infective endocarditis **[B]**[7].

**Valvular heart disease and valvular surgery increase the risk of infective endocarditis**

| Outcome | Risk factor | PEER | OR (95% CI) | NNH (95% CI) |
|---|---|---|---|---|
| Infective endocarditis **[B]**[6] | Severe valvular heart disease (mixed or prosthetic valves) | 0.050% | 131 (6.9 to 2489) | 160 (9 to 3400) |
| Infective endocarditis **[B]**[6] | Cardiac valvular surgery | 0.050% | 74.6 (12.5 to 447) | 270 (46 to 1700) |
| Infective endocarditis **[B]**[6] | Previous episode of endocarditis | 0.050% | 37.2 (4.4 to 317) | 550 (64 to 5900) |
| Infective endocarditis **[B]**[6] | Known mitral valve prolapse | 0.050% | 19.4 (6.4 to 58.4) | 1100 (350 to 3700) |
| Infective endocarditis **[B]**[6] | Any cardiac valvular abnormality | 0.050% | 16.7 (7.4 to 37.4) | 1300 (550 to 3100) |
| Infective endocarditis **[B]**[6] | Rheumatic fever | 0.050% | 13.4 (4.5 to 39.5) | 1600 (520 to 5700) |
| Infective endocarditis **[B]**[7] | Infectious episode | 0.021% | 3.9 (2.1 to 7.3) | 1600 (760 to 4300) |
| Infective endocarditis **[B]**[7] | Skin wound | 0.021% | 3.9 (1.6 to 9.6) | 1600 (560 to 7900) |
| Infective endocarditis **[B]**[6] | Congenital heart disease | 0.050% | 6.7 (2.3 to 19.4) | 3500 (1100 to 15 000) |
| Infective endocarditis **[B]**[6] | Heart murmur | 0.050% | 4.2 (2.0 to 8.9) | 6300 (2500 to 20 000) |
| Infective endocarditis **[B]**[6] | Any dental procedure | 0.050% | 1.4 (0.7 to 2.7) | 50 000 (−67000 to 12 000) |

**Superficial wound infections and active endocarditis following prosthetic valve surgery increase the risk infective endocarditis**

| Patient **[A]**[3] | Prognostic factor | Outcome | Control rate | RR (95% CI) | NNF+ (95% CI) |
|---|---|---|---|---|---|
| Prosthetic valve replacement in last 2 months | Preoperative hypoxia ($Po_2 < 80$ mmHg) | Infective endocarditis at 8 years | 1.3% | 7.9 | 11 |
| Prosthetic valve replacement in last 2 months | Active endocarditis | Infective endocarditis at 8 years | 1.3% | 6.8 | 13 |
| Prosthetic valve replacement in last 2 months | Superficial wound infection | Infective endocarditis at 8 years | 1.3%) | 3.5 | 9 |
| Prosthetic valve replacement in last 2 months | Resident as primary surgeon | Infective endocarditis at 8 years | 1.3% | 3.2 | 34 |
| Prosthetic valve replacement in last 2 months | Preoperative valve lesion | Infective endocarditis at 8 years | 1.3% | ? | ? |

Look for [C]² [C]⁹ [C]¹⁰:

- fever
- rigors
- a new or changed heart murmur

**Note**
- 24% of patients with infective endocarditis have no murmur.
- Very few patients with infective endocarditis are afebrile.

- complications
  - neurological involvement (headache, mental state changes)
  - emboli: strokes, petechiae (including palatal, Janeway lesions, conjunctival haemorrhages, Roth spots)
  - evidence of heart failure or dyspnoea
  - hepatomegaly
  - splenomegaly.

**Note**
- Splinter haemorrhages are not very helpful in diagnosing infective endocarditis.

**Why?**
- Splinter haemorrhages are common (occurring in 10% of medical patients) [C]¹¹.
- No patients with splinter haemorrhages in one study had infective endocarditis [C]¹¹.

**Sensitivity of clinical features in infective endocarditis**

| [C]² [C]⁸ [C]⁹ [C]¹⁰ | Sweden | USA | Denmark | France |
|---|---|---|---|---|
| Fever | 100% | | 94% | 94% |
| Rigors | 68% | | | |
| Heart murmur | 68% | | | |
|   new or changed murmur | | 39% | 47% | |
|   no murmur | | 24% | | |
| CNS involvement (headache, mental state changes) | 53% | | | |
| Heart failure | 44% | | | |
| Dyspnoea | 39% | | 44% | |
| CNS emboli | 33% | | | 24% |
| Skin infection | 27% | | | |
| Petechiae/splinters/Janeway lesions | 27% | | 8.1% | |
| Splinter haemorrhages | | | 8.1% | |
| Hepatomegaly | 20% | | | |
| Splenomegaly | 3% | | | 15% |
| Conjunctival haemorrhages | 3% | | | |

## INVESTIGATIONS

- Draw blood cultures **[A]**: take three separate sets **[C]**[12].

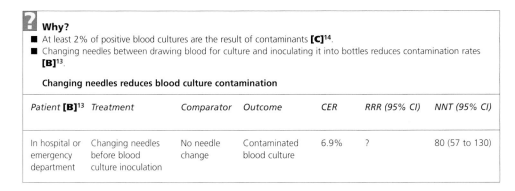

| ? **Why?** | |
|---|---|
| Serial blood cultures increase the chance of culturing an organism | |
| **[C]**[12] | *Sensitivity 95% CI)* |
| First blood culture | 92% (88% to 95%) |
| Second blood culture | 99% (98% to 100%) |
| Third blood culture | 100% (99% to 100%) |

Remember to change the needle before inoculating culture bottles! **[B]**[13]

| ? **Why?** |
|---|
| ■ At least 2% of positive blood cultures are the result of contaminants **[C]**[14]. |
| ■ Changing needles between drawing blood for culture and inoculating it into bottles reduces contamination rates **[B]**[13]. |

**Changing needles reduces blood culture contamination**

| Patient **[B]**[13] | Treatment | Comparator | Outcome | CER | RRR (95% CI) | NNT (95% CI) |
|---|---|---|---|---|---|---|
| In hospital or emergency department | Changing needles before blood culture inoculation | No needle change | Contaminated blood culture | 6.9% | ? | 80 (57 to 130) |

- Blood count **[C]**[15].
- CRP **[C]**[15].
- Urea and electrolytes, creatinine **[C]**[15].
- Liver function tests **[C]**[15].

| ? **Why?** | |
|---|---|
| A raised CRP, ESR and white cell count are common in infective endocarditis | |
| *Test* | *Sensitivity (95% CI)* |
| CRP (> Upper level of normal) | 96% (91% to 100%) |
| ESR (> Upper level of normal) | 74% (65% to 83%) |
| Differential count | 73% (64% to 83%) |
| Leucocyte count abnormal | 60% (51% to 67%) |
| Serum creatinine (> Upper level of normal) | 50% (40% to 59%) |
| Liver function tests | 45% (35% to 54%) |
| Haemoglobin low | 33% (24% to 42%) |

- Save blood for serological investigation of 'culture negative' endocarditis **[C]**[16]

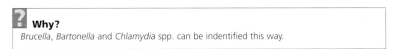

> **Why?**
> *Brucella*, *Bartonella* and *Chlamydia* spp. can be indentified this way.

- Test urine for haematuria using a dipstick **[C]**[9].

> **Why?**
> **Haematuria on dipstick helps diagnose infective endocarditis**
>
> | Patient **[C]**[9] | Target disorder (reference standard) | Diagnostic test | LR+ (95% CI) | Post-test probability | LR− (95% CI) | Post-test probability |
> | --- | --- | --- | --- | --- | --- | --- |
> | Suspected infective endocarditis (pre-test probability 56%) | Infective endocarditis (von Reyn criteria) | Haematuria on urine dipstick | 4.5 (2.2 to 9.0) | 86% | 0.35 (0.23 to 0.52) | 33% |

- ECG **[B]**[17].

> **Why?**
> **Conduction abnormalities increase the chance of perivalvular abscesses being present**
>
> | Patient **[B]**[17] | Target disorder (reference standard) | Diagnostic test | LR+(95% CI) | Post-test probability | LR−(95% CI) | Post-test probability |
> | --- | --- | --- | --- | --- | --- | --- |
> | Suspected infective endocarditis (pre-test probability 56%) | Perivalvular abscesses (pathological evidence) | Atrioventricular and/or bundle-branch or fascicular blocks on ECG | 4.5 (1.2 to 17) | 86% | 0.61 (0.45 to 0.84) | 44% |

- Chest X-ray **[C]**[2].

> **Why?**
> ■ Chest X-ray is moderately sensitive for infective endocarditis: sensitivity 47% (38% to 56%).

- Echocardiography **[B]**[17] (preferably transoesophageal), looking for vegetations.

**Why?**

■ Transoesophageal echocardiography is better at diagnosing and excluding perivalvular abscesses than transthoracic **[B]**[17] **[C]**[18].

**Echocardiography for perivalvular abscesses in infective endocarditis**

| Patient | Target disorder (reference standard) | Diagnostic test | LR+ (95% CI) | Post-test probability | LR– (95% CI) | Post-test probability |
|---|---|---|---|---|---|---|
| Infective endocarditis (pre-test probability 38%) **[B]**[17] | Perivalvular abscesses (pathological evidence) | 2-D transthoracic echocardiogram | 5.4 (1.9 to 15) | 77% | 0.23 (0.11 to 0.46) | 27% |
| Infective endocarditis (pre-test probability 38%) **[C]**[18] | Perivalvular abscesses (pathological evidence) | Transoesophageal echocardiogram | 16 (6.2 to 42) | 91% | 0.14 (0.065 to 0.29) | 8% |

 **Note**

■ The left heart is affected more than the right (88% compared with 7% of cases) **[C]**[10].
■ The aortic valve is affected in 25–36% of cases and the mitral valve in 29–33% **[B]**[19] **[B]**[20].
■ Patients with vegetations are not clearly at increased risk of emboli **[B]**[21].

● Use the Duke criteria to establish the diagnosis **[C]**[4].

**Why?**

■ They rule out infective endocarditis better than the von Reyn criteria, and are as effective at making the diagnosis.

**Duke criteria for infective endocarditis**

| Patient **[C]**[4] | Target disorder (reference standard) | Diagnostic test | LR+(95% CI) | Post-test probability |
|---|---|---|---|---|
| Suspected infective endocarditis (pre-test probability 48%) | Infective endocarditis (pathological diagnosis) | Definite on Duke | 29 (7.3 to 120) | 92% |
| | | Possible on Duke | 2.3 (0.83 to 6.2) | 46% |
| | | Rejected on Duke | 0.0 (0.0 to 0.12) | 0% |

## Duke criteria
### Definite
Any of

● Pathological criteria:
  – microorganism: demonstrated by culture or histology in a vegetation, or in a vegetation that has embolised or in an intracardiac abscess; or

  - pathological lesions: vegetation or intracardiac abscess present confirmed by histology showing active endocarditis.
- Clinical criteria: any of (Box 1):
  - two major criteria
  - one major and three minor criteria
  - five minor criteria.

Possible

Findings consistent with infective endocarditis that fall short of 'definite' but not 'rejected'.

Rejected

Any of

- firm alternative diagnosis explaining evidence of infective endocarditis
- resolution of infective endocarditis syndrome with antibiotic treatment for ≤ 4 days
- no pathological evidence of infective endocarditis at surgery or autopsy with antibiotic therapy for ≤ 4 days.

---

**Box 1  Duke Criteria**

*Major criteria*

1. Positive blood culture for infective endocarditis
   (a) typical microorganisms for infective endocarditis from two separate blood cultures
      ■ Viridans streptococci, *Streptococcus bovis*, HACEK* group
      ■ commonly acquired *Staphylococcus aureus* or enterococci in absence of primary focus
   (b) persistently positive blood culture defined as a microorganism consistent with infective endocarditis from
      ■ blood cultures drawn more than 12 h apart
      ■ all three, or a majority of four or more blood cultures with first and last drawn at least 1 h apart
2. Evidence of endocardial involvement: positive echocardiogram for infective endocarditis
   ■ oscillating intracardiac mass on valve or supporting structure in the path of regurgitant stream or on iatrogenic devices in the absence of an alternative anatomical explanation
   ■ abscess
   ■ new partial dehiscence of prosthetic valve or new valvular regurgitation (worsening or changing of pre-existing murmur not sufficient)

*Minor criteria*

1. Predisposing heart condition or iv drug use
2. Fever ≥ 38°C
3. Vascular phenomena: arterial embolism, septic pulmonary infarcts, mycotic aneurysm, intracranial haemorrhage, Janeway lesions
4. Immunological phenomena: glomerulonephritis, Osler's nodes, Roth spots
5. Echocardiogram consistent with infective endocarditis but not meeting major criteria as noted previously, or serological evidence of active infection with organism consistent with infective endocarditis

*HACEK = *Haemophilus, Actinobacillus, Cardiobacterium, Eikenella* and *Kingella* spp.

## THERAPY

Give antibiotics [A]:
- immediately if endocarditis strongly suspected [A] otherwise
- once there is a positive blood culture [C][22].

---

**? Why do this?**

■ Patients suspected of having bacterial endocarditis partially treated with antibiotics are less likely to have positive blood cultures [C][22].

**Starting therapy for infective endocarditis**

| Patient [C][22] | Treatment | Comparator | Outcome | CER | RRI(%) (95% CI) | NNH (95% CI) |
|---|---|---|---|---|---|---|
| Suspected infective endocarditis | Antibiotics before a positive blood culture | No antibiotics | Any positive blood culture after 3 weeks | 97% | 6 (1 to 10) | 18 (10 to 70) |

---

**‖ Note**

■ The commonest infective organisms are staphylococcus and streptococci (20%) [B][17] [B][21].

**Proportion of organisms causing endocarditis**

| Organism [B][17] [B][21] | Prevalence |
|---|---|
| Viridans streptococci | 42% |
| *Staphylococcus aureus* | 18%–23% |
| All streptococci | 20% |
| Enterococci | 8% |
| Other streptococci | 8% |
| HACEK group | 6% |
| 'Culture negative' | 2% |

---

Give combination therapy (commonly an aminoglycoside and a broad-spectrum pencillin)[C][23] [C][24] preferably iv [C][25] for at least 2 weeks [C][23] [C][24] (and probably for longer).

**Note**
- 70% of patients with right-sided endocarditis are cured following 2 weeks of iv cloxacillin and gentamicin **[C]**[23].
- 94% of selected patients with right-sided staphylococcal endocarditis are treated safely and effectively with a 2 week course of nafcillin plus tobramycin **[C]**[24].
- Oral antibiotics are not clearly as effective as iv antibiotics in iv drug users with right-sided staphylococcal endocarditis, although patients have less liver damage and kidney damage **[C]**[25].

**Antibiotics for infective endocarditis**

| Patient **[C]**[22] | Treatment | Comparator | Outcome | CER | RRI (95% CI) | NNH (95% CI) |
|---|---|---|---|---|---|---|
| Right-sided infective endocarditis | Oral antibiotics | Intravenous antibiotics | Treatment failure at 1 month | 12 | 56% (−290% to 95%) | 15 (NNT = 4 to infinity; NNH = 11 to infinity) |
| Right-sided infective endocarditis | Oral antibiotics | Intravenous antibiotics | Hepatotoxicity during hospital stay | 33 | 92% (39% to 99%) | 3 (2 to 7) |
| Right-sided infective endocarditis | Oral antibiotics | Intravenous antibiotics | Nephrotoxicity during hospital stay | 26 | 100% | 4 (3 to 8) |

Ask a cardiac surgeon for an opinion if any of the following are present: **[B]**[26]

- left ventricular failure
- recurrent embolism
- uncontrolled infection.

## PREVENTION

Use antibiotic prophylaxis for high-risk patients (valvular heart disease, prosthetic heart valves, previous rheumatic fever or infective endocarditis) during dental surgery **[A]**[27] and invasive procedures **[C]**[28].

**Why do this?**
- Antibiotic prophylaxis to prevent infective endocarditis in patients at high risk undergoing dental extraction saves money **[A]**[27].
- Antibiotic prophylaxis following an invasive procedure reduces the risk of infective endocarditis in patients with prosthetic heart valves **[C]**[28].

**Antibiotic prophylaxis for patients at risk of infective endocarditis**

| Patient **[C]**[22] | Treatment | Comparator | Outcome | CER | RRR (95% CI) | NNT (95% CI) |
|---|---|---|---|---|---|---|
| Prosthetic heart valve | Oral antibiotic prophylaxis | No antibiotics | Infective endocarditis at 2 weeks | 2.0% | 100% | 51 (28 to 240) |

In addition, for prosthetic valve insertion, avoid **[A]**[3]:

- pre-operative hypoxia
- surgery during active infection if possible
- an inexperienced surgeon.

**Why do this?**
Prognostic factors for infective endocarditis following prosthetic valve surgery

| Patient [A][3] | Prognostic factor | Outcome | Control rate | RR (95% CI) | NNF+ (95% CI) |
|---|---|---|---|---|---|
| Prosthetic valve replacement in last 2 months | Pre-operative hypoxia ($Po_2 < 80$ mmHg) | Infective endocarditis at 8 years | 1.3% (0.7% to 2.0%) | 7.9 | 11 |
| Prosthetic valve replacement in last 2 months | Active endocarditis | Infective endocarditis at 8 years | 1.3% (0.7% to 2.0%) | 6.8 | 13 |
| Prosthetic valve replacement in last 2 months | Resident as primary surgeon | Infective endocarditis at 8 years | 1.3% (0.7% to 2.0%) | 3.2 | 34 |

## PROGNOSIS

10–20% die in hospital [B][26] [B][28].
The risk is increased with:

- infected prosthetic valve [A][3]
- systemic embolisation [B][26]
- *Staphylococcus aureus* infection [B][26]
- neurological complications [C][29].

**Note**
- Two-thirds of patients with prosthetic valve infective endocarditis die [A][3].

**Death and neurological complications in infective endocarditis**

| Patient [C][29] | Prognostic factor | Outcome | Control rate | RR (95% CI) | NNF (95% CI) |
|---|---|---|---|---|---|
| Infective endocarditis | Neurological complication *not independent* | Death at 3 months | 56% | 1.31 (1.09 to 1.57) | 6 (3 to 19) |

50% will require surgery [B][26].
25% develop neurological complications [C][29].

**Note**
- 26% have surgery for heart failure, 9% for recurrent embolism and 6% for uncontrolled infection.
- 50% have a stroke, 25% with toxic confusion, 20% with meningitis [C][29].

15% develop embolic events [B][21].

**Note**

■ These are not predicted by vegetations on echocardiography **[B]**[21].
■ The risk decreases on starting antibiotic therapy **[B]**[21].

**Guideline writers**: Carl Heneghan, Sumit Dhingra, Christopher Ball
**CAT writers**: Carl Heneghan, Sumit Dhingra, Christopher Ball

## REFERENCES

| No | Level | Citation |
|---|---|---|
| 1 | 2c | Berlin JA et al. Incidence of infective endocarditis in the Delaware Valley, 1988–1990. Am J Cardiol 1995; 76: 933–6 |
| 2 | 4 | Espersen F et al. *Staphylococcus aureus* endocarditis. Arch Intern Med 1986; 146: 1118–21 |
| 3 | 1b | Grover FL et al. Determinants of the occurrence of and survival from prosthetic valve endocarditis: experience of the Veterans Affairs Cooperative Study on Valvular Heart Disease. J Thorac Cardiovasc Surg 1994; 108: 207–14 |
| 4 | 4 | Cecchi E et al. New diagnostic criteria for infective endocarditis: a study of sensitivity and specificity. Eur Heart J 1997; 18: 1149–56 |
| 5 | 1b | Irani W N et al. A negative transthoracic echocardiogram obviates the need for trans-oesophageal echocardiography in patients suspected with native valve active endocarditis. Am J Cardiol 1996; 78: 101–3 |
| 6 | 3b | Strom BL, Abrutyn E, Berlin JA et al. Dental and cardiac risk factors for infective endocarditis: a population-based case-control study. Ann Intern Med 1998; 129: 761–9 |
| 7 | 3b | Lacassin F, Hoen B, Leport C et al. Procedures associated with infective endocarditis in adults: a case control study. Eur Heart J 1995; 16: 1968–74 |
| 8 | 4 | Hogevik H et al. Epidemiolgic aspects of infective endocarditis in an urban population. Medicine 1995; 74: 324–9 |
| 9 | 4 | Benn M et al. Infective endocarditis, 1984 through 1993: a clinical and microbiological survey. J Intern Med 1997; 242: 15–22 |
| 10 | 4 | Delahaye et al. Characteristics of infective endocarditis in France in 1991. A 1 year survey. 1995 European Heart Journal: 16: 394–401 |
| 11 | 4 | Kilpatrick ZM et al. Splinter haemorrhages: their clinical significance. Arch Intern Med 1965; 115: 730–5 |
| 12 | 4 | Weinstein MP et al. The clinical significance of positive blood cultures: a comprehensive analysis of 500 episodes of bacteraemia and fungaemia in adults. Rev Infect Dis 1983; 5: 35–53 |
| 13 | 2a | Spitalnic SJ, Woolard RH, Mermel LA. The significance of changing needles when inoculating blood cultures. Clin Infect Dis 1995; 21: 1103–6 |
| 14 | 4 | Wilson WR et al. Incidence of bacteraemia in adults without infection. J Clin Microbiol 1975; 2: 94–5 |
| 15 | 4 | Hogevik H, Olaison L, Anderson R et al. C-reactive protein is more sensitive than erythrocyte sedimentation rate for diagnosis of infective endocarditis. Infection 1997; 25: 82–5 |

| No | Level | Citation |
|----|-------|----------|
| 16 | 4 | Bayer AS et al. Diagnosis and management of infective endocarditis and its complications. Circulation 1998; 98: 2936–48 |
| 17 | 2b | Aguado JM et al. Perivalvular abscesses associated with endocarditis: clinical features and diagnostic accuracy of two-dimensional echocardiography. Chest 1993; 104: 88–93 |
| 18 | 4 | Daniel WG, Mugge A, Martin RP et al. Improvement in the diagnosis of abscesses associated with endocarditis by transoesophageal echocardiography. N Engl J Med 1991; 324: 795–800 |
| 19 | 2c | Van der Meer Jan TM et al. Epidemiology of bacterial endocarditis in the Netherlands. I. Patient characteristics. Arch Intern Med 1992; 152: 1863–9 |
| 20 | 4 | DiNuble M et al. Cardiac conduction abnormalities complicating native valve infective endocarditis. Am J Cardiol 1986; 58: 1213–17 |
| 21 | 2b | Steckelberg JM, Murphy JG, Ballard D et al. Emboli in infective endocarditis: the prognostic value of echocardiography. Ann Intern Med 1991; 114: 635–40 |
| 22 | 4 | Werner AS et al. Studies of the bacteraemia of bacterial endocarditis. JAMA 1967; 202: 199–203 |
| 23 | 4 | Ribera E et al. Effectiveness of cloxacillin with and without gentamicin in short-term therapy for right-sided *Staphylococcus aureus* endocarditis. A randomized controlled trial. Ann Intern Med 1996; 125: 969–74 |
| 24 | 4 | Chambers HF et al. Right-Sided *Staphylococcus aureus* Endocarditis in Intavenous Drug Abusers: Two-Week Combination Therapy. Annals of Internal Medicine 1988; 109: 9619–624 |
| 25 | 4c | Heldman AW et al. Oral antibiotic treatment of right-sided staphylococcal endocarditis in injection drug users: prospective randomized comparison with parenteral therapy. Am J Med 1996; 101: 68–76 |
| 26 | 2b | Jaffe WM et al. Infective endocarditis, 1983–1988: echocardiographic findings and factors influencing morbidity and mortality 1990: 15; 1221–6 |
| 27 | 1b | Gould et al. Cost effectiveness of prophylaxis in dental practice to prevent infective endocarditis. Br Heart J 1993; 70: 79–83 |
| 28 | 4 | Horstkotte et al. Contribution for choosing the optimal prophylaxis of bacterial endocarditis. Eur Heart J 1987; 8 (suppl): 379–81 |
| 29 | 4 | Roder BL et al. Neurologic manifestations in *Staphylococcus aureus* endocarditis: a review of 260 bacteraemic cases in nondrug addicts. Am J Med 1997; 102: 379–86 |

## PREVALENCE

New-onset Crohn's disease **[B]**[1] and ulcerative colitis are rare **[D]**, but relapses are common in patients with known disease **[B]**[2] **[B]**[3].

### Note
- The prevalence of Crohn's disease in one US county was 0.14% **[B]**[1].
- 50% of patients with prolonged colitis (diarrhoea and rectal inflammation on sigmoidoscopy) have inflammatory bowel disease (95% CI: 40% to 58%) **[C]**[4].
- A third of patients with Crohn's disease have active disease: 32% (95% CI: 24% to 41%) **[C]**[5].

## CLINICAL FEATURES

### First attack of colitis
Ask about:
- speed of onset **[C]**[6]

### Why?
An insidious onset makes inflammatory bowel disease more likely, and an acute one less, likely

| Patient **[C]**[6] | Target disorder (reference standard) | Diagnostic test | LR+ (95% CI) | Post-test probability |
|---|---|---|---|---|
| Colitis (pre-test probability 50%) | IBD (stool culture, histology, follow-up) | Insidious onset | 18 (2.6 to 120) | 95% |
| | | Acute deterioration, previous slight symptoms | 5.5 (0.74 to 42) | 84% |
| | | Subacute onset | 1.5 (0.53 to 4.5) | 58% |
| | | Acute onset | 0.095 (0.036 to 0.25) | 9% |

- number of bowel movements per day at onset **[C]**[6]

### Why?
Few bowel movements a day at onset make inflammatory bowel disease more likely

| Patient **[C]**[6] | Target disorder (reference standard) | Diagnostic test | LR+ (95% CI) | Post-test probability |
|---|---|---|---|---|
| Colitis (pre-test probability 50%) | IBD (stool culture, histology, follow-up) | Bowel movements at onset: | | |
| | | < 4 per day | 15 (2.2 to 110) | 94% |
| | | 4–6 per day | 3.9 (1.3 to 12) | 79% |
| | | 7–9 per day | 0.37 (0.095 to 1.4) | 27% |
| | | 10–12 per day | 0.26 (0.10 to 0.66) | 20% |
| | | > 12 per day | 0.0 (0.0 to 0.15) | 0% |

- any fever [C][6]

| Patient [C][12] | Target disorder (reference standard) | Diagnostic test | LR+ (95% CI) | Post-test probability |
|---|---|---|---|---|
| Colitis (pre-test probability 50%) | IBD (stool culture, histology, follow-up) | No fever | 4.2 (1.6 to 11) | 80% |
| | | Late fever > 38°C | 3.3 (1.0 to 10) | 76% |
| | | Early fever, previous slight symptoms | 3.7 (0.47 to 29) | 78% |
| | | Early fever | 0.077 (0.025 to 0.24) | 7% |

**Why?**
A fever early in the illness makes inflammatory bowel disease much less likely

- any recent travel abroad [C][6].

**Why?**
Recent foreign travel makes inflammatory bowel disease less likely

| Patient [C][6] | Target disorder (reference standard) | Diagnostic test | LR+ (95% CI) | Post-test probability | LR– (95% CI) | Post-test probability |
|---|---|---|---|---|---|---|
| Colitis (pre-test probability 50%) | IBD (stool culture, histology, follow-up) | Travelling abroad | 0.45 (0.24 to 0.86) | 31% | 1.5 (1.0 to 2.1) | 60% |

Look for [C][6]:
- macroscopically bloody stool
- severe abdominal pain
- vomiting.

**Why?**
Severe abdominal pain or vomiting makes inflammatory bowel disease less likely

| Patient [C][6] | Target disorder (reference standard) | Diagnostic test | LR+ (95% CI) | Post-test probability | LR– (95% CI) | Post-test probability |
|---|---|---|---|---|---|---|
| Colitis (pre-test probability: 50%) | IBD (stool culture, histology, follow-up) | Macroscopically bloody stool | 1.8 (1.2 to 2.5) | 64% | 0.23 (0.10 to 0.53) | 18% |
| | | Severe abdominal pain | 0.26 (0.073 to 0.95) | 20% | 1.2 (0.99 to 1.5) | 54% |
| | | Vomiting | 0.34 (0.14 to 0.82) | 25% | 1.5 (1.0 to 1.8) | 60% |

## Known Crohn's disease

Ask patients about [C][7]:
- their general well-being in the last 24 hours
- any abdominal pain in the last 24 hours
- the number of liquid stools per day

and look for [C][7]:
- an abdominal mass
- any complications
  - arthralgia
  - uveitis
  - erythema nodosum, pyoderma gangrenosum
  - aphthous ulcers
  - anal fissure
  - new fistula
  - abscess.

### Why?
- Use the following index as an objective measure of relapse [C][7].
- It correlates with the Crohn's disease activity index (widely used to monitor disease activity in studies) [B][8] but is simpler to use [C][7].

**A disease activity index can be used to monitor relapse and remission in Crohn's disease**

| Harvey-Bradshaw index [C][7] | Score |
|---|---|
| ● General well-being in the last 24 hours | 0 = very well, 1 = slightly below par, 2 = poor, 3 = very poor, 4 = terrible |
| ● Abdominal pain in the last 24 hours | 0 = none, 1 = mild, 2 = moderate, 3 = severe |
| ● Number of liquid stools per day | 1 point per episode |
| ● Abdominal mass | 0 = none, 1 = dubious, 2 = definite, 3 = definite and tender |
| ● Complications: arthralgia, uveitis, erythema nodosum, aphthous ulcers, pyoderma gangrenosum, anal fissure, new fistula, abscess | 1 point per item |

**The Harvey-Bradshaw index helps diagnose and exclude relapse in Crohn's disease**

| Patient [C][7] | Target disorder (reference standard) | Diagnostic test | LR+ (95% CI) | Post-test probability |
|---|---|---|---|---|
| Crohn's disease (pre-test probability 32%) | Relapse (CDAI index > 150) | ≥ 7<br>4–6<br>≤ 3 | 38 (5.3 to 270)<br>3.0 (1.6 to 5.6)<br>0.034 (0.0048 to 0.23) | 95%<br>59%<br>1.6% |

Watch out for [C][9]:
- weight loss > 2.5 kg
- lower gastrointestinal bleeding
- anal fissures or abscesses.

> **? Why?**
> ■ All are common in active disease.
>
> | Clinical features [C][9] | Patients with active disease |
> |---|---|
> | Weight loss (> 2.5 kg) | 85% |
> | Lower GI bleeding | 41% |
> | Anal fistula, abscess | 36% |

## Known ulcerative colitis

Ask patients about:

- number of bowel motions per day, and whether there was any blood [C][10].

Look for [C][10]:

- tachycardia
- fever
- anaemia
- raised ESR.

> **? Why?**
> **The Truelove criteria can help rank disease severity**
>
> | Disease severity [C][10] | Criteria |
> |---|---|
> | Severe | ≥ 6 motions a day with macroscopic blood<br>Fever > 37.8°C on 2 out of 4 days<br>Pulse > 90 beats/min<br>Anaemia < 75% predicted<br>ESR > 30 mm/h |
> | Moderate | Not severe or mild |
> | Mild | ≤ 4 motions a day with no more than small amounts of macroscopic blood<br>No fever<br>Pulse < 90 beats/min<br>Anaemia not severe<br>ESR ≤ 30 mm/h |
>
> **Severe clinical disease makes severe endoscopic disease slightly more likely**
>
> | Patient [C][10] | Target disorder (reference standard) | Diagnostic test | LR+ (95% CI) | Post-test probability | LR– (95% CI) | Post-test probability |
> |---|---|---|---|---|---|---|
> | Active ulcerative colitis (pre-test probability 54%) | Severe colitis (endoscopy) | Severe disease on Truelove criteria | 1.6 (1.03 to 2.5) | 65% | 0.59 (0.37 to 0.95) | 41% |

*Remember*
- Deep ulceration is common, but clinical features cannot predict which patients have it **[C]**[12]. Further investigations are required **[C]**[13].

> **?** **Why?**
> - 62% of patients with active colitis have deep ulceration (95% CI: 46% to 77%) **[C]**[12].
> - Patients with acute colitis who have deep ulceration are more likely to develop dilatation of the colon. The effect on perforations is unclear **[C]**[12].
>
> **Severe ulceration increases the risk of dilatation of the colon**
>
> | Patient **[C]**[12] | Prognostic factor | Outcome | Control rate | OR (95% CI) | NNF (95% CI) |
> | --- | --- | --- | --- | --- | --- |
> | Active colitis | Severe ulceration *independent* | Colonic dilatation at ?discharge | 58% | 2.48 (1.12 to 5.48) | 2 (1 to 23) |

## DIFFERENTIAL DIAGNOSIS

The commonest causes of a first prolonged attack of colitis are **[C]**[6]:
- inflammatory bowel disease
- infectious colitis
- non-specific colitis.

> **?** **Why?**
> **Half of patients with colitis have inflammatory bowel disease**
>
> | Cause of colitis **[C]**[6] | % (95% CI) |
> | --- | --- |
> | IBD | 50% (40% to 58%) |
> | Infectious colitis | 31% (22% to 39%) |
> | Non-specific colitis | 20% (12% to 28%) |

Alternatives to inflammatory bowel disease include **[D]**:
- bacterial and amoebic colitis
- pseudomembranous colitis
- diverticular disease
- ischaemic colitis
- bowel cancer
- radiation colitis.

## INVESTIGATIONS

- Blood count **[C]**[10]
- ESR **[C]**[10].

**? Why?**

**A normal ESR makes inflammatory bowel disease slightly less likely**

| Patient [C][14] | Target disorder (reference standard) | Diagnostic test | LR+ (95% CI) | Post-test probability | LR– (95% CI) | Post-test probability |
|---|---|---|---|---|---|---|
| Children with suspected IBD (pre-test probability 50%) | IBD (histology) | ESR > 20 mm/h | 1.31 (0.89 to 1.94) | 57% | 0.38 (0.10 to 1.35) | 41% |

- CRP [B][15].

**? Why?**

**Ulcerative colitis: a CRP that remains elevated increases the risk of colectomy**

| Patient [B][15] | Prognostic factor | Outcome | Control rate | OR (95% CI) | NNF+ (95% CI) |
|---|---|---|---|---|---|
| Active ulcerative colitis | > 8 bowel actions and a CRP > 45 on day 3 of admission *not independent* | Colectomy at discharge | 8.5% | 8.75 (2.86 to 26.8) | 2 (1 to 6) |

- Urea, electrolytes, creatinine [D].
- Glucose [D].
- Calcium, magnesium [D].
- Liver function tests [B][16] [C][17].
- Group and save/cross-match blood [D].
- p-ANCA in new cases [C][18]

**? Why?**

**A positive p-ANCA diagnoses inflammatory bowel disease**

| Patient [C][18] | Target disorder (reference standard) | Diagnostic test | LR+ (95% CI) | Post-test probability | LR– (95% CI) | Post-test probability |
|---|---|---|---|---|---|---|
| IBD | IBD (radiology, endoscopy and histology, negative culture) | p-ANCA | Infinity (4.3 to infinity) | 100% | 0.61 (0.57 to 0.66) | 39% |

- Stool culture and microscopy [D].
- *Clostridium difficile* toxin assay [D].
- Erect chest X-ray [D]
- Abdominal X-ray [C][19] [C][20]

Look for:

- extent of colitis (extent of faecal residue, evidence of mucosal ulceration and alteration of haustral pattern) **[C]**[19]
- small bowel distention: presence of ≥ three loops of gas-filled small bowel **[C]**[19] **[C]**[20].

**Why?**

Ulcerative colitis: small bowel distention and pancolitis increases the risk that medical therapy will fail

| Outcome | Risk factor | PEER | OR (95% CI) | NNH (95% CI) |
|---|---|---|---|---|
| Colectomy **[C]**[19] | Small bowel distention *not independent* | 30% | 3.56 (1.33 to 9.47) | 3 (2 to 16) |
| | Pancolitis *not independent* | 30% | 6.38 (2.12 to 19.18) | 2 (2 to 6) |
| Toxic megacolon **[C]**[20] | Increased small-bowel gas on supine plain abdominal film (> 74 cm²) *not independent* | 39% | 2.58 (1.89 to 3.53) | 2 (1 to 3) |

Consider performing:

- colonoscopy **[C]**[11] with biopsies **[D]** – it is a better test than sigmoidoscopy followed by barium enema **[A]**[21]

**Why?**

- It is safe in acute disease: 1.2% of patients with acute colitis suffer toxic dilatation following colonoscopy performed by experienced operators (95% CI: 0.0% to 3.5%) **[C]**[11].
- It is a better test than sigmoidoscopy followed by barium enema in patients with suspected large bowel disease: there are more complete examinations and fewer additional investigations, but no clear difference in the number of diagnoses made nor patient satisfaction **[A]**[21].

**Colonoscopy leads to more complete examinations and fewer further investigations**

| Patient **[A]**[21] | Treatment | Comparator | Outcome | CER | RRR | NNT |
|---|---|---|---|---|---|---|
| Suspected large bowel disease | Colonoscopy | Sigmoidoscopy and barium enema | Complete examination | 36% | 87% (36% to 160%) | 3 (2 to 6) |
| | | | Further investigation required | 27% | 72% (35% to 88%) | 5 (3 to 12) |

**A normal colonoscopy makes inflammatory bowel disease much less likely**

| Patient **[C]**[22] | Target disorder (reference standard) | Diagnostic test | LR+ (95% CI) | Post-test probability | LR– (95% CI) | Post-test probability |
|---|---|---|---|---|---|---|
| Children with suspected IBD (pre-test probability 50%) | IBD (histology) | Abnormal colonoscopy | 2.7 (1.2 to 5.8) | 73% | 0.056 (0.0078 to 0.40) | 5% |

- an air enema **[B]**[13]. Look for severe changes (irregular mucosal contour, > 2 mm deep ulceration, or ulceration undermining the mucosa).

| ? Why? Ulcerative colitis: lack of severe changes on air enema reduces the risk of deep ulceration | | | | | | |
|---|---|---|---|---|---|---|
| Patient **[B]**[13] | Target disorder (reference standard) | Diagnostic test | LR + (95% CI) | Post-test probability | LR – (95% CI) | Post-test probability |
| Suspected deep ulceration (pre-test probability 68%) | Deep ulceration (histology) | Air enema | 3.6 (1.6 to 8.6) | 88% | 0.12 (0.040 to 0.37) | 20% |

Consider the following in first episodes of colitis:
- abdominal ultrasound scan **[B]**[23]; look for:
  - target appearance of bowel (strong echogenic centre with a sonolucent rim ≥ 0.5 cm diameter) ± stenosis
  - distended fluid-filled loops, luminal narrowing, movement of echogenic particles or stiff loops

| ? Why? A normal abdominal ultrasound scan makes Crohn's disease less likely | | | | | | |
|---|---|---|---|---|---|---|
| Patient **[B]**[23] | Target disorder (reference standard) | Diagnostic test | LR + (95% CI) | Post-test probability | LR – (95% CI) | Post-test probability |
| Suspected IBD (pre-test probability 50%) | Crohn's disease (histology, endoscopy, radiology and clinical findings) | Abdominal ultrasound scan | 4.9 (3.1 to 7.6) | 83% | 0.19 (0.12 to 0.31) | 16% |

- white cell scanning **[C]**[22].

| ? Why? A normal white cell scan makes inflammatory bowel disease less likely | | | | | | |
|---|---|---|---|---|---|---|
| Patient **[C]**[22] | Target disorder (reference standard) | Diagnostic test | LR + (95% CI) | Post-test probability | LR – (95% CI) | Post-test probability |
| Children with suspected IBD (pre-test probability 50%) | IBD (histology) | White cell scanning: positive if activity seen in the gut in early stages | 2.8 (1.1 to 7.1) | 74% | 0.10 (0.024 to 0.41) | 9% |

Barium follow-through studies are unhelpful **[C]**[22].

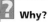

**Why?**

It is unable usefully to diagnose or exclude inflammatory bowel disease **[C]**[22].

Monitor the following:
● vital signs **[C]**[10]
● number of stools passed per day **[B]**[24] **[C]**[7]
● blood count **[C]**[10]
● inflammatory markers **[B]**[24] **[C]**[10]
● urea and electrolytes **[D]**

**Why?**

**Continued frequent diarrhoea and elevated inflammatory markers increase the risk of colectomy**

| Patient **[B]**[24] | Prognostic factor | Outcome | Control rate | RR (95% CI) | NNF + (95% CI) |
|---|---|---|---|---|---|
| Active ulcerative colitis | > 8 bowel actions and a CRP > 45 on day 3 of admission *not independent* | Colectomy at discharge | 8.5% | 8.75 (2.86 to 26.8) | 2 (1 to 6) |

● abdominal film for small bowel distension **[C]**[20].

## THERAPY

● Resuscitate the patient **[A]**.
● Give steroids. Options include:
  – hydrocortisone 200 mg iv three times a day
  – prednisolone 30 mg daily by mouth
  – prednisone 30 mg daily by mouth.

**Why?**

■ Steroids increase the rate of remission in active ulcerative colitis **[A]**[10] **[A]**[25] or Crohn's disease **[A]**[27] **[A]**[28].

**Steroids induce remission in active inflammatory bowel disease**

| Patient | Treatment | Comparator | Outcome | CER | RRR | NNT |
|---|---|---|---|---|---|---|
| Active ulcerative colitis **[A]**[25] | Oral prednisone | Placebo | Remission at 28 days | 17% | 310% (40% to 1100%) | 2 (1 to 4) |
| Active Crohn's disease **[B]**[26] | Oral prednisone | Placebo | Remission at 17 weeks | 26% | 100% (33 to 210%) | 4 (2 to 8) |

An alternative is budesonide **[B]**[26] **[A]**[30].

**? Why?**
- It induces remission in active Crohn's disease if given in daily dose of 9 mg or more **[B]**[26].
- It is slightly less effective than prednisolone at Improving symptoms, but causes fewer steroid side-effects. **[A]**[30].
- It is more effective than mesalazine, and causes fewer patients to stop medication because of side-effects **[A]**[31].

**Crohn's disease: budesonide increases remission and causes fewer side-effects than mesalazine or prednisolone**

| Patient | Treatment | Comparator | Outcome | CER | RRR | NNT |
|---------|-----------|------------|---------|-----|-----|-----|
| Active Crohn's disease **[B]**[26] | Oral budesonide | Placebo | Remission at 10 weeks | 20% | 160% (49% to 350%) | 3 (2 to 7) |
| Active Crohn's disease **[A]**[30] | Oral budesonide | Oral prednisone | Side-effects at 10 weeks | 55% | 40%(14% to 58%) | |
| Active Crohn's disease **[A]**[31] | Oral budesonide | Oral mesalazine | Remission at 16 weeks | 52% | 61% (38% to 75%) | 3 (2 to 5) |
| | | | Withdrawal at 16 weeks | 14% | 180% (60% to 400%) | 4 (3 to 8) |

Use rectal steroids for mild-to-moderate distal ulcerative colitis.

**? Why?**
- Rectal steroids improve symptoms and increase remission rates **[A]**[32].
- Rectal steroids are more effective than oral prednisolone **[A]**[33], though not clearly better than rectal budesonide **[A]**[33].
- The combination of oral and rectal steroids is not clearly better than rectal steroids alone **[D]**[33].

**Ulcerative colitis: rectal steroids improve symptoms and increase remission**

| Patient **[A]**[32] | Treatment | Comparator | Outcome | CER | OR | NNT |
|---------|-----------|------------|---------|-----|-----|-----|
| Distal ulcerative colitis | Rectal corticosteroids | Placebo | Symptomatic improvement at 2–3 weeks | 34% | 0.21 (0.07 to 0.71) | 4 (3 to 14) |
| | | | Symptomatic remission at 2–3 weeks | 9% | 0.07 (0.02 to 0.29) | 12 (11 to 16) |

**Ulcerative colitis: rectal steroids lead to more remissions than oral steroids**

| Patient **[A]**[33] | Treatment | Comparator | Outcome | CER | RBI | NNT |
|---------|-----------|------------|---------|-----|-----|-----|
| Distal ulcerative colitis | Rectal corticosteroid | Oral steroids | Clinical remission at 2 weeks | 35% | 110% (30% to 230%) | 3 (2 to 6) |

- Give 5-Aminosalicylates (e.g. mesalamine).

 **Why?**
- It increases remission in mild-to-moderate disease **[A]**[34] **[B]**[35].
- Newer 5-aminosalicylates are as effective as sulfasalazine but cause fewer side-effects **[A]**[34].

**5-Aminosalicylates increase remission in mild-to-moderate Crohn's disease**

| Patient **[B]**[35] | Treatment | Comparator | Outcome | CER | RRR | NNT |
|---|---|---|---|---|---|---|
| Mild-to-moderate Crohn's disease | Mesalazine 1–4 g daily by mouth | Placebo | Remission at 16 weeks | 36% | 62% (4% to 150%) | 5 (3 to 21) |

**5-Aminosalicylates increase remission in mild-to-moderate ulcerative colitis**

| Patient **[A]**[34] | Treatment | Comparator | Outcome | CER | OR | NNT |
|---|---|---|---|---|---|---|
| Mild-to-moderate ulcerative colitis | 5-ASA | Placebo | Remission or improvement at 4 weeks | 22% | 0.48 (0.35 to 0.66) | 11 (7 to 22) |
| | Newer 5-ASA | Sulfasalazine | Withdrawal due to adverse effects | 18% | 0.19 (0.07 to 0.54) | 7 (6 to 14) |

Give patients with distal ulcerative colitis rectal **[A]**[32] and oral 5-Aminosalicylate **[A]**[36].

**Why?**
- Rectal aminosalicylates lead to more remission than low-dose rectal steroids or rectal budesonide, but are not clearly better than high-dose rectal steroids **[A]**[32].
- Combining rectal and oral aminosalicylates stops rectal bleeding in more patients and sooner (on average by 13 days) than either alone **[A]**[36].

**Ulcerative colitis: combining oral and rectal mesalamine stops rectal bleeding better than either alone**

| Patient **[A]**[36] | Treatment | Comparator | Outcome | CER | RRR | NNT |
|---|---|---|---|---|---|---|
| Distal ulcerative colitis | Daily oral mesalazine and twice weekly rectal mesalazine | Oral or rectal mesalamine | Cessation of rectal bleeding at 6 weeks | 60% | 40% (1% to 96%) | 4 (2 to 88) |

**Ulcerative colitis: rectal 5-ASA is more effective than low-dose rectal steroids at inducing remission**

| Patient **[A]**[32] | Treatment | Comparator | Outcome | CER | OR | NNT |
|---|---|---|---|---|---|---|
| Distal ulcerative colitis | Low-dose rectal corticosteroids | Rectal 5-ASA | Symptomatic remission at 2–7 weeks | 9% | 2.42 (1.72 to 3.41) | −10 (−18 to −6) |
| | Rectal 5-ASA | Budesonide | Symptomatic remission at 4 weeks | 9% | 0.41 (0.18 to 0.94) | 20 (14 to 200) |

- Give antibiotics:
  - ciprofloxacin in ulcerative colitis [A][37]

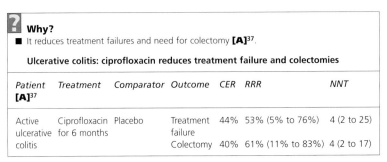

> **Why?**
> ■ It reduces treatment failures and need for colectomy [A][37].
>
> **Ulcerative colitis: ciprofloxacin reduces treatment failure and colectomies**
>
> | Patient [A][37] | Treatment | Comparator | Outcome | CER | RRR | NNT |
> |---|---|---|---|---|---|---|
> | Active ulcerative colitis | Ciprofloxacin for 6 months | Placebo | Treatment failure | 44% | 53% (5% to 76%) | 4 (2 to 25) |
> | | | | Colectomy | 40% | 61% (11% to 83%) | 4 (2 to 17) |

  - metronidazole in perianal and colonic Crohn's disease [A][38].

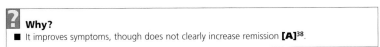

> **Why?**
> ■ It improves symptoms, though does not clearly increase remission [A][38].

There is no clear benefit from:
- vancomycin [D][39]
- antituberculosis therapy for Crohn's disease [A][40].

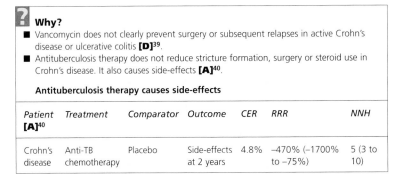

> **Why?**
> ■ Vancomycin does not clearly prevent surgery or subsequent relapses in active Crohn's disease or ulcerative colitis [D][39].
> ■ Antituberculosis therapy does not reduce stricture formation, surgery or steroid use in Crohn's disease. It also causes side-effects [A][40].
>
> **Antituberculosis therapy causes side-effects**
>
> | Patient [A][40] | Treatment | Comparator | Outcome | CER | RRR | NNH |
> |---|---|---|---|---|---|---|
> | Crohn's disease | Anti-TB chemotherapy | Placebo | Side-effects at 2 years | 4.8% | −470% (−1700% to −75%) | 5 (3 to 10) |

  - ciprofloxacin in Crohn's disease [D][41].
  - metronidazole in ulcerative colitis [D][42].
- Consider using nicotine patches for patients with ulcerative colitis who have relapsed on therapy [A][43].

**Why?**

■ It increases the rate of remission for patients who relapsed on steroids and ASA compounds. **[A]**[43].

■ However, side-effects are common (nausea, light-headedness, headache, sleep disturbance, dizziness, skin irritation, sweating, vomiting and tremor) **[A]**[43].

**Nicotine patches increase remission in relapsed ulcerative colitis**

| Patient [A][43] | Treatment | Comparator | Outcome | CER | RRR | NNT |
|---|---|---|---|---|---|---|
| Relapsed ulcerative colitis | Nicotine patches | Placebo | Remission at 6 weeks | 24% | −100% (−290% to 3%) | 4 (2 to 37) |
| | | | Side-effects at 6 weeks | 30% | −120% (−280% to −28%) | −3 (−7 to −2) |

Ask for a surgical opinion if there are any of the following **[D]**:

● toxic megacolon; while waiting, ask the patient to roll on to the abdomen for 10–15 min every 2–3 h, and then try and pass gas or liquid stool after lying prone for another 10–15 min **[C]**[14]

 **Why?**

■ Medical decompression may be an option in toxic megacolon **[C]**[44].

● free perforation of the colon
● massive haemorrhage
● sepsis/septic shock
● severe metabolic disturbance/secondary organ failure
● failure to improve on medical therapy.

Avoid using:
● antidiarrhoeal drugs **[D]**[45]

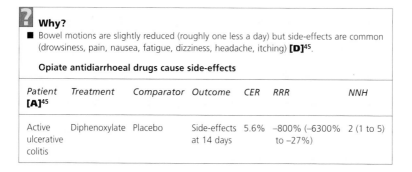 **Why?**

■ Bowel motions are slightly reduced (roughly one less a day) but side-effects are common (drowsiness, pain, nausea, fatigue, dizziness, headache, itching) **[D]**[45].

**Opiate antidiarrhoeal drugs cause side-effects**

| Patient [A][45] | Treatment | Comparator | Outcome | CER | RRR | NNH |
|---|---|---|---|---|---|---|
| Active ulcerative colitis | Diphenoxylate | Placebo | Side-effects at 14 days | 5.6% | −800% (−6300% to −27%) | 2 (1 to 5) |

- enteral nutrition **[A]**[46] **[A]**[47].

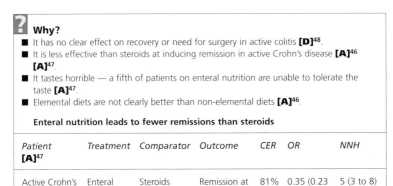

**? Why?**
- It has no clear effect on recovery or need for surgery in active colitis **[D]**[48].
- It is less effective than steroids at inducing remission in active Crohn's disease **[A]**[46] **[A]**[47].
- It tastes horrible — a fifth of patients on enteral nutrition are unable to tolerate the taste **[A]**[47].
- Elemental diets are not clearly better than non-elemental diets **[A]**[46].

**Enteral nutrition leads to fewer remissions than steroids**

| Patient **[A]**[47] | Treatment | Comparator | Outcome | CER | OR | NNH |
|---|---|---|---|---|---|---|
| Active Crohn's disease | Enteral nutrition | Steroids | Remission at 4–8 weeks | 81% | 0.35 (0.23 to 0.53) | 5 (3 to 8) |

Withdraw steroids gradually once clinical symptoms and inflammatory markers are improving. **[A]**[49] Do not reduce the dose based on colonoscopic signs alone **[A]**[50].

**? Why?**
- Fewer patients fail to achieve remission or relapse when steroids are reduced on the basis of symptoms and inflammatory markers, but more remain on steroids **[A]**[49].
- Continuing steroid therapy in asymptomatic patients with active lesions on colonoscopy increases steroid side-effects without preventing relapse **[A]**[50].

**Steroid tapering using symptoms and inflammatory markers reduces failure to achieve remission or relapse**

| Patient | Treatment | Comparator | Outcome | CER | RRR | NNT |
|---|---|---|---|---|---|---|
| IBD **[A]**[49] | Steroid tapering based on symptoms and orosomucoid levels | Steroid tapering based on symptoms alone | Stopped steroids at 1 year | 63% | −61% (−78% to −31%) | −3 (−5 to −2) |
| | | | Failure to achieve remission or relapse at 1 year | 61% | 56% (24% to 74%) | 3 (2 to 7) |

**Crohn's disease: treating asymptomatic lesions on colonoscopy leads to steroid side-effects**

| Patient **[A]**[50] | Treatment | Comparator | Outcome | CER | RRR | NNT |
|---|---|---|---|---|---|---|
| Asymptomatic Crohn's on steroids with active lesions on colonoscopy | Continuing steroids for 5 weeks | Immediate steroid tapering | Steroid side-effects at 5 weeks | 22% | −140% (−350% to −25%) | −3 (−9 to −2) |

For active disease that fails to respond to steroids, consider:
- antimetabolites **[A]**[51] **[A]**[52]
  - azathioprine
  - methotrexate
  - 6-mercaptopurine

side-effects are common and careful monitoring is required **[A]**[51] **[A]**[53].

**Why?**
- Antimetabolites increase the rate of remission **[A]**[51] and reduce the steroid doses **[A]**[51] **[A]**[52]; however, patients need to be treated for up to 4 months before there is any clear benefit **[A]**[51].
- Adverse effects are common (including pancreatitis, leucopenia, nausea, abnormal LFTs and infection) **[A]**[51] **[A]**[53].

**Antmetabolites increase remission and reduce steroid doses but cause side-effects**

| Patient | Treatment | Comparator | Outcome | CER | OR | NNT |
|---|---|---|---|---|---|---|
| Active Crohn's disease **[A]**[51] | Azathioprine or 6-mercaptopurine | Placebo | Remission at 2–12 months | 33% | 2.43 (1.62 to 3.64) | 5 (3 to 9) |
| | | | Steroid-sparing at 2–12 months | 33% | 3.69 (2.12 to 6.42) | 3 (2 to 5) |
| | | | Adverse effects at 2–12 months | 33% | 3.44 (1.52 to 7.77) | −19 (−86 to −8) |

- ciclosporin **[A]**[54] **[A]**[55]

**Why?**
- It improves symptoms, but adverse effects are common (particularly paraesthesia, temperature intolerance and hypertension) **[A]**[54] **[A]**[55].

**Ciclosporin improves symptoms in steroid-resistant disease**

| Patient | Treatment | Comparator | Outcome | CER | RRR | NNT |
|---|---|---|---|---|---|---|
| Active ulcerative colitis **[A]**[55] | Ciclosporin for up to 14 days | Placebo | Improvement at 7 days | 0.0% | | 1 (1 to 2) |
| Active chronic Crohn's disease **[A]**[54] | Ciclosporin for 3 months | Placebo | Symptom improvement at 6 months | 14 | 160% (4% to 540%) | 4 (2 to 29) |
| | | | Adverse effects at 3 months | | −270% (−890% to −36%) | −3 (−8 to −2) |

- infliximab **[A]**[56] **[A]**[57] for Crohn's disease.

> **?** **Why?**
> - It improves symptoms and rates of remission in chronic active disease **[A]**[56].
> - It helps chronic abdominal or perianal fistulas heal **[A]**[57].
>
> **Infliximab increases remission in chronic active disease**
>
> | Patient | Treatment | Comparator | Outcome | CER | RRR | NNT |
> |---------|-----------|------------|---------|-----|-----|-----|
> | Chronic active Crohn's disease **[A]**[56] | Single infusion of infliximab | Placebo | Remission at 12 weeks | 8.0% | 200% (−24% to 1100%) | 6 (3 to 49) |
> | | | | Symptom improvement at 12 weeks | 12% | 240% (14% to 920%) | 3 (2 to 8) |
> | Crohn's disease with chronic abdominal or perianal fistulas **[A]**[57] | Three infusions of infliximab | Placebo | Complete healing | 13% | 257% (38% to 825%) | 3 (2 to 6) |
> | | | | 50% reduction in fistulas | 26% | 140% (28% to 349%) | 3 (2 to 6) |

## PREVENTION

## Crohn's disease

- Advise patients to stop smoking **[C]**[58].

> **?** **Why?**
> - Smoking increases the risk of surgery **[C]**[58].
>
> **Smoking increases the risk of further surgery**
>
> | Patient [C]58 | Prognostic factor | Outcome | Control rate | OR (95% CI) | NNF+(95% CI) |
> |---------------|-------------------|---------|--------------|-------------|--------------|
> | Crohn's disease following surgery | Smoking *not independent* | Further surgery at 11 years | 48% | 1.7 (1.03 to 2.79) | 7 (3 to 140) |

- Give fish oil **[A]**[59].

> **?** **Why?**
> - It reduces relapse **[A]**[59]. There is no clear increase in severe diarrhoea.
>
> **Crohn's disease: fish oil reduces relapse**
>
> | Patient [A]59 | Treatment | Comparator | Outcome | CER | RRR | NNT |
> |---------------|-----------|------------|---------|-----|-----|-----|
> | Crohn's disease in remission | Fish oil | Placebo | Relapse at 1 year | 69% | 59% (30% to 76%) | 2 (2 to 5) |

In patients with frequent relapses **[D]** give:
- budesonide 6 mg daily **[B]**[60]

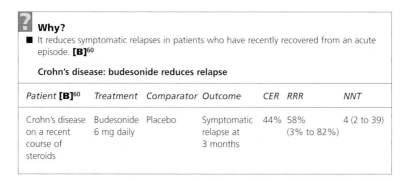

**?** **Why?**

■ It reduces symptomatic relapses in patients who have recently recovered from an acute episode. **[B]**[60].

**Crohn's disease: budesonide reduces relapse**

| Patient **[B]**[60] | Treatment | Comparator | Outcome | CER | RRR | NNT |
|---|---|---|---|---|---|---|
| Crohn's disease on a recent course of steroids | Budesonide 6 mg daily | Placebo | Symptomatic relapse at 3 months | 44% | 58% (3% to 82%) | 4 (2 to 39) |

- azathioprine (≥ 2.0 mg/kg daily) **[A]**[61].

**?** **Why?**

■ It reduces relapse and steroid use, but adverse effects are common (pancreatitis, leucopenia, nausea, 'allergy' and infection) **[A]**[61].

**Azathioprine helps maintain remission but causes adverse effects**

| Patient **[A]**[61] | Treatment | Comparator | Outcome | CER | OR | NNT |
|---|---|---|---|---|---|---|
| Crohn's disease | Azathioprine | Placebo | Still in remission at 6–12 months | 53% | 2.16 (1.35 to 3.47) | 6 (4 to 14) |
| | | | On 10 mg prednisolone or less per day at 6–12 months | 53% | 5.22 (1.06 to 25.68) | 3 (2 to 69) |
| | | | Adverse effects | 1.6% | 4.36 (1.63 to 11.67) | −20 (−100 to −7) |

Following surgery:
- give mesalamine **[A]**[62]

**?** **Why?**

■ It reduces symptomatic relapse after surgery. There is no clear benefit for patients on medical therapy **[A]**[62].

**Crohn's disease: mesalamine reduces relapse after surgery**

| Patient **[A]**[62] | Treatment | Comparator | Outcome | ARR | NNT |
|---|---|---|---|---|---|
| Crohn's disease in remission following surgery | Mesalamine | Placebo | Relapse at 2 years | 13.1% (4.5% to 22%) | 8 (5 to 22) |

- give cimetidine (400 mg qds) following extensive ileal resection **[A]**[63].

**Why?**
- Cimetidine leads to a clinically-useful reduction in stool volume (22% less) following extensive ileal resection **[A]**[63].

There is no clear benefit from:
- other steroids **[A]**[64]
- ciclosporin **[A]**[65].

**Why?**
- Steroids fail to reduce relapse rates **[A]**[64].
- Cyclosporine causes side-effects without clearly reducing relapse **[A]**[65].

**Crohn's disease: cyclosporine causes adverse effects**

| Patient [B][65] | Treatment | Comparator | Outcome | CER | RRR | NNT |
|---|---|---|---|---|---|---|
| Crohn's disease in remission | Cyclosporine | Placebo | Withdrawal due to adverse effects | 3.3% | −350% (−1100% to −74%) | −9 (−20 to −6) |

## Ulcerative colitis

Give:
- 5-aminosalicylates (preferably sulfasalazine) **[A]**[34] as tablets and enemas.

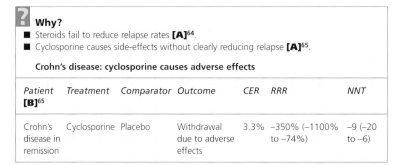

**Why?**
- 5-aminosalicylates reduce relapse **[A]**[34].
- Sulfasalazine is more effective than newer compounds **[A]**[34].
- The combination of enemas and tablets prevents more relapses than tablets alone **[A]**[66].

**Ulcerative colitis: 5-aminosalicylates reduce relapse**

| Patient [A][34] | Treatment | Comparator | Outcome | CER | OR | NNT |
|---|---|---|---|---|---|---|
| Ulcerative colitis in remission | 5-ASA | Placebo | Relapse at 6–12 months | 65% | 0.48 (0.37 to 0.62) | 6 (4 to 9) |
| | Newer 5-ASAs | Sulfasalazine | Relapse at 6–12 months | 44% | 1.29 (1.05 to 1.57) | −16 (−83 to −9) |

**Ulcerative colitis: combining 5-ASA tablets and enemas reduces relapses**

| Patient [A][66] | Treatment | Comparator | Outcome | CER | RRR | NNT |
|---|---|---|---|---|---|---|
| Ulcerative colitis in remission | 5-ASA enemas and tablets | 5-ASA tablets | Relapse at 12 months | 65% | 38% (−1% to 62%) | 4 (2 to 62) |

There is no clear benefit from using:

- fish oil **[A]**[67]
- azathioprine **[D]**[68].

 **Why?**

- Fish oil does not increase remission in active disease, and does not clearly reduce relapses **[A]**[67].
- Withdrawing azathioprine in patients with ulcerative colitis in remission does not clearly increase the relapse rate **[D]**[68].

Consider screening patients with inflammatory bowel disease for cancer by annual assessment with endoscopy (or radiography if endoscopy not available) **[C]**[69] **[C]**[70].

 **Why?**

- Patients with inflammatory bowel disease who have adequate treatment and surveillance are not more likely to die or have any intestinal cancer than the general population **[C]**[69] **[C]**[70].

## PROGNOSIS

- Monitor inpatients with severe colitis for toxic megacolon **[C]**[71].

Look for **[C]**[71]:

- abdominal distension
- localised or generalised peritonitis
- fever $\geq 38°C$
- tachycardia > 120 beats/min
- leucocytosis > $11 \times 10^9$/l
- small bowel distension on plain abdominal X-ray **[C]**[20].

 **Why?**

- 10% of patients with acute ulcerative colitis develop toxic dilatation (95% CI: 7.6% to 12%), compared with 2% of patients with acute Crohn's disease **[C]**[71].
- 16% die (95% CI: 7.7% to 24%) **[C]**[71].

**Small bowel distension increases the risk of toxic megacolon**

| Outcome | Risk factor | PEER | OR (95% CI) | NNH (95% CI) |
|---|---|---|---|---|
| Toxic megacolon **[C]**[20] | Increased small bowel gas on supine plain abdominal film (> 74 cm²) *not independent* | 39% | 2.58 (1.89 to 3.53) | 2 (1 to 3) |

- Colectomy is common in acute colitis **[B]**[15] **[B]**[16].

> **Note**
> ■ 30% of patients with acute colitis have a colectomy (95% CI: 17% to 42%) **[B]**[15] **[B]**[16].

Patients are at increased risk with:
- ≥ 6 bowel motions on the day of admission **[B]**[16]
- > 8 bowel actions and a CRP > 45 on the third day of admission **[B]**[15]
- fever ≥ 38°C or pulse ≥ 90 beats/min on any day **[B]**[16]
- serum albumin level ≤ 35 g/dl **[B]**[16]
- pancolitis or small bowel distention on abdominal X-ray **[C]**[19]
- severe endoscopic colitis **[C]**[11]
  - extensive deep ulcerations or well-like ulcerations
  - mucosal detachment on the edge of these ulcerations
  - large mucosal abrasions.

> **Why?**
>
> **Continued frequent diarrhoea and a raised CRP increase the risk of colectomy**
>
> | Patient **[B]**[15] | Prognostic factor | Outcome | Control rate | RR (95% CI) | NNF + (95% CI) |
> |---|---|---|---|---|---|
> | Active ulcerative colitis | > 8 bowel actions and a CRP > 45 on day 3 of admission *not independent* | Colectomy at discharge | 8.5% | 8.75 (2.86 to 26.8) | 2 (1 to 6) |
>
> **Small bowel distention and pancolitis on abdominal X-ray increase the risk of colectomy**
>
> | Outcome | Risk factor | PEER | OR (95% CI) | NNH (95% CI) |
> |---|---|---|---|---|
> | Colectomy **[C]**[217] | Small bowel distention *not independent* | 30% | 3.56 (1.33 to 9.47) | 3 (2 to 16) |
> | | Pancolitis *not independent* | 30% | 6.38 (2.12 to 19.18) | 2 (2 to 6) |
>
> **Severe colitis on endoscopy increases the risk of colectomy**
>
> | Patient **[C]**[11] | Prognostic factor | Outcome | Control rate | RR (95% CI) | NNF + (95% CI) |
> |---|---|---|---|---|---|
> | Acute colitis | Severe colitis on endoscopy *not independent* | Surgery at discharge | 23% | 4.05 (2.27 to 7.22) | 1 (1 to 3) |

- Relapse and subsequent surgery are common following discharge **[B]**[72] **[B]**[73] **[B]**[74], but death is uncommon **[B]**[74].

| ? Why? Most patients relapse and many require surgery | |
|---|---|
| Outcome **[B]**[72] **[B]**[73] **[B]**[74] | % (95% CI) |
| Crohn's disease relapse at 10 years **[B]**[72] | 99% (97% to 100%) |
| Crohn's disease surgery at 6 years **[B]**[72] | 55% (48% to 62%) |
| Definite ulcerative colitis relapse at 7 years **[B]**[73] | 75% (70% to 80%) |
| Indeterminate colitis relapse at 7 years **[B]**[73] | 83% (74% to 91%) |
| Ulcerative colitis: surgery at 13 years **[B]**[74] | 38% (35% to 41%) |
| Ulcerative colitis: toxic, fulminant or severe colitis at 13 years **[B]**[74] | 13% (11% to 15%) |
| Ulcerative colitis: bleeding at 13 years **[B]**[74] | 17% (15% to 19%) |
| Ulcerative colitis: death at 13 years **[B]**[74] | 1.0% (0.4% to 1.6%) |

- Disease extension is common in ulcerative colitis. **[B]**[74] The risk is increased with **[B]**[74]:
  - toxic, fulminant or severe colitis
  - joint symptoms
  - left-sided disease at diagnosis.

| Note |
|---|
| ■ 61% of patients with ulcerative colitis have disease extension (95% CI: 58% to 64%). |

Ulcerative colitis: severe colitis, left-sided disease and joint symptoms increase the risk of disease extension

| Patient **[B]**[74] | Prognostic factor | Outcome | Control rate | OR (95% CI) | NNF+(95% CI) |
|---|---|---|---|---|---|
| Ulcerative colitis | Toxic, fulminant or severe colitis *independent* | Disease extension at 13 years | 61% | 14.8 (3.5 to 63.1) | 2 (2 to 4) |
| | Left-sided disease extent at diagnosis *independent* | Disease extension at 13 years | 61% | 2.5 (1.6 to 3.9) | 5 (4 to 9) |
| | Joint symptoms *independent* | Disease extension at 13 years | 61% | 3.7 (1.6 to 8.6) | 4 (3 to 9) |

- Systemic manifestations are uncommon **[B]**[74].

**Note**

The commonest systemic manifestations of ulcerative colitis are joint disease and kidney stones.

| [B][74] | Ulcerative colitis |
|---------|-------------------|
| Joints | 8.5% (6.9% to 10%) |
| Skin | 3.4% (2.3% to 4.5%) |
| Liver | 1.3% (0.7% to 2.0%) |
| Retarded growth | 1.3% (0.7% to 2.0%) |
| Urolithiasis | 6.5% (5.0% to 7.9%) |
| Cholelithiasis | 4.1% (3.0% to 5.3%) |

- Many patients have multiple manifestations [C][75].
- No manifestation is clearly commoner in Crohn's disease than ulcerative colitis, except for malabsorption (10% of patients with Crohn's disease in one study) [C][75].

- Cancer is uncommon.

**Note**

- 0.5% of patients with Crohn's disease develop cancer (0.0% to 1.6%) over 10 years [B][72].
- 12% of patients with ulcerative colitis have cancer or dysplasia on initial surveillance colonoscopy (95% CI: 10% to 15%) [B][76].

The risk is increased in patients with ulcerative colitis who have a first-degree relative with colorectal cancer [B][77].

**Why?**

Ulcerative colitis: first-degree relative with colorectal cancer increases the risk of colorectal cancer

| Outcome [B][77] | Risk factor | PEER | OR (95% CI) | NNH (95% CI) |
|-----------------|-------------|------|-------------|--------------|
| Colorectal cancer | First-degree relative with colorectal cancer *independent* | 6.7% | 2.31 (1.06 to 5.14) | 13 (5 to 270) |

**Guideline writer**: Christopher Ball
**CAT writers**: David Ford, Christopher Ball

## REFERENCES

| No | Level | Citation |
|----|-------|----------|
| 1 | 2c | Loftus EV et al. Crohn's disease in Olmsted County, Minnesota, 1940–1993: incidence, prevalence and survival. Gastroenterology 1998; 114: 1161–8 |
| 2 | 2b | Stewenius J et al. Risk of relapse in new cases of ulcerative colitis and indeterminate colitis. Dis Colon Rectum 1996; 39: 1019–25 |

| No | Level | Citation |
|----|-------|----------|
| 3 | 2c | Binder V et al. Prognosis in Crohn's disease – based on results from a regional patient group from the county of Copenhagen. Gut 1985; 26: 146–50 |
| 4 | 4 | Schumacher G et al. A prospective study of first attacks of inflammatory bowel disease and infectious colitis: clinical findings and early diagnosis. Scand J Gastroenterol 1994; 29: 265–74 |
| 5 | 4 | Harvey RF, Bradshaw JM. A simple index of Crohn's disease activity. Lancet 1980; i: 514 |
| 6 | 4 | Schumacher G et al. A prospective study of first attacks of inflammatory bowel disease and infectious colitis: clinical findings and early diagnosis. Scand J Gastroenterol 1994; 29: 265–74 |
| 7 | 4 | Harvey RF, Bradshaw JM. A simple index of Crohn's disease activity. Lancet (1980); i: 514 |
| 8 | 2b | Best WR et al. Development of a Crohn's disease activity index: National Cooperative Crohn's Disease Study. Gastroenterology 1976; 70: 439–44 |
| 9 | 4 | Mekhjian HS et al. Clinical features and natural history of Crohn's disease. Gastroenterology 1979; 77: 898–906 |
| 10 | 4 | Truelove SC, Witts LJ. Cortisone in ulcerative colitis: final report on a therapeutic trial. BMJ 1955; 1041–8 |
| 11 | 4 | Carbonnel F et al. Colonoscopy of acute colitis: a safe and reliable tool for assessment of severity. Dig Dis Sci 1994; 39: 1550–7 |
| 12 | 4 | Bucknell NA et al. Depth of ulceration with outcome and clinical and radiologic features. Gastroenterology 1980; 79: 19–25 |
| 13 | 2b | Almer S et al. Use of air enema radiography to assess depth of ulceration during acute attacks of ulcerative colitis. Lancet 1996; 1731–5 |
| 14 | 4 | Jobling JC et al. Investigating inflammatory bowel disease: white cell scanning, radiology and colonoscopy. Arch Dis Child 1996; 74: 22–6 |
| 15 | 2a | Travis SP et al. Predicting outcome in severe ulcerative colitis. Gut 1996; 38: 905–10 |
| 16 | 2b | Lennard-Jones JE et al. Assessment of severity in colitis: a preliminary study. Gut 1975; 16: 579–84 |
| 17 | 4 | Greenstein AJ et al. Outcome of toxic dilatation in ulcerative and Crohn's colitis. J Clin Gastroenterol 1985; 7: 137–44 |
| 18 | 4 | Freeman H et al. Prospective evaluation of neutrophil autoantibodies in 500 consecutive patients with inflammatory bowel disease. Can J Gastroenterol 1997; 11: 203–7 |
| 19 | 4 | Chew CN et al. Small bowel gas in severe ulcerative colitis. Gut 1991; 1535–6 |
| 20 | 4 | Caprilli R et al. Early recognition of toxic megacolon. J Clin Gastroenterol 1988; 9: 160–4 |
| 21 | 1b | Lindsay et al. Should colonoscopy be the first investigation for colonic disease? BMJ 1988; 296: 167–9 |
| 22 | 4 | Jobling JC et al. Investigating inflammatory bowel disease: white cell scanning, radiology and colonoscopy. Arch Dis Child 1996; 74: 22–6 |
| 23 | 3b | Pera A et al. Ultrasonography in the detection of Crohn's disease and in the differential diagnosis of inflammatory bowel disease. Digestion 1988; 41: 180–4 |
| 24 | 2a | Travis SP et al. Predicting outcome in severe ulcerative colitis. Gut 1996; 38: 905–10 |
| 25 | 1a | Kornbluth AA et al. Meta-analysis of the effectiveness of current drug therapy of ulcerative colitis. J Clin Gastroenterol 1993; 16: 215–8 |

| No | Level | Citation |
|----|-------|----------|
| 26 | 1b | Summers RW et al. National Cooperative Crohn's Disease Study: results of drug treatment. Gastroenterology 1979; 77: 847–69 |
| 27 | 1b | Winship DH et al. National Cooperative Crohn's disease study: study design and conduct of the study. Gastroenterology 1979; 77: 829–42 |
| 28 | 1b | Malchow H et al. European Cooperative Crohn's disease study (ECCDS): results of drug treatment. Gastroenterology 1984; 86: 249–66 |
| 29 | 2b | Oral budesonide was effective for Crohn disease. ACP J Club 1995; 112: 15. Summary of Greenberg GR et al. Oral budesonide for active Crohn's disease. N Engl J Med 1994; 331: 836–41 |
| 30 | 1b | Oral budesonide was less effective, less toxic than prednisolone for Crohn's disease: ACP J Club 1995; 122: 14. Summary of Rutgeerts P et al. A comparison of budesonide with prednisolone for active Crohn's disease. N Engl J Med 1994; 331: 842–5 |
| 31 | 1b | Thomsen OO et al. A comparison of budesonide and mesalamine for active Crohn's disease. N Engl J Med 1998; 339: 370–4 |
| 32 | 1a | Marshall JK & Irvine EJ. Rectal corticosteroids versus alternative treatments in ulcerative colitis: a meta-analysis. Gut 1997; 40: 775–81 |
| 33 | 1b | Truelove SC. Systemic and local corticosteroid therapy in ulcerative colitis. BMJ 1960; i: 464–7 |
| 34 | 1a | Sutherland L, Roth D, Beck P et al. Systematic review of the use of oral 5-aminosalicylic acid in the induction of remission in ulcerative colitis (Cochrane Review). In: The Cochrane Library, Issue 3, 1998. Oxford: Update Software |
| 35 | 2b | Singleton JW et al. Mesalamine capsules for the treatment of active Crohn's disease: results of a 16 week trial. Gastroenterology 1993; 104: 1293–1301 |
| 36 | 1b | Safdi M, DeMicco M, Sninisky C et al. A double-blind comparison of oral versus rectal mesalamine versus combination therapy in the treatment of distal ulcerative colitis. Am J Gastroenterol 1997; 92: 1867–71 |
| 37 | 1b | Turunen UM, Farkkila MA, Hakala K et al. Long-term treatment of ulcerative colitis with ciprofloxacin: a prospective double-blind, placebo-controlled study. Gastroenterology 1998; 115: 1072–8 |
| 38 | 1b | Sutherland L et al. Double-blind placebo-controlled trial of metronidazole in Crohn's disease. Gut 1990; 32: 1071–5 |
| 39 | 1b – | Dickinson RJ et al. Double blind controlled trial of oral vancomycin as adjunctive treatment in acute exacerbations of idiopathic colitis. Gut 1985; 26: 1380–4 |
| 40 | 1b | Swift GL et al. Controlled trial of anti-tuberculous chemotherapy for two years in Crohn's disease. Gut 1994; 35: 363–8 |
| 41 | 1b – | Prantera C et al. An antibiotic regimen for the treatment of active Crohn's disease: a randomised controlled trial of metronidazole plus ciprofloxacin. Am J Gastroenterol 1996; 91: 328–32 |
| 42 | 1b – | Chapman RW et al. Controlled trial of intravenous metronidazole as an adjunct to corticosteroids in severe ulcerative colitis. Gut 1986; 27: 1210–12 |
| 43 | 1b | Transdermal nicotine improved symptoms in ulcerative colitis. ACP J Club 1994 July-Aug; 121: 17. Summary of Pullan RD, Rhodes J, Ganesh S et al. Transdermal nicotine for active ulcerative colitis. N Engl J Med 1994; 330: 811–5 |

| No | Level | Citation |
|----|-------|----------|
| 44 | 4 | Present DH et al. Medical decompression of toxic megacolon by 'rolling': a new technique of decompression with favorable long-term follow-up. J Clin Gastroenterol 1988; 10: 485–90 |
| 45 | 1b | Engbaek J et al. The constipating effect of diphenoxylate (Retardin®) in ulcerative colitis. Scand J Gastroenterol 1975; 10: 695–8 |
| 46 | 1a | Fernandez-Banares F et al. How effective is enteral nutrition in inducing clinical remission in active Crohn's disease: a meta-analysis of the randomised controlled trials. J Parenter Eneter Nutr 1995; 19: 356–64 |
| 47 | 1a | Griffiths AM et al. Meta-analysis of enteral nutrition as a primary treatment of active Crohn's disease. Gastroenterology 1995; 108: 1056–67 |
| 48 | 1b – | McIntyre P et al. A controlled trial of bowel rest in the treatment of severe acute colitis. Gut 1986; 27: 481–5 |
| 49 | 1b | Kjeldsen J et al. Serum concentrations of orosomucoid: improved decision-making for tapering prednisolone therapy in patients with inflammatory bowel disease? Scand J Gastroenterol 1997; 32: 933–41 |
| 50 | 1b | Landi B et al. Endoscopic monitoring of Crohn's disease treatment: a prospective randomised clinical trial. Gastroenterology 1992; 102: 1647–53 |
| 51 | 1a | Sandborn W, Sutherland L, Pearson D et al. Azathioprine or 6-mercaptopurine therapy for induction of remission in active Crohn's disease (Cochrane Review). In: The Cochrane Library, Issue 3, 1998. Oxford: Update Software |
| 52 | 1b | Rosenberg JL et al. A controlled trial of azathioprine in the management of chronic ulcerative colitis. Gastroenterology 1975; 69: 96–9 |
| 53 | 1b | Feagan BG et al. Methotrexate for the treatment of Crohn's disease. N Engl J Med 1995; 332: 292–7 |
| 54 | 1b | Brynskov JB et al. A placebo-controlled double-blind randomized trial of cyclosporine therapy in active chronic Crohn's disease. 1989; 321: 845–50 |
| 55 | 1b | Cyclosporine was effective for corticosteroid-resistant ulcerative colitis. ACP Club 1994; 121: 68. Summary of Lichtger S et al. Cyclosporine in severe ulcerative colitis refractory to steroid therapy. N Engl J Med 1994; 330: 1841–5 |
| 56 | 1b | Targan SR, Hanauer SB, van Deventer SJ et al. A short-term study of chimeric monoclonal antibody cA2 to tumor necrosis factor alpha for Crohn's disease. N Engl J Med 1997; 337: 1029–35 |
| 57 | 1b | Present DH et al. Infliximab for the treatment of fistulas in patients with Crohn's disease. N Engl J Med 1999; 340: 1398–1406 |
| 58 | 4 | Sutherland LR, Ramcharan S, Bryant H et al. Effect of cigarette smoking on recurrence of Crohn's disease. Gastroenterology 1990; 98: 1123–8 |
| 59 | 1b | Fish oil reduced relapse and maintained remission in Crohn disease. ACP J Club 1996 Nov-Dec; 125: 66. Evidence-Based Med 1996 Nov-Dec; 1: 214. Summary of Belluzzi A, Brignola C, Campieri M et al. Effect of an enteric-coated fish-oil preparation on relapses in Crohn's disease. N Engl J Med 1996; 334: 1557–60 |
| 60 | 2b | Lofberg R, Rutgeerts P, Malchow H et al. Budesonide prolongs time to relapse in ileal and ileocaecal Crohn's disease. A placebo-controlled one year study. Gut 1996; 39: 82–6 |
| 61 | 1a | Pearson DC, May GR, Fick G et al. Azathioprine for maintenance of remission of Crohn's disease (Cochrane Review). In: The Cochrane Library, Issue 3, 1998. Oxford: Update Software |

| No | Level | Citation |
|----|-------|----------|
| 62 | 1a | Camma C, Giunta M, Rosselli M et al. Mesalamine in the maintenance treatment of Crohn's disease: a meta-analysis adjusted for confounding variables. Gastroenterology 1997; 113: 1465–73 |
| 63 | 1b | Aly A et al. Effect of an $H_2$-receptor blocking agent on diarrhoeas after extensive small bowel resection in Crohn's disease: Acta Med Scand 1980; 207: 119–22 |
| 64 | 1a | Steinhart AH, Ewe K, Griffiths AM. Corticosteroid therapy for maintenance of remission in Crohn's disease (Cochrane Review). In: The Cochrane Library, Issue 3, 1999. Oxford: Update Software |
| 65 | 2b | Feagan BG et al. Low-dose cyclosporine for the treatment of Crohn's disease. N Engl J Med 1994; 330: 1846–51 |
| 66 | 1b | d'Albasio G, Pacini F, Camarri E. Combined therapy with 5-aminosalicylic acid tablets and enemas for maintaining remission in ulcerative colitis: a randomized double-blind study. Am J Gastroenterol 1997; 92: 1143–7 |
| 67 | 1b | Hawthorne AB et al. Treatment of ulcerative colitis with fish oil supplementation: a prospective 12 month randomised controlled trial. Gut 1992; 33: 992–8 |
| 68 | 1b – | Hawthorne AB et al. Randomised controlled trial of azathioprine withdrawal in ulcerative colitis. BMJ 1992; 305: 20–2 |
| 69 | 4 | Munkholm P et al. Intestinal cancer risk and mortality in patients with Crohn's disease. Gastroenterology 1993; 105: 1716–23 |
| 70 | 4 | Langholz E et al. Colorectal cancer risk and mortality in patients with ulcerative colitis. Gastroenterology 1992; 103: 1444–51 |
| 71 | 4 | Greenstein AJ et al. Outcome of toxic dilatation in ulcerative and Crohn's colitis. J Clin Gastroenterol 1985; 7: 137–44 |
| 72 | 2c | Binder V et al. Prognosis in Crohn's disease – based on results from a regional patient group from the county of Copenhagen. Gut 1985; 26: 146–50 |
| 73 | 2b | Stewenius J et al. Risk of relapse in new cases of ulcerative colitis and indeterminate colitis. Dis Colon Rectum 1996; 39: 1019–25 |
| 74 | 2b | Farmer RG et al. Clinical patterns, natural history and progression of ulcerative colitis: a long-term follow-up of 1116 patients. Dig Dis Sci 1993; 38: 1137–46 |
| 75 | 4 | Greenstein AJ et al. The extra-intestinal complications of Crohn's disease and ulcerative colitis: a study of 700 patients. Medicine 1976; 55: 401–12 |
| 76 | 2a | Bernstein CN et al. Are we telling patients the truth about surveillance colonoscopy in ulcerative colitis? Lancet 1994; 343: 71–4 |
| 77 | 3b | Nuako KW, Ahlquist DA, Mahoney DW et al. Familial predisposition for colorectal cancer in chronic ulcerative colitis: a case-control study. Gastroenterology 1998; 115: 1079–83 |

## PREVALENCE

Meningitis is common in patients with suspected meningitis [A][1] [B][2].

**Note**
- Half of children with suspected meningitis have it (55%; 95% CI: 49% to 62%) [A][1].
- 60% of patients with a recent-onset headache and a fever have CSF pleocytosis (63%; 95% CI: 51% to 76%) [B][2].

Bacterial meningitis is uncommon in patients undergoing 'routine' lumbar puncture [B][3].

**Note**
- One in twenty patients undergoing lumbar puncture has a bacterial meningitis (4.8%; 95% CI: 3.4% to 6.1%) [B][3].

Viral meningitis is uncommon [C][4].

**Note**
- One in thirteen patients with suspected meningitis has a viral meningitis (7.5%; 95% CI: 6.4% to 8.7%) [C][4].

Most cases occur out of hospital [B][5].

**Note**
- 60% of cases of bacterial meningitis are community-acquired (62%; 95% CI: 57% to 66%) [B][5].

## CAUSES

Common causes include [B][5] [B][6] [B][7]:

- *Neisseria meningitidis*
- *Streptococcus pneumoniae*
- Gram-negative bacilli

Remember [D]:

- *Listeria monocytogenes*
- *Haemophilus Haemophilus influenzae*
- Group B streptococcus (mainly neonates)
- tuberculosis
- *Cryptococcus*
- viral infections (coxsackie, echovirus, mumps, polio) [C][8].

> ⬛ **Note**
>
> **Meningococcus and pneumococcus are common causes of meningitis**
>
> | Causes of bacterial meningitis **[B]**[5] **[B]**[6] **[B]**[7] | % |
> |---|---|
> | Neisseria meningitidis | 7.1% to 56% |
> | Streptococcus pneumoniae | 21% to 47% |
> | Gram-negative bacilli | 21% |
> | Listeria monocytogenes | 6% to 8% |
> | Haemophilus influenzae | 5% to 7% |
> | Group B streptococcus (mainly neonatal cases) | 13% |

## CLINICAL FEATURES

Ask about:

- fever **[B]**[9]
- nausea and vomiting **[B]**[9]
- headache **[B]**[9]
- neck stiffness **[B]**[9]
- photophobia **[D]**.

Look for:

- fever **[B]**[9]
- neck stiffness **[B]**[2]

> ❓ **Why?**
>
> **Lack of neck stiffness does not rule out meningitis**
>
> | Patient | Target disorder and reference standard | Diagnostic test | LR+ (95% CI) | Post-test probability | LR− (95% CI) | Post-test probability |
> |---|---|---|---|---|---|---|
> | Recent-onset headache and fever **[B]**[9] (pre-test probability %) | CSF pleocytosis (5 or more white cells per mm $^3$ of CSF) | Neck stiffness | − (1.1 to infinity) | 100% | 0.85 (0.75 to 0.98) | 59% |
>
> ⬛ Neck stiffness is common in elderly patients without meningitis (35%) **[B]**[9].

- altered mental state **[B]**[9]
- focal neurological signs **[B]**[9]
- photophobia **[D]**
- rash **[B]**[9]

? **Why?**
**Fever, neck stiffness and altered mental state are common findings with meningitis**

| Clinical feature | % (95% CI) |
|---|---|
| Fever [B][9] | 85% (78% to 91%) |
| Neck stiffness | 70% (58% to 82%) |
| Altered mental state | 67% (52% to 82%) |
| Headache | 50% (32% to 68%) |
| Fever, neck stiffness and altered mental state | 46% (22% to 69%) |
| Nausea and vomiting | 30% (22% to 38%) |
| Focal neurologic neurological findings | 23% (15% to 31%) |
| Rash | 22% (1% to 43%) |

- Kernig's sign [B][2]
  Positive if the patient's headache worsens on flexing the patient's
  legs at the hip and extending them at the knees.

**Why?**
**An absent Kernig's sign does not rule out meningitis**

| Patient | Target disorder and reference standard | Diagnostic test | LR+ (95% CI) | Post-test probability | LR– (95% CI) | Post-test probability |
|---|---|---|---|---|---|---|
| Recent-onset headache and fever [B][2] (pre-test probability 63%) | CSF pleocytosis (5 or more white cells per mm$^3$ of CSF) | Positive Kernig's sign | – (0.62 to infinity) | 100% | 0.91 (0.82 to 1.0) | 61% |

- jolt accentuation [B][2]
  Positive if the patient's headache worsens on rotating the head
  horizontally 2 or 3 times.

**Why?**
**No jolt accentuation makes meningitis less likely**

| Patient | Target disorder and reference standard | Diagnostic test | LR+ (95% CI) | Post-test probability | LR– (95% CI) | Post-test probability |
|---|---|---|---|---|---|---|
| Recent-onset headache and fever [B][2] (pre-test probability 63%) | CSF pleocytosis (5 or more white cells per mm$^3$ of CSF) | Jolt accentuation | 2.4 (1.4 to 4.2) | 80% | 0.049 (0.0069 to 0.35) | 8% |

## DIFFERENTIAL DIAGNOSIS

Remember **[D]**:

- subarachnoid haemorrhage
- encephalitis
- other causes of raised intracranial pressure
- migraine.

## INVESTIGATIONS

- Blood count **[D]**.
- Clotting studies **[D]**.
- Urea, electrolytes, creatinine **[D]**.
- Glucose **[D]**.
- Blood cultures **[D]**.
- Chest X-ray **[A]**.
- Throat swab **[D]**.
- Lumbar puncture **[A]**
  - considering arranging a CT brain before performing the lumbar puncture

## ? Why?

- One in seven patients requiring an urgent lumbar puncture has an intracranial lesion on CT scan (15%: 95% CI: 8.6% to 22%)**[A]**[10] and one in forty have a contraindication (2.7%: 95% CI: 0.0% to 5.7%) **[A]**[10].

**Papilloedema, focal neurologic signs, and altered mentation make an intracranial lesion more likely [A][10]**

| Patient | Target disorder and reference standard | Diagnostic test | LR+ (95% CI) | Post-test probability | LR– (95% CI) | Post-test probability |
|---|---|---|---|---|---|---|
| Urgent need for lumbar puncture (pre-test probability 15%) | Intracranial mass (CT head) | Papilloedema | 11 (1.1 to 120) | 67% | 0.89 (0.75 to 1.1) | 14% |
| Urgent need for lumbar puncture (pre-test probability 15%) | Intracranial mass (CT head) | Focal neurological signs | 4.3 (1.9 to 10) | 44% | 0.64 (0.38 to 1.0) | 10% |
| Urgent need for lumbar puncture (pre-test probability 15%) | Intracranial mass (CT head) | Altered mentation | 2.2 (1.5 to 3.2) | 28% | 0.36 (0.15 to 0.90) | 6% |
| Urgent need for lumbar puncture (pre-test probability 15%) | Intracranial mass (CT brain) | 1 or more abnormality present | 1.6 (1.2 to 1.9) | 22% | 0.0 (0.0 to 0.6) | 0% |
| Urgent need for lumbar puncture (pre-test probability 15%) | Intracranial mass (CT brain) | Physician's prediction of a new lesion | 9.1 (2.4 to 34) | 62% | 0.63 (0.40 to 1.0) | 10% |

**A physician's prediction of no contraindication to lumbar puncture makes a contraindication less likely but does not clearly rule one out [A][10]**

| Patient | Target disorder and reference standard | Diagnostic test | LR+ (95% CI) | Post-test probability | LR– (95% CI) | Post-test probability |
|---|---|---|---|---|---|---|
| Urgent need for lumbar puncture (pre-test probability 2.7%) | Contraindication (CT of brain) | Physician's prediction of a contraindication | 19 (4.8 to 43) | 34% | 0.0 (0.0 to 0.7) | 0% |

> **Note**
> ■ None of the following features were found to predict intracranial lesions **[A]**[10]:
>   – HIV positive or HIV risk factors
>   – immunosuppressed
>   – malignant neoplasm
>   – head trauma within previous 72 hours
>   – known CNS mass
>   – seizures within previous 72 hours.
> ■ Few patients suffer complications following lumbar puncture (0% to 5%) **[C]**[11].
> ■ Warning patients about a post-lumbar puncture headache leads to more patients having one **[A]**[12]
>
> **Warning about post-lumbar puncture headaches makes symptoms more likely**
>
> | Patient | Treatment | Comparison | Outcome | CER | RRR (95% CI) | NNT (95% CI) |
> |---------|-----------|------------|---------|-----|--------------|--------------|
> | Adults undergoing lumbar puncture **[A]**[12] | No warning about headache | Warning about headache | Post-lumbar puncture headache at ? days | 46% | 91% | 3 (1 to 10) |

– use a narrow gauge, non-cutting needle **[A]**[13] through a bleb of local anaesthetic **[C]**[14]

> **?** **Why?**
> **Narrow gauge needles and non-cutting needles reduce post-lumbar puncture headache**
>
> | Patient | Treatment | Comparison | Outcome | CER | RRR (95% CI) | NNT (95% CI) |
> |---------|-----------|------------|---------|-----|--------------|--------------|
> | Adults undergoing lumbar puncture **[A]**[13] | Small gauge needle | Large gauge needle | Post-lumbar puncture headache at ? weeks | 11% | 0.30 (0.20 to 0.41) | 13 (12 to 16) |
> | Adults undergoing lumbar puncture | Non-cutting needles | Cutting tip needles | Post-lumbar puncture headache at ? weeks | 6.8% | 0.50 (0.27 to 0.68) | 31 (21 to 49) |

**Note**

- Non-cutting needles (with round tip) require an introducer needle to break the skin.
- Back pain and failure rates do not clearly differ with small, large, cutting or non-cutting needles **[D]**[13].
- A bleb of lignocaine does not clearly reduce the success rate for first lumbar puncture attempt **[C]**[14].

– replace the stylet before withdrawing the needle **[A]**[15]

**Why?**
Replacing the stylet reduces post-lumbar puncture headache

| Patient | Treatment | Comparison | Outcome | CER | RRR (95% CI) | NNT (95% CI) |
|---------|-----------|------------|---------|-----|--------------|--------------|
| Adult undergoing lumbar puncture **[A]**[15] | Replacing stylet | No replacement | Post-lumbar puncture headache at 7 days | 16% | 69% (47% to 82%) | 9 (6 to 15) |

– there is no clear benefit from bedrest post-lumbar puncture **[D]**[16] **[D]**[17]

**Why?**

- Patients who lie supine for four hours following lumbar puncture compared with getting up immediately are not clearly less likely to develop post-lumbar puncture headache **[D]**[16] **[D]**[17].

Send CSF for:

– Gram stain and cell count **[C]**[18]

**Note**

| Positive CSF Gram stains | % (95% CI) |
|--------------------------|------------|
| Bacterial meningitis **[C]**[18] | 71% (65% to 77%) |
| Viral meningitis | 1.0% (0.0% to 2.3%) |

- CSF leukocyte counts in bacterial meningitis are higher than in viral meningitis (1.2 × $10^9$/1 compared with 0.1 × $10^9$/l) **[C]**[18].

- culture **[A]**
- glucose and protein **[C]**[18]

> **?** **Why?**
> ■ Protein levels in bacterial meningitis are higher than in viral meningitis (1.7 g/l compared with 0.45 g/l) **[C]**[18].
> ■ Glucose levels are lower in bacterial meningitis compared with viral meningitis (0.29 g/l compared with 0.61 g/l) **[C]**[18].

Consider:
- using reagent strips (e.g. urine dipsticks) **[A]**[1] **[B]**[19] to look for leucocyte esterase, glucose and protein levels.

> **?** **Why?**
> **Reagent strips can help diagnose meningitis**
>
> | Patient | Target disorder and reference standard | Diagnostic test | LR+ (95% CI) | Post-test probability | LR– (95% CI) | Post-test probability |
> |---|---|---|---|---|---|---|
> | Children with suspected meningitis **[A]**[1] (pre-test probability 55%) | Bacterial or viral meningitis (laboratory values of CSF glucose, protein and leucocytes) | Positive reagent strips to CSF glucose, protein or leucocytes | 52 (13 to 200) | 98% | 0.016 (0.0040 to 0.063) | 2% |
> | Undergoing lumbar puncture in the emergency department **[B]**[19] (pre-test probability 5%) | Bacterial meningitis (CSF culture or 'clinical' meningitis) | Positive or trace on leukocyte-esterase dipstick | 19 (14 to 28) | 49% | 0.23 (0.13 to 0.40) | 1.1% |

- blood for PCR for meningococcus **[B]**[20]

> **?** **Why?**
> **Blood PCR can help diagnose meningococcal disease**
>
> | Patient | Target disorder and reference standard | Diagnostic test | LR+ (95% CI) | LR– (95% CI) |
> |---|---|---|---|---|
> | Meningitis **[B]**[20] (pre-test probability %) | Meningococcal disease (culture) | Blood PCR | 3.5 (1.5 to 8.3) | 0.16 (0.19 to 0.61) |

– CSF for PCR for meningococcus [B][21] or viruses [C][4]

**?** **Why?**

**PCR of cerebrospinal fluid can help diagnose meningococcal meningitis**

| Patient | Target disorder and reference standard | Diagnostic test | LR+ (95% CI) | LR– (95% CI) |
|---------|----------------------------------------|-----------------|--------------|--------------|
| Undergoing lumbar puncture [B][21] (pre-test probability: %) | Meningococcal meningitis (CSF culture or microscopy) | PCR | 9.7 (3.7 to 25) | 0.10 (0.015 to 0.65) |

**Viral PCR can help diagnose viral meningitis**

| Patient | Target disorder and reference standard | Diagnostic test | LR+ (95% CI) | Post-test probability | LR– (95% CI) | Post-test probability |
|---------|----------------------------------------|----------------|--------------|----------------------|--------------|----------------------|
| Suspected meningitis [C][4] (pre-test probability 7.5%) | Viral meningitis (viral load in culture media and clinical corroboration) | viral PCR | – (240 to infinity) | 100% | 0.01 (0.00 to 0.05) | 0% |

– Latex agglutination tests for diagnosing meningococcal, pneumococcal or *H. influenzae* b infections [C][22] [C][23]

**?** **Why?**

**Latex agglutination tests can help diagnose specific types of bacterial meningitis**

| Patient | Target disorder and reference standard | Diagnostic test | LR+ (95% CI) | LR– (95% CI) |
|---------|----------------------------------------|-----------------|--------------|--------------|
| Suspected meningitis or meningococcal septicaemia [C][23] (pre-test probability –%) | Meningococcal infection (CSF or blood culture, serology for *N. meningitides*) | Agglutination using test card | – (3.0 to infinity) | 0.69 (0.57 to 0.83) |
| Suspected meningitis or meningococcal septicaemia (pre-test probability –%) | Meningococcal infection (CSF or blood culture, serology for *N. meningitides*) | Agglutination following ultrasound | 9.4 (2.4 to 36) | 0.38 (0.26 to 0.56) |

**Why?**

Latex agglutination tests can help diagnose specific types of bacterial meningitis

| Patient | Target disorder and reference standard | Diagnostic test | LR+ (95% CI) | Post-test probability | LR– (95% CI) | Post-test probability |
|---|---|---|---|---|---|---|
| Children with suspected septicaemia or meningitis **[C]**[22] (pre-test probability 18%) | Infection with *Neisseria meningitidis*, *Streptococcus pneumoniae* or *Haemophilus influenzae* (culture) | Latex agglutination tests | 29 (16 to 54) | 86% | 0.0 (0.0 to 0.47) | 0.0% |

## THERAPY

Resuscitate and seek help if needed.
Give:

- antibiotics **[A]** once suspected **[D]** (e.g. ceftriaxone 2 to 4 g iv daily) **[B]**[24] **[B]**[25].

**Why?**

■ Ceftriaxone is effective – one in seven die, (13%: 95% CI: 5.9% to 20%) and toxicity is rare (0.0%: 95% CI: 0.0% to 3.6%) **[B]**[24].

Consider giving:
- ampicillin 500 mg iv to elderly patients
- acyclovir 10 mg/kg iv over 1 hour every 8 hours if Herpes simplex encephalitis is a possibility

- analgesia
- treat sepsis – patients may require:
  - central venous access
  - urinary catheter
  - transfer to intensive care unit.

There is no clear benefit from dexamethasone in adults **[D]**[26]

**Why?**

■ Adults with meningitis who receive dexamethasone compared with no steroids are not clearly less likely to die or develop neurological sequelae **[D]**[24].

- Give dexamethasone to children with proven H. *influenzae* b meningitis **[A]**[27].

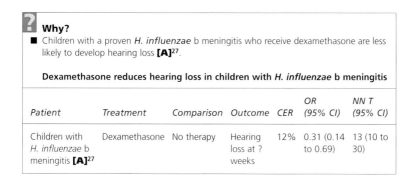

> **Why?**
> ■ Children with a proven *H. influenzae* b meningitis who receive dexamethasone are less likely to develop hearing loss **[A]**[27].
>
> **Dexamethasone reduces hearing loss in children with *H. influenzae* b meningitis**

| Patient | Treatment | Comparison | Outcome | CER | OR (95% CI) | NN T (95% CI) |
|---|---|---|---|---|---|---|
| Children with H. influenzae b meningitis **[A]**[27] | Dexamethasone | No therapy | Hearing loss at ? weeks | 12% | 0.31 (0.14 to 0.69) | 13 (10 to 30) |

## PREVENTION

- Arrange chemoprophylaxis for household contacts of patients with *Neisseria meningitidis* meningitis **[A]**.
  - Use a single dose of ceftriaxone 250 mg im **[A]**[29] or ciprofloxacin 600 mg orally **[A]**[28].

> **Why?**
> **Ceftriaxone and ciprofloxacin are more effective than rifampicin at eradicating nasopharyngeal meningococcus**

| Patient | Treatment | Comparison | Outcome | CER | RR (95% CI) | NNT (95% CI) |
|---|---|---|---|---|---|---|
| Household contacts of confirmed cases of meningococcal meningitis with positive nasal cultures **[A]**[29] | Single dose of im ceftriaxone | Oral rifampicin for 2 days | Eradication at 6 days | 75% | 29% (7% to 57%) | 5 (3 to 14) |
| Close household contact of patient with confirmed meningococcal meningitis, with nasopharyngeal meningococci **[A]**[28] | Single oral dose of ciprofloxacin 750 mg | Oral rifampicin for 2 days | Eradication at 2 weeks | 89% | 8% (−0.20% to 16%) | 13 6 to 5900) |

- There is no clear benefit from prophylactic antibiotics for base of skull fractures **[A]**[30].

**Why?**
■ Patients with basilar skull fractures who receive prophylactic antibiotics compared with those who do not are not clearly less likely to develop meningitis **[A]**[36].

## PROGNOSIS

### Bacterial meningitis

Mortality with bacterial meningitis is high **[A]**[31] **[B]**[32] **[B]**[5] **[B]**[33].

 **Note**
■ 19% to 27% of patients with bacterial meningitis die **[B]**[32] **[B]**[5] **[C]**[34]. More patients over 60 die (38%: 95% CI: 24% to 51%) **[A]**[31]. Fewer patients with meningococcal meningitis die (7.5%: 95% CI: 4.2% to 11%) **[B]**[5].

Seizures are common **[C]**[34] **[B]**[5].

 **Note**
■ One in four patients has seizures (23%: 95% CI: 19% to 27%) **[C]**[34] **[B]**[5].

Neurological sequelae are common; some will be disabled by their illness **[C]**[34] **[A]**[35].

 **Note**
■ Almost half of patients fail to make a complete recovery (44%: 95% CI: 34% to 54%) **[C]**[35].
■ One in four has focal neurologic signs (28%: 95% CI: 18% to 37%) **[C]**[35].
■ One in nine has severe disability or are in a vegetative state (11%: 95% CI: 4% to 17%) **[C]**[33].

- The risk of dying or suffering neurologic disability is increased with **[A]**[31] **[B]**[32] **[B]**[33]:
  - neck or back stiffness **[A]**[31]
  - hypotension **[B]**[32]
  - seizures **[B]**[32]
  - altered mental state **[B]**[32] **[C]**[35]
  - stenosis of intracranial arteries **[A]**[36]
  - anaemia on admission (Hb < 11 g/dl) **[B]**[33]

**Why?**

| Patient | Prognostic factor | Outcome | CER | OR (95% CI) | NNF+ (95% CI) |
|---|---|---|---|---|---|
| Patients aged 60 or more with meningitis [A][31] | Neck or back stiffness *independent* | Death at ? | 38% | 2.3 (1.6 to 3.4) | 4 (3 to 45) |
| Community-acquired meningitis [B][32] | Hypotension *Independent* | Death or neurological disability at ? | 35% | 2.75 (1.22 to 6.18) | 5 (2 to 30) |
| Community-acquired meningitis [B][32] | Seizures *independent* | Death or neurological disability at ? | 35% | 4.42 (1.56 to 12.5) | 4 (2 to 17) |
| Community-acquired meningitis [B][32] | Altered mental status *independent* | Death or neurological disability at ? | 10% | 6.56 (1.71 to 25.2) | 7 (6 to 16) |
| Community-acquired meningitis [A][36] | Stenosis of intracranial arteries *independent* | Death or severe disability at weeks | 55% | 7.4 (1.1 to 45.6) | 3 (2 to 43) |

- Increasing age and anaemia increase the risk of dying or severe disability [B][33].

## Viral meningitis
Viral meningitis is less severe [C][35]

 **Why?**
- Although half of patients have objective motor signs (54%: 95% CI: 48% to 59%) [C][35] only one in nine has a serious illness (11%: 95% CI: 8.4% to 15%) [C][35].

**Guideline writers**: Robert Phillips, Christopher Ball
**CAT writers**: Christopher Ball, Robert Phillips, Clare Wotton

## REFERENCES

| No | Level | Citation |
|---|---|---|
| 1 | 1b | Moosa AA, Quortum HA. Rapid diagnosis of bacterial meningitis with reagent strips. Lancet 1995; 345: 1290–1 |
| 2 | 2b | Uchihara T, Tsukagoshi H. Jolt accentuation of headache: the most sensitive sign of CSF pleocytosis. Headache 1990; 31: 167–171 |
| 3 | 2b | DeLozier JS, Auerbach PS. The leukocyte esterase test for detection of cerebrospinal fluid leukocytosis and bacterial meningitis. Ann Emerg Med 1989; 18: 1191–8 |
| 4 | 4 | Read SJ, Jeffery KJM, Bangham CRM. Aseptic meningitis and enchephalitis: the role of PCR in the diagnostic laboratory. J Clin Microbiol 1997; 35: 691–6 |
| 5 | 2c | Durand ML, Calderwood SB, Weber DJ et al. Acute bacterial meningitis in adults: a review of 493 episodes. N Engl J Med 1993; 328: 21–8 |

| No | Level | Citation |
|----|-------|----------|
| 6 | 2c | Sigurdardottir B, Bjornsson OM, Jonsdottir KE et al. Acute bacterial meningitis in adults: a 20-year overview. Arch Intern Med 1997; 157: 425–30 |
| 7 | 2c | Schuchat A, Robinson K, Wenger JD et al. Bacterial meningitis in the United States in 1995. N Engl J Med 1997; 337: 970–6 |
| 8 | 4 | Lepow ML, Carver DH, Wright HT et al. Clinical, epidemiologic and laboratory investigation of aseptic meningitis during the four-year period, 1955–1958 (I and II). N Engl J Med 1962; 266: 1181–7, 1188–93 |
| 9 | 2a | Attia J, Hatala R, Wong JG et al. Does this adult patient have acute meningitis? JAMA 1999; 282: 175–81 |
| 10 | 1b | Gopal AK, Whitehouse JD, Simel DL, et al. Cranial computed tomography before lumbar puncture: a prospective clinical evaluation. Archives of Internal Medicine 1999; 159: 2681–2685 |
| 11 | 3a | Archer BD. CT before LP in acute menigits: a review of the risks and benefits. Can Med Assoc J 1993; 148: 961–5 |
| 12 | 1b | Daniels AM. Headache, lumbar puncture, and expectation. Lancet 1981; (i): 1003 |
| 13 | 1a | Halpern S, preston R. Postdural puncture headache and spinal needle design: metaanalyses. Anesthesiology 1994; 81: 1376–83 |
| 14 | 4 | Carraccio C, Feinberg P, Sinclair L et al. Lidocaine for lumbar puncture: a help not a hindrance. Arch Pediatr Adolesc Med 1996; 150: 1044–6 |
| 15 | 1b | Strupp M, Brandt T. Should one reinsert the stylet during lumbar puncture? N Engl J Med 1997; 1190 |
| 16 | 1b– | Spriggs DA, Burn DJ, French J, et al. Is bed rest useful after diagnostic lumbar puncture? Postgraduate Medical Journal 1992; 68: 581–583 |
| 17 | 1b– | Handler CE, Smith FR, Perkin GD et al. Posture and lumbar puncture headache: a controlled trial in 50 patients. J R Soc Med 1982; 75: 404–7 |
| 18 | 2c | Spanos A, Harrell FE, Durack DT. Differential diagnosis of acute meningitis: an analysis of the predictive value of initial observations. JAMA 1989; 262: 2700–7 |
| 19 | 2b | DeLozier JS, and Auerbach PS. The leukocyte esterase test for detection of cerebrospinal fluid leukocytosis and bacterial meningitis. Annals of Emergency Medicine 1989; 18: 1191–1198 |
| 20 | 2b | Newcombe J, Cartwright K, Palmer WH et al. PCR of peripheral blood for diagnosis of meningococcal disease. J Clin Microbiol 1996; 34: 1637–40 |
| 21 | 4 | Ni H-L, Knight Al, Cartwright K et al. Polymerase chain reaction for diagnosis of meningococcal meningtis. Lancet 1992; 340: 1432–4 |
| 22 | 4 | Barnes RA, Jenkins P, Coakley WT. Preliminary clinical evaluation of meningococcal disease and bacterial meningitis by ultrasonic enhancement. Arch Dis Child 1998; 78: 58–60 |
| 23 | 4 | Williams G, Hart CA. Rapid identification of bacterial antigen in blood cultures and cerebrospinal fluid. J Clin Pathol 1988; 41: 691–3 |
| 24 | 2b | Cabellos C, Viladrich PF, Verdaguer R et al. A single daily dose of ceftriaxone for bacterial meningitis in adults: experience with 84 patients and review of the literature. Clin Infect Dis 1995; 20: 1164–8 |
| 25 | 2b | Girgis NI, Farid Z, Bishay E. Ceftriaxone in bacterial meningitis. Lancet 1989; 2: 510 |

| No | Level | Citation |
|----|-------|----------|
| 26 | 1b | Thomas R, Le Tulzo Y, Bouget J et al. Trial of dexamethasone treatment for severe bacterial meningitis in adults. Intensive Care Med 1999; 25: 475–80 |
| 27 | 1a | Mcintyre PB, Berkey CS, King SM et al. Dexamethasone as adjunctive therapy in bacterial meningitis: a meta-analysis of randomized clinical trials since 1988. JAMA 1997; 278: 925–31 |
| 28 | 1b | Cuevas LE, Kazembe P, Mughogho GK et al. Eradication of nasopharyngeal carriage of *Neisseria meningitidis* in children and adults in rural Africa: a comparison of ciprofloxacin and rifampicin. J Infect Dis 1995; 171: 728–31 |
| 29 | 1b | Schwartz B, Al-Tobaiqi A, Al-Ruwais A et al. Comparative efficacy of ceftriazone and rifampicin in eradicating pharyngeal carriage of group. A *Neisseria meningitidis*. Lancet 1988; (i): 1239–42 |
| 30 | 1a | Villalobos T, Arango C, Kubilis P, et al. Antibiotic prophylaxis after basilar skull fracture: a meta-analysis. Clinical Infectious Diseases 1998; 27: 364–369 |
| 31 | 1b | Rasmussen HH, Sorensen HT, Moller-Petersen J et al. Bacterial meningitis in elderly patients: clinical picture and course. Age Ageing 1992; 21: 216–20 |
| 32 | 2b | Aronin SI, Peduzzi P, Quagliarello VJ. Community-acquired bacterial meningitis: risk stratification for adverse clinical outcome and effect of antibiotic timing. Ann Intern Med 1998; 129: 862–9 |
| 33 | 2b | Andersen J, Backer V, Voldsgaard P et al. Acute meningococcal meningitis: analysis of features of the disease according to the age of 255 patients. J Infect 1997; 34: 227–35 |
| 34 | 4 | Pfister H-W, Feiden W, Einhaupl K-M: Spectrum of complications during bacterial meningitis: results of a prospective clinical study. Arch Neurol 1993; 50: 575–81 |
| 35 | 1b– | Schutte C-M, van der Meyden CH. A prospective study of Glasgow Coma Scale (GCS), age, CSF-neutrophil count, and CSF-protein and glucose levels as prognostic indicators in 100 adults patients with meningitis. J Infect 1998; 37: 112–15 |
| 36 | 1a | Muller M, Merkelbach S, Hermes M et al. Relationship between short-term outcome and occurrence of cerebral artery stenosis in survivors of bacterial meningitis. J Neurol 1998; 245: 87–92 |

## PREVALENCE

Myocardial infarction is a common cause of chest pain **[A]**[1] **[A]**[2].

>
> **Note**
> - One in six patients with chest pain has an MI (14% to 20%) **[A]**[1] **[A]**[2].
> - The risk is higher in elderly patients (20%; 95% CI: 19% to 22%) **[A]**[1] and patients with a typical history **[A]**[1].

It is defined as two of **[D]**:
- prolonged chest pain (> 20 min)
- characteristic rise and fall of cardiac enzymes
- characteristic changes on ECG.

## CLINICAL FEATURES

Ask about:

- Pain, specifically:
  - its position **[B]**[3]

**Why?**
Chest or left arm pain makes an MI more likely

| Patient **[B]**[3] | Target disorder (reference standard) | Diagnostic test | LR+ (95% CI) | Post-test probability |
|---|---|---|---|---|
| Attending emergency department with chest pain (pre-test probability 20%) | MI (ECG and cardiac enzyme changes) | Pain in chest or left arm | 2.7 | 40% |

  - its duration **[A]**[4] **[B]**[5] **[C]**[6]

**Why?**
Chest pain that began 48 h or more ago makes an MI more likely **[A]**[4].

Episodes of chest pain for over 1 year make coronary artery disease more likely

| Patient **[C]**[6] | Target disorder (reference standard) | Diagnostic test | LR+ (95% CI) | Post-test probability | LR− (95% CI) | Post-test probability |
|---|---|---|---|---|---|---|
| Intermittent chest pain referred for investigation (pre-test probability 67%) | Coronary artery disease (angiography and exercise test) | Chest pain for over 1 year | Infinity (3.5 to infinity) | 100% | 0.37 (0.23 to 0.59) | 43% |

> **?**
>
> **Constant pain makes a myocardial infarction more likely**
>
> | Patient **[B]**[5] | Target disorder (reference standard) | Diagnostic test | LR+ (95% CI) | Post-test probability | LR– (95% CI) | Post-test probability |
> |---|---|---|---|---|---|---|
> | Anterior chest pain (pre-test probability 12%) | MI (cardiac enzymes, ECG) | Constant pain | 1.7 (1.3 to 2.1) | 19% | 0.58 (0.41 to 0.82) | 8% |

– its nature **[A]**[2] **[A]**[4] **[B]**[3] **[B]**[5]

> **?**
>
> **Why?**
> **Pressure makes coronary artery disease more likely, but sharp or stabbing pain makes it less likely**
>
> | Patient **[A]**[2] | Target disorder (reference standard) | Diagnostic test | LR+ (95% CI) | Post-test probability | LR– (95% CI) | Post-test probability |
> |---|---|---|---|---|---|---|
> | Central or left-sided chest pain (pre-test probability 41%) | MI or unstable angina (ECG, cardiac enzymes, stress tests) | Pressure | 1.7 (1.4 to 2.0) | 54% | 0.67 (0.57 to 0.78) | 32% |
> | | | Sharp or stabbing pain | 0.41 (0.29 to 0.63) | 22% | 1.3 (1.2 to 1.5) | 48% |
>
> **A pleuritic chest pain makes unstable angina or a myocardial infarction unlikely**
>
> | Patient **[A]**[20] | Target disorder (reference standard) | Diagnostic test | LR+ (95% CI) | Post-test probability |
> |---|---|---|---|---|
> | Central or left-sided chest pain (pre-test probability 41%) | MI or unstable angina (ECG, cardiac enzymes, stress tests) | Pleuritic pain | 0.0 (0.0 to 0.12) | 0% |
> | | | Partly pleuritic pain | 0.22 (0.13 to 0.39) | 14% |
> | | | Pain not pleuritic | 1.4 (1.3 to 1.6) | 50% |
>
> **Positional chest pain makes unstable angina or a myocardial infarction less likely**
>
> | Patient **[A]**[21] | Target disorder (reference standard) | Diagnostic test | LR+ (95% CI) | Post-test probability |
> |---|---|---|---|---|
> | Central or left-sided chest pain (pre-test probability 41%) | MI or unstable angina (ECG, cardiac enzymes, stress tests) | Positional pain | 0.13 (0.030 to 0.54) | 8% |
> | | | Pain partly positional | 0.31 (0.20 to 0.48) | 18% |
> | | | Pain not positional | 1.4 (1.3 to 1.5) | 49% |

> ⏸ **Note**
> ■ Aching or burning pain is not helpful at diagnosing or excluding MI or unstable angina **[A]**[2].

– any radiation **[A]**[4], particularly to the right arm or shoulder **[B]**[3] **[B]**[5]

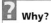 **Why?**
**Chest pain that radiates to the arms makes an MI more likely**

| Patient | Target disorder (reference standard) | Diagnostic test | LR+ (95% CI) | Post-test probability | LR– (95% CI) | Post-test probability |
|---|---|---|---|---|---|---|
| Anterior chest pain (pre-test probability 12%) **[B]**[5] | MI (cardiac enzymes, ECG) | Chest pain radiation to right shoulder | 2.9 (1.4 to 6.0) | 29% | 0.90 (0.81 to 1.0) | 11% |
| Attending emergency department with chest pain (pre-test probability 20%) **[B]**[3] | MI (ECG and cardiac enzyme changes) | Chest pain radiation to left arm | 2.3 (1.7 to 3.1) | 37% | | |
| | | Chest pain radiation to both left and right arms | 7.1 (3.6 to 14) | 64% | | |

– any similarity to previous infarcts on angina attacks **[A]**[4]

 **Why?**
■ Pain similar to previous MI or angina attacks makes an MI more likely **[A]**[4].

– any exacerbating or relieving factors **[B]**[7].

**Why?**
■ Pain brought on by exertion, or relieved by nitrates or rest, makes significant coronary artery disease more likely **[B]**[7].

● Nausea or vomiting **[B]**[3] **[B]**[5].

**? Why?**

**Nausea and vomiting make an MI more likely**

| Patient | Target disorder (reference standard) | Diagnostic test | LR+ (95% CI) | Post-test probability | LR− (95% CI) | Post-test probability |
|---|---|---|---|---|---|---|
| Attending emergency department with chest pain [B][3] (pre-test probability 20%) | MI (ECG and cardiac enzyme changes) | Nausea or vomiting | 1.9 (1.7 to 2.3) | 32% | | |
| Anterior chest pain [B][5] (pre-test probability 12%) | MI (cardiac enzymes, ECG) | History of associated nausea | 1.9 (1.4 to 2.4) | 21% | 0.63 (0.47 to 0.84) | 8% |

– Sweating [B][5].

**? Why?**

**Sweating makes an MI more likely**

| Patient [B][5] | Target disorder (reference standard) | Diagnostic test | LR+ (95% CI) | Post-test probability | LR− (95% CI) | Post-test probability |
|---|---|---|---|---|---|---|
| Anterior chest pain (pre-test probability 12%) | MI (cardiac enzymes, ECG) | History of sweating | 2.5 (2.0 to 3.3) | 26% | 0.52 (0.38 to 0.71) | 7% |

● History of:
  – angina or MI [A][4] [A][8] [B][3] [B][5]

**? Why?**

**Previous unstable angina or an MI makes a further episode more likely**

| Patient [A][2] | Target disorder (reference standard) | Diagnostic test | LR+ (95% CI) | Post-test probability | LR− (95% CI) | Post-test probability |
|---|---|---|---|---|---|---|
| Central or left-sided chest pain (pre-test probability 41%) | MI or unstable angina (ECG, cardiac enzymes, stress tests) | Previous history of MI or angina | 2.3 (1.9 to 2.7) | 62% | 0.37 (0.30 to 0.47) | 21% |

– heart failure [A][8]

**Why?**

■ Heart failure increases the risk of an MI **[A]**[8] and subsequent mortality **[A]**[9] **[A]**[10] **[B]**[11] **[B]**[12].

– an acute respiratory infection in the previous 10 days **[B]**[13].

**Why?**

**A respiratory infection within the previous 10 days slightly increases the risk of an MI**

| Outcome **[B]**[13] | Risk factor | PEER (%) | OR (95% CI) | NNH (95% CI) |
|---|---|---|---|---|
| MI | Respiratory tract infection within previous 10 days *independent* | 0.1% | 3.0 (1.1 to 2.4) | 500 (300 to 910) |

- Cardiovascular risk factors:
  – hypertension **[A]**[8] **[B]**[11] **[B]**[14] **[B]**[15]
  – smoking **[B]**[14]
  – diabetes mellitus **[A]**[8] **[A]**[16] **[B]**[14]
  – elevated total cholesterol or triglycerides **[A]**[8] **[B]**[17].

**Why?**

■ Cardiovascular risk factors increase the risk of dying **[A]**[16] **[B]**[11] **[B]**[14] or having a recurrent MI **[B]**[15] **[B]**[17].
■ Cardiovascular risk factors (smoking, hypertension, diabetes, etc.) are not clearly helpful at diagnosing an MI **[B]**[3].

**Cardiovascular disease increases the risk of an MI**

| Patient **[A]**[8] | Prognostic factor | Outcome | Control rate | OR (95% CI) | NNF+ (95% CI) |
|---|---|---|---|---|---|
| Aged 65 years or more | Clinical cardiovascular disease *independent* | MI at 5 years | 6.1% | 189 (1.47 to 2.42) | 18 (12 to 35) |

- Usual levels of activity **[A]**[18].

**Why?**

■ People with a sedentary lifestyle are at increased risk of having an MI or dying from coronary heart disease **[A]**[18].

- Parental history of angina or MI before the age of 60 years **[A]**[19].

**Why?**

■ A parental history of ischaemic heart disease before the age of 60 years increases the risk of MI **[A]**[19].

Look for:

- sweating [B][5]

| Why? Sweating makes an MI more likely | | | | | | |
|---|---|---|---|---|---|---|
| Patient [B][5] | Target disorder (reference standard) | Diagnostic test | LR+ (95% CI) | Post-test probability | LR– (95% CI) | Post-test probability |
| Anterior chest pain (pre-test probability 12%) | MI (cardiac enzymes, ECG) | Sweating | 4.6 (2.7 to 8.0) | 40% | 0.77 (0.66 to 0.90) | 10% |

- hypotension [B][5]

| Why? Hypotension makes an MI more likely | | | | |
|---|---|---|---|---|
| Patient | Target disorder (reference standard) | Diagnostic test | LR+ (95% CI) | Post-test probability |
| Attending emergency department with chest pain [B][3] (pre-test probability 20%) | MI (ECG and cardiac enzyme changes) | Hypotension (systolic BP ≤ 80 mmHg) | 3.1 (1.8 to 5.2) | 44% |

- Kussmaul's sign (JVP rising during quiet inspiration) [C][20]

| Why? | | | | | | |
|---|---|---|---|---|---|---|
| ■ It makes right ventricular infarction more likely in inferior MI [C][20]. | | | | | | |
| Inferior MI: Kussmaul's sign helps diagnose right ventricular failure | | | | | | |
| Patient [C][20] | Target disorder (reference standard) | Diagnostic test | LR+ (95% CI) | Post-test probability | LR– (95% CI) | Post-test probability |
| Acute inferior MI (pre-test probability 15%) | Right ventricular infarction (atrial pressure) | Kussmaul's sign | Infinity (5.9 to infinity) | 100% | 0.0 (0.0 to 0.73) | 0% |

- a third [B][5] or fourth heart sound [C][21]

**?** **Why?**
**A third heart sound makes an MI more likely**

| Patient | Target disorder (reference standard) | Diagnostic test | LR+ (95% CI) | Post-test probability | LR– (95% CI) | Post-test probability |
|---|---|---|---|---|---|---|
| Anterior chest pain [B][5] (pre-test probability 12%) | MI (cardiac enzymes, ECG) | Third heart sound on auscultation | 3.2 (1.6 to 6.5) | 31% | 0.88 (0.79 to 0.99) | 11% |

**A clearly audible S4 increases the risk of dying**

| Patient [C][21] | Prognostic factor | Outcome | Control rate | OR (95% CI) | NNF+ (95% CI) |
|---|---|---|---|---|---|
| MI | Clearly audible S4 ? independent | Death at 5 years | 12% | 4.29 (1.10 to 16.75) | 4 (4 to 96) |

- chest pain that is reproduced on palpation [A][2] [A][4] [B][3] [B][5]

**?** **Why?**
**Pain reproduced on palpation makes unstable angina or an MI less likely**

| Patient [A][2] | Target disorder (reference standard) | Diagnostic test | LR+ (95% CI) | Post-test probability |
|---|---|---|---|---|
| Central or left-sided chest pain (pre-test probability 41%) | MI or unstable angina (ECG, cardiac enzymes, stress tests) | Pain reproduced by chest wall palpation | 0.11 (0.057 to 0.21) | 7% |
| | | Pain partially reproduced by chest wall palpation | 0.43 (0.20 to 0.94) | 24% |
| | | Pain not reproduced by chest wall palpation | 1.6 (1.4 to 1.7) | 53% |

- pulmonary crackles [B][5].

**?** **Why?**
**Pulmonary crackles make an MI more likely**

| Patient | Target disorder (reference standard) | Diagnostic test | LR+ (95% CI) | Post-test probability | LR– (95% CI) | Post-test probability |
|---|---|---|---|---|---|---|
| Anterior chest pain [B][5] (pre-test probability 12%) | MI (cardiac enzymes, ECG) | Pulmonary crackles on auscultation | 2.1 (1.5 to 3.1) | 23% | 0.76 (0.62 to 0.92) | 10% |

> **Note**
> ■ In the elderly, the following features are less helpful at diagnosing an MI **[A]**[1]:
>   – male sex
>   – pain location and similarity to previous MI or angina
>   – ECG changes in the emergency department.

## DIFFERENTIAL DIAGNOSIS

Other common causes of chest pain include **[C]**[22]:

- angina
- pulmonary embolism
- chest infection
- musculoskeletal pain
- pericarditis.

Rarer causes include **[D]:**
- aortic dissection
- oesophageal spasm.

> **Note**
> **MI, angina and PE are common causes of chest pain**
>
> | Chest pain in emergency department **[A]**[1] **[A]**[2] **[C]**[22] | % |
> |---|---|
> | MI | 12% to 20% |
> | Unstable angina | 24% (21% to 27%) |
> | Stable angina | 9.0% (5.6% to 12%) |
> | PE | 5.8% (3.0% to 8.5%) |
> | Other pulmonary disease | 5.8% (3.0% to 8.5%) |
> | Chest wall pain | 5.4% (2.7% to 8.1%) |
> | Pericarditis | 5.0% (2.5% to 7.6%) |
> | Psychogenic | 2.9% (0.9% to 4.8%) |
> | Other heart disease | 1.1% (0.0% to 2.3%) |
> | Other disease | 1.1% (0.0% to 2.3%) |
> | Unknown | 11% (7.5% to 15%) |

## INVESTIGATIONS

Consider performing simple investigations (ECG, cardiac enzymes), even in low-risk patients **[A]**[23].

**Why?**

- Physicians are good at predicting which patients are at high risk for acute MI, but are less good at excluding it **[B]**[5] **[C]**[24].
- Patients at low risk for ischaemic heart disease who have an ECG and cardiac enzymes measured feel better, and have improved activity at 3 weeks **[A]**[23].

**Basic investigations make patients feel better**

| Patient **[A]**[23] | Treatment | Comparator | Outcome | CER | RRR | NNT |
|---|---|---|---|---|---|---|
| Chest pain at low risk for ischaemic heart disease | Basic investigations | No basic investigations | Activity same or less than before at 3 weeks | 20% | 120% (37% to 260%) | 4 (3 to 9) |
| | | | 'feel sick all the time' at 3 weeks | 11% | 130% (10% to 370%) | 7 (4 to 44) |

Perform:

- a blood count **[B]**[25]

 **Why?**

**A high leucocyte count or low relative lymphocyte percentage makes an MI more likely**

| Patient **[B]**[25] | Target disorder (reference standard) | Diagnostic test | LR+ (95% CI) | Post-test probability | LR– (95% CI) | Post-test probability |
|---|---|---|---|---|---|---|
| Central or left-sided chest pain (pre-test probability 18%) | MI (CK-MB at 24 hours) | Elevated leucocyte count | 6.8 (4.3 to 11) | 60% | 0.56 (0.45 to 0.70) | 11% |
| | | Decreased relative lymphocyte percentage | 6.3 (4.2 to 9.4) | 58% | 0.46 (0.35 to 0.61) | 9% |

- urea, electrolytes and creatinine **[D]**.
- glucose **[A]**[26]
- lipid levels **[A]**[27] **[A]**[28]
- serial cardiac enzymes, ideally CK-MB **[C]**[24] **[C]**[29].

**❓ Why?**

**Early CK-MB rise diagnoses an MI and normal levels at 20 h rule it out**

| Patient [C][24] | Target disorder (reference standard) | Diagnostic test | LR+ (95% CI) | Post-test probability | LR– (95% CI) | Post-test probability |
|---|---|---|---|---|---|---|
| Suspected MI (pre-test probability 18%) | MI (history, ECG, CK-MB$_{act}$) | Elevated CK-MB$_{mass}$ at 3 h after symptom onset: | Infinity (16 to infinity) | 100% | 0.68 (0.61 to 0.75) | 13% |
| | | at 4 h | 28 (19 to 42) | 86% | 0.45 (0.39 to 0.52) | 9% |
| | | at 6 h | 29 (19 to 44) | 86% | 0.13 (0.11 to 0.16) | 3% |
| | | at 8 h | 19 (13 to 27) | 81% | 0.063 (0.053 to 0.076) | 1% |
| | | at 12 h | 14 (11 to 18) | 75% | 0.032 (0.027 to 0.039) | 0.7% |
| | | at 20 h | 11 (8 to 16) | 71% | 0.00 (0.0 to 0.020) | 0% |

Less helpful alternatives include:

- troponin T [A][30] [A][31] [C][24] [C][29] or troponin I [C][29]

**❓ Why?**

**A normal troponin T at 20 h makes an MI unlikely**

| Patient [C][24] | Target disorder (reference standard) | Diagnostic test | LR+ (95% CI) | Post-test probability | LR– (95% CI) | Post-test probability |
|---|---|---|---|---|---|---|
| Suspected MI (pre-test probability) 18%) | MI (history, ECG, CK-MB$_{act}$) | Elevated troponin T at 3 h after symptom onset: | 6 (4 to 9) | 57% | 0.67 (0.59 to 0.76) | 13% |
| | | at 4 h | 11 (7 to 16) | 71% | 0.59 (0.52 to 0.67) | 9% |
| | | at 6 h | 7 (4 to 10) | 61% | 0.37 (0.31 to 0.43) | 8% |
| | | at 8 h | 9 (6 to 13) | 66% | 0.23 (0.19 to 0.27) | 5% |
| | | at 12 h | 9 (7 to 12) | 66% | 0.078 (0.064 to 0.094) | 2% |
| | | at 20 h | 9 (6 to 13) | 66% | 0.022 (0.019 to 0.027) | 0.5% |

**Why?**

**Normal CK-MB and troponin I can help rule out MI**

| Patient [C]29 | Target disorder (reference standard) | Diagnostic test | LR+ (95% CI) | Post-test probability | LR– (95% CI) | Post-test probability |
|---|---|---|---|---|---|---|
| Chest pain lasting for at least 15 min within previous 24 h [C]29 (pre-test probability 37%) | MI (CK-MB$_{mass}$ at 24 h) | Troponin I at 6 h | 10 (7.3 to 14) | 59% | 0.45 (0.37 to 0.56) | 6% |
| | | Troponin I at 18 h | 15 (11 to 19) | 67% | 0.045 (0.019 to 0.11) | 1% |

- myoglobin [C]24

**Why?**

**An elevated myoglobin diagnoses an MI, but normal levels cannot safely rule it out**

| Patient [C]24 | Target disorder (reference standard) | Diagnostic test | LR+ (95% CI) | Post-test probability | LR– (95% CI) | Post-test probability |
|---|---|---|---|---|---|---|
| Suspected MI (pre-test probability 18%) | MI (history, ECG, CK-MB$_{act}$) | Elevated myoglobin at 3 h after symptom onset: | 34 (23 to 49) | 88% | 0.33 (0.28 to 0.38) | 7% |
| | | at 4 h | 26 (17 to 38) | 85% | 0.24 (0.20 to 0.28) | 5% |
| | | at 6 h | 26 (17 to 39) | 85% | 0.23 (0.19 to 0.27) | 5% |
| | | at 8 h | 25 (17 to 36) | 85% | 0.26 (0.22 to 0.30) | 5% |
| | | at 12 h | 23 (16 to 31) | 83% | 0.33 (0.28 to 0.39) | 7% |
| | | at 20 h | 13 (8 to 20) | 74% | 0.63 (0.56 to 0.71) | 12% |

- serial creatine kinase (CK) [B]25 [C]32, aspartate transaminase (AST) [A]2, lactate dehydrogenase (LDH) [A]2 taken over 24 h [A]33

**Why?**

■ 96% of MIs can be diagnosed at 24 h using CK-MB, LDH, CK and ECG changes (95% to 98%)[A]33.

**Elevated creatine kinase levels diagnose MI**

| Patient [C]32 | Target disorder (reference standard) | Diagnostic test | LR+ (95% CI) | Post-test probability |
|---|---|---|---|---|
| Suspected MI (pre-test probability 64%) | MI (ECG changes) | Highest CK ≥ 280 iu/l | 54 (7.7 to 380) | 99% |
| | | CK 80–279 iu/l | 4.5 (2.7 to 7.3) | 89% |
| | | CK 40–79 iu/l | 0.30 (0.16 to 0.56) | 35% |
| | | CK < 40 iu/l | 0.013 (0.0032 to 0.051) | 2.0% |

## ? Why?

**Elevated AST levels taken 12 h or more after symptom onset help diagnose MI**

| Patient [A][2] | Target disorder (reference standard) | Diagnostic test | LR+ (95% CI) | Post-test probability |
|---|---|---|---|---|
| Central or left-sided chest pain (pre-test probability 41%) | MI (ECG, cardiac enzymes, stress tests) | AST taken more than 12 h after chest pain onset: | | |
| | | ≥ 100 iu/l | 30 | 89% |
| | | 80 iu/l | 2.3 | 39% |
| | | 60 iu/l | 5.6 | 60% |
| | | 50 iu/l | 0.40 | 10% |
| | | 40 iu/l | 0.59 | 14% |
| | | 30 iu/l | 0.32 | 8% |
| | | < 30 iu/l | 0.078 | 2% |

■ CK [A][2] [B][25], AST [A][2] or LDH [A][2] taken within 12 h of symptom onset cannot safely exclude an MI.

**Cardiac enzymes taken in the emergency department cannot diagnose or exclude an MI**

| Patient [A][2] | Target disorder (reference standard) | Diagnostic test | LR+ (95% CI) | Post-test probability | LR– (95% CI) | Post-test probability |
|---|---|---|---|---|---|---|
| Central or left-sided chest pain (pre-test probability 17%) | MI (ECG, cardiac enzymes) | CK> 180 iu | 1.8 (1.3 to 2.5) | 27% | 0.77 (0.65 to 0.91) | 14% |
| | | AST > 60 iu | 6.1 (3.5 to 10) | 56% | 0.43 (0.29 to 0.64) | 8% |
| | | AST > 47 iu | 3.4 (2.3 to 5.1) | 41% | 0.44 (0.29 to 0.68) | 8% |
| | | LDH > 200 iu | 2.0 | 29% | 0.59 | 11% |
| | | CK or AST abnormal | 1.7 (1.3 to 2.2) | 26% | 0.65 (0.51 to 0.82) | 12% |

**CK levels alone taken at 24 h cannot safely diagnose or exclude MI**

| Patient [B][25] | Target disorder (reference standard) | Diagnostic test | LR+ (95% CI) | Post-test probability | LR- (95% CI) | Post-test probability |
|---|---|---|---|---|---|---|
| Central or left-sided chest pain (pre-test probability 18%) | MI (CK-MB at 24 hours) | Elevated creatine kinase | 6.0 (3.7 to 9.8) | 57% | 0.62 (0.50 to 0.76) | 12% |

● a 12-lead ECG **[A]**[4] **[B]**[3] **[B]**[5] **[B]**[25] – read it carefully! **[A]**[34]

**? Why?**

ECG features suggestive of an MI make an MI or unstable angina more likely

| Patient [A][2] | Target disorder (reference standard) | Diagnostic test | LR+ (95% CI) | Post-test probability |
|---|---|---|---|---|
| Central or left-sided chest pain (pre-test probability 41%) | MI (ECG, cardiac enzymes, stress tests) | Probable MI | 8.7 (4.8 to 16) | 86% |
| | | Ischaemia or strain not known to be old | 3.1 (2.1 to 4.4) | 68% |
| | | Ischaemia or strain or infarction but changes known to be old | 1.7 (1.1 to 2.8) | 55% |
| | | Abnormal but not diagnostic of ischaemia | 0.47 (0.28 to 0.78) | 25% |
| | | Non-specific ST or T wave changes | 0.48 (0.35 to 0.67) | 25% |
| | | Normal | 0.078 (0.035 to 0.18) | 5% |

- Emergency physicians can misread ECGs for patients with cardiac chest pain – missing 12% of ST elevation and 12% of T wave inversion [A][34].

Look for features suggestive of cardiac ischaemia:

- any ST elevation, particularly if in two or more leads or not known to be old [A][4] [B][3] [B][5] [B][25]
- any ST depression, particularly if not known to be old [B][3] [B][5]
- any Q waves, particularly if in two leads or more or not known to be old [A][4] [B][3] [B][5]
- any T wave inversion, particularly if not known to be old [B][3] [B][5]
- any conduction defect, particularly if not known to be old [B][3] [B][5]

**? Why?**

ST elevation or depression, Q waves and T wave inversion help diagnose MI

| Patient | Target disorder (reference standard) | Diagnostic test | LR+ (95% CI) | Post-test probability | LR– (95% CI) | Post-test probability |
|---|---|---|---|---|---|---|
| Central or left-sided chest pain [B][25] (pre-test probability 18%) | MI (CK-MB at 24 h) | ST elevation in two contiguous leads | 62 (15 to 250) | 93% | 0.61 (0.51 to 0.74) | 12% |
| Attending emergency department with chest pain [B][3] (pre-test probability 20%) | MI (ECG and cardiac enzyme changes) | New ST segment elevation ≥ 1 mm | 5.7 to 54 | 59% to 93% | | |
| Anterior chest pain [B][5] (pre-test probability 12%) | | Any ST segment elevation | 11 (7.1 to 18) | 61% | 0.45 (0.34 to 0.60) | 6% |
| Attending emergency department with chest pain [B][3] (pre-test probability 20%) | | New ST depression | 3.0 to 5.2 | 43% | | |

**Why?**

**ST elevation or depression, Q waves and T wave inversion help diagnose MI (*contd.*)**

| Patient | Target disorder (reference standard) | Diagnostic test | LR+ (95% CI) | Post-test probability | LR– (95% CI) | Post-test probability |
|---|---|---|---|---|---|---|
| Anterior chest pain **[B]**[5] (pre-test probability 12%) | | Any ST segment depression | 3.2 (2.5 to 4.1) | 31% | 0.38 (0.26 to 0.56) | 5% |
| Attending emergency department with chest pain **[B]**[3] (pre-test probability 20%) | | New Q wave | 5.3 to 25 | 57% to 86% | | |
| Anterior chest pain **[B]**[5] (pre-test probability 12%) | | Any Q wave | 3.9 (2.7 to 5.7) | 36% | 0.60 (0.47 to 0.76) | 8% |
| | | T wave peaking and/or inversion ≥ 1 mm | 3.1 | 44% | | |
| | | New T wave inversion | 2.4 to 2.8 | 38% to 41% | | |
| Attending emergency department with chest pain **[B]**[3] (pre-test probability 20%) | | New conduction defect | 6.3 (2.5 to 16) | 61% | | |
| Anterior chest pain **[B]**[5] (pre-test probability 12%) | | Any conduction defect | 2.7 (1.4 to 5.4) | 28% | 0.89 (0.79 to 1.00) | 11% |
| | | Normal ECG | 0.1 to 0.3 | 2% to 7% | | |

**Note**

■ Few patients with a normal ECG go on to have life-threatening complications (1.3%; 95% CI: 0.0 to 3.0%) **[C]**[35].

**An abnormal admission ECG makes life-threatening complications more likely**

| Patient **[C]**[36] | Prognostic factor | Outcome | Control rate | RR (95% to CI) | NNF+ (95% CI) |
|---|---|---|---|---|---|
| Suspected MI | Abnormal admission ECG *not independent* | VT, VF or heart block at discharge | 1% | 23.7 (3.29 to 171) | 7 (1 to 73) |

● followed by serial ECGs **[A]**[37]

**Why?**

**Abnormalities on serial ECGs help diagnose an MI**

| Patient **[A]**[37] | Target disorder (reference standard) | Diagnostic test | LR+ (95% CI) | Post-test probability | LR– (95% CI) | Post-test probability |
|---|---|---|---|---|---|---|
| Chest pain (pre-test probability 20%) | MI (ECG at 24 hours, cardiac enzymes) | Initial ECG | 10 (7.5 to 14) | 72% | 0.47 (0.40 to 0.55) | 11% |
| | | Serial ECG | 13 (9.7 to 18) | 77% | 0.34 (0.27 to 0.41) | 8% |

- a chest X-ray[A].

Use the clinical prediction rule in Table 1 to rank your patient for risk of an MI [A]⁴.

**Table 1 Ranking a patient for risk of an MI**

| If clinical finding not present, go on to next question [A]⁴ | | | LR (95% CI) | Probability of MI (95% CI) |
|---|---|---|---|---|
| ST elevation or Q waves in ≥ 2 leads, not known to be old ⇓ | | | 22 (17 to 27) | 75% (70% to 79%) |
| Chest pain began ≥ 48 h ago | ⇒ | ST-T changes of ischaemia or strain, not known to be old ⇓ | 2.0 (1.5 to 2.9) | 22% (15% to 28%) |
| ⇓ | | No changes or old | 0.12 (0.076 to 0.19) | 1.6% (0.9% to 2.4%) |
| Previous history of angina or MI | ⇒ | ST-T changes of ischaemia or strain, not known to be old | 2.6 (2.0 to 3.2) | 26% (21% to 31%) |
| | | longest pain episode < 1 h | 0.30 (0.18 to 0.49) | 4.0% (2.1% to 5.9%) |
| ⇓ | | Pain worse than prior angina or the same as a prior MI ⇓ | 0.92 (0.65 to 1.3) | 11% (7.6% to 1.5%) |
| | | Pain not as bad | 0.076 (0.019 to 0.31) | 1.0% (0.0% to 2.5%) |
| Pain radiates to neck, left shoulder or left arm | ⇒ | Aged < 40 years | 0.18 (0.058 to 0.57) | 2.4% (0.0% to 5.1%) |
| | | ⇓ | | |
| | | Chest pain reproduced by palpation | 0.093 (0.013 to 0.67) | 1.3% (0.0% to 3.7%) |
| ⇓ | | Pain radiates to back, abdomen or legs ⇓ | 0.60 (0.25 to 1.5) | 7.7% (1.2% to 14%) |
| | | Chest pain stabbing ⇓ | 0.13 (0.018 to 0.94) | 1.8% (0.0% to 5.2%) |
| | | Chest pain not stabbing | 1.5 (1.1 to 2.0) | 1.7% (13% to 22%) |
| ST-T changes of ischaemia or strain, not known to be old ⇓ | | | 2.3 (1.7 to 3.3) | 26% (19% to 33%) |
| No changes or old | | | 0.15 (0.099 to 0.22) | 2.0% (1.2% to 2.8%) |

**? Why do this?**

- A third of patients can be classified as low risk (36%; 95% CI: 34% to 38%) – 1% will die in hospital (95% CI: 0.3% to 1.8%) and 0.4% have life-threatening complications (95% CI: 0.0% to 0.8%)

Patients at low risk for an MI can be assessed in a rapid evaluation unit [B]³⁸ by:

- CK-MB at 0, 4, 8, 12 h
- serial 12-lead ECGs
- clinical assessment at 0, 6, 12 h
- exercise ECG: if all the above negative.

**Why?**

**Patients at low risk for an MI who have no CK-MB rise or further pain within 12 h are unlikely to have one**

| Patient [B][39] | Target disorder (reference standard) | Diagnostic test | LR+ (95% CI) | Post-test probability | LR− (95% CI) | Post-test probability |
|---|---|---|---|---|---|---|
| Low-risk for MI (pre-test probability 7%) | MI (typical change in cardiac enzymes or cardiac arrest) | Cardiac enzyme rise or recurrent chest pain within 12 h | 6.8 (5.7 to 8.1) | 34% | 0.069 (0.027 to 0.18) | 0.5% |

■ Patients admitted to a rapid assessment unit are not clearly less likely to be diagnosed with an MI or unstable angina [D][40], but spend on average 40 h less in hospital [D][40].
■ Half of patients are still admitted to hospital (45%; 95% CI: 34% to 56%) [A][41].

Use the clinical prediction rule (Table 2) to help determine admission to coronary care units [A][42]. Look for the following risk factors:

- pain worse than prior angina or the same as the pain associated with a prior MI
- systolic blood pressure < 110 mmHg
- crackles above the bases bilaterally
- ST elevation or Q waves, not known to be old, in two or more leads
- ST segment or T wave changes, not known to be old, indicative of myocardial ischaemia.

**Table 2 Risk of major complications**

| Group [A][42] | Risk of major complication at 4 days |
|---|---|
| Suspected MI on ECG or Suspected ischaemia on ECG and ≥ 2 risk factors | High |
| Suspected ischaemia on ECG and 1 or no risk factor | Moderate |
| One risk factor with no MI or ischaemia on ECG | Low |
| No risk factors | Very low |

**Why do this?**

**A clinical prediction rule can help identify patients at risk of having major complications**

| Group [A][42] | Risk of major complication at 4 days | % (95% CI) | NNF (95% CI) |
|---|---|---|---|
| Suspected MI on ECG or Suspected ischaemia on ECG and ≥ 2 risk factor | High | 16% (12% to 20%) | 6 (5 to 8) |
| Suspected ischaemia on ECG and 1 or no factor | Moderate | 7.8% (6.0% to 9.6%) | 13 (11 to 17) |
| One risk factor with no MI or ischaemia | Low | 3.9% (2.7% to 5.2%) | 26 (19 to 37) |
| No risk factors | Very low | 0.58% (0.29% to 0.87%) | 170 (110 to 340) |

## THERAPY

Give:
- oxygen **[D]**
- analgesia **[A]**
- nitrous oxide **[B]**[43].

**Why do this?**
**Nitrous oxide added to oxygen helps reduce pain**

| Patient **[B]**[43] | Treatment | Comparator | Outcome | CER | RRR | NNT |
|---|---|---|---|---|---|---|
| Suspected MI | Nitrous oxide and oxygen | Oxygen | Reduction in pain at 1 year | 29% | 44% (61% to 28%) | 2 (2 to 4) |

- opiate analgesia **[A]**[44].

**Note**
- There is no clear difference for pain relief between 5 mg morphine, 5 mg pethidine or 5 mg nicomorphine **[D]**[44].

Give aspirin **[A]**[45].

**Why do this?**
- It reduces death, strokes and MIs **[A]**[45].
- Patients who continue to take aspirin have benefit for up to 3 years **[A]**[45].
- 75–325 mg of aspirin daily is as effective as higher doses **[A]**[45].

**Antiplatelet medication reduces death, stroke and recurrent MI**

| Patient **[A]**[45] | Treatment | Comparator | Outcome | CER | OR | NNT |
|---|---|---|---|---|---|---|
| Acute MI | Antiplatelet drug | Placebo | Death, stroke, MI at 1 to 2 years | 14% | 0.29 (0.23 to 100) | 26 (21 to 35) |

Alternatives include:
- clopidrogel **[A]**[46].

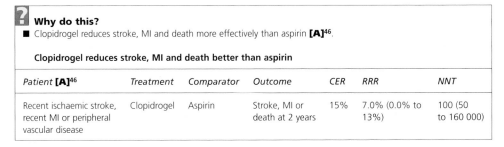

**Why do this?**
- Clopidrogel reduces stroke, MI and death more effectively than aspirin **[A]**[46].

**Clopidrogel reduces stroke, MI and death better than aspirin**

| Patient **[A]**[46] | Treatment | Comparator | Outcome | CER | RRR | NNT |
|---|---|---|---|---|---|---|
| Recent ischaemic stroke, recent MI or peripheral vascular disease | Clopidrogel | Aspirin | Stroke, MI or death at 2 years | 15% | 7.0% (0.0% to 13%) | 100 (50 to 160 000) |

There is no clear benefit from:

- adding fixed-dose warfarin to aspirin **[D]**[47].

> **Why?**
> ■ Patients are not clearly less likely to die or to have a non-fatal MI or an ischaemic stroke **[D]**[47].

For patients with ≥ 1 mm ST elevation in two contiguous limb leads or ≥ 2 mm in two contiguous precordial leads **[A]**[48]:

- offer primary angioplasty if available **[A]**[49].

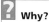

> **Why do this?**
> ■ It is more effective than thrombolysis (even tPA) – fewer patients die or have another infarction, recurrent ischaemia or a stroke.
> ■ There is no clear difference for major bleeding, subsequent need for bypass surgery or long-term mortality.
> ■ It is more cost-effective than thrombolysis **[C]**[50].
>
> **Primary angioplasty is more effective than thrombolysis at reducing death, reinfarction and stroke**

| Patient **[A]**[49] | Treatment | Comparator | Outcome | CER | OR | NNT |
|---|---|---|---|---|---|---|
| MI | Primary angioplasty | Thrombolysis | Death at ?months | 6.5% | 0.67 (0.48 to 0.94) | 49 (30 to 270) |
| | | | Reinfarction at ?months | 7.2% | 0.47 (0.32 to 0.69) | 27 (21 to 47) |
| | | | Any stroke at ?months | 2.4% | 0.35 (0.18 to 0.68) | 64 (50 to 130) |
| | | | Recurrent ischaemia at ?months | 15% | 0.42 (0.31 to 0.57) | 12 (10 to 17) |

There is no clear benefit from offering urgent angioplasty after thrombolysis **[D]**[51] **[D]**[52].

> **Why?**
> ■ Patients with a first MI who receive urgent angioplasty after thrombolysis compared with thrombolysis alone are not clearly less likely to die or have another MI **[D]**[51] or require subsequent revascularisation **[D]**[52].

Avoid using:

■ prophylactic intra-aortic balloon counterpulsation following primary angioplasty **[A]**[53].

**? Why?**

■ More patients develop strokes, but there is no clear reduction in mortality, reinfarction or heart failure **[A]**[53].

**Prophylactic intra-aortic balloon counterpulsation causes stroke**

| Patient **[A]**[53] | Treatment | Comparator | Outcome | CER | RRR | NNH |
|---|---|---|---|---|---|---|
| MI treated with primary angioplasty | Prophylactic intra-aortic balloon counterpulsation | No treatment | Stroke at ? weeks | 0.0% | | 42 (23 to 320) |

Otherwise give thrombolysis **[A]**[54] as soon as possible **[A]**[55] if there are no contraindications such as:

● active bleeding **[A]**
● recent surgery or trauma **[C]**
● recent stroke **[A]**[56]
● active peptic ulcer disease **[D]**
● evidence of aortic dissection **[D]**.

**? Why do this?**

■ Thrombolysis reduces mortality, but there is a small increased risk of stroke **[A]**[54]. Fewer patients have ventricular arrhythmias **[A]**[57].
■ It is cost-effective **[A]**[58] **[A]**[59].

**Thrombolysis reduces mortality but slightly increases the risk of stroke**

| Patient **[A]**[54] | Treatment | Comparator | Outcome | CER | RRR | NNT |
|---|---|---|---|---|---|---|
| Suspected MI | Thrombolysis | No thrombolysis | Death at 1 month | 12% | 16% (12% to 20%) | 54 (43 to 74) |
| | | | Any stroke at 1 month | 0.76% | 52% (79% to 28%) | 250 (120 to 180) |

**Thrombolysis reduces VT and VF**

| Patient **[A]**[57] | Treatment | Comparator | Outcome | CER | ARR | NNT |
|---|---|---|---|---|---|---|
| MI | Thrombolysis | No thrombolysis | Ventricular tachycardia or fibrillation at discharge | — | 2.7% (0.5% to 4.8%) | 37 (21 to 200) |

■ Patients receive benefit from thrombolysis for up to 12 h, but the reduction in mortality decreases the longer thrombolysis is delayed **[A]**[60].

**Early thrombolysis saves lives**

| Thrombolysis given within | NNT (95% CI) |
|---|---|
| 1 h | 15 (11 to 26) |
| 2–3 h | 27 (18 to 50) |
| 3–6 h | 38 (27 to 71) |
| 6–12 h | 34 (25 to 52) |
| 12–24 h | 110 (NNT = 45 to infinity, NNH = 200 to infinity) |

Consider using alteplase (tPA) **[A]**[48] **[A]**[61] **[A]**[62] rather than streptokinase, particularly for:

- older patients **[A]**[63] **[A]**[64]
- patients with an anterior MI **[A]**[63] **[A]**[64]
- patients who have received streptokinase or anistreplase in the previous 5 days to 6 months **[D].**

 **Why do this?**

- Alteplase reduces death **[A]**[48] **[A]**[61] and reinfarction better than streptokinase, but causes more strokes **[A]**[48] **[A]**[61] **[A]**[65].
- Fewer patients on alteplase suffer allergic reactions or profound hypotension **[A]**[62].
- However, alteplase costs more than streptokinase – it is most cost-effective in elderly patients and patients with anterior MI **[A]**[63] **[A]**[64]. It is not clearly cost-effective for patients aged <40-years with an anterior MI, or patients aged <60-years with an inferior MI **[A]**[64].

**Alteplase reduces death and reinfarction compared with streptokinase, but causes more strokes**

| Patient | Treatment | Comparator | Outcome | CER | RRR | NNT |
|---|---|---|---|---|---|---|
| MI **[A]**[48] **[A]**[61] | tPA | Streptokinase | Death at 1 year | 10% | 12% (5% to 20%) | 80 (49 to 230) |
| | | | Stroke at 1 month | 1.2% | −28% (−63% to −11%) | −290 (−5000 to −150) |
| MI **[A]**[62] | tPA | Streptokinase | Reinfarction at 1 month | 3.5% | 16% (4% to 26%) | 180 (100 to 800) |
| | | | Allergic reaction at 1 month | 3.6% | 78% (73% to 82%) | 35 (32 to 40) |
| | | | Profound hypotension at 1 month | 12% | 40% (35% to 44%) | 21 (19 to 25) |

 **Note**

- Combining alteplase and streptokinase is less effective than using alteplase alone **[A]**[48] **[A]**[61]

Alternatives that may be easier to give than alteplase include:

- reteplase **[A]**[66]
- tenecteplase **[A]**[67].

 **Why?**

- Patients who receive reteplase and tenecteplase compared with alteplase are not less likely to die or have a stroke **[A]**[66] **[A]**[67].

## Note

- One in eight patients have moderate or severe bleeding after thrombolysis (13%; 95% CI: 13% to 14%) **[A]**[68]; 5.0% have a major bleed (95% CI: 3.9% to 6.0%) **[B]**[69].
- Ocular haemorrhage is extremely rare (0.03%; 95% CI: 0.01% to 0.05%) **[B]**[70].
- Few patients develop a cardiac tamponade following thrombolysis (1%; 95% CI: 0.03% to 2.02%) **[C]** [71].
- 1.1% of patients given thrombolysis will have a stroke (95% CI 0.99% to 1.3%) **[B]**[65].
- The risk of major bleeding is increased with **[A]**[68]:
  - female sex
  - African ancestry
  - increasing age.

**Women, persons African ancestry and older patients are at increased risk of bleeding**

| Patient **[A]**[68] | Prognostic factor | Outcome | Control rate | OR (95% CI) | NNF+ (95% CI) |
|---|---|---|---|---|---|
| MI given thrombolysis | Female *independent* | Moderate or severe bleeding at 30 days | 7.8% | 1.42 (1.31 to 1.53) | 34 (27 to 46) |
| | African ancestry *independent* | | | 1.33 (1.12 to 1.57) | 29 (17 to 77) |
| | Increasing age *independent* | | | 1.30 (1.26 to 1.35) | |

- The risk of stroke is increased with **[B]**[65]:
  - severe hypertension
  - increasing age
  - heart failure
  - use of alteplase
  - an anterior MI.

**Severe hypertension, increasing age and heart failure increase the risk of a stroke after thrombolysis**

| Patient **[B]**[65] | Prognostic factor | Outcome | Control rate | OR (95% CI) | NNF+ (95% CI) |
|---|---|---|---|---|---|
| MI | Alteplase (versus streptokinase) *independent* | Stroke at ? days | 1.1% | 1.42 (1.09 to 1.84) | 210 (110 to 1000) |
| | Aged 60–70 years *independent* | | | 1.67 (1.15 to 2.41) | 130 (64 to 590) |
| | Aged >70 years *independent* | | | 2.72 (1.85 to 4.00) | 53 (31 to 110) |
| | Anterior site of MI *independent* | | | 1.38 (1.06 to 1.79) | 240 (110 to 1500) |
| | Killip class 2 at admission *independent* | | | 1.49 (1.10 to 2.03) | 182 (87 to 890) |
| | Killip class 3 or 4 at admission *independent* | | | 1.87 (1.14 to 3.09) | 110 (45 to 660) |
| | Diastolic blood pressure >110 mmHg *independent* | | | 2.88 (1.11 to 7.49) | 48 (15 to 810) |

## Note

- Cardiac enzyme levels post-thrombolysis cannot usefully identify failed reperfusion **[C]**[72].

Consider:
- anticoagulating patients with anterior MI who do not receive thrombolysis **[A]**[73]

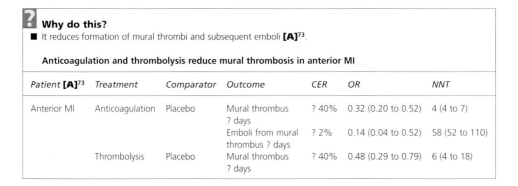

**?** **Why do this?**
- It reduces formation of mural thrombi and subsequent emboli **[A]**[73].

**Anticoagulation and thrombolysis reduce mural thrombosis in anterior MI**

| Patient **[A]**[73] | Treatment | Comparator | Outcome | CER | OR | NNT |
|---|---|---|---|---|---|---|
| Anterior MI | Anticoagulation | Placebo | Mural thrombus ? days | ? 40% | 0.32 (0.20 to 0.52) | 4 (4 to 7) |
| | | | Emboli from mural thrombus ? days | ? 2% | 0.14 (0.04 to 0.52) | 58 (52 to 110) |
| | Thrombolysis | Placebo | Mural thrombus ? days | ? 40% | 0.48 (0.29 to 0.79) | 6 (4 to 18) |

- giving LMWH long-term **[A]**[74].

**?** **Why do this?**
Patients on LMWH for 6 months are less likely to die from heart disease, reinfarct or develop angina **[A]**[74].

**LMWH reduces death, reinfarction and angina**

| Patient **[A]**[74] | Treatment | Comparator | Outcome | CER | RRR | NNT |
|---|---|---|---|---|---|---|
| MI | Clexane | No therapy | MI, angina or cardiac death at 6 months | 45% | 69% (31% to 86%) | 3 (2 to 7) |

There is no clear benefit from:
- heparin **[A]**[62] **[A]**[75–77]

**?** **Why?**
- Adding heparin to aspirin reduces the risk of dying slightly, but increases the risk of severe bleeding (requiring a transfusion) **[A]**[62] **[A]**[75–77].
- The effect on stroke is unclear **[A]**[77].

**Adding heparin to aspirin slightly reduces death and slightly increases severe bleeding**

| Patient | Treatment | Comparator | Outcome | CER | OR | NNT |
|---|---|---|---|---|---|---|
| MI **[A]**[77] | Aspirin and heparin | Aspirin | Death at ? months | 9% | 0.94 (0.9 to 1.0) | 200 (120 to infinity) |
| | | | Severe bleeding at ? months | 1.1% | 1.4 (1.2 to 1.7) | −230 (−60 to −430) |
| MI **[A]**[75] | Heparin | No heparin | Any bleeding at ? | 16% | 1.55 (1.21 to 1.98) | 15 (9 to 36) |

- hirudin [D][78].

**Why?**

■ It is not clearly more effective than heparin at reducing death, reinfarction or severe heart failure, nor less likely to cause severe bleeding [D][78].

Give:

- an insulin–glucose infusion [A][26] for 24 h followed by subcutaneous insulin, four times daily for at least 3 months to patients with an admission glucose > 11.0 mmol/l [A][79]

**Why do this?**

■ Patients with an acute MI and an admission glucose > 11.0 mmol/l who receive an intensive insulin regimen compared with standard treatment are less likely to die [A][79] [A][80].

**Intensive insulin treatment reduces mortality for patients with a glucose > 11.0 mmol/l**

| Patient [A][79] [A][80] | Treatment | Comparator | Outcome | CER | RRR | NNT |
|---|---|---|---|---|---|---|
| MI and admission glucose >11.0 mmol/l | iv insulin infusion for 24 h followed by sc insulin 4 times daily for 3 months | Standard treatment | Death at 3.4 years | 44% | 24% (7% to 38%) | 9 (5 to 33) |

- beta-blockers [A][81–83] as soon as possible [A][84]

**Why do this?**

■ Long-term beta-blockers reduce death and reinfarction better than placebo, but patients are more likely to stop medication. There is no clear benefit from short-term beta-blockers [A][81].
■ Patients who receive beta-blockers immediately compared with after 6 days are less likely to develop recurrent chest pain within 6 days or reinfarct within 6 weeks. There is no clear effect on mortality [A][84].

**Beta-blockers reduce death and reinfarction**

| Patient [A][81] | Treatment | Comparator | Outcome | CER | OR | NNT |
|---|---|---|---|---|---|---|
| Acute or recent MI | Beta-blockers | Control | Death at 2 years | 11% | 0.77 (0.69 to 0.85) | 44 (32 to 68) |
| | | | Reinfarction at 2 years | 8% | ? | 110 (63 to 330) |

**Patients on beta-blockers are more likely to stop medication**

| Patient [A][81] | Treatment | Comparator | Outcome | CER | ARR | NNH |
|---|---|---|---|---|---|---|
| Acute or recent MI | Beta-blockers | Control | Withdrawal at 2 years | 22% | −1.16% (−1.76% to −0.56%) | 86 (57 to 180) |

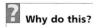

**Why do this?**

**Beta-blockers given early reduce recurrent chest pain and reinfarction**

| Patient [A][84] | Treatment | Comparator | Outcome | CER | RRR | NNT |
|---|---|---|---|---|---|---|
| MI [A][84] | Beta-blockers immediately | Beta-blockers at 6 days | Fatal or non-fatal reinfarction at 6 days | 5.0% | 48% (10% to 70%) | 42 (23 to 430) |
| | | | Recurrent chest pain at 6 days | 24% | 22% (4% to 36%) | 19 (11 to 100) |
| | | | Fatal or non-fatal infarction at 6 weeks | 7.1% | 38% (4% to 60%) | 37 (20 to 350) |

● an ACE inhibitor [A][85], particularly for patients with a reduced left ventricular ejection fraction (< 40%) [A][86] [A][87] unless patients have cardiogenic shock or a systolic blood pressure of < 100 mmHg [C][89].

**Why do this?**

- ACE inhibitors reduce death and non-fatal heart failure, but increase the risk of persistent hypotension, renal dysfunction and cardiogenic shock [A][85].
- It is cost-effective [A][88].
- Fewer patients with LV dysfunction die [A][89–91], reinfarct [A][90] or develop heart failure [A][89] [A][90] or atrial fibrillation [A][92], but the risk of hypotension and renal failure is increased [A][89].

**ACE inhibitors started within 36 h reduce death and heart failure**

| Patient [A][85] | Treatment | Comparator | Outcome | CER | RRR | NNT |
|---|---|---|---|---|---|---|
| MI | ACE inhibitor started within 36 h and continued for 4–6 h | No ACE inhibitor | Death at 30 days | 7.6% | 6% (2% to 10%) | 210 (130 to 660) |
| | | | Non-fatal heart failure at 30 days | 14% | 3% (0.4% to 6%) | 200 (110 to 1600) |
| | | | Persistent hypotension at 30 days | 9.2% | −90% (−97% to −84%) | −12 (−13 to −11) |
| | | | Renal dysfunction at 30 days | 0.64% | −98% (−126% to −73%) | −160 (−200 to −30) |
| | | | Cardiogenic shock at 30 days | 3.5% | −13% (−21% to −6%) | −220 (−450 to −140) |

**ACE inhibitors reduce death, heart failure and reinfarction in patients with reduced LV function**

| Patient | Treatment | Comparator | Outcome | CER | RRR | NNT |
|---|---|---|---|---|---|---|
| MI and clinical heart failure [A][89] | Ramipril | Placebo | Death at 6 months | 23% | 25% (10% to 37%) | 18 (11 to 46) |
| | | | Severe or resistant heart failure at 6 months | 18% | 3.9% (0.65% to 7.1%) | 26 (14 to 160) |
| | | | Severe adverse effects (hypotension, renal failure, syncope) at 6 months | 64% | 5.6% (1.5% to 10%) | 17 (10 to 67) |

**❓ Why?**

**ACE inhibitors reduce death, heart failure and reinfarction in patients with reduced LV function (*contd.*)**

| Patient | Treatment | Comparator | Outcome | CER | RRR | NNT |
|---|---|---|---|---|---|---|
| MI and asymptomatic LV dysfunction [A][90] | Captopril | Placebo | Death at 3.5 years | 25% | 17% (3% to 29%) | 24 (13 to 140) |
| | | | Severe heart failure at 3.5 years | 16% | 34% (18% to 47%) | 18 (12 to 38) |
| | | | Hospitalised with heart failure at 3.5 years | 17% | 20% (2% to 34%) | 29 (16 to 260) |
| | | | Recurrent MI at 3.5 years | 15% | 22% (3% to 37%) | 30 (16 to 220) |
| MI and impaired LV function [A][92] | Trandolapril | Placebo | Atrial fibrillation at 2 years | 5.3% | 48% (13% to 69%) | 39 (22 to 170) |

Continue ACE inhibitors in all patients with one other cardiovascular risk factor (hypertension, elevated total cholesterol levels, low high-density lipoprotein cholesterol levels, cigarette smoking or documented microalbuminuria) [A][93].

**❓ Why do this?**

- Patients at high-risk for cardiovascular disease who take ramipril are less likely to die or to have a stroke, MI or cardiac arrest or to develop heart failure [A][93].
- Many patients stop therapy, particularly due to cough [A][93].

**Ramipril reduces death and cardiovascular complications in patients at high-risk for cardiovascular disease**

| Patient | Treatment | Comparator | Outcome | CER | RRR | NNT |
|---|---|---|---|---|---|---|
| Previous stroke, MI or peripheral vascular disease and at least one other cardiovascular risk factor | Ramipril | Placebo | Death from any cause at 5 years | 12% | 15% (5% to 24%) | 55 (32 to 180) |
| | | | MI at 5 years | 12% | 19% (9% to 28%) | 44 (28 to 99) |
| | | | Stroke at 5 years | 4.9% | 30% (15% to 43%) | 68 (44 to 150) |
| | | | Heart failure at 5 years | 12% | 22% (12% to 31%) | 39 (26 to 77) |
| | | | Cardiac arrest at 5 years | 1.3% | 36% (4% to 58%) | 220 (120 to 2400) |
| | | | Discontinued therapy permanently at 5 years | 31% | −6% (−3% to −0.086%) | −52 (−3500 to −26) |
| | | | Treatment discontinued due to cough at 5 years | 1.9% | −300% (−410% to −220%) | −18 (−22 to −16) |

There is no clear benefit from:

- calcium-channel blockers [A]⁸³ [A]⁹⁴ [A]⁹⁵

**Why?**
- Nifedipine has no clear effect on mortality [A]⁹⁴ [A]⁹⁵ [D]⁹⁶, but causes side-effects [A]⁹⁷.
- Verapamil and diltiazem reduce rates of reinfarction, but have no clear effect on mortality [A]⁸³ [A]⁹⁴ [A]⁹⁸ or development of heart failure [D]⁹⁹.

**Verapamil or diltiazem reduces reinfarction**

| Patient [A]⁹⁴ [A]⁹⁵ | Treatment | Comparator | Outcome | CER | OR | NNT |
|---|---|---|---|---|---|---|
| MI or unstable angina | Verapamil or diltiazem | Control | Reinfarction at 2 days to 6 weeks | 7.5% | 0.79 (0.67 to 0.94) | 68 (43 to 240) |

**Nifedipine causes side-effects**

| Patient [A]⁹⁷ | Treatment | Comparator | Outcome | CER | RRR | NNT |
|---|---|---|---|---|---|---|
| MI | Nifedipine | Placebo | Side-effects at 28 days | 4.2% | 2% (1% to 4%) | 43 (27 to 98) |

- magnesium sulphate [A]⁸⁶

**Why?**
- Patients given magnesium sulphate have no clear reduction in mortality, reinfarction or arrhythmias, but are at increased risk of developing heart failure, cardiogenic shock and severe hypotension [A]⁸⁶ [A]¹⁰⁰.

**Magnesium sulphate increases the risk of heart failure and severe hypotension**

| Patient | Treatment | Comparator | Outcome | CER | RRR | NNH |
|---|---|---|---|---|---|---|
| MI | Magnesium sulphate | Placebo | Heart failure at 5 weeks | 16% | −7% (−11% to −3%) | −84 (−56 to −170) |
| | | | Cardiogenic shock at 5 weeks | 4.0% | −11% (−20% to −3%) | −220 (−130 to −750) |
| | | | Treatment withdrawal due to severe hypotension at 24 h | 4.7% | −110% (−120% to −96%) | −20 (−18 to −21) |

- nitrates [A]⁸⁶ [A]¹⁰¹.

**Why?**
Patients given nitrates compared with placebo are not clearly less likely to die [A]⁸⁶ [A]¹⁰¹, reinfarct or develop heart failure, but more stop medication due to severe hypotension [A]⁸⁶.

Observe patients for at least 5 days **[D]**[102].

**Why do this?**
- Discharging patients within 3 days of an infarction is not clearly as safe as remaining in hospital for at least 5 days **[D]**[103].

Provide cardiac rehabilitation **[A]**[103] involving:

- a structured exercise programme **[A]**[104]
- psychosocial interventions **[A]**[105] – encourage patients to be realistic about their illness **[C]**[106].

**Why do this?**
- Cardiac rehabilitation reduces death, particularly from cardiovascular causes **[A]**[103].
- A structured exercise programme reduces death, but there is no clear effect on reinfarction rates **[A]**[104].

**Cardiac rehabilitation reduces mortality**

| Patient | Treatment | Comparator | Outcome | CER | OR | NNT |
|---|---|---|---|---|---|---|
| MI **[A]**[103] | Cardiac rehabilitation | No cardiac rehabilitation | Death at >2 years | 16% | 0.76 (0.63 to 0.92) | 30 (19 to 91) |
| MI **[A]**[104] | Structured exercise programme | Usual daily activity | Death at 3 years | 13% | 0.80 (0.66 to 0.96) | 43 (25 to 220) |

- Rehabilitation programmes with a formal psychosocial component help reduce mortality and morbidity **[A]**[105].
- Patients are more likely to return to work if they view their illness as less severe **[C]**[106].

## PREVENTION

Encourage patients to eat a Mediterranean-style diet **[A]**[107].

**Why do this?**
- Patients who eat more bread, more root and green vegetables, more fish, less meat (beef, lamb and pork to be replaced with poultry), have no day without fruit and replaced butter and cream with margarine, rapeseed and olive oils are less likely to have another MI than patients who continue their usual diet **[A]**[107].
**A Mediterranean-style diet reduces further MI and cardiovascular death**

| Patient **[A]**[107] | Treatment | Comparator | Outcome | CER | RRR | NNT |
|---|---|---|---|---|---|---|
| MI | Mediterranean-style diet | Usual diet | Cardiovascular death at 3 years | 5.3% | 81% (36% to 94%) | 23 (14 to 65) |
| | | | Non-fatal MI at 3 years | 5.6% | 70% (21% to 89%) | 25 (14 to 100) |

Lower cholesterol levels **[A]**[108], even for patients with average levels (cholesterol 4.0–6.2 mmol/l) **[A]**[109] **[A]**[110]

**Why do this?**

■ Patients with coronary artery disease who have cholesterol-lowering therapy are less likely to die, particularly from heart disease **[A]**[108].

**Lowering cholesterol reduces mortality**

| Patient **[A]**[108] | Treatment | Comparator | Outcome | CER | RRR | NNT |
|---|---|---|---|---|---|---|
| Coronary artery disease | Cholesterol-lowering therapy | No therapy | Deathat > 2 years | 10% | 16% (12% to 19%) | 63 (51 to 81) |
| | | | Death from coronary heart disease at > 2 years | 6.4% | 28% (24% to 32%) | 56 (48 to 67) |

■ Patients with cholesterol levels < 6.2 mmol/l who take pravastatin are less likely to have another MI or die from heart disease, or require invasive therapy **[A]**[109] **[A]**[110].

**Pravastatin reduces MI or invasive therapy in patients with cholesterol levels < 6.2 mmol/l**

| Patient | Treatment | Comparator | Outcome | CER | RRR | NNT |
|---|---|---|---|---|---|---|
| MI and cholesterol levels < 6.2 mmol/l **[A]**[109] | Pravastatin | Placebo | Non-fatal MI at 5 years | 8.3% | 28% (9% to 47%) | 43 (26 to 140) |
| | | | CABG or PTCA at 5 years | 19% | 26% (14% to 37%) | 21 (14 to 39) |
| MI or unstable angina and cholesterol levels 4.0–7.0 mmol/l **[A]**[110] | | | Death at 6 years | 14% | 22% (12% to 30%) | 33 (23 to 60) |
| | | | Hospitalisation with unstable angina at 6 years | 25% | 9% (2% to 16%) | 44 (25 to 180) |

using:

● diet modification **[A]**[111]: encourage patients to eat less fat **[A]**[112] (particularly cholesterol **[A]**[113]) and more oats **[A]**[114], fish **[A]**[115] and soy protein **[A]**[116]

**Why do this?**

■ Diet modification can lower cholesterol levels slightly, but there is no clear effect on blood pressure levels **[A]**[111].
■ Low-fat diets help reduce cholesterol levels **[A]**[112] – on average by 0.6 mmol/l. Triglycerides fall on average by 0.2 mmol/l **[A]**[113].
■ Patients who eat oat products have a small fall in cholesterol levels (0.13 mmol/l; 95% CI: 0.017 to 0.19) **[A]**[114].
■ Eating around 50 g of soy protein a day reduces cholesterol level by roughly 0.6 mmol/l, and triglyceride levels by 0.2 mmol/l **[A]**[116].
■ Patients who eat more fish (at least two weekly portions of fatty fish) are less likely to die **[A]**[115].

**Eating more fish reduces mortality**

| Patient **[A]**[115] | Treatment | Comparator | Outcome | CER | RRR | NNT |
|---|---|---|---|---|---|---|
| MI | Increased fish intake | Usual diet | Death at 2 years | 13% | 27% (7% to 44%) | 28 (16 to 130) |

- a statin **[A]**[117] **[A]**[118]

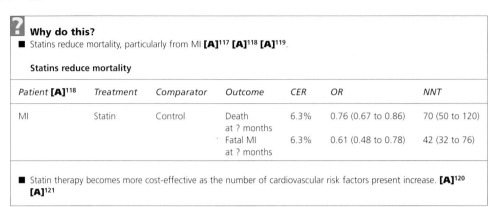

- Statins reduce mortality, particularly from MI **[A]**[117] **[A]**[118] **[A]**[119].

**Statins reduce mortality**

| Patient **[A]**[118] | Treatment | Comparator | Outcome | CER | OR | NNT |
|---|---|---|---|---|---|---|
| MI | Statin | Control | Death at ? months | 6.3% | 0.76 (0.67 to 0.86) | 70 (50 to 120) |
| | | | Fatal MI at ? months | 6.3% | 0.61 (0.48 to 0.78) | 42 (32 to 76) |

- Statin therapy becomes more cost-effective as the number of cardiovascular risk factors present increase. **[A]**[120] **[A]**[121]

- gemfibrozil for patients with a low HDL level **[A]**[122].

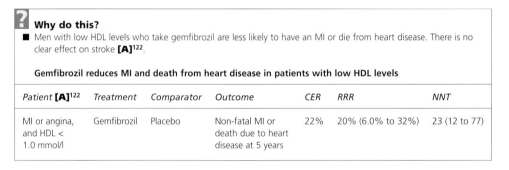

**?** **Why do this?**
- Men with low HDL levels who take gemfibrozil are less likely to have an MI or die from heart disease. There is no clear effect on stroke **[A]**[122].

**Gemfibrozil reduces MI and death from heart disease in patients with low HDL levels**

| Patient **[A]**[122] | Treatment | Comparator | Outcome | CER | RRR | NNT |
|---|---|---|---|---|---|---|
| MI or angina, and HDL < 1.0 mmol/l | Gemfibrozil | Placebo | Non-fatal MI or death due to heart disease at 5 years | 22% | 20% (6.0% to 32%) | 23 (12 to 77) |

Consider giving patients:
- n-3 polyunsaturated fatty acid supplements **[A]**[123]

**?** **Why do this?**
- Patients given n-3 polyunsaturated fatty acids are less likely to die, have an MI or a stroke **[A]**[123].

**n-3 polyunsaturated fatty acids reduce death, MI or stroke**

| Patient | Treatment | Comparator | Outcome | CER | RRR | NNT |
|---|---|---|---|---|---|---|
| MI | n-3 polyunsaturated fatty acids | Placebo | Death, MI or stroke at 3.5 years | 15% | 14% (2.0% to 25%) | 48 (26 to 330) |

- vitamin E supplements (alpha-tocopherol) **[A]**[124].

**Why do this?**

Alpha-tocopherol reduces non-fatal MI **[A]**[124]. There is no clear effect on mortality or stroke **[A]**[123] **[A]**[124].

**Vitamin E reduces non-fatal MI in proven coronary artery disease**

| Patient **[A]**[124] | Treatment | Comparator | Outcome | CER | RRR | NNT |
|---|---|---|---|---|---|---|
| Proven coronary artery disease | Alpha-tocopherol | Placebo | Non-fatal MI at 1.4 years | 4.2% | 68% (42% to 82%) | 35 (23 to 70) |

Avoid giving:
- beta-carotene **[A]**[125].

**Why?**

It increases mortality, despite reducing non-fatal MI **[A]**[125]

**Beta-carotene reduces non-fatal MI but increases mortality**

| Patient **[A]**[125] | Treatment | Comparator | Outcome | CER | RRR | NNT |
|---|---|---|---|---|---|---|
| MI | Beta-carotene | Placebo | Non-fatal MI at 6 years | 13% | 33% (1% to 54%) | 24 (12 to 1200) |
| | | | Death at 6 years | 8.9% | −80% (−160% to −25%) | −14 (−35 to −9) |

There is no clear benefit from giving postmenopausal women oestrogen and progestin **[D]**[126].

**Why?**

- There is no significant reduction in MI or death from heart disease **[D]**[126].

Treat hypertension **[A]**[127].

**Why do this?**

- Treating hypertension with low-dose diuretics or beta-blockers reduces stroke, cardiovascular disease and heart failure **[A]**[127].
- The benefits are greater for elderly patients **[A]**[128], particularly with diuretics **[A]** [129].

**Hypertension: beta-blockers and low-dose diuretics reduce stroke and heart failure**

| Patient **[A]**[127] | Treatment | Comparator | Outcome | CER | OR | NNT |
|---|---|---|---|---|---|---|
| Hypertension | Low-dose diuretics | Placebo | Stroke at 5 years | 6.8% | 0.66 (0.55 to 0.78) | 42 (32 to 65) |
| | | | Coronary heart disease at 5 years | 7.1% | 0.71 (0.59 to 0.86) | 120 (81 to 240) |
| | Beta-blockers | Placebo | Heart failure at 5 years | 2.6% | 0.72 (0.61 to 0.85) | 51 (37 to 95) |
| | | | Stroke at 5 years | 2.8% | 0.58 (0.44 to 0.76) | 91 (68 to 160) |
| | | | Heart failure at 5 years | 1.4% | 0.58 (0.40 to 0.84) | 170 (120 to 430) |

Encourage patients to stop smoking **[A]**¹³⁰, and ask nurses **[A]**¹³¹ and other staff **[B]**¹³² to provide further advice.

**Why do this?**

■ Patients who continue to smoke are at increased risk of dying or having another MI **[A]**¹³³.

**Patients who keep smoking are at increased risk of dying or reinfarcting**

| Patient [A]¹³³ | Prognostic factor | Outcome | Control rate | RR (95% CI) | NNF+ (95% CI) |
|---|---|---|---|---|---|
| MI | Continuing to smoke *independent* | Death at 10 years | 23% | 1.60 (1.26 to 2.02) | 9 (6 to 21) |
| | | Non-fatal MI at 10 years | 24% | 1.50 (1.20 to 1.88) | 10 (6 to 27) |

■ Patients who receive advice from doctors are more likely to stop **[A]**¹³⁰, and from nurses are more likely to stay off cigarettes **[A]**¹³¹.
■ A nurse-run smoking cessation programme is cost-effective **[A]**¹³⁴.

**Physician advice helps patients stop smoking**

| Patient [A]¹³⁰ | Treatment | Comparator | Outcome | ARR | NNT |
|---|---|---|---|---|---|
| MI | Physician advice | No advice | Stopped smoking at ? months | 36% (23% to 48%) | 3 (2 to 4) |

**Nursing advice helps smokers stop cigarettes long-term**

| Patient [A]¹³¹ | Treatment | Comparator | Outcome | CER | OR | NNT |
|---|---|---|---|---|---|---|
| Adult smoker | Nursing advice | No advice | Sustained smoking cessation at ? | 13% | 1.43 (1.24 to 1.66) | 22 (15 to 39) |

■ Two-thirds of men with an MI who receive repeated advice to stop smoking will quit (63%; 95% CI: 55% to 72%). A sixth will continue smoking at the same rate (15%; 95% CI: 8.9% to 22%) **[B]**¹³¹.

Offer nicotine patches **[A]**¹³⁵ or gum **[A]**¹³⁰.

**Why do this?**

■ Nicotine replacement patches help patients with coronary artery disease quit **[A]**¹³⁵ without clearly causing cardiac disease or severe adverse effects **[D]**¹³⁶. Patches are cost-effective **[A]**¹³⁷.
■ Nicotine gum helps smokers quit **[A]**¹³⁰.

**Nicotine patches help smokers quit**

| Patient [A]¹³⁵ | Treatment | Comparator | Outcome | CER | RRR | NNT |
|---|---|---|---|---|---|---|
| Smokers with coronary artery disease | Nicotine patches | Placebo | Stopped smoking at 5 weeks | 22% | 15% (0.1% to 29%) | 7 (3 to 130) |

**Why do this?**
Nicotine gum helps smokers quit

| Patient [A][130] | Treatment | Comparator | Outcome | ARR | NNT |
|---|---|---|---|---|---|
| Smoker | Nicotine gum | No gum | Stopped smoking at ? months | 3% (2% to 5%) | 30 (20 to 50) |

There is no clear benefit from:
● a vigorous exercise programme [D][138].

**Why?**
■ Women who undergo a vigorous exercise programme are not clearly less likely to stop smoking [D][138].

Consider:
● giving amiodarone [A][139] [A][140], particularly to patients with ventricular arrhythmias [A][141].

**Why do this?**
■ Patients with an acute MI or congestive heart failure who take prophylactic amiodarone are less likely to die, particularly from arrhythmias [A][139].

**Amiodarone reduces death**

| Patient [A][139] | Treatment | Comparator | Outcome | CER | OR | NNT |
|---|---|---|---|---|---|---|
| Acute MI or congestive heart failure | Amiodarone | Placebo or usual care | Death at ? months | 8.6% | 0.87 (0.78 to 0.99) | 97 (57 to 1300) |
|  |  |  | Arrhythmic or sudden death at ? months | 4.0% | 0.71 (0.59 to 0.85) | 90 (63 to 180) |

Avoid using:
● class I antiarrhythmic agents [A][140], particularly class Ic drugs [A][142] [A][143] and lidocaine [A][144] [A][145]

**Why?**
Patients at risk of sudden cardiac death who receive class I antiarrhythmics are more likely to die [A][140].

**Class I antiarrhythmic drugs increase mortality**

| Patient | Treatment | Comparator | Outcome | CER | OR | NNH |
|---|---|---|---|---|---|---|
| At risk of sudden cardiac death [A][140] | Class I antiarrhythmic agent | Control | Death at ? months | 5.0% | 1.13 (1.01 to 1.27) | 160 (79 to 2100) |
| MI [A][146] | Class I antiarrhythmic agent | Control | Death at ? months | 5.0% | 1.14 (1.01 to 1.28) | 150 (76 to 2100) |

**Why?**

**Encainide and flecainide increase mortality**

| Patient [A]142 [A]143 | Treatment | Comparator | Outcome | CER | RRR | NNH |
|---|---|---|---|---|---|---|
| MI poor ejection fraction and mildly symptomatic arrhythmias | Encainide or flecainide | Placebo | Death or cardiac arrest at 10 months | 3.5% | −140% (−270% to −53%) | 21 (14 to 40) |

■ Prophylactic lidocaine does not clearly reduce death or occurrence of ventricular fibrillation [A]145. Lidocaine given only to patients with early ventricular arrhythmias is not clearly better than prophylactic lidocaine [D]147.

• sotalol [A]148.

**Why?**

■ Patients with LV dysfunction who receive prophylactic sotalol compared with placebo are at increased risk of dying [A]148.

**Sotalol increases mortality with heart failure**

| Patient | Treatment | Comparator | Outcome | CER | RRR | NNH |
|---|---|---|---|---|---|---|
| MI and heart failure | Sotalol | Placebo | Death at 5 months | 3.1% | 65% (140% to 16%) | 50 (30 to 170) |

Perform stress testing using any of:
• Myocardial perfusion imaging [B]149
• echocardiography [B]149
• a symptom-limited [B]150 exercise tolerance test looking for [B]149:
  – limited exercise duration
  – impaired systolic blood pressure changes
  – ST segment depression > 1 mm.

**Why do this?**

■ Patients who have symptom-limited tolerance tests compared with low-level tests are more likely to show signs of ischaemia [B]150.
■ Abnormal exercise tolerance tests slightly increase the risk of dying from heart disease [B]149.
■ ST segment depression on exercise test increases the risk of recurrent MI [A]151.

**Abnormal stress testing slightly increases the risk of dying from heart disease**

| Patient [B]149 | Prognostic factor | Outcome | Control rate | OR (95% CI) | NNF+ (95% CI) |
|---|---|---|---|---|---|
| MI | Exercise ECG: ST depression > 1 mm | Death from heart disease at ? months | 4.4% | 1.7 (1.2 to 2.5) | 35 (17 to 120) |
| | Exercise ECG: impaired systolic BP | Death from heart disease at ? months | 4.4% | 4.0 (2.5 to 6.3) | 9 (6 to 17) |

**? Why do this?**
**Abnormal stress testing slightly increases the risk of dying from heart disease (*contd.*)**

| Patient [B][149] | Prognostic factor | Outcome | Control rate | OR (95% CI) | NNF+ (95% CI) |
|---|---|---|---|---|---|
| | Exercise ECG: limited exercise duration | | 4.4% | 4.0 (1.9 to 8.4) | 9 (4 to 27) |
| | Myocardial perfusion imaging; Exercise testing: reversible perfusion defect | | | 3.1 (1.6 to 4.6) | 12 (8 to 41) |
| | Ventricular function; exercise stress: ejection fraction < 40% | | | 3.2 | 12 |
| | Ventricular function; exercise stress: ejection fraction change < 5% | | | 4.2 | 8 |
| | Ventricular function; exercise stress: new dyssynergy | | | 1.2 | 120 |
| | Ventricular function; pharmacological stress: new dyssynergy | | | 2.7 (1.4 to 5.2) | 15 (7 to 60) |

Refer all patients for arteriography (followed by PTCA or CABG as required) if they develop [A][152]:

- symptomatic angina pectoris during predischarge exercise test
- ST changes during exercise, compatible with ischaemia.

**? Why do this?**

■ Performing angiography followed by PTCA or CABG on all patients with post-infarction ischaemia reduces subsequent reinfarction and unstable angina compared with conservative management unless patients have severe angina. There is no clear effect on mortality [A][152].

**Invasive therapy following MI reduces reinfarction and unstable angina compared with conservative therapy**

| Patient [A][152] | Treatment | Comparator | Outcome | CER | RRR | NNT |
|---|---|---|---|---|---|---|
| MI | Invasive therapy (arteriography and PTCA or CABG) | Medical therapy | Unstable angina at 12 months | 39% | 39% (24% to 52%) | 9 (6 to 16) |
| | | | Reinfarction at 12 months | 11% | 47% (18% to 66%) | 20 (12 to 63) |

## PROGNOSIS

### Complications
Watch out for [B][153]:

- arrhythmias
- mitral regurgitation
- ventricular septal rupture
- signs of heart failure
- post-infarct angina.

**Why?**
- Complications are common, particularly arrhythmias and cardiogenic shock [B][153].
- Half of patients with inferior MI have complications (47%; 95% CI: 40 to 54%) [A][154].

**Common complications include AV block, cardiogenic shock and ventricular fibrillation**

| Complication [B][153] | % (95% CI) | NNF at 30 days (95% CI) |
|---|---|---|
| AV block | 8.2% (7.9% to 8.5%) | 12 (12 to 13) |
| Ventricular fibrillation | 6.6% (6.4% to 6.9%) | 15 (15 to 16) |
| Sustained ventricular tachycardia | 6.1% (5.9% to 6.3%) | 16 (16 to 17) |
| Asystole | 5.7% (5.4% to 5.9%) | 18 (17 to 18) |
| Cardiogenic shock | 7.2% (7.0% to 7.5%) | 14 (13 to 14) |
| Acute mitral regurgitation | 1.4% (1.3% to 1.5%) | 72 (66 to 78) |
| Ventricular septal defect | 0.48% (0.41% to 0.54%) | 210 (190 to 250) |

### Arrhythmias
Ventricular arrhythmias are common post-arrest [B][153] for up to 6 months [B][155].
Watch out for cardiac arrests[B][156].

**Note**
- 5.6% of patients will have an episode of VF within 6 months (95% CI: 5.1% to 6.1%) [B][155]. One in five dies (19%; 95% CI: 12% to 26%) [B][157].
- 2.9% of patients will have a cardiac arrest (95% CI: 2.1% to 3.7%) [B][156].

The risk of VF is increased with [B][155]:

- young age
- admission bradycardia
- hypotension
- current smoking
- an inferioposterior infarct
- widespread ST elevation
- hypokalaemia.

**Why?**

Hypokalaemia, hypotension and smoking increase the risk of VF

| Patient | Prognostic factor | Outcome | Control rate | OR (95% CI) | NNF+ (95% CI) |
|---------|-------------------|---------|--------------|-------------|---------------|
| First MI **[B]**[155] | Serum K+ < 3.6 mmol/l *independent* | VF at 6 months | 5.6% | 1.97 (1.51 to 2.56) | 270 (13 to 38) |
| | Systolic BP < 120 mmHg *independent* | | | 1.74 (1.34 to 2.26) | 27 (16 to 57) |
| | Current smoking *independent* | | | 1.66 (1.15 to 2.41) | 30 (14 to 130) |
| | > Three leads with ST elevation *independent* | | | 1.66 (1.24 to 2.23) | 30 (16 to 80) |
| | Age < 71 years *independent* | | | 1.61 (1.08 to 2.40) | 32 (15 to 240) |
| | inferioposterior infarct *independent* | | | 1.45 (1.10 to 1.91) | 43 (22 to 190) |
| | Admission bradycardia (< 60 beats/minute) *independent* | | | 1.39 (1.05 to 1.84) | 50 (24 to 380) |

Bradycardias are common within the first 24 h **[B]**[158], but are more problematic with inferior MI **[A]**[159].

**Note**

- A fifth of patients have bradycardia within 4 h of symptom onset 21% (95% CI; 17% to 25%), but many settle – only a tenth have bradycardia after this time (9.0%; 95% CI: 4.2% to 13%) **[B]**[158].
- One in ten patients with an inferior MI go on to develop complete heart block (9.4%; 95% CI: 7.1% to 11%) **[A]**[159].
- Second- or third-degree heart block within 24 h of admission is not clearly associated with death **[B]**[160].

## Heart failure and cardiogenic shock

Look for evidence of heart failure **[B]**[12], particularly cardiogenic shock **[A]**[153]**[A]**[161].

Cardiogenic shock is relatively common and often fatal **[A]**[153]**[A]**[161].

**Why?**

- 3.9% will develop congestive heart failure (95% CI: 3.5% to 4.3%) **[B]**[12].
- One in 14 patients develops cardiogenic shock in hospital (7.5%; 95% CI: 6.8% to 8.3%) **[A]**[153] **[A]**[161] **[A]**[162].
- Over half of patients with cardiogenic shock die (55% to 77%) **[A]**[153] **[A]**[161].

The risk of developing heart failure is increased with:

- a dilated heart [B][12]
- a reduced ejection fraction [B][12].

| Why? | | | | | |
|------|--|--|--|--|--|
| **A dilated heart and a reduced ejection fraction increase the risk of congestive heart failure** | | | | | |
| Patient [B][12] | Prognostic factor | Outcome | Control rate (%) | RR (95% CI) | NNF+ (95% CI) |
| MI; survived 6 weeks | 10% decrease in ejection fraction | Death or congestive heart failure at 6 months | — | 1.59 (1.48 to 1.71) | |
| | 10 ml increase in end-systolic volume | | — | 1.34 (1.28 to 1.41) | |
| | 10 ml increase in end-diastolic volume | | — | 1.16 (1.12 to 1.20) | |

Rank your patient's severity using the Killip classification (Table 3).

| Table 3 Killip classification | |
|-------------------------------|--|
| Killip class [C][163] | Signs |
| I | No clinical signs of heart failure |
| II | Crackles, S3 gallop and elevated JVP |
| III | Frank pulmonary oedema |
| IV | Cardiogenic shock – hypotension (systolic BP < 90 mmHg) and evidence of peripheral vasoconstriction (oliguria, cyanosis, sweating) |

| Why? | | | | | |
|------|--|--|--|--|--|
| **Worsening Killip class increases the risk of dying** | | | | | |
| Patient | Prognostic factor | Outcome | Control rate | OR (95% CI) | NNF+ (95% CI) |
| MI [B][164] | Killip class IV v. I independent | Death at 1 month | 5.1% | 7.86 (5.88 to 10.49) | 4 (3 to 5) |
| | Killip class III v. I independent | | | 4.37 (3.34 to 5.71) | 7 (5 to 10) |
| MI [A][165] | Killip class II or more independent | Death at 18 months | 4.0% | 6.16 (2.01 to 18.83) | 6 (3 to 27) |
| **Cardiogenic shock greatly increases the risk of dying** | | | | | |
| Patient [A][161] | Prognostic factor | Outcome | Control rate | OR (95% CI) | NNF+ (95% CI) |
| MI | Cardiogenic shock independent | Death at discharge | 14% | 11.3 (8.22 to 15.5) | 1 (1 to 1) |

The risk of dying from cardiogenic shock is increased with [B]162:

- old age (> 65 years)
- reduced left ventricular ejection fraction (< 35%)
- elevated CK-MB (> 160 iu)
- diabetes mellitus
- previous MI.

There is no clear benefit from:

- intra-aortic balloon counterpulsation for cardiogenic shock [D]166.

**Why?**
- Patients with early heart failure who receive intra-aortic balloon counterpulsation are not clearly less likely to die [D]166.

## Pericarditis and pericardial effusions
Listen for a pericardial rub [C]167.

**Note**
- Pericardial effusions are common (25%; 95% CI: 21% to 30%) [C]167 [C]168, but less than half have an associated pericardial rub (46%; 95% CI: 35 to 57%) [C]167.

**A pericardial rub increases the risk of dying**

| Patient | Prognostic factor | Outcome | Control rate | RR (95% CI) | NNF+ (95% CI) |
|---------|-------------------|---------|--------------|-------------|---------------|
| MI [C]169 | Clinical pericardial rub *not independent* | Death at discharge | 6% | 5 (2 to 10) | 4 (2 to 12) |

Give NSAIDs if there is evidence of pericarditis [D]170.

**Why do this?**
- NSAIDs reduce pain, but watch out for side-effects [D]170.

## Ventricular rupture
Look for evidence of ventricular rupture [C]171 – it is often fatal [B]172:

- cardiac tamponade
- pulseless electrical activity
- a large pericardial effusion (> 5 mm diameter on echocardiography)
- haemopericardium on pericardiocentesis.

**Note**
**Ventricular rupture is uncommon**

| Complication [C][171] | % (95% CI) | NNF at 30 days (95% CI) |
|---|---|---|
| Ventricular rupture | 0.89% (0.41% to 1.4%) | 110 (73 to 240) |

■ One in 50 patients develops ventricular septal rupture (2.0%; 95% CI: 1.2% to 2.7%) **[B]**[172]. Over half die from it (56%; 95% CI: 37 to 76%) **[B]**[172].

**Cardiac tamponade and a large pericardial effusion increase the risk of ventricular rupture**

| Patient [C][171] | Target disorder (reference standard) | Diagnostic test | LR+ (95% CI) | Post-test probability | LR– (95% CI) | Post-test probability |
|---|---|---|---|---|---|---|
| MI (pre-test probability 0.9%) | Subacute ventricular rupture (surgery or autopsy) | Cardiac tamponade | 140 | 56% | 0.30 | 0.3% |
| | | Pericardial effusion >5 mm | 14 | 11% | 0.0 | 0.0% |
| | | Electromechanical dissociation | 71 | 39% | 0.79 | 0.7% |
| | | Haemopericardium (pericardiocentesis) | 4.3 | 4% | 0.0 | 0.0% |

## Reinfarction

Further MIs can occur **[A]**[173] **[B]**[174].

**Note**
■ 2.6% have a recurrent infarction within 1 year (95% CI: 0.5% to 4.6%) **[A]**[173]; 31% have a reinfarction within 10 years (95% CI: 27% to 36%) **[B]**[174].
■ One in five patients will have unstable angina or MI in the next year (18%; 95% CI: 16% to 21%) **[B]**[175].

The risk of reinfarction is increased with:

- hypertension **[B]**[174]
- elevated total cholesterol or triglycerides **[B]**[176]
- angina before MI **[A]**[173]
- a non-Q wave MI **[B]**[174]
- worsening angiographic findings **[A]**[173]
- ST segment depression on exercise test **[A]**[173].

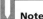

**Why?**
Hypertension and a non-Q wave MI increase the risk of reinfarction

| Patient [B][174] | Prognostic factor | Outcome | Control rate | OR (95% CI) | NNF+ (95% CI) |
|---|---|---|---|---|---|
| MI | Hypertension *independent* | Reinfarction at 10 years | 48% | 1.80 (1.10 to 3.20) | 7 (4 to 42) |
| | Non-Q wave MI *independent* | | | 1.80 (1.10 to 3.10) | 8 (18 to 52) |

## Angina

Post-infarct angina is relatively common **[A]**[173].

**Note**
■ One in nine patients develops angina within 12 months (12%; 95% CI: 7.5% to 16%) **[A]**[173].

Refer all patients with symptomatic angina pectoris presenting spontaneously >36 h after admission for arteriography, followed by PTCA or CABG as required **[A]**[177].

**Why do this?**
■ Performing angiography followed by PTCA or CABG on all patients with post-infarction ischaemia reduces subsequent reinfarction and unstable angina compared with conservative management unless patients have severe angina. There is no clear effect on mortality **[A]**[177].

**Invasive therapy following MI reduces reinfarction and unstable angina compared with conservative therapy**

| Patient [A][177] | Treatment | Comparator | Outcome | CER | RRR | NNT |
|---|---|---|---|---|---|---|
| MI | Invasive therapy (arteriography and PTCA or CABG) | Medical therapy | Unstable angina at 12 months | 39% | 39% (24% to 52%) | 9 (6 to 16) |
| | | | Reinfarction at 12 months | 11% | 47% (18% to 66%) | 20 (12 to 63) |

See chapter on **Unstable angina** for more details on therapy.

## Left ventricular aneurysms

Look for evidence of ventricular aneurysms **[B]**[178].

**Why do this?**
■ Ventricular aneurysms increase the risk of systemic emboli; 1.3% will have systemic emboli within 5 years (95% CI: 0.0% to 3.9%) **[B]**[178].
■ A third of patients with ventricular aneurysms will die within 5 years (37%; 95% CI: 26% to 48%) **[B]**[178].

Start anticoagulation if patients have an aneurysm **[B]**[178].

**Why do this?**
■ Anticoagulation reduces this risk of systemic emboli **[B]**[178].

## Mitral regurgitation
Listen for mitral regurgitation **[A]**[179].

**Why?**
■ It is common, though rarely clinically detectable **[A]**[179].
■ One in eight patients develops mitral regurgitation within 7 h (13%; 95% CI: 8.5% to 18%) – one in 40 has moderate to severe regurgitation (2.4%; 95% CI: 0.33% to 4.5%) **[A]**[179].
■ One in five patients with LV dysfunction develops mitral regurgitation within 2 weeks (19%; 95% CI: 17% to 22%) **[B]**[180].

**Mitral regurgitation increases the risk of dying**

| Patient | Prognostic factor | Outcome | Control rate | OR (95% CI) | NNF+ (95% CI) |
|---|---|---|---|---|---|
| MI **[B]**[180] | Mitral regurgitation *independent* | Death from heart disease at 2 years | 12% | 2.00 (1.28 to 3.04) | 11 (6 to 35) |

## Death
Some patients will die **[A]**[179].

**Why?**
■ One in 30 dies within 10 days (3.4%; 95% CI: 0.92% to 5.9%) **[A]**[179].
■ The risk is higher in elderly patients (15%; 95% CI: 15% to 16%) **[A]**[181], and lower in patients with an inferior MI (3 to 4%) **[B]**[182] **[B]**[183].

The risk of dying remains high long-term **[A]**[165] **[A]**[173] **[A]**[179] **[B]**[174] **[B]**[180].

**Why?**
■ 4 to 8% die within 12 months **[B]**[12] **[A]**[165] **[A]**[173] **[A]**[179].
■ One in 30 who survive 6 weeks will die in the next 6 months (3.1%; 95% CI: 3.5% to 4.3%) **[B]**[12].
■ 15% die from heart disease within 2 years **[B]**[180], and over 60% die within 10 years (95% CI: 58% to 68%) **[B]**[174].

The risk of dying is increased with:

● increasing age **[A]**[159] **[A]**[179] **[A]**[184] **[B]**[164] **[B]**[165] **[B]**[186] **[B]**[187]
● female sex **[A]**[188] **[B]**[185]
● hospitals that admit few cases of MI **[A]**[181]

**Why?**
Female sex and increasing age increase the risk of dying

| Patient | Prognostic factor | Outcome | Control rate | OR (95% CI) | NNF+ (95% CI) |
|---|---|---|---|---|---|
| MI [A][188] | Female *independent* | Death at ? months | 14% | 1.18 (1.16 to 1.20) | 26 (23 to 28) |
| First MI [B][187] | Advanced age (> 70 years) *independent* | Death at discharge | 4.0% | 7.0 (4.8 to 10.2) | 5 (4 to 8) |

- previous cardiovascular disease
  - previous MI [A][165] or subsequent recurrent infarction [A][184] [B][185] [B][187]
  - previous angina [A][173] [A][189] [B][185] or early post-infarction angina [A][173]
  - a previous stroke [B][164] [B][185]
  - an increasing number of stenosed coronary vessels [B][180] or previous CABG [B][164]

❓ **Why?**
Cardiovascular disease increases the risk of dying

| Patient | Prognostic factor | Outcome | Control rate | OR (95% CI) | NNF+ (95% CI) |
|---|---|---|---|---|---|
| MI [A][165] | Previous MI *independent* | Death at 18 months | 3.6% | 5.20 (1.50 to 17.97) | 8 (3 to 59) |
| MI [B][185] | Recurrent MI within 1 year *independent* | Death at 1 year | 20% | 4.76 (4.06 to 5.57) | 3 (3 to 3) |
| First MI [B][189] | Angina for > 1 month before MI *independent* | Death at discharge | 12% | 1.30 (1.10 to 1.53) | 33 (19 to 96) |
| MI [B][185] | Previous stroke *independent* | Death at 1 year | 20% | 1.93 (1.56 to 2.38) | 8 (6 to 12) |
| MI [B][180] | Increasing number of vessels with 70% stenosis or more *independent* | Death from heart disease at 2 years | 12% | 1.90 (1.48 to 2.44) | |

- cardiovascular risk factors
  - hypertension [B][164] [B][180]
  - smoking [B][164]
  - diabetes mellitus [A][190] [B][164]

**?** **Why?**
Cardiovascular risk factors increase the risk of dying

| Patient | Prognostic factor | Outcome | Control rate | OR (95% CI) | NNF+ (95% CI) |
|---|---|---|---|---|---|
| MI **[B]**[180] | Hypertension *independent* | Death from heart disease at 2 years | 15% | 2.04 (1.36 to 3.05) | 9 (5 to 23) |
| MI **[A]**[190] | Male and diabetes *independent* | Death at 1 year | 26% | 1.38 (1.18 to 1.61) | 15 (10 to 31) |
| | Female and diabetes *independent* | Death at 1 year | 26% | 1.86 (1.40 to 2.46) | 7 (5 to 14) |

- an anterior MI **[A]**[184] **[A]**[191] **[B]**[164] **[B]**[187]
- a Q wave infarct **[B]**[187]

**?** **Why?**
An anterior MI or Q wave MI increases the risk of dying

| Patient | Prognostic factor | Outcome | Control rate | OR (95% CI) | NNF+ (95% CI) |
|---|---|---|---|---|---|
| MI **[A]**[191] | Anterior MI *independent* | Death at discharge | 11% | 1.57 (1.26 to 1.96) | 19 (12 to 40) |
| First MI **[B]**[187] | Non-Q wave infarct *independent* | Death at discharge | 4.0% | 0.08 (0.03 to 0.23) | −27 (−33 to −26) |

- an abnormal admission ECG (the more abnormalities present, the greater the risk of dying) **[A]**[192]
  - abnormal QRS complexes **[A]**[193]
  - ST elevation **[B]**[194], particularly if present in many leads **[B]**[187]
  - bundle-branch block **[B]**[194] **[B]**[195]

**?** **Why?**
ST elevation and bundle-branch block increase the risk of dying in hospital

| Patient | Prognostic factor | Outcome | Control rate | OR (95% CI) | NNF+ (95% CI) |
|---|---|---|---|---|---|
| MI **[B]**[194] | ST elevation without bundle-branch block *independent* | Death at discharge | 13% | 1.53 (1.49 to 1.58) | 18 (16 to 19) |
| First MI **[B]**[187] | Increased number of leads with ST elevation (6–7) *independent* | Death at discharge | 4.0% | 1.86 (1.26 to 2.74) | 31 (16 to 100) |
| MI **[B]**[194] | Left bundle-branch block *independent* | Death at discharge | 13% | 1.34 (1.28 to 1.39) | 27 (24 to 33) |
| | Right bundle-branch block *independent* | | | 1.64 (1.57 to 1.71) | 15 (14 to 17) |

- specifically for an inferior MI
  - precordial ST depression [B][196]
  - evidence of right ventricular infarction (ST segment elevation ≥ 0.1 mV in lead $V_{4R}$ [A][197]

| ? Why? | | | | | |
|---|---|---|---|---|---|
| A right ventricular infarction increases the risk of dying | | | | | |
| Patient | Prognostic factor | Outcome | Control rate | OR (95% CI) | NNF+ (95% CI) |
| Inferior MI [A][197] | Right ventricular infarction *independent* | Death at discharge | 19% | 7.70 (2.60 to 23.0) | 1 (1 to 3) |

- complications
  - evidence of heart failure [A][159] [A][184] [B][185] [B][187], particularly cardiogenic shock [A][161]
    - worsening Killip class [A][165] [A][197] [B][164] [B][186] [B][198]
    - reduced ejection fraction [A][173] [A][179] [B][12] [B][180]
    - reduced LV end-diastolic pressure [A][173]
  - increased heart rate [B][164]
  - hypotension [B][164]
  - mitral regurgitation [B][180], particularly if early [A][179]

| ? Why? | | | | | |
|---|---|---|---|---|---|
| Heart failure and mitral regurgitation increase the risk of dying | | | | | |
| Patient | Prognostic factor | Outcome | Control rate | OR (95% CI) | NNF+ (95% CI) |
| First MI [B][187] | Heart failure *independent* | Death at discharge | 4.0% | 2.47 (1.84 to 3.33) | 19 (12 to 32) |
| MI [B][164] | Killip class IV v. I *independent* | Death at 1 month | 5.1% | 7.86 (5.88 to 10.49) | 4 (3 to 5) |
| | Killip class III v. I *independent* | | | 4.37 (3.34 to 5.71) | 7 (5 to 10) |
| MI [A][165] | Killip class II or more *independent* | Death at 18 months | 4.0% | 6.16 (2.01 to 18.83) | 6 (3 to 27) |
| MI [B][180] | Mitral regurgitation *independent* | Death from heart disease at 2 years | 12% | 2.00 (1.28 to 3.04) | 11 (6 to 35) |

- arrhythmias
  - 10 or more premature ventricular contractions per hour [A][165] [B][199]
  - VF (particularly after 48 h) [B][187]
  - Second- [A][187] or third-degree heart block [A][159] [B][187] after 24 h
  - cardiac arrest [A][184] [B][187]

**❓ Why?**

**Ventricular arrhythmias and heart block increase the risk of dying**

| Patient | Prognostic factor | Outcome | Control rate | OR (95% CI) | NNF+ (95% CI) |
|---|---|---|---|---|---|
| MI [A][165] | 10 or more premature ventricular contractions per hour *independent* | Death at 18 months | 5.8% | 6.06 (1.90 to 19.4) | 5 (2 to 21) |
| MI [B][199] | Complex ventricular arrhythmias *independent* | Death at 6 months | 3.0% | 2.55 (1.96 to 3.32) | 23 (16 to 37) |
| First MI [B][187] | VF within 4 h of infarction *independent* | Death at discharge | 4.0% | 2.47 (1.48 to 4.13) | 19 (9 to 55) |
| | VF > 4 h but <48 h after infarction *independent* | | | 3.97 (1.51 to 10.5) | 10 (4 to 52) |
| | VF > 48 h after infarction *independent* | | | 20.2 (11.5 to 35.5) | 2 (2 to 4) |
| MI [B][199] | 2nd- or 3rd-degree heart block *independent* | Death at discharge | 4.0% | 2.89 (2.03 to 4.09) | 15 (9 to 26) |
| Inferior MI [A][159] | Complete heart block *independent* | Death at 1 year | 16% | 2.7 (1.3 to 5.5) | 5 (3 to 25) |

- psychosocial factors
  - depression [A][165]
  - lack of social support [A][200], e.g. living alone [B][198]
  - failure to take medication [B][201]
  - education for <12 years [B][198].

**❓ Why?**

**Depression, living alone and poor adherence to medication increase the risk of dying**

| Patient | Prognostic factor | Outcome | Control rate | OR (95% CI) | NNF+ (95% CI) |
|---|---|---|---|---|---|
| MI [A][165] | Depression *independent* | Death at 18 months | 2.7% | 6.06 (1.90 to 19.4) | 9 (3 to 44) |
| MI [B][198] | Living alone *independent* | Recurrent cardiac event at 1 year | 12% | 1.54 (1.04 to 2.29) | 19 (9 to 241) |
| Women with an MI [B][201] | Poor adherence to medication *independent* | Death at 2 years | 8.7% | 2.4 (1.1 to 5.6) | 13 (4 to 180) |
| MI [B][198] | Education <12 years *independent* | Recurrent cardiac event at 1 year | 12% | 1.76 (1.24 to 2.50) | 16 (9 to 49) |

**Guideline writers**: Chris Ball, Nick Shenker
**CAT writers**: Clare Wotton, Nick Shenker, Bob Phillips, Chris Ball

# REFERENCES

| No. | Level | Citation |
|-----|-------|----------|
| 1 | 1b | Solomon CG et al. Comparison of clinical presentation of acute myocardial infarction in patients older than 65 years of age to younger patients: the multicenter chest pain study experience. Am J Cardiol 1989; 63: 772–6 |
| 2 | 1b | Lee TH et al. Acute chest pain in the emergency room: identification and examination of low-risk patients. Arch Intern Med 1985; 145: 65–9 |
| 3 | 2a | Panju AA et al. Is this patient having a myocardial infarction? JAMA 1998; 280: 1256–63 |
| 4 | 1a | Goldman L et al. A computer protocol to predict myocardial infarction in emergency department patients with chest pain. N Engl J Med 1988; 318: 797–803 |
| 5 | 2b | Tierney WM et al. Physicians' estimates of the probability of myocardial infarction in the emergency room patient with chest pain. Med Decis Making 1986; 6: 12–17 |
| 6 | 4 | Lux G et al. Ambulatory pressure, pH and ECG recording in patients with normal and pathological coronary angiography and intermittent chest pain. Neurogastroenterol. Motil 1995; 7: 23–30 |
| 7 | 2a | Diamond GA, Forrester JS. Analysis of probability as an aid in the clinical diagnosis of coronary artery disease. N Engl J Med 1979; 300: 1350–8 |
| 8 | 1b | Psaty BM, Furberg CD, Kuller LH et al. Traditional risk factors and subclinical disease measures as predictors of first myocardial infarction in older adults: the cardiovascular health study. Arch Intern Med 1999; 159: 1339–47 |
| 9 | 1b | Galjee MA, Visser FC, De Cock CC et al. The prognostic value, clinical and angiographic characteristics of patients with early postinfarction angina after a first myocardial infarction. Am Heart J 1992; 125: 48–55 |
| 10 | 1b | Lehmann KG, Francis CK, Dodge HT et al. Mitral regurgitation in early myocardial infarction: incidence, clinical detection and prognostic implications. Ann Intern Med 1992; 117: 10–17 |
| 11 | 2b | Lamas GA, Mitchell GF, Flaker GC et al. Clinical significance of mitral regurgitation after acute myocardial infarction. Circulation 1997; 96: 827–33 |
| 12 | 2b | Nicolosi GL, Latini R, Marino P et al. The prognostic value of predischarge quantitative two-dimensional echocardiographic measurements and the effects of early lisinopril treatment on left ventricular structure and function after acute myocardial infarction in the GISSI-3 trial (Gruppo Italiano per lo Studio della Sopravvivenza Nell' Infarto Miocardico). Eur Heart J 1996; 17: 1646–56 |
| 13 | 3b | Meier CR, Jick SS, Derby LE et al. Acute respiratory-tract infections and risk of first-time acute myocardial infarction. Lancet 1998; 351: 1467–71 |
| 14 | 2b | Lee KL, Woodlief LH, Topol EJ et al. Predictors of 30-day mortality in the era of reperfusion for acute myocardial infarction: results from an international trial of 41 021 patients. Circulation 1995; 91: 1659–68 |
| 15 | 2b | Berger CJ, Murabito JM, Evans JC et al. Prognosis after first myocardial infarction: comparison of Q-wave and non-Q-wave myocardial infarction in the Framingham Heart Study. JAMA 1992; 268: 1545–51 |
| 16 | 1b | Miettinen H, Haffner SM, Lehto S et al. Impact of diabetes on mortality after the first myocardial infarction. Diabetes Care 1998; 21: 69–75 |

| No. | Level | Citation |
| --- | --- | --- |
| 17 | 3b | Stampfer MJ, Krauss RM, Ma J et al. A prospective study of triglyceride level, low-density lipoprotein particle diameter, and risk of myocardial infarction. JAMA 1996; 276: 882–8 |
| 18 | 1a | Berlin JA, Colditz GA. A meta-analysis of physical activity in the prevention of coronary heart disease. Am J Epidemiol 1990; 132: 612–8 |
| 19 | 1b | Jousilahti P, Puska P, Vartiainen E et al. Parental history of premature coronary heart disease: an independent risk factor of myocardial infarction. J Clin Epidemiol 1996; 49: 497–503 |
| 20 | 4 | Dell'Italia LJ, Starling MR, O'Rourke RA. Physical examination for exclusion of haemodynamically important right ventricular infarction. Ann Intern Med 1983; 99: 608–11 |
| 21 | 4 | Ishikawa M, Sataka K, Maki A et al. Prognostic significance of a clearly audible fourth heart sound detected a month after an acute myocardial infarction. Am J Cardiol 1997; 80: 617–21 |
| 22 | 4 | Berger JP et al. Right arm involvement and pain extension can help to differentiate coronary disease from chest pain of other origin: a prospective emergency ward study of 278 consecutive patients admitted for chest pain. J Intern Med 1990; 227: 165–72 |
| 23 | 1b | Sox HC et al. Psychologically-mediated effects of diagnostic tests. Ann Intern Med 1981; 95: 680–5 |
| 24 | 4 | de Winter RJ et al. Value of myoglobin, troponin T and CK-MB (mass) in ruling out an acute myocardial infarction in the emergency room. Circulation 1995; 92: 3401–7 |
| 25 | 2b | Thomsen SP, Gibbons RJ, Smars PA et al. Incremental value of the leukocyte differential and the creatine kinase-MB isoenzyme for the early diagnosis of myocardial infarction. Ann Intern Med 1995; 122: 335–41 |
| 26 | 1a | Fath-Ordoubadi F, Beatt KJ. Glucose–insulin–potassium therapy for treatment of acute myocardial infarction. Circulation 1997; 96: 1152–6 |
| 27 | 1a | Rembold CM. Number-needed-to-treat analysis of the prevention of myocardial infarction and death by antidyslipidemic therapy. J Fam Pract 1996; 42: 577–86 |
| 28 | 1a | Ross SD, Allen IE, Connelly JE et al. Clinical outcomes in statin trials. Arch Intern Med 1999; 159: 1793–802 |
| 29 | 4 | Zimmerman J, Fromm R, Meyer D et al. Diagnostic Marker Cooperative Study for the diagnosis of myocardial infarction. Circulation 1999; 99: 1671–7 |
| 30 | 1b | Antman EM et al. Evaluation of a rapid bedside assay for detection of serum cardiac troponin T. JAMA 1995; 273: 1279–82 |
| 31 | 2b | Sayre MR et al. Measurement of cardiac troponin T is an effective method for predicting complications among emergency department patients with chest pain. Ann Emerg Med 1998; 31: 539–49 |
| 32 | 4 | Smith AF. Diagnostic value of serum-creatine-kinase in a coronary-care unit. Lancet 1967; i: 178–82 |
| 33 | 1b | Lee TH, Rouan GW, Weisberg MC et al. Sensitivity of routine clinical criteria for diagnosing myocardial infarction within 24 hours of hospitalization. Ann Intern Med 1987; 106: 181–6 |
| 34 | 1b | Jayes RL, Larsen GC, Beshansky JR et al. Physician electrocardiogram reading in the emergency department – accuracy and effect on triage decisions: findings from a multicenter study. J Gen Intern Med 1992; 7: 387–92 |
| 35 | 4 | Stark JL, Vacek JL. The initial electrocardiogram during admission for myocardial infarction: use as a predictor of clinical course and facility utilization. Arch Intern Med 1987; 147: 843–6 |

| No. | Level | Citation |
| --- | --- | --- |
| 36 | 4 | Brush JE, Brand DA, Acampora D et al. Use of the initial electrocardiogram to predict in-hospital complications of acute myocardial infarction. N Eng J Med 1985; 312: 1137–41 |
| 37 | 1b | Fesmire FM et al. Usefulness of automated serial 12-lead ECG monitoring during initial emergency department evaluation of patients with chest pain. Ann Emerg Med 1998; 31: 3–11 |
| 38 | 2b | Zalenski RJ et al. Evaluation of a chest pain diagnostic protocol to exclude acute cardiac ischemia in the emergency department. Arch Intern Med 1997; 157: 1085–91 |
| 39 | 1a | Lee TH, Juarez G, Cook EF et al. Ruling out acute myocardial infarction: prospective multicenter validation of a 12-hour strategy for patients at low risk. N Eng J Med 1991; 324: 1239–46 |
| 40 | 1b– | Gomez MA et al. An emergency department-based protocol for rapidly ruling out myocardial ischaemia decreases hospital time and expense: results of a randomised study (ROMIO). J Am Coll Cardiol 1996; 28:25–33 |
| 41 | 1b | Roberts RR, Zalenski RJ, Mensah EK et al. Costs of an emergency department-based accelerated diagnostic protocol vs hospitalization in patients with chest pain: a randomized controlled trial. JAMA 1997; 278: 1670–6 |
| 42 | 1a | Goldman L, Cook F, Johnson PA et al. Prediction of the need for intensive care in patients who come to emergency departments with acute chest pain. New Engl J Med 1996; 334: 1498–1504 |
| 43 | 2b | Thompson PL, Lown B. Nitrous oxide as an analgesic in acute myocardial infarction. JAMA 1976; 235: 924–7 |
| 44 | 1b– | Nielsen LR, Pedersen KE, Dahlstrom CG et al. Analgetic treatment in acute myocardial infarction. Acta Med Scand 1984; 215: 349–54 |
| 45 | 1a | Antiplatelet Trialists' Collaboration. Collaborative overview of randomised trials of antiplatelet therapy I: prevention of death, MI and stroke by prolonged antiplatelet therapy in various categories of patients. BMJ 1994; 308: 81–106 |
| 46 | 1b | CAPRIE Steering Committee. A randomised, blinded, trial of clopidogrel versus aspirin in patients at risk of ischaemic events (CAPRIE). Lancet 1996; 348: 1329–39 |
| 47 | 1b | Coumadin Aspirin Reinfarction Study (CARS) Investigators. Randomised double-blind trial of fixed low-dose warfarin with aspirin after myocardial infarction. Lancet 1997; 350: 389–96 |
| 48 | 1b | The GUSTO Investigators. An international randomized trial comparing four thrombolytic strategies for acute myocardial infarction. N Engl J Med 1993; 329: 673–82 |
| 49 | 1a | Cucherat M, Bonnefoy E, Tremeau G. Primary angioplasty versus intravenous thrombolysis for acute myocardial infarction (Cochrane Review). In: The Cochrane Library, Issue 2, 1999. Oxford: Update Software |
| 50 | 4 | Stone GW, Grines CL, Rothbaum D et al. Analysis of the relative costs and effectiveness of primary angioplasty versus tissue-type plasminogen activator: the Primary Angioplasty in Myocardial infarction (PAMI) trial. J Am Coll Cardiol 1997; 29: 901–7 |
| 51 | 1b– | SWIFT Group. SWIFT trial of delayed elective intervention vs conservative treatment after thrombolysis with anistreplase in acute myocardial infarction. BMJ 1991; 302: 555–60 |
| 52 | 1b– | Ellis SG, Ribeiro da Silva E, Heyndrickx G et al. Randomized comparison of rescue angioplasty with conservative management of patients with early failure of thrombolysis for acute anterior myocardial infarction (RESCUE). Circulation 1994; 90: 2280–4 |

| No. | Level | Citation |
| --- | --- | --- |
| 53 | 1b | Stone GW, Marsalese D, Brodie BR et al. A prospective, randomized evaluation of prophylactic intraaortic balloon counterpulsation in high risk patients with acute myocardial infarction treated with primary angioplasty. J Am Coll Cardiol 1997; 29: 1459–67 |
| 54 | 1a | Fibrinolytic Therapy Trialists' (FTT) Collaborative Group. Indications for fibrinolytic therapy in suspected acute myocardial infarction: collaborative overview of early mortality and major morbidity results from all randomised trials of more than 1000 patients. Lancet 1994; 343: 311–22 |
| 55 | 1a | Boersma E, Maas AC, Deckers JW et al. Early thombolytic treatment in acute myocardial infarction: reappraisal of the golden hour. Lancet 1996; 348: 771–5 |
| 56 | 1a | Wardlaw JM, Yamaguchi T, del Zappo G. Thrombolysis for acute ischaemic stroke (Cochrane Review). In: The Cochrane Library, Issue 2, 1999. Oxford: Update Software. |
| 57 | 1a | Solomon SD, Ridker PM, Antman EM. Ventricular arrhthymias in trials of thrombolytic therapy for acute myocardial infarction. A meta-analysis. Circulation 1993; 88: 2575–81 |
| 58 | 1b | Castillo PA, Palmer CS, Halpern MT et al. Cost-effectiveness of thrombolytic therapy for acute myocardial infarction. Ann Pharmacother 1997; 31: 596–603 |
| 59 | 1b | Krumholz HM, Pasternak RC, Weinstein MC et al. Cost effectiveness of thrombolytic therapy with streptokinase in elderly patients with suspected acute myocardial infarction. N Engl J Med 1992; 327: 7–13. |
| 60 | 1a | Boersma E, Maas AC, Deckers JW et al. Early thombolytic treatment in acute myocardial infarction: reappraisal of the golden hour. Lancet 1996: 348: 771–5 |
| 61 | 1b | Califf RM, White HD, Van de Werf F et al. One-year results from the Global Utilization of Streptokinase and TPA for Occluded Coronary Arteries (GUSTO-1) Trial. Circulation 1996; 94: 1233–8 |
| 62 | 1b | ISIS-3 (Third International Study of Infarct Survival) Collaborative Group. ISIS-3: a randomised comparison of streptokinase vs tissue plasminogen activator vs anistreplase and of aspirin plus heparin vs aspirin alone among 41 299 cases of suspected myocardial infarction. Lancet 1992; 339: 753–70 |
| 63 | 1b | Kalish SC, Gurwitz JH, Krumholz HM et al. A cost-effectiveness model of thrombolytic therapy for acute myocardial infarction. J Gen Intern Med 1995; 10: 321–30 |
| 64 | 1b | Mark DB, Hlatky MA, Califf RM et al. Cost-effectiveness model of thrombolytic therapy with tissue plasminogen activator as compared with streptokinase for acute myocardial infarction. N Engl J Med 1995; 332: 1418–24 |
| 65 | 1b | Maggioni AP, Franzosi MG, Santoro E et al. The risk of stroke in patients with acute myocardial infarction after thrombolytic and antithrombotic treatment. N Engl J Med 1992; 327: 1–6 |
| 66 | 1b | The Global Use of Strategies to Open Occluded Coronary Arteries (GUSTO-III) Investigators. comparison of reteplase with alteplase for acute myocardial infarction. N Engl J Med 1997; 337: 1118–23 |
| 67 | 1b | Assessment of the Safety and Efficacy of a New Thrombolytic (ASSENT-2) Investigators. Single-bolus tenecteplase compared with front-loaded alteplase in acute myocardial infarction: The ASSENT-2 double-blind randomised trial. Lancet 1999; 354: 716–22 |
| 68 | 1b | Berkowitz SD, Granger CB, Pieper KS et al. Incidence and predictors of bleeding after contemporary thrombolytic therapy for myocardial infarction. Circulation 1997; 95: 2508–16 |

| No. | Level | Citation |
|-----|-------|----------|
| 69 | 2c | Selker HP, Griffith JL, Beshansky JR et al. Patient-specific predictions of outcomes in myocardial infarction for real-time emergency use: a thrombolytic predictive instrument. Ann Intern Med 1997; 127: 538–56 |
| 70 | 2c | Mahaffey KW, Granger CB, Toth CA et al. Diabetic retinopathy should not be a contraindication to thrombolytic therapy for acute myocardial infarction: review of ocular hemorrhage incidence and location in the GUSTO-I trial. J Am Coll Cardiol 1997; 30: 1606–10 |
| 71 | 4 | Renkin J, De Bruyne B, Benit E et al. Cardiac tamponade early after thrombolysis for acute myocardial infarction: a rare but not reported hemorrhagic complication. J Am Coll Cardiol 1991; 17: 280–5 |
| 72 | 4 | Stewart JT, French JK, Theroux P et al. Early noninvasive identification of failed reperfusion after intravenous thrombolytic therapy in acute myocardial infarction. J Am Coll Cardiol 1998; 31: 1499–505 |
| 73 | 1a | Vaitkus PT, Barnathan ES. Embolic potential, prevention and management of mural thrombus complicating anterior myocardial infraction: a meta-analysis. J Am Coll Cardiol 1993; 22: 1004–9 |
| 74 | 1b | Glick A, Kornowski R, Michowich Y et al. Reduction of reinfarction and angina with use of low-molecular-weight heparin therapy after streptokinase (and heparin) in acute myocardial infarction. Am J Cardiol 1996; 77: 1145–8 |
| 75 | 1a | Mahaffrey KW, Granger CB, Collins R et al. Overview of randomized trial of intravenous heparin in patients with acute myocardial infarction treated with thrombolytic therapy. Am J Cardiol 1996; 77: 551–6. |
| 76 | 1b | Gruppo Italiano per lo Studio della Sopravvienza Nell' Infarcto Miocardico. GISSI-2: a factorial randomized trial of alteplase versus streptokinase and heparin versus no heparin among 12 490 patients with acute myocardial infarction. Lancet 1990; 336: 65–71 |
| 77 | 1a | Collins R, MacMahon S, Flather M et al. Clinical effects of anticoagulant therapy in suspected acute myocardial infarction: systematic overview of randomised trials. BMJ 1996; 313: 652–9 |
| 78 | 1b– | Antman EM and the TIMI 9B investigators. Hirudin in acute myocardial infarction. Circulation 1996; 94: 911–21 |
| 79 | 1b | Malmberg K for the DIGAMI (Diabetes Mellitus, Insulin Glucose Infusion in Acute Myocardial Infarction) Study Group. Prospective randomised study of intensive insulin treatment on long term survival after acute myocardial infarction in patients with diabetes mellitus. BMJ 1997; 314: 1512–5 |
| 80 | 1b | Malmberg K, Ryden L, Efendic S et al. Randomized trial of insulin–glucose infusion followed by subcutaneous insulin treatment in diabetic patients with acute myocardial infarction (DIGAMI Study): effect on mortality at 1 year. J Am Coll Cardiol 1995; 26: 57–63 |
| 81 | 1a | Freemantle N, Cleland J, Young P et al. Beta-blockade after myocardial infarction: systematic review and meta regression analysis. BMJ 1999; 318: 1730–7 |
| 82 | 1a | McAlister FA, and Teo KK. Antiarrhythmic therapies for the prevention of sudden cardiac death. Drugs 1997; 54 (2): 235–252 |
| 83 | 1a | Teo KK, Yusuf S, Furberg CD. Effects of prophylactic antiarrhythmic drug therapy in acute myocardial infarction. JAMA 1993; 270: 1589–95 |

| No. | Level | Citation |
|-----|-------|----------|
| 84 | 1b | Roberts R, Rogers WJ, Mueller HS et al. Immediate versus deferred beta-blockade following thrombolytic therapy in patients with acute myocardial infarction: results of thrombolysis in myocardial infarction (TIMI) II-B study. Circulation 1991; 83: 422–37 |
| 85 | 1a | ACE inhibitor Myocardial infarction Collaborative Group. Indications for ACE inhibitors in the early treatment of acute myocardial infarction: systematic overview of the individual data from 100 000 patients in randomized trials. Circulation 1998; 97:202–12 |
| 86 | 1b | ISIS-4 (Fourth International Study of Infarct Survival) Collaborative Group. ISIS-4: a randomised factorial trial assessing early oral captopril, oral mononitrate, and intravenous magnesium sulphate in 58 050 patients with suspected acute myocardial infarction. Lancet 1995; 345: 669–85 |
| 87 | 1a | Kober L, Torp-Pedersen C, Carlsen JE et al. A clinical trial of the angiotensin-converting-enzyme inhibitor trandolapril in patients with left ventricular dysfunction after myocardial infarction (TRACE). N Engl J Med 1995;333: 1670–6 |
| 88 | 1b | Tsevat J, Duke D, Goldman L et al. Cost-effectiveness of captopril therapy after myocardial infarction. J Am Coll Cardiol 1995; 26:914–19 |
| 89 | 1b | The Acute Infarction Ramipril Efficacy (AIRE) Study Investigatiors. Effect of ramipril on mortality and morbidity of survivors of acute myocardial infarction with clinical evidence of heart failure. Lancet 1993;342:821–8. |
| 90 | 1b | Pfeffer MA, Braunwald E, Moye LA et al. Effect of captopril on mortaility and morbidity in patients with left ventricular dysfunction after myocardial infarction: results of the Survival and Ventricular Enlargement (SAVE) trial. N Engl J Med 1992; 327: 669–77 |
| 91 | 1b | Kober L, Torp-Pedersen C, Carlsen JE, et al. A clinical trial of the angiotensin-converting-enzyme inhibitor trandolapril in patients with left ventricular dysfunction after myocardial infarction (TRACE). New England Journal of Medicine 1995;333: 1670–1676 |
| 92 | 1b | Pedersen OG, Bagger H, Kober L et al. Trandolapril reduces the incidence of atrial fibrillation after acute myocardial infarction in patients with left ventricular dysfunction. Circulation 1999; 100: 376–80 |
| 93 | 1b | The Heart Outcomes Prevention Evaluation Study Investigators. Effects of an angiotensin-converting-enzyme inhibitor, ramipril, on death from cardiovascular causes, myocardial infarction, and stroke in high-risk patients. N Engl J Med 2000; 334 |
| 94 | 1a | Held PH et al. Calcium channel blockers in acute myocardial infarction and unstable angina: an overview. BMJ 1989; 299: 1187–92 |
| 95 | 1a | Yusuf S et al. Update of effects of calcium antagonists in myocardial infarction or angina in light of the second Danish Verapamil Infarction Trial (DAVIT-II) and other recent studies. Am J Cardiol 1991; 67: 1295–7 |
| 96 | 1b– | Goldbourt U, Behar S, Reicher-Reioss H et al. Early administration of nifedipine in suspected acute myocardial infarction. Arch Intern Med 1993; 153: 345–53 |
| 97 | 1b | Willcox RG, Hampton JR, Banks DC et al. Trial of early nifedipine in acute myocardial infarction: the Trent Study. BMJ 1986; 293: 1204–8 |
| 98 | 1a | McAlister FA, Teo KK. Antiarrhythmic therapies for the prevention of sudden cardiac death. Drugs 1997; 54: 235–52. |
| 99 | 1b– | Goldstein RE, Boccuzzi SJ, Cruess D et al. Diltiazem increases late-onset congestive heart failure in postinfarction patients with early reduction in ejection fraction. Circulation 1991; 83: 52–60 |

| No. | Level | Citation |
|-----|-------|----------|
| 100 | 1a | Visser PJ, Bredero AC, Hoekstra JBL. Magnesium therapy in acute myocardial infarction. Neth J Med 1995; 46: 156–65 |
| 101 | 1b | Gruppo Italiano per lo Studio della Soprativenza nell'Infarto Miocardico. GISSI-3: effects of lisinopril and transdermal glyceryl trinitrate singly and together on 6-week mortality and ventricular function after acute myocardial infarction. Lancet 1994; 343:1115–22 |
| 102 | 1b– | Grines CL, Marsalese DL, Brodie B et al. Safety and cost-effectiveness of early discharge after primary angioplasty in low risk patients with acute myocardial infarction. J Am Coll Cardiol 1998; 31: 967–72 |
| 103 | 1a | Oldridge NB, Guyatt GH, Fischer ME et al. Cardiac rehabilitation after myocardial infarction: combined experience of randomized clinical trials. JAMA 1988; 260: 945–50 |
| 104 | 1a | O'Connor GT, Buring JE, Yusuf S et al. An overview of randomized trials of rehabilitation with exercise after myocardial infarction. Circulation 1989; 80: 234–44 |
| 105 | 1a | Linden W, Stossel C, Maurice J. Psychosocial interventions for patients with coronary artery disease. A meta analysis. Arch Intern Med 1996; 156: 745–52 |
| 106 | 4 | Petrie KJ, Weinman J, Sharpe N. Patient's views of their illness in predicting return to work and functioning after myocardial infarction: a longitudinal study. BMJ 1996; 312: 1191–4 |
| 107 | 1b | de Lorgeril M, Renaud S, Mamelle N et al. Mediterranean alpha-linolenic acid-rich diet in secondary prevention of coronary heart disease. Lancet 1994; 343: 1454–9 |
| 108 | 1a | Gould AL, Rossouw JE, Santanello NC et al. Cholesterol reduction yields clinical benefit: impact of statin trials. Circulation 1998; 97: 946–952 |
| 109 | 1b | Sacks FM et al. The effect of pravastatin on coronary events after myocardial infarction in patients with average cholesterol levels. N Engl J Med 1996; 335: 1001–9 |
| 110 | 1b | The Long-term Intervention with Pravastatin in Ischaemic Disease (LIPID) Study Group. Prevention of cardiovascular events and death with pravastatin in patients with coronary heart disease and a broad range of initial cholesterol levels. N Engl J Med 1998; 339: 1349–57 |
| 111 | 1a | Brunner E, White I, Thorogood M et al. Can dietary interventions change diet and cardiovascular risk factors? A meta-analysis of randomized controlled trials. Am J Public Health 1997; 87: 1415–22 |
| 112 | 1a | Tang JL, Armitage JM, Lancaster T et al. Systematic review of dietary intervention trials to lower blood cholesterol in free-living subjects. BMJ 1998; 316: 1213–20 |
| 113 | 1a | Yu-Poth S, Zhao G, Etherton T et al. Effects of the national cholesterol education program's step I and step II dietary intervention programs on cardiovascular disease risk factors: a meta-analysis. Am J Clin Nutr 1999; 69: 632–46 |
| 114 | 1a | Ripsin CM, Keenan JM, Jacobs Dr et al. Oat products and lipid lowering: a meta-analysis JAMA 1992; 267:3317–25 |
| 115 | 1b | Burr ML, Fehily AM, Gilbert JF et al. Effects of changes in fat, fish and fibre intakes on death and myocardial infarction: diet and reinfarction trial (DART). Lancet 1989: ii: 757–61 |
| 116 | 2a | Anderson JW, Johnstone BM, Cook-Newall ME. Meta-analysis of the effects of soy protein intake on serum lipids. N Engl J Med 1995; 333: 276–82 |
| 117 | 1a | Rembold CM. Number-needed-to-treat analysis of the prevention of myocardial infarction and death by antidyslipidemic therapy. J Fam Pract 1996; 42: 577–86 |

| No. | Level | Citation |
|-----|-------|----------|
| 118 | 1a | Ross SD, Allen IE, Connelly JE et al. Clinical outcomes in statin trials. Arch Intern Med 1999; 159: 1793–802 |
| 119 | 1b | Scandinavian Simvastatin Survival Study Group. Randomized trial of cholesterol lowering in 4444 patients with coronary heart disease: the Scandinavian Simvastatin Survival Study (4S). Lancet 1994; 344: 1383–9 |
| 120 | 1b | Johannesson M, Jonsson B, Kjekshus J et al. Cost effectiveness of simvastatin treatment to lower cholesterol levels in patients with coronary heart disease. N Engl J Med 1997; 336: 332–6 |
| 121 | 2b | Pharoah PDP, Hollingworth W. Cost effectiveness of lowering cholesterol concentration with statins in patients with and without pre-existing coronary heart disease: life table method applied to a health authority population. BMJ 1996; 312: 1443–8 |
| 122 | 1b | Rubins HB, Robins SJ, Collins D et al. Gemfibrozil for the secondary prevention of coronary heart disease in men with low levels of high-density lipoprotein cholesterol. N Engl J Med 1999; 341: 410–8 |
| 123 | 1b | GISSI-Prevenzione Investigators. Dietary supplementation with n-3 polyunsaturated fatty acids and vitamin E after myocardial infarction: results of the GISSI-Prevenzione trial. Lancet 1999; 354: 447–55 |
| 124 | 1b | Stephens NG, Parsons A, Schofield PM et al. Randomised controlled trial of vitamin E in patients with coronary disease: Cambridge Heart Antioxidant Study (CHAOS). Lancet 1996; 347: 781–6 |
| 125 | 1b | Rapola JM, Virtamo J, Ripatti S et al. Randomised trial of alpha-tocopherol and beta-carotene supplements on incidence of major coronary events in men with previous myocardial infarction. Lancet 1997; 349: 1715–20 |
| 126 | 1b– | Hulley S, Grady D, Bush T et al. Randomized trial of estrogen plus progestin for secondary prevention of coronary heart disease in postmenopausal women. JAMA 1998; 280: 605–13 |
| 127 | 1a | Psaty BM, Smith NL, Siscovick DS et al. Health outcomes associated with antihypertensive therapies used as first-line agents: a systematic review and meta-analysis. JAMA 1997; 277: 739–45 |
| 128 | 1a | Mulrow CD, Cornell JA, Herrera CR et al. Hypertension in the elderly; implications and generalizability of randomized trials. JAMA 1994; 272: 1932–8 |
| 129 | 1a | Messerli FH, Grossman E, Goldbourt U. Are β-blockers efficacious as first-line therapy for hypertension in the elderly? A systematic review. JAMA. 1998; 279: 1903–7 |
| 130 | 1a | Law M, Tang JL. An analysis of the effectiveness of interventions intended to help people stop smoking. Arch Intern Med 1995; 155: 1933–41 |
| 131 | 1a | Rice VH, Stead LF. Nursing interventions for smoking cessation (Cochrane Review). In: The Cochrane Library, Issue 3, 1999. Oxford: Update Software |
| 132 | 2c | Burt A, Thornley P, Illingworth D et al. Stopping smoking after myocardial infarction. Lancet 1974; i: 304–6 |
| 133 | 1b | Aberg A, Bergstrand R, Johansson Saga et al. Cessation of smoking after myocardial infarction: effects on mortality after 10 years. Br Heart J 1983; 49: 416–22 |
| 134 | 1b | Krumholz HM, Cohen BJ, Tsevat J et al. Cost-effectiveness of a smoking cessation program after myocardial infarction. J Am Coll Cardiol 1993; 22: 1697–702 |

| No. | Level | Citation |
|-----|-------|----------|
| 135 | 1b | Working Group for the Study of Transdermal Nicotine. Nicotine replacement therapy for patients with coronary artery disease. Arch Intern Med 1994; 154: 989–95 |
| 136 | 1b– | Joseph AM, Norman SM, Ferry LH et al. The safety of transdermal nicotine as an aid to smoking cessation in patients with cardiac disease. N Engl J Med 1996; 335: 1792–8 |
| 137 | 1b | Stapleton JA, Lowin A, Russell MAH. Prescription of transdermal nicotine patches for smoking cessation in general practice: evaluation of cost-effectiveness. Lancet 1999; 354: 210–15 |
| 138 | 1b– | Marcus BH, Albrecht AE, King TK, et al. The efficacy of exercise as an aid for smoking cessation in women: a randomized controlled trial. Arch Intern Med 1999; 159: 1229–34 |
| 139 | 1a | Amiodarone Trials Meta-Analysis Investigators. The effect of prophylactic amiodarone on mortality after acute myocardial infarction and in congestive heart failure: a meta-analysis of individual data from 6500 patients in 13 randomised trials. Lancet 1997; 350: 1417–24 |
| 140 | 1a | McAlister FA, Teo KK. Antiarrhythmic therapies for the prevention of sudden cardiac death. Drugs 1997; 54 (2): 235–252 |
| 141 | 1a | Sim I, McDonald KM, Lavori PW et al. Quantitative overview of randomised trials of amiodarone to prevent sudden cardiac death. Circulation 1997; 96: 2823–9 |
| 142 | 1b | Echt DS et al. Mortality and morbidity of patients receiving encainide, flecainide, or placebo: the Cardiac Arrhythmia Suppression Trial. N Engl J Med 1991; 324: 781–8 |
| 143 | 1b | CAST Investigators. Special report. Preliminary report: effect of encainide and flecainide on mortality in a randomized trial of arrhythmia suppression after myocardial infarction. N Engl J Med 1989; 321: 406–12 |
| 144 | 1a | Hine LK, Laird N, Hewitt P et al. Meta-analytic evidence against prophylactic use of lidocaine in acute myocardial infarction. Arch Intern Med 1989; 149: 2694–8 |
| 145 | 1a | Sadowski ZP, Alexander JH, Skrabucha B et al. Multicentre randomised trial and a systematic overview of lidocaine in acute myocardial infarction. Am J Cardiol 1999; 137: 792–8 |
| 146 | 1a | Teo KK, Yusuf S, Furberg CD. Effects of prophylactic antiarrhythmic drug therapy in acute myocardial infarction. JAMA 1993; 270: 1589–95 |
| 147 | 1b– | Wyse G, Kellen J, Rademaker AW. Prophylactic versus selective lidocaine for early ventricular arrhythmias of myocardial infarction. J Am Coll Cardiol 1988; 12: 507–13 |
| 148 | 1b | Waldo AL, Camm AJ, deRuyter H et al. Effect of d-sotalol on mortality in patients with left ventricular dysfunction after recent and remote myocardial infarction. Lancet 1996; 348: 7–12 |
| 149 | 2a | Shaw LJ, Peterson ED, Kesler K et al. A meta-analysis of predischarge risk stratification after acute myocardial infarction with stress echocardiography, myocardial perfusion and ventricular function imaging. Am J Cardiol 1996; 78: 1327–37 |
| 150 | 2b | Jain A, Myers H, Sapin PM et al. Comparison of symptom-limited and low level exercise tolerance tests early after myocardial infarction. J Am Coll Cardiol 1993; 22: 1816–20 |
| 151 | 1b | Galjee MA, Visser FC, De Cock CC et al. The prognostic value, clinical and angiographic characteristics of patients with early postinfarction angina after a first myocardial infarction. Am Heart J 1992; 125: 48–55 |
| 152 | 1b | Madsen JK, Grande P, Saunamaki K et al. Danish multicenter randomized study of invasive versus conservative treatment in patients with inducible ischemia after thrombolysis in acute myocardial infarction (DANAMI). Circulation 1997; 96: 748–55 |

| No. | Level | Citation |
|-----|-------|----------|
| 153 | 2c | Holmes DR, Bates ER, Kleiman NS et al. Contemporary reperfusion therapy for cardiogenic shock. J Am Coll Cardiol 1995; 26: 668–76 |
| 154 | 1b | Zehender M, Kasper W, Kauder E et al. Right ventricular infarction as an independent predictor of prognosis after acute inferior myocardial infarction. N Engl J Med 1993; 328: 981–8 |
| 155 | 2b | Volpi A, Cavalli A, Santoro L et al. Incidence and prognosis of early primary ventricular fibrillation in acute myocardial infarction: results of the GISSI-2 database. Am J Cardiol 1998; 82: 265–71 |
| 156 | 2c | Selker HP, Griffith JL, Beshansky JR et al. Patient-specific predictions of outcomes in myocardial infarction for real time emergency use: a thrombolytic predictive instrument. Am Intern Med 1997; 127: 538–56 |
| 157 | 2b | Behar S, Goldbourt U, Reicher-Reiss H et al. Prognosis of acute myocardial infarction complicated by primary ventricular fibrillation. Am J Cardiol 1990; 66: 1208–11 |
| 158 | 2c | Adgey AAJ, Geddes JS, Mulholland HC et al. Incidence, significance, and management of early bradyarrhythmia complicating acute myocardial infarction. Lancet 1968; ii: 1097–1101 |
| 159 | 1b | Moreno AM, Tomas JG, Alberola AG et al. Significacion pronostica del bloqueo auriculoventricular completo en pacientes con infarto agudo de miocardio inferior. Un estudio en la era trombolitica. Rev Esp Cardiol 1997; 50: 397–405 |
| 160 | 2b | Berger PB, Ruocco NA, Ryan TJ et al. Incidence and prognostic implications of heart block complicating inferior myocardial infarction treated with thrombolytic therapy: results from TIMI II. J Am Coll Cardiol 1992; 20: 533–40 |
| 161 | 1b | Goldberg RJ, Gore JM, Alpert JS et al. Cardiogenic shock after acute myocardial infarction: incidence and mortality from a community-wide perspective, 1975 to 1988. N Engl J Med 1991; 325: 1117–22 |
| 162 | 2b | Hands ME, Rutherford JD, Muller JE et al. The in-hospital development of cardiogenic shock after myocardial infarction: incidence, predictors of occurrence, outcome and prognostic factors. J Am Coll Cardiol 1989; 14: 40–6 |
| 163 | 4 | Killip T, Kimball JT. Treatment of myocardial infarction in a coronary care unit: a two year experience of 250 patients. Am J Cardiol 1967; 20: 457–64 |
| 164 | 2b | Lee KL, Woodlief LH, Topol EJ et al. Predictors of 30-day mortality in the era of reperfusion for acute myocardial infarction: results from an international trial of 41 021 patients. Circulation 1995; 91: 1659–68 |
| 165 | 1b | Frasure-Smith N, Lesperance F, Talajic M. Depression and 18-month prognosis after myocardial infarction. Circulation 1995; 91: 999–1005 |
| 166 | 2b– | O'Rourke MF, Norris RM, Campbell TJ et al. Randomized controlled trial of intraaortic balloon counterpulsation in early myocardial infarction with acute heart failure. Am J Cardiol 1981; 47: 815–20 |
| 167 | 4 | Sugiura T, Iwasaka T, Takayama Y et al. Factors associated with pericardial effusion in acute Q wave myocardial infarction. Circulation 1990; 81: 477–81 |
| 168 | 4 | Pierard LA, Albert A, Henrard L et al. Incidence and significance of pericardial effusion in acute myocardial infarction as determined by two-dimensional echocardiography. J Am Coll Cardiol 1986; 8: 517–20 |

| No. | Level | Citation |
|---|---|---|
| 169 | 4 | Wall TC, Califf RM, Harrelson-Woodlief L et al. Usefulness of a pericardial friction rub after thrombolytic therapy during acute myocardial infarction in predicting amount of myocardial damage. Am J Cardiol 1990; 66: 1418–21 |
| 170 | 1b– | Berman J, Haffajee CI, Alpert JS. Therapy for symptomatic pericarditis after myocardial infarction: retrospective and prospective studies of aspirin, indomethacin, prednisolone, and spontaneous resolution. Am Heart J 1981; 101: 750–3 |
| 171 | 4 | Lopez-Sendon J, Gonzalez A, Lopez E et al. Diagnosis of subacute ventricular wall rupture after acute myocardial infarction: sensitivity and specificity of clinical, hemodynamic and echocardiographic criteria. J Am Coll Cardiol 1992; 19: 1145–53 |
| 172 | 2b | Moore CA, Nygaard TW, Kaiser DL et al. Postinfarction ventricular septal rupture: the importance of location of infarction and right ventricular function in determining survival. Circulation 1986; 74: 45–55 |
| 173 | 1b | Galjee MA, Visser FC, De Cock CC et al. The prognostic value, clinical and angiographic characteristics of patients with early postinfarction angina after a first myocardial infarction. Am Heart J 1992; 125: 48–55 |
| 174 | 2b | Berger CJ, Murabito JM, Evans JC et al. Prognosis after first myocardial infarction: comparison of Q-wave and non-Q-wave myocardial infarction in the Framingham Heart Study. JAMA 1992; 267: 515–19 |
| 175 | 2b | Case RB, Moss AJ, Case N et al. Living alone after myocardial infarction: impact on prognosis. JAMA 1992; 268: 1545–51 |
| 176 | 3b | Stampfer MJ, Krauss RM, Ma J et al. A prospective study of triglyceride level, low-density lipoprotein particle diameter, and risk of myocardial infarction. JAMA 1996; 276: 882–8 |
| 177 | 1b | Madsen JK, Grande P, Saunamaki K et al. Danish multicenter randomized study of invasive versus conservative treatment in patients with inducible ischemia after thrombolysis in acute myocardial infarction (DANAMI). Circulation 1997; 96: 748–55 |
| 178 | 2c | Lapeyre AC, Steele PM, Kazmier FJ et al. Systemic embolism in chronic left ventricular aneurysm: incidence and the role of anticoagulation: J Am Coll Cardiol 1985; 6: 534–8 |
| 179 | 1b | Lehmann KG, Francis CK, Dodge HT et al. Mitral regurgitation in early myocardial infarction: incidence, clinical detection and prognostic implications. Ann Intern Med 1992; 117: 10–17 |
| 180 | 2b | Lamas GA, Mitchell GF, Flaker GC et al. Clinical significance of mitral regurgitation after acute myocardial infarction. Circulation 1997; 96: 827–33 |
| 181 | 1b | Thiemann DR, Coresh J, Oetgen WJ et al. The association between hospital volume and survival after acute myocardial infarction in elderly patients. N Engl J Med 1999; 340: 1640–8 |
| 182 | 2b | Peterson ED, Hathaway WR, Zabel KM et al. Prognostic significance of precordial ST segment depression during inferior myocardial infarction in the thrombolytic era: results in 16 521 patients. J Am Coll Cardiol 1996; 28: 305–12 |
| 183 | 2b | Berger PB, Ruocco NA, Ryan TJ et al. Incidence and prognostic implications of heart block complicating inferior myocardial infarction treated with thrombolytic therapy: results from TIMI II. J Am Coll Cardiol 1992; 20: 533–40 |
| 184 | 1b | Willems AR, Tijssen JGP, van Capelle FJL et al. Determinants of prognosis in symptomatic ventricular tachycardia or ventricular fibrillation late after myocardial infarction. J Am Coll Cardiol 1990; 16: 521–30 |

| No. | Level | Citation |
|---|---|---|
| 185 | 2b | Kornowski R, Goldbourt U, Zion M et al. Predictors and long-term prognostic significance of recurrent infarction in the year after a first myocardial infarction. Am J Cardiol 1993; 72: 883–8 |
| 186 | 2b | Stone GW, Grines CL, Browne KF et al. Predictors of in-hospital and 6-month outcome after acute myocardial infarction in the reperfusion era: the Primary Angioplasty in Myocardial Infarction (PAMI) Trial. J Am Coll Cardiol 1995; 25: 370–7 |
| 187 | 2b | Volpi A, Cavalli A, Santoro L et al. Incidence and prognosis of early primary ventricular fibrillation in acute myocardial infarction: results of the GISSI-2 database. Am J Cardiol 1998; 82: 265–71 |
| 188 | 1b | Vaccarino V, Parsons L, Every NR et al. Sex-based differences in early mortality after myocardial infarction. N Engl J Med 1999; 341: 217–25 |
| 189 | 1b | Behar S, Reicher-Ross H, Abinader E et al. The prognostic significance of angina pectoris preceding the occurrence of a first myocardial infarction in 4166 consecutive hospitalized patients. Am Heart J 1992; 123: 1481–6 |
| 190 | 1b | Miettinen H, Haffner SM, Lehto S et al. Impact of diabetes on mortality after the first myocardial infarction. Diabetes Care 1998; 21: 69–75 |
| 191 | 1b | Behar S, Rabinowitz B, Zion M et al. Immediate and long-term prognostic significance of a first anterior vs inferior wall Q-wave actue myocardial infarction. Am J Cardiol 1993; 72: 1366–70 |
| 192 | 1b | van Domburg RT, Klootwijk P, Deckers JW et al. The cardiac infarction injury score as a predictor for long-term mortality in survivors of a myocardial infarction. Eur Heart J 1998; 19: 1034–41 |
| 193 | 1b | Birnbaum Y, Sclarovsky S, Blum A et al. Prognostic significance of the initial electrocardiographic pattern in a first acute anterior wall myocardial infarction. Chest 1993; 103: 1681–7 |
| 194 | 2b | Go AS, Barron HV, Rundle AC et al. Bundle-branch block and in-hospital mortality in acute myocardial infarction. Ann Intern Med 1998; 129: 690–7 |
| 195 | 2b | Ricou F, Nicod P, Gilpin E et al. Influence of right bundle-branch block on short-and long-term survival after acute anterior myocardial infarction. J Am Coll Cardiol 1991; 17: 858–63 |
| 196 | 2b | Peterson ED, Hathaway WR, Zabel KM et al. Prognostic significance of precordial ST segment depression during inferior myocardial infarction in the thrombolytic era: results in 16 521 patients. J Am Coll Cardiol 1996; 28: 305–12 |
| 197 | 1b | Zehender M, Kasper W, Kauder E et al. Right ventricular infarction as an independent predictor of prognosis after acute inferior myocardial infarction. N Engl J Med 1993; 328: 981–8 |
| 198 | 2b | Case RB, Moss AJ, Case N et al. Living alone after myocardial infarction: impact on prognosis. JAMA 1992; 267: 515–19 |
| 199 | 2b | Maggioni AP, Zuanetti G, Franzosi MG et al. Prevalence and prognostic significance of ventricular arrhythmias after acute myocardial infarction in the fibrinolytic era: GISSI-2 results. Circulation 1993; 87: 312–22 |
| 200 | 1a | Bucher HC. Social support and prognosis following first myocardial infarction. J Gen Intern Med 1994; 9: 409–17 |
| 201 | 2b | Gallagher EJ, Viscoli CM, Horwitz RI. The relationship of treatment adherence to the risk of death after myocardial infarction in women. JAMA 1993; 270: 742–4 |

## CAUSES

Common causes of pleural effusions include **[B]**[1] **[B]**[2] **[C]**[3] **[C]**[4]:

- transudates
  - congestive heart failure
  - liver cirrhosis
  - nephrotic syndrome
  - hypoalbuminaemia

- exudates
  - malignant effusions
  - parapneumonic effusions
  - tuberculosis
  - pulmonary embolism.

**Note**

The commonest causes of pleural effusions are malignancy, heart failure and infection

| Cause | Wards **[B]**[1] **[B]**[2] **[C]**[3] | Intensive care unit **[C]**[4] |
|---|---|---|
| *Transudates* | | |
| Congestive heart failure | 10–27% | |
| Liver cirrhosis | 3% | |
| Nephrotic syndrome | 2% | |
| Hypoalbuminaemia | | 8% |
| *Exudates* | | |
| Malignant effusions | 30–48% | 3% |
| Parapneumonic effusions | 11–17% | 11% |
| TB | 15–20% | |
| PE | 3–6% | |
| Collagen vascular disease | 1% | |
| Trauma | 1% | |
| Pancreatitis | 0.3% | |
| Other | 5% | |

## CLINICAL FEATURES

Ask about:
- weight loss **[C]**[5]
- fever **[C]**[5]

| | | | | | | |
|---|---|---|---|---|---|---|
| **? Why?** | | | | | | |
| Weight loss and fever make malignant or granulomatous disease more likely | | | | | | |
| Patient **[C]**[5] | Target disorder (reference standard) | Diagnostic test | LR+ (95% CI) | Post-test probability | LR− (95% CI) | Post-test probability |
| Pleural effusion (pre-test probability 39%) | Malignancy or granulomatous disease (culture or biopsy) | Weight loss > 4.5 kg | 4.2 (2.2 to 7.8) | 7.3% | 0.35 (0.21 to 0.60) | 19% |
| | | Fever > 38°C | 4.3 (1.5 to 12) | 73% | 0.73 (0.57 to 0.93) | 32% |

- previous diagnoses **[D]**.

Look for the following on chest examination:

- reduced expansion **[D]**
- a change in dullness on auscultatory percussion above the 12th rib **[B]**[2]

**Examination**

1. Ask your patient to sit upright or stand for 5 min to allow any free pleural fluid to drain to the lung base.
2. Place the stethoscope diaphragm 3 cm below the 12th rib in the midclavicular line.
3. Percuss directly with your free hand (by finger flicking or with the pulp of a finger) along three or more parallel lines from the apex of each hemithorax perpendicularly down toward the base.
4. Pleural effusions can be confirmed by asking a patient to lean to one side and then reassessing the fluid level to see whether it had shifted.

| | | | | |
|---|---|---|---|---|
| **? Why?** | | | | |
| Auscultatory percussion can help diagnose a pleural effusion | | | | |
| Patient **[C]**[5] | Target disorder (reference standard) | Diagnostic test | LR+ (95% CI) | LR − (95% CI) |
| Suspected pleural effusion | Pleural effusion (chest X-ray) | Dullness on auscultatory percussion | 19 (9.8 to 35) | 0.045 (0.019 to 0.11) |

- 'stony dullness' on percussion **[D]**
- decreased air entry **[D]**.

## INVESTIGATIONS

### Step 1

- Take a chest X-ray and perform thoracentesis [C][6].

>  **Why?**
> - 35% of diagnoses are made on history, examination, chest X-ray, macroscopic examination and first cytological study of pleural fluid [C][6].

- Chest X-ray or ultrasound scan [C][7].

> **Why?**
> A chest X-ray or ultrasound scan can help diagnose an effusion
>
> | Patient [C][7] | Target disorder (reference standard) | Diagnostic test | LR+ (95% CI) | Post-test probability | LR– (95% CI) | Post-test probability |
> | --- | --- | --- | --- | --- | --- | --- |
> | Pleural disease and suspected pleural effusion (pre-test probability 69%) | Pleural effusion (thoracentesis) | Effusion on chest X-ray | 4.2 (2.2 to 7.8) | 73% | 0.35 (0.21 to 0.60) | 19% |
> | | | Effusion on ultrasound scan | 4.3 (1.5 to 12) | 73% | 0.73 (0.57 to 0.93) | 32% |

A large effusion ($> \frac{1}{2}$ hemithorax) increases the risk of malignancy or TB. [C][7]

> **Why?**
> A large effusion increases the risk of malignancy or TB but cannot rule them out
>
> | Patient [C][7] | Target disorder (reference standard) | Diagnostic test | LR+ (95% CI) | Post-test probability | LR– (95% CI) | Post-test probability |
> | --- | --- | --- | --- | --- | --- | --- |
> | Pleural effusion (pre-test probability 39%) | Malignancy or granulomatous disease (culture or biopsy) | Large effusion | 6.2 (1.9 to 21) | 80% | 0.69 (0.53 to 89) | 31% |

- Thoracentesis:
  - preferably using ultrasound guidance [A][8]
  - otherwise a 20G needle and syringe [A][8]; watch out for subsequent pneumothorax [C][8].

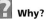 **Why?**

■ It reduces complications, particularly dry taps (inadequate tap, pain, subcutaneous haematoma or pneumothorax) **[A]**[8].

■ It is safer than using a 20G needle and syringe, or using a 14G as an introducer for a 16G needle, catheter and syringe **[A]**[8].

**Ultrasound-guided thoracentesis is safer using a needle and syringe**

| Patient | Treatment | Comparator | Outcome | CER | RRR | NNT |
|---------|-----------|------------|---------|-----|-----|-----|
| Pleural effusion **[A]**[8] | Needle and catheter | Needle | Any complication at 48 h | 47% | −110% (−270% to −25%) | −2 (−4 to −1) |
| Pleural effusion **[A]**[8] | Ultrasound-guided | Needle | Any complication at 48 h | 47% | 66% (−9% to 90%) | 3 (2 to 130) |

● Look at the fluid collected.
A milky appearance helps diagnose a chylous effusion **[C]**[7].

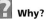 **Why?**

**A milky appearance makes a chylous effusion more likely**

| Patient **[C]**[7] | Target disorder (reference standard) | Diagnostic test | LR+ (95% CI) | Post-test probability | LR− (95% CI) | Post-test probability |
|--------|------|------|------|------|------|------|
| Pleural effusion (pre-test probability 27%) | Chylous fluid (chylomicrons in pleural fluid) | Milky appearance | 25 (6.0 to 100) | 90% | 0.54 (0.40 to 0.73) | 16% |

**Note**

■ Chylous fluid increases the chance of lymphoma (~ 50% of patients). Other common causes are post-operative/traumatic (24%) or idiopathic 13%.

● Send the fluid for **[C]**[6]:
  – cytology
  – biochemistry
  – bacteriology
  – microscopic examination of fluid
  – tumour markers

**Why?**

■ 36% of diagnoses are made using these investigations **[C]**[6].
**Cytology can help diagnose malignancy or TB, but does not safely exclude it**

| Patient | Target disorder (reference standard) | Diagnostic test | LR+ (95% CI) | Post-test probability (%) | LR– (95% CI) | Post-test probability |
|---|---|---|---|---|---|---|
| Pleural effusion (pre-test probability 68%) **[C]**[9] | Malignancy (other biopsies, clinical features, operation or autopsy) | Cytology | Infinity (22 to infinity) | 100% | 0.52 (0.46 to 0.58) | 47% |
| Pleural effusion (pre-test probability 39%) **[C]**[7] | Malignancy or granulomatous disease (culture or biopsy) | >95% lymphocytes in pleural fluid | 2.0 (1.0 to 3.8) | 56% | 0.74 (0.54 to 1.0) | 32% |

- Biochemistry:
  - glucose **[C]**[10]
  - amylase **[C]**[10]
  - LDH **[B]**[1]
  - albumin **[B]**[1]
  - protein **[B]**[1]
  - triglycerides (≥ 1.0 mmol/l): chylous **[C]**[11]

**Note**

■ Biochemical tests can help distinguish exudates and transudates, but remember up to 1% of patients with malignancy have transudative pleural effusions **[C]**[12].

**Why?**

| Patient | Target disorder (reference standard) | Diagnostic test | LR+ (95% CI) | Post-test probability | LR– (95% CI) | Post-test probability |
|---|---|---|---|---|---|---|
| Pleural effusion (pre-test probability 74%) **[B]**[1] | Exudate (biopsy, imaging, follow-up) | LDH>0.45 upper limit of normal | 4.8 | 93% | 0.15 | 30% |
| | | protein > 2.9 g/dl | 5.4 | 94% | 0.10 | 22% |
| Pleural effusion (pre-test probability 85%) **[C]**[3] | Exudate (biopsy, cytology) | Light's criteria: any abnormal LDH, LDH ratio or protein ratio | 4.3 (2.5 to 7.4) | 96% | 0.036 (0.017 to 0.076) | 17% |

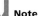

### Why?

| Patient | Target disorder (reference standard) | Diagnostic test | LR+ (95% CI) | Post-test probability | LR– (95% CI) | Post-test probability |
|---|---|---|---|---|---|---|
| Pleural effusion (pre-test probability 49%) [C][10] | Exudate (final diagnosis) | Glucose ≤ 6.0 mmol/l | 5.0 (2.8 to 8.8) | 83% | 0.31 (0.21 to 0.47) | 23% |
| Pleural effusion (pre-test probability 49%) [C][10] | Exudate (final diagnosis) | Amylase≥ 1000 units/l | 8.5 (2.0 to 35) | 89% | 0.80 (0.70 to 0.91) | 43% |

### Elevated triglyceride levels make a chylous effusion more likely

| Patient | Target disorder (reference standard) | Diagnostic test | LR+ (95% CI) | Post-test probability | LR– (95% CI) | Post-test probability |
|---|---|---|---|---|---|---|
| Pleural effusion (pre-test probability 27%) | Chylous fluid (chylomicrons in pleural fluid) | Triglyceride ≥ 1.0 mmol/l | 13 (6.2 to 27) | 83% | 0.14 (0.062 to 0.32) | 5% |

- Bacteriology.

### Note
■ 64% of infections are due to aerobic organisms, 23% mixed, 13% anaerobic [C][13].

- Consider taking the following blood tests:
  - blood count [D]
  - urea and electrolytes [D]
  - glucose [C]
  - protein [B][1]
  - liver function tests [B][1]
  - albumin [B][1]
  - calcium [D].

## Step 2
If considering the following conditions, consider these tests.

### Pneumonia and an effusion
These tests can help diagnose a complicated parapneumonic effusion:
- glucose [B][14]
- LDH [B][14]
- pH [B][14].

? **Why?**
A low glucose increases the risk of a complicated parapneumonic effusion

| Patient [B][14] | Target disorder (reference standard) | Diagnostic test | LR+ (95% CI) | Post-test probability |
|---|---|---|---|---|
| Parapneumonic effusion (pre-test probability 40%) | Complicated effusion (frank pus or requiring drainage) | Glucose <2.0 mmol/l | 16 (5.2 to 50) | 91% |
| | | 2.0–5.0 mmol/l | 0.92 (0.47 to 1.8) | 38% |
| | | <5.0 mmol/l | 0.28 (0.16 to 0.47) | 15% |

A raised LDH increases the risk of a complicated parapneumonic effusion

| Patient [B][14] | Target disorder (reference standard) | Diagnostic test | LR+ (95% CI) | Post-test probability |
|---|---|---|---|---|
| Parapneumonic effusion (pre-test probability 40%) | Complicated effusion (frank pus or requiring drainage) | LDH < 1600 units/ml | 8.1 (3.3 to 20) | 81% |
| | | 600–1600 units/ml | 1.0 (0.53 to 2.0) | 36% |
| | | < 600 units/ml | 0.29 (0.15 to 0.55) | 14% |

A pH > 7.3 reduces the risk of a complicated parapneumonic effusion

| Patient [B][14] | Target disorder (reference standard) | Diagnostic test | LR+ (95% CI) | Post-test probability |
|---|---|---|---|---|
| Parapneumonic effusion (pre-test probability 40%) | Complicated effusion (frank pus or requiring drainage) | pH ≤ 7.2 | 9.9 (5.7 to 17) | 87% |
| | | 7.2–7.3 | 1.2 (0.63 to 2.4) | 45% |
| | | >7.3 | 0.086 (0.042 to 0.18) | 5% |

Possible malignancy
First look for:

- weight loss > 4.5 kg
- fever > 38°C
- large effusion (> $\frac{1}{2}$ hemithorax)
- positive tuberculin test
- >95% lymphocytes in pleural fluid

The presence of two or more of these increases the risk of malignancy or TB; if there are none, malignancy or TB is far less likely.

| ? Why?<br>Five simple tests can help rule malignancy or TB in and out | | | | | | |
|---|---|---|---|---|---|---|
| Patient [C][9] | Target disorder (reference standard) | Diagnostic test | LR+ (95% CI) | Post-test probability | LR– (95% CI) | Post-test probability |
| Pleural effusion (pre-test probability 39%) | Malignancy or granulomatous disease (culture or biopsy) | Any two present | 7.2 (3.0 to 17) | 82% | 0.36 (0.22 to 0.59) | 19% |
| | | Any present | 2.3 (1.7 to 3.2) | 60% | 0.050 (0.0072 to 0.35) | 3% |

- carcinoembryonic antigen [C][15] [C][16]

| ? Why?<br>High levels of carcinoembryonic antigen can diagnose malignancy | | | | | | |
|---|---|---|---|---|---|---|
| Patient | Target disorder (reference standard) | Diagnostic test | LR+ (95% CI) | Post-test probability | LR– (95% CI) | Post-test probability |
| Pleural effusion (pre-test probability 31%) [C][15] | Malignancy (histology or cytology) | CEA> 40 ng/ml | Infinity (21 to inf) | 100% | 0.57 (0.46 to 0.70) | 21% |
| Pleural effusion (pre-test probability 34%) [C][16] | Malignancy (histology or cytology) | CEA> 10 ng/ml | 5.0 (3.0 to 8.2) | 72% | 0.59 (0.49 to 0.72) | 23% |

– serum tests are an alternative [C][6]

| ? Why?<br>Raised CEA and serum tissue polypeptide levels make malignancy more likely | | | | | | |
|---|---|---|---|---|---|---|
| Patient | Target disorder (reference standard) | Diagnostic test | LR+ (95% CI) | Post-test probability | LR– (95% CI) | Post-test probability |
| Pleural effusion (pre-test probability 44%) [C][15] | Malignancy (cytology, pleural biopsy specimen or autopsy) | Serum CEA> 8.0 mg/dl | 5.4 (2.0 to 14) | 90% | 0.70 (0.60 to 0.82) | 55% |
| | | Serum tissue polypeptide> 100 units/ml | 4.8 (2.8 to 8.3) | 89% | 0.19 (0.12 to 0.30) | 25% |

- complement (C3, C4) **[C]**[17]
- alpha-l-antitrypsin **[C]**[17]

| ? Why? Low complement and alpha-l-antitrypsin reduce the chance of malignancy | | | | | | |
| --- | --- | --- | --- | --- | --- | --- |
| Patient **[C]**[17] | Target disorder (reference standard) | Diagnostic test | LR+ (95% CI) | Post-test probability | LR– (95% CI) | Post-test probability |
| Pleural effusion (pre-test probability 47%) | Malignancy (histology or follow-up) | C3 > 300 mg/dl | 1.7 (1.3 to 2.1) | 59% | 0.15 (0.047 to 0.46) | 12% |
| | | C4 > 700 mg/dl | 2.0 (1.6 to 2.7) | 64% | 0.00 (0.00 to 0.13) | 0% |
| | | alpha-1-antitrypsin > 150 mg/dl | 1.4 (1.2 to 1.7) | 55% | 0.00 (0.00 to 0.086) | 0% |

## Possible tuberculosis

First look for:
- weight loss > 4.5 kg
- fever > 38°C
- large effusion (> $\frac{1}{2}$ hemithorax)
- positive tuberculin test
- > 95% lymphocytes in pleural fluid

The presence of two or more increases the risk of malignancy or TB; if there are none, malignancy or TB are far less likely.

| ? Why? Five simple tests can help rule malignancy or TB in and out | | | | | | |
| --- | --- | --- | --- | --- | --- | --- |
| Patient **[C]**[5] | Target disorder (reference standard) | Diagnostic test | LR+ (95% CI) | Post-test probability | LR– (95% CI) | Post-test probability |
| Pleural effusion (pre-test probability 39%) | Malignancy or granulomatous disease (culture or biopsy) | Any two present | 7.2 (3.0 to 17) | 82% | 0.36 (0.22 to 0.59) | 19% |
| | | Any present | 2.3 (1.7 to 3.2) | 60% | 0.050 (0.0072 to 0.35) | 3% |

- culture **[A]**.

Consider:
- interferon gamma (positive if > 140 pg/ml) **[C]**[18]
- adenosine deaminase (positive if > 45 units/l) **[A]**[19] **[C]**[18].

**Why?**

- A tuberculin test alone cannot safely diagnose or exclude TB **[C]**[9].
- Adenosine deaminase has variable reported test characteristics **[A]**[19] **[C]**[17].

**Interferon gamma may rule TB out, unlike a tuberculin test and adenosine deaminase**

| Patient | Target disorder (reference standard) | Diagnostic test | LR+ (95% CI) | Post-test probability | LR– (95% CI) | Post-test probability |
|---------|------|------|------|------|------|------|
| Pleural effusion **[A]**[19] (pre-test probability 23%) | Tuberculous effusion (biopsy, histology or culture) | Adenosine deaminase (> 45 units/l) | 4.5 (2.4 to 8.7) | 86% | 0.27 (0.17 to 0.44) | 26% |
| Pleural effusion **[C]**[17] (pre-test probability 23%) | Tuberculous pleurisy (biopsy) | Adenosine deaminase (> 47 units/l) | 20 (12 to 32) | 85% | 0.00 (0.0 to 0.034) | 0% |
| Pleural effusion **[C]**[17] (pre-test probability 23%) | Tuberculous pleurisy (biopsy) | Interferon gamma (> 140 pg/ml) | 12 (6.1 to 21) | 79% | 0.062 (0.016 to 0.24) | 2% |
| Pleural effusion **[C]**[17] (pre-test probability 39%) | Malignancy or granulomatous disease (culture or biopsy) | Positive tuberculin test | 2.0 (1.0 to 3.8) | 56% | 0.74 (0.54 to 1.0) | 32% |

## Possible systemic lupus erythematosus
- Antinuclear antibodies **[C]**[20].

**Why?**
A positive ANA test increases the chance of SLE

| Patient **[C]**[20] | Target disorder (reference standard) | Diagnostic test | LR+ (95% CI) | Post-test probability | LR– (95% CI) | Post-test probability |
|---------|------|------|------|------|------|------|
| Pleural effusion (pre-test probability 9.8%) | SLE (American Rheumatology Association criteria for SLE) | ANA positive | 6.9 (3.2 to 15) | 43% | 0.28 (0.084 to 0.93) | 3% |

## Step 3
If there is still no clear diagnosis, consider **[C]**[6]:
- needle biopsy **[C]**[9] **[C]**[21] **[C]**[22]
- spiral CT, lung scan (or pulmonary angiography if neither available) **[D]**
- bronchoscopy **[C]**[23].

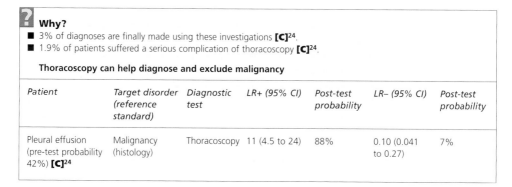

**? Why?**

■ Up to 27% of diagnoses are made using these investigations **[C]**[6].

**Needle biopsy and bronchoscopy can help diagnose malignancy or TB but not safely exclude them**

| Patient | Target disorder (reference standard) | Diagnostic test | LR+ (95% CI) | Post-test probability | LR– (95% CI) | Post-test probability |
|---|---|---|---|---|---|---|
| Pleural effusion (pre-test probability 48%) **[C]**[9]**[C]**[21]**[C]**[22] | Malignancy or TB (culture or histology) | Needle biopsy | 69 (9.8 to 490) | 98% | 0.33 (0.24 to 0.44) | 23% |
| Pleural effusion (pre-test probability 68%) **[C]**[23] | Malignancy (histology) | Bronchoscopy | Infinity (8.5 to infinity) | 100% | 0.45 (0.36 to 0.56) | 49% |

## Step 4

If there is still no clear diagnosis, consider **[C]**[6]:

● thoracoscopy **[C]**[24].

**? Why?**

■ 3% of diagnoses are finally made using these investigations **[C]**[24].
■ 1.9% of patients suffered a serious complication of thoracoscopy **[C]**[24].

**Thoracoscopy can help diagnose and exclude malignancy**

| Patient | Target disorder (reference standard) | Diagnostic test | LR+ (95% CI) | Post-test probability | LR– (95% CI) | Post-test probability |
|---|---|---|---|---|---|---|
| Pleural effusion (pre-test probability 42%) **[C]**[24] | Malignancy (histology) | Thoracoscopy | 11 (4.5 to 24) | 88% | 0.10 (0.041 to 0.27) | 7% |

## THERAPY

### Malignancy

● Insert a chest drain and perform pleurodesis **[A]** in recurrent cases **[D]**.

**? Note**

● Patients find small-bore chest drains (gauge 10) more comfortable and no worse than thoracentesis **[A]**[25].
● However, small-bore chest drains are not clearly as effective as standard sizes at preventing recurrent effusions **[D]**[26].

Perform pleurodesis once **[D]**[27] after the chest tube is draining < 150 ml of fluid per day **[D]**[8] and a chest X-ray shows no remaining fluid **[D]**. The effect of rotating the patient immediately after insertion of the sclerosant on successful pleurodesis is unclear.

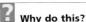

**Why do this?**
- Multiple instillations of tetracycline are not clearly better than a single instillation at preventing recurrence of malignant pleural effusions **[D]**[27].
- Pleurodesis following a short period of drainage is not clearly better than waiting until < 150 ml drains a day, and may well be worse **[D]**[28].
- Patients who roll around during chemical pleurodesis do not clearly have a less chance of recurrence of the effusion than those who do not **[D]**[29].

- An alternative is surgical pleurodesis using thoracoscopy **[D]**[30].

**Why do this?**
- Surgical pleurodesis is probably at least as effective as medical pleurodesis in patients with malignant pleural effusions **[D]**[30].

Use talc slurry **[B]**[31] when performing surgical pleurodesis.

**Why do this?**
- It is the cheapest and most effective sclerosant but requires pleurodesis **[B]**[31] **[D]**[32].

Use any of the following when performing medical pleurodesis:
- tetracycline **[B]**[33] and bleomycin **[A]**[4]
- doxycycline **[B]**[33]
- minocycline **[B]**[33]
- mepacrine **[A]**[35].

**Why do this?**
**Talc, tetracycline and doxycycline are effective sclerosants**

| Complete resolution of pleural effusion **[B]**[32] | % (95% CI) |
| --- | --- |
| Talc insufflation 2.5–10 g (requires thoracoscopy) | 93% (89% to 97%) |
| Minocycline 300 mg | 86% (53% to 100%) |
| Doxycycline 500 mg | 71% (60% to 83%) |
| Tetracycline 500 mg–20 mg/kg | 67% (62% to 72%) |
| Fluorouracil 2–3 g | 66% (50% to 81%) |
| Bleomycin 15–240 units | 54% (47% to 61%) |

- Mepacrine prevents recurrent effusions more effectively than bleomycin **[A]**[35].

**Mepacrine prevents recurrent effusion better than bleomycin**

| Patient | Treatment | Comparator | Outcome | CER | RRR | NNT |
| --- | --- | --- | --- | --- | --- | --- |
| Malignant pleural effusion **[A]**[35] | Mepacrine pleurodesis | Bleomycin pleurodesis | Repeat thoracentesis required at 1 month | 55% | 73% (17% to 91%) | 3 (1 to 8) |

**Why do this?**

- A combination of tetracycline and bleomycin is better than either alone at preventing recurrence. There is no clear difference in the side-effects between combination or single therapy **[A]**[34].

**Bleomycin and tetracycline prevent recurrent effusion better than either alone**

| Patient | Treatment | Comparator | Outcome | CER | RRR | NNT |
|---------|-----------|------------|---------|-----|-----|-----|
| Malignant pleural effusion **[A]**[34] | Tetracycline and bleomycin pleurodesis | Tetracycline pleurodesis | Recurrent effusion at 6 months | 50% | 60% (–7% to 85%) | 3 (2 to 52) |

Pain and fever are common after pleurodesis **[B]**[33], so give prophylactic analgesia **[D]** — options include opiates **[D]** and intrathecal lidocaine **[D]**.

 **Note**

**A quarter of patients have pain, and a fifth fever, following pleurodesis**

| Adverse effect | % (95% CI) |
|----------------|------------|
| Pain | 23% (17% to 22%) |
| Fever | 19% (17% to 22%) |

## Parapneumonic effusion

Drain a parapneumonic effusion if it is purulent or loculated **[D]**.

 **Note**

- 40% of parapneumonic effusions require drainage **[B]**[14].

- Insert a chest drain **[A]**
- Instill streptokinase **[A]**[36] or urokinase **[D]**[37] through the drain (e.g. 250 000 units streptokinase in 20 ml daily).

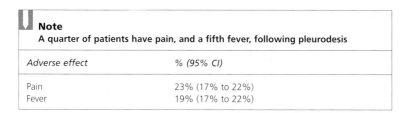 **Why do this?**

- Patients who have streptokinase compared with saline instilled daily into their chest drain pass more fluid (–1.5 l more) and more have at least a 50% reduction in the effusion at discharge **[A]**[36].
- Patients are less likely to require surgery **[A]**[36].
- Streptokinase and urokinase are probably equally effective in treating parapneumonic effusions. Both increase the fluid drained from the chest **[D]**[36].

**Streptokinase increases drainage and reduces need for surgery**

| Patient | Treatment | Comparator | Outcome | CER | RRR | NNT |
|---------|-----------|------------|---------|-----|-----|-----|
| Parapneumonic effusion **[A]**[36] | Streptokinase | Saline | Reduction in volume > 50% at discharge | 58% | 71% (–177% to –6%) | 2 (1 to 7) |
| | | | Surgery at discharge | 25% | 100% | 4 (2 to 200) |

Refer patients for ultrasound–guided drainage or surgery if drainage is unsuccessful **[D]**[37].

**Note**

- Around 10% of patients with parapneumonic effusions require surgery to clear them **[D]**[37].

## Tuberculosis

- Give antituberculous chemotherapy **[A]**.
  If TB is prevalent, consider empiric treatment in patients in whom no clear cause can be found **[D]**.
- Insert a chest drain **[D]**.
- There is no clear role for steroids once the effusion has been drained **[D]**[38] **[D]**[39].

**Why?**

- Steroids do not clearly reduce symptoms or prevent pleural thickening in patients with TB pleurisy and effusions which have been drained **[D]**[38] **[D]**[39].

## PROGNOSIS

- Malignant effusions often recur **[D]**[40] and mortality is high **[B]**[28].

**Note**

- Half of patients with a malignant effusion have a recurrence within 6 months (47%; 95% CI: 34 to 59%) **[D]**[40].
- Most patients are dead within 26 months (92%; 95% CI: 81% to 100%) **[D]**[28].

The commonest primaries are lung and breast, but no primary can be found in 10% of effusions.

**Note**

**Common cancers cause malignant pleural effusions**

| Men **[C]**[41] **[C]**[42] | % (95% CI) | Women | % (95% CI) |
|---|---|---|---|
| Lung | 49% (43% to 55%) | Breast | 37% (31% to 44%) |
| Lymphoma/leukaemia | 21% (16% to 26%) | Female genital tract | 20% (15% to 26%) |
| GI tract | 7.0% (4.1% to 10%) | Lung | 15% (9.9% to 20%) |
| GU tract | 6.0% (3.2% to 8.7%) | Lymphoma/leukaemia | 8.0% (4.1% to 12%) |
| Melanoma | 1.4% (0.0% to 2.8%) | GI tract | 4.3% (1.4% to 7.2%) |
| Mesothelioma | 1.1% (0.0% to 2.2%) | Melanoma | 3.2% (0.7% to 5.7%) |
| Other tumours | 3.5% (1.4% to 5.6%) | Urinary tract | 1.1% (0.0% to 2.5%) |
| Primary site unknown | 11% (7.3% to 15%) | Other tumours | 1.6% (0.0% to 3.4%) |
| | | Primary site unknown | 9.1% (5.0% to 13%) |

- If no definite cause can be found, the prognosis is good **[C]**[43].

> **Note**
> - In one series of patients with non-specific pleural effusions, all effusions eventually resolved (half within 6 months) **[C]**[43].
> - A cause is subsequently found in a fifth (20%; 95% CI: 7.6% to 32%) **[C]**[43].
> - Only a sixth relapse (13%; 95% CI: 2.3% to 23%) **[C]**[43].

**Guideline writer**: Christopher Ball
**CAT writers**: Don Stanley, Christopher Ball

## REFERENCES

| No. | Level | Citation |
| --- | --- | --- |
| 1 | 2a | Heffner JE et al. Diagnostic value of tests that discriminate between exudative and transudative pleural effusions. Chest 1997; 111: 970–80 |
| 2 | 2b | Guarino JR et al. Auscultatory percussion: a simple method to detect pleural effusion: J Gen Intern Med 1994; 9: 71–4 |
| 3 | 4 | Romero S et al. Evaluation of different criteria for the separation of pleural transudates from exudates. Chest 1993; 104: 399–404 |
| 4 | 4 | Mattison LE et al. Pleural effusion in the medical ICU: prevalence, causes and clinical implications. Chest 1997; 111: 1018–23 |
| 5 | 4 | Leslie WK et al. Clinical characteristics of patients with non-specific pleuritis. Chest 1988; 94: 603–8 |
| 6 | 4 | Marel M et al. Diagnosis of pleural effusions: experience with clinical studies, 1986 to 1990. Chest 1995; 107: 1598–03 |
| 7 | 4 | Gryminski J et al. The diagnosis of pleural effusion by ultrasonic and radiologic techniques. Chest 1976; 70: 33–7 |
| 8 | 1b | Grogan DR et al. Complications associated with thoracentesis: a prospective randomised study comparing three different Methods. Arch Intern Med 1990; 150: 873–7 |
| 9 | 4 | Prakash UB, Reiman HM. Comparison of needle biopsy with cytologic analysis for the evaluation of pleural effusion: analysis of 414 cases. Mayo Clin Proc 1985; 60: 158–64 |
| 10 | 4 | Light RW, Ball WC. Glucose and amylase in pleural effusions. JAMA 1973; 225: 257–60 |
| 11 | 4 | Staats BA et al. The lipoprotein profile of chylous and nonchylous pleural effusion. Mayo Clin Proc 1980; 55: 700–4 |
| 12 | 4 | Assi Z et al. Cytologically proved malignant pleural effusions: distribution of transudates and exudates. Chest 1998; 113: 1302–4 |
| 13 | 4 | Brook I, Frazier EH. Aerobic and anaerobic microbiology of empyema: a retrospective review in two military hospitals. Chest 1993; 103: 1502–7 |
| 14 | 2a | Heffner JE et al. Pleural fluid chemical analysis in parapneumonic effusion: a meta-analysis. Am J Respir Crit Care Med 1995; 151: 1700–8 |

| No. | Level | Citation |
|-----|-------|----------|
| 15 | 4 | Villena V et al. Diagnostic value of CA 72–4, carcinoembryonic antigen, CA 15–3 and CA 19–9 assay in pleural fluid. Cancer 1996; 78: 736–40 |
| 16 | 4 | Garcia-Pachon E et al. Elevated level of carcinoembryonic antigen, in non-malignant pleural effusion. Chest 1997; 111: 643–7 |
| 17 | 4 | Alexandrakis M et al. Diagnostic value of ferritin, haptoglobin, $\alpha_1$-antitrypsin, lactate dehydrogenase and complement factors $C_3$ and $C_4$ in pleural effusion differentiation. Respir Med 1997; 91: 517–23 |
| 18 | 4 | Valdes L et al. Diagnosis of tuberculous pleurisy using the biologic parameters adenosine deaminase, lysozyme and interferon gamma. Chest 1993; 102(3): 458–65 |
| 19 | 1b | Marrtens G, Bateman ED. Tuberculous pleural effusion: increased culture yield with bedside innoculation of pleural fluid and poor diagnostic value of adenosine deaminase. Thorax 1991; 46: 96–9 |
| 20 | 4 | Khare V et al. Antinuclear antibodies in pleural fluid. Chest 1994; 106: 866–71 |
| 21 | 4 | Poe RH et al. Sensitivity, specificity and predictive values of closed pleural biopsy. Arch Intern Med 1994; 144: 325–8 |
| 22 | 4 | Mungall IPF, Cowen PN, Cooke NT et al. Multiple pleural biopsies with the Abrams needle. Thorax 1980; 35: 600–2 |
| 23 | 4 | Chang & Peong. The role of fiberoptic bronchoscopy in evaluating the causes of pleural effusion. Arch Intern Med 1989; 149: 855–7 |
| 24 | 4 | Menzies R et al. Thoracoscopy for the diagnosis of pleural disease. Ann Intern Med 1991; 114: 271–6 |
| 25 | 1b– | Clementsen P et al. Treatment of malignant pleural effusion: pleurodesis using a small percutaneous catheter: a prospective randomized study. Respir Med 1998; 92: 593–6 |
| 26 | 1b– | Clementsen P et al. Treatment of malignant pleural effusion: pleurodesis using a small percutaneous catheter: a prospective randomized study: Respiratory Medicine 1998: 92(3): 593–596 |
| 27 | 1b– | Landvater L et al. Malignant pleural effusion treated by tetracycline sclerotherapy: a comparison of single versus repeated instillation. Chest 1988; 93: 1196–8 |
| 28 | 1b– | Villenueva AG et al. Efficacy of short-term versus long-term tube thoracostomy drainage before tetracycline pleurodesis in the treatment of malignant pleural effusion. Thorax 1994; 49: 23–5 |
| 29 | 1b– | Dryzer SR et al. Comparison of rotation and nonrotation in tetracycline pleurodesis. Chest 1993; 104: 1763–66 |
| 30 | 1b– | Evans TRJ et al. A randomised prospective trial of surgical against medical tetracycline pleurodesis in the management of malignant pleural effusions secondary to breast cancer. Eur J Cancer 1993; 291: 316–19 |
| 31 | 2a | Walker-Renard PW et al. Chemical pleurodesis for malignant pleural effusions. Ann Intern Med 1994; 120: 56–64 |
| 32 | 1b– | Zimmer PW et al. Prospective randomized trial of talc slurry vs bleomycin in pleurodesis for symptomatic malignant pleural effusions. Chest 1997; 112: 430–4 |
| 33 | 2a | Walker-Renard PW et al. Chemical pleurodesis for malignant pleural effusions. Ann Intern Med 1994; 120: 56–64 |

| No. | Level | Citation |
|-----|-------|----------|
| 34 | 1b | Emad A, Rezaian GR. Treatment of malignant pleural effusions with a combination of bleomycin and tetracycline: a comparison of bleomycin or tetracycline alone versus a combination of bleomycin and tetracycline. Cancer 1996; 78: 498–501 |
| 35 | 1b | Koldsland S et al. Chemical pleurodesis in malignant pleural effusions: a randomised prospective study of mepacrine versus bleomycin. Thorax 1993; 48: 790–3 |
| 36 | 1b | Davies RJ et al. Randomised controlled trial of intrapleural streptokinase in community acquired pleural infection. Thorax 1997; 52: 416–21 |
| 37 | 1b– | Bouros D et al. Intrapleural streptokinase versus urokinase in the treatment of complicated parapneumonic effusions: a prospective double-blind study. Am J Respir Crit Care Med 1997; 155: 291–5 |
| 38 | 1b– | Wyser C et al. Corticosteroids in the treatment of tuberculous pleurisy: a double-blind, placebo-controlled, randomized study. Chest 1996; 100: 333–8 |
| 39 | 1b– | Fleishman SJ et al. Antituberculous therapy combined with adrenal steroids in the treatment of pleural effusions: a controlled therapeutic trial. Lancet 1960: 199–201 |
| 40 | 1b– | Emad A & Rezaian GR. Treatment of malignant pleural effusions with a combination of bleomycin and tetracycline: a comparison of bleomycin or tetracycline alone versus a combination of bleomycin and tetracycline: Cancer 1996: 78: 498–501 |
| 41 | 4 | Johnston WW. The malignant pleural effusion: a review of cytopathologic diagnoses of 584 specimens from 472 consecutive patients. Cancer 1985; 56: 905–9 |
| 42 | 4 | Chernow B, Sahn SA. Carcinomatous involvement of the pleura: an analysis of 96 patients. Am J Med 1977; 63: 695–701 |
| 43 | 4 | Ferrer JS et al. Evolution of idiopathic pleural effusion: a prospective long-term follow-up study. Chest 1996; 109: 1508–13 |

## PREVALENCE

Community-acquired pneumonia is relatively common in suspected cases.

 **Note**
- 15%–28% of patients attending hospital with suspected pneumonia have it **[A]**[1].

## CAUSES

Common causes of community-acquired pneumonia are **[C]**[2] **[C]**[3]:
- *Streptococcus pneumoniae*
- *Mycoplasma pneumoniae*.

Remember less common causes **[C]**[2] **[C]**[3]:
- *Influenza A* virus
- *Haemophilus influenzae*
- *Chlamydia psittaci*
- *Legionella pneumophila*
- *Coxiella burnetii*
- *Staphylococcus aureus*.

**Note**

*S. pneumoniae* causes at least a third of pneumonias

| Infecting organism **[C]**[2] **[C]**[3] | Prevalence (95% CI) |
|---|---|
| Streptococcus pneumoniae | 32% (28% to 37%) |
| Mycoplasma pneumoniae | 17% (13% to 20%) |
| Influenza A virus | 5.4% (3.3% to 7.6%) |
| Haemophilus influenzae | 4.1% (2.2% to 5.9%) |
| Chlamydia psittaci | 2.3% (0.9% to 3.7%) |
| Legionella pneumophila | 1.6% (0.4% to 2.8%) |
| Coxiella burnetii | 1.1% (0.1% to 2.1%) |
| Staphylococcus aureus | 0.9% (0.02% to 1.8%) |
| Other known causes | 3.6% (1.9% to 5.4%) |
| Unknown microbiology | 34% (29% to 38%) |

## CLINICAL FEATURES

Ask about:
- age **[C]**[3]

 **Why?**
- Patients aged under 40 are more likely to have a *Mycoplasma pneumoniae* infection **[C]**[3].

- duration of illness **[C]**[3]

**Why?**
- Patients who have been unwell for 9 or more days are more likely to have a *Mycoplasma pneumoniae* infection **[C]**[3].

- any recent diarrhoea **[C]**[4]

**Why?**
**Diarrhoea makes *Legionella* pneumonia more likely**

| Patient **[C]**[4] | Target disorder (reference standard) | Diagnostic test | LR+(95% CI) | Post-test probability |
|---|---|---|---|---|
| Possible *Legionella* infection (pre-test probability 12%) | *Legionella* pneumonia (microscopy or serology) | Diarrhoea | 5.8 (1.5 to 22) | 44% |

- pleuritic chest pain **[B]**[5]
- chills **[B]**[5]

**Why?**
**Pleuritic chest pain or chills reduce the risk of dying from pneumonia**

| Patient **[B]**[5] | Prognostic factor | Outcome | Control rate | OR (95% CI) | NNF+ (95% CI) |
|---|---|---|---|---|---|
| Community-acquired pneumonia | Pleuritic chest pain | Death at ?discharge | 14% | 0.5 (0.3 to 0.8) | −16 (−41 to −11) |
| | Chills | Death at ?discharge | 14% | 0.4 (0.2 to 0.7) | −13 (−27 to −9) |

- a history of:
  - asthma **[A]**[1]
  - dementia **[A]**[6]
  - any immunosuppression **[A]**[6]

**Why?**
**Dementia and immunosuppression increase the risk of pneumonia**

| Patient **[A]**[6] | Target disorder (reference standard) | Diagnostic test | LR+ (95% CI) | Post-test probability | LR− (95% CI) | Post-test probability |
|---|---|---|---|---|---|---|
| Suspected pneumonia (pre-test probability 5%) | Pneumonia (chest X-ray) | History of dementia | 3.4 | 15% | 0.94 | 5% |
| | | History of immunosuppression | 2.2 | 10% | 0.85 | 4% |

- any underlying lung disease [C][4]

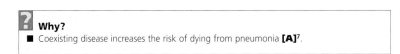

| ? **Why?** Underlying disease makes *Legionella* pneumonia less likely | | | | |
|---|---|---|---|---|
| *Patient [C][4]* | *Target disorder (reference standard)* | *Diagnostic test* | *LR–(95% CI)* | *Post-test probability* |
| Possible *Legionella* infection (pre-test probability 12%) | *Legionella* pneumonia (microscopy or serology) | Underlying disease | 0.22 (0.069 to 0.72) | 3% |

- coexisting disease [A][7]:
  - neoplastic disease
  - liver disease
  - congestive heart failure
  - cerebrovascular disease
  - renal disease

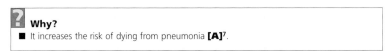

| ? **Why?** |
|---|
| ■ Coexisting disease increases the risk of dying from pneumonia [A][7]. |

- any pets [D].

Look for:
- altered mental status [A][7]

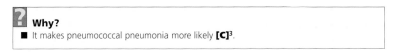

| ? **Why?** |
|---|
| ■ It increases the risk of dying from pneumonia [A][7]. |

- bloody sputum [C][3]

| ? **Why?** |
|---|
| ■ It makes pneumococcal pneumonia more likely [C][3]. |

- a cough [B][8]
- fever [A][1] [B][8]
- respiratory rate > 30 per minute [B][8]
- tachycardia [A][1] [B][8]

**Why?**
**No cough and normal vital signs make pneumonia less likely**

| Patient [B][8] | Target disorder (reference standard) | Diagnostic test | LR+(95% CI) | Post-test probability | LR-(95% CI) | Post-test probability |
|---|---|---|---|---|---|---|
| Suspected pneumonia (pre-test probability 5%) | Pneumonia (chest X-ray) | Cough | 1.8 | 9% | 0.31 | 2% |
| | | Fever | 2.1 (1.4 to 2.9) | 10% | 0.59 | 3% |
| | | Respiratory rate > 30/min | 2.6 | 12% | 0.80 | 4% |
| | | Any of respiratory rate > 30/min, heart rate > 100 beats/min, temperature > 37.8°C | 1.2 | 6% | 0.18 (0.07 to 46) | 0.9% |

- asymmetric respiration [B][8]
- dullness to percussion [B][8]
- decreased breath sounds [A][1] [B][8]
- bronchial breathing [B][8]
- crackles [A][1]
- aegophony [B][8].

**Why?**
**Abnormal chest findings make pneumonia more likely**

| Patient [B][8] | Target disorder (reference standard) | Diagnostic test | LR+ (95% CI) | Post-test probability | LR- (95% CI) | Post-test probability |
|---|---|---|---|---|---|---|
| Suspected pneumonia (pre-test probability 5%) | Pneumonia (chest X-ray) | Asymmetric respiration | Infinity (3.2 to inf) | 100% | 0.96 | 5% |
| | | Dullness to percussion | 2.2 | 10% | 0.92 | 5% |
| | | Decreased breath sounds | 2.3 | 11% | 0.78 | 4% |
| | | Bronchial breath sounds | 3.5 | 16% | 0.90 | 5% |
| | | Crackles | 1.6 | 8% | 0.83 | 4% |
| | | Aegophony | 2.0 | 10% | 0.96 | 5% |

 **Note**
- Other clinical features are not particularly helpful at diagnosing pneumonia [A][6].
- Clinicians agree moderately about dullness to percussion, reduced chest movement, wheeze and crackles, but agree poorly about whispering pectoriloquy and increased tactile fremitus [A][6].

Rank your patient for risk of a pulmonary infiltrate on chest X-ray.
Score one point for [A][1]:
- absence of asthma
- temperature >37.8°C
- pulse > 100 beats/min
- crackles
- decreased breath sounds.

| Box 1 A high score makes pneumonia more likely | |
| --- | --- |
| Score | Risk of pneumonia |
| 4 or 5 | high |
| 2 or 3 | moderate |
| 0 or 1 | low |

**Why?**

**Clinicians are not very good at diagnosing or excluding pneumonia**

| Patient [B][8] | Target disorder (reference standard) | Diagnostic test | LR+ (95% CI) | Post-test probability | LR– (95% CI) | Post-test probability |
| --- | --- | --- | --- | --- | --- | --- |
| Suspected pneumonia (pre-test probability 5%) | Pneumonia (chest X-ray) | Clinician's prediction | 2.0 (1.5 to 2.4) | 10% | 0.25 (0.09 to 0.61) | 1% |

**This clinical prediction rule can help rank patients for risk of pneumonia**

| Patient [A][1] | Target disorder (reference standard) | Diagnostic test | LR+ (95% CI) | Post-test probability |
| --- | --- | --- | --- | --- |
| Suspected pneumonia (pre-test probability 15%) | Pneumonia (pulmonary infiltrate on chest X-ray) | Score: 5 | 17 (6.5 to 47) | 75% |
| | | 4 | 7.2 (4.6 to 11) | 55% |
| | | 3 | 1.6 (1.2 to 2.2) | 22% |
| | | 2 | 0.70 (0.50 to 0.99) | 11% |
| | | 1 | 0.20 (0.11 to 0.36) | 3% |
| | | 0 | 0.12 (0.017 to 0.87) | 2% |

## DIFFERENTIAL DIAGNOSIS

### Dyspnoea

Think about other causes of breathlessness. Common causes include **[B]**[9]:

- asthma
- heart failure
- COPD
- arrhythmia
- interstitial lung disease
- anaemia.

**Why?**

**Asthma and heart failure are common causes of dyspnoea**

| Causes of dyspnoea **[B]**[9] | % |
| --- | --- |
| Asthma | 33% |
| Heart failure | 31% |
| COPD | 9% |
| Arrhythmia | 7% |
| Infection | 5% |
| Interstitial lung disease | 4% |
| Anaemia | 2% |
| PE | <2% |

## INVESTIGATIONS

- Pulse oximetry **[C]**[10].

**Why?**

- Significant hypoxia produces minimal changes in vital signs in healthy people **[C]**[10].

- Blood count **[C]**[3].

**Why?**

- A white cell count > 14.4 × 10[9]/ml makes a pneumococcal infection more likely **[C]**[3].
- Leucopenia **[B]**[5] or a haematocrit <30% increases the risk of dying in the next month **[A]**[7].

**Leucopenia increases the risk of dying**

| Patient **[B]**[5] | Prognostic factor | Outcome | Control rate | OR (95% CI) | NNF+ (95% CI) |
| --- | --- | --- | --- | --- | --- |
| Community-acquired pneumonia | Leucopenia | Death | 14% | 2.5 (1.6 to 3.7) | 13 (7 to 100) |

- Urea, electrolytes and creatinine **[A]**[7].
- Glucose **[A]**[7].

> **?**
> **Why?**
> ■ Urea ≥ 11 mmol/l, sodium < 130 mmol/l or glucose ≥ 14 mmol/l increases the risk of dying in the next month **[A]**[7].

- Creatine kinase **[C]**[4].

> **?**
> **Why?**
> **A raised creatine kinase makes *Legionella* pneumonia more likely**
>
> | Patient **[C]**[4] | Target disorder (reference standard) | Diagnostic test | LR+ (95% CI) | Post-test probability |
> |---|---|---|---|---|
> | Possible *Legionella* infection (pre-test probability 12%) | *Legionella* pneumonia (microscopy or serology) | CK >232 U/l | 5.8 (1.5 to 22) | 44% |

- Blood culture **[C]**[11].
- Sputum Gram stain **[D]**[12] and culture **[C]**[11].

> **U**
> **Note**
> ■ Only 70% of patients were able to produce a purulent sputum sample **[D]**[12].
> ■ Routine microbial investigations often fail to detect a causative agent (74%; 95% CI: 65% to 82%) **[C]**[13] and even with extensive screening a third of patients will have no specific pathogen identified (34%; 95% CI: 29% to 38%) **[C]**[2] **[C]**[3].
> ■ Few patients have antibiotics changed on the basis of microbial results (7.6%; 95% CI: 2.5% to 13%) **[C]**[13].
>
> **Specimen culture in pneumonia often fails to detect a causative organism**
>
> | Specimen **[C]**[11] | Organism cultured |
> |---|---|
> | Sputum smear | 52% (43% to 61%) |
> | Sputum culture | 35% (26% to 43%) |
> | Blood culture | 11% (6.3% to 16%) |
>
> ■ Bacteraemia increases the risk of dying in the next month **[B]**[5].
>
> **Bacteraemia increases the risk of dying**
>
> | Patient **[B]**[5] | Prognostic factor | Outcome | Control rate | OR (95% CI) | NNF+ (95% CI) |
> |---|---|---|---|---|---|
> | Community-acquired pneumonia | Bacteraemia | Death at ? discharge | 14% | 2.8 (2.3 to 3.6) | 7 (5 to 10) |

- Serology if atypical organisms are suspected **[A]**:
  - *Influenza A* and *B* viruses
  - *Coxiella burnetii*
  - *Chlamydia psittaci*
  - *Mycoplasma pneumoniae*
  - *Legionella pneumophila*
- Urine for *Legionella* antigen **[C]**[14].

 **Why?**
- Urine *Legionella* antigen is the most sensitive test for detecting *Legionella* (sensitivity 80%; 95% CI: 68% to 92%) **[C]**[14].

- Arterial blood gas **[A]**[7].

 **Why?**
- An arterial pH<7.35 or a $Po_2$<8.0 pKa increases the risk of dying in the next month **[A]**[7].

- Chest X-ray **[A]**.

  Look for:
  - a lobar infiltrate **[C]**[3]

 **Why?**
- A lobar infiltrate makes pneumococcal pneumonia more likely **[C]**[3].
- A multilobar infiltrate increases the risk of dying before discharge **[B]**[5].

**A multilobar infiltrate increases the risk of dying**

| Patient **[B]**[5] | Prognostic factor | Outcome | Control rate | OR (95% CI) | NNF + (95% CI) |
|---|---|---|---|---|---|
| Community-acquired pneumonia | Multilobar radiographic pulmonary infiltrate | Death ? at discharge. | 14% | 3.9 (1.9 to 5.1) | 7 (4 to 30) |

  - pleural effusion **[A]**[7].

 **Why?**
- A pleural effusion increases the risk of dying in the next month **[A]**[7].

 **Note**
- Radiographic shadowing, lobar distribution and changes over time do not usefully help to distinguish infecting organisms **[C]**[15].
- Radiologists agreed moderately well about the presence of an infiltrate and a pleural effusion on chest radiographs of patients with pneumonia, but fail to agree about the presence of lobar pneumonia or air bronchograms **[A]**[16].

- Consider bronchoalveolar lavage **[A]**[17] if the diagnosis remains uncertain.

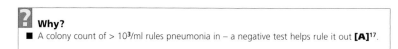

> **Why?**
> ■ A colony count of > 10³/ml rules pneumonia in – a negative test helps rule it out **[A]**[17].

## THERAPY

- Give oxygen to hypoxic patients **[A]**.
- Give antibiotics **[A]** intravenously to patients who are any of the following:
  - acutely confused
  - immunocompromised
  - critically ill
  - requiring inotropic or respiratory support
  - septicaemic
  - unable to tolerate oral medication
  - pregnant or lactating.

Uncomplicated cases can have oral antibiotics **[A]**[18].

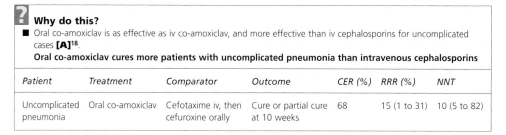

> **Why do this?**
> ■ Oral co-amoxiclav is as effective as iv co-amoxiclav, and more effective than iv cephalosporins for uncomplicated cases **[A]**[18].
> **Oral co-amoxiclav cures more patients with uncomplicated pneumonia than intravenous cephalosporins**

| Patient | Treatment | Comparator | Outcome | CER (%) | RRR (%) | NNT |
|---------|-----------|------------|---------|---------|---------|-----|
| Uncomplicated pneumonia | Oral co-amoxiclav | Cefotaxime iv, then cefuroxine orally | Cure or partial cure at 10 weeks | 68 | 15 (1 to 31) | 10 (5 to 82) |

Give elderly patients any of:
- second-or third-generation cephalosporins with a macrolide **[B]**[19]
- fluoroquinolone **[B]**[19].

### Why do this?

■ Elderly patients who receive second-or third-generation cephalosporins with a macrolide or fluoroquinolone are less likely to die **[B]**[19].

■ Patients who receive beta-lactam/beta-lactamase inhibitors plus macrolide or an aminoglycoside plus any other antimicrobial agent are at increased risk of dying **[B]**[19].

**Fluoroquinolones and second-or third-generation cephalosporins with a macrolide reduce mortality in the elderly**

| Patient **[B]**[19] | Prognostic factor | Outcome | Control rate | OR (95% CI) | NNF+ (95% CI) |
|---|---|---|---|---|---|
| Elderly with pneumonia | Fluoroquinolones only *independent* | Death at 30 days | 25% | 0.64 (0.43 to 0.94) | −20 (−130 to −12) |
| | Second-generation cephalosporin plus macrolide *independent* | | | 0.71 (0.52 to 0.96) | −25 (−190 to −15) |
| | Non-pseudomonal third-generation cephalosporin plus macrolide *independent* | | | 0.74 (0.60 to 0.92) | −29 (−95 to −18) |
| | Beta-lactam/ beta-lactamase inhibitors plus macrolide *independent* | | | 1.77 (1.28 to 2.46) | 11 (6 to 29) |
| | Aminoglycoside plus any other antimicrobial agent(s) *independent* | | | 1.21 (1.02 to 1.43) | 38 (19 to 390) |

■ More patients on levofloxacin improve or are cured than ceftriaxone or cefuroxime **[A]**[20].

■ Fewer patients relapse on sparfloxacin than on amoxicillin **[A]**[21].

**Fluoroquinolones cure more patients**

| Patient | Treatment | Comparator | Outcome | CER | RRR (%) | NNT |
|---|---|---|---|---|---|---|
| Community-acquired pneumonia **[A]**[20] | Levofloxacin | Ceftriaxone or cefuroxime | Clinical success at 7 days | 90% | −7 (−12 to −1) | 17 (9 to 73) |
| Community-acquired pneumonia **[A]**[21] | Sparfloxacin | Amoxicillin | Relapse at follow-up visit | 6.5% | 71 (−3 to 92) | 22 (11 to 310) |

Monitor your patient's response **[C]**[11] and repeat investigations if there is no improvement after 72 h **[D].**

**Why do this?**
- One in seven patients fails to respond to the first antibiotic regimen (14%; 95% CI: 8.6% to 19%) **[C]**[11].
- Pneumococcal pneumonia resistant to penicillins and cephalosporins is becoming more common, particularly for patients **[C]**[22]:
  - with two or more comorbidities
  - aged 65 or more.

**Old age and multiple comorbidities increase the risk of antibiotic-resistant infection**

| Outcome | Risk factor | PEER | OR (95% CI) | NNH (95% CI) |
|---|---|---|---|---|
| Cephalosporin-resistant pneumonia | Aged 65 or more *not independent* | 28% | 5.0 (1.3 to 18.8) | 3 (2 to 5) |
| Penicillin-resistant pneumonia | 2 or more comorbidities *not independent* | 38% | 4.7 (1.2 to 19.1) | 3 (2 to 23) |

- Give analgesia for pleuritic pain, e.g. a NSAID.

**Why do this?**
- Indometacin reduces severe pleuritic chest pain compared with placebo **[A]**[23].
- Indometacin increases FVC and $FEV_1$ and reduces the respiratory rate **[A]**[23].

**Indometacin gives effective pain relief for severe pleuritic chest pain**

| Patient **[A]**[23] | Treatment | Comparator | Outcome | CER | RRR | NNT |
|---|---|---|---|---|---|---|
| Severe pleuritic chest pain | Indometacin | Placebo | Pain relief good or excellent at 2 hours | 34% | 140% (39% to 320%) | 2 (1 to 4) |

- Consider transferring patients with any of the following to intensive care **[D]**:
  - severe pneumonia
  - severe hypoxia despite high-flow oxygen, hypercapnia
  - exhausted, drowsiness or unconscious
  - respiratory or cardiac arrest
  - shock.

## Parapneumonic effusion
Drain a parapneumonic effusion if it is purulent or loculated **[D]**.

**Note**
- 40% of parapneumonic effusions require drainage **[B]**[24].

- Insert a chest drain **[A]**.
- Instill streptokinase **[A]**[25] or urokinase **[D]**[26] through the drain (e.g. 250 000 units streptokinase in 20 ml daily).

**Why do this?**
- Patients who have streptokinase compared with saline instilled daily into their chest drain pass more fluid (~ 1.5:l more) and more have at least a 50% reduction in the effusion at discharge **[A]**[25].
- Patients are less likely to require surgery **[A]**[25].
- Streptokinase and urokinase are probably equally effective in treating parapneumonic effusions. Both increase the fluid drained from the chest **[D]**[26].

**Streptokinase increases drainage and reduces need for surgery**

| Patient | Treatment | Comparator | Outcome | CER | RRR | NNT |
|---|---|---|---|---|---|---|
| Parapneumonic effusion **[A]**[25] | Streptokinase | Saline | Reduction in volume > 50% at discharge | 58% | −71% (−177% to −6%) | 2 (1 to 7) |
| | | | Surgery at discharge | 25% | 100% | 4 (2 to 200) |

Refer patients for surgery if drainage is unsuccessful **[D]**[26].

**Note**
- Around 10% of patients with parapneumonic effusions require surgery to clear them **[D]**[26].

## PREVENTION

Give elderly patients **[B]**[27] and patients with lung disease **[D]:**
- influenza vaccine (preferably combined live and inactivated **[A]**[28].

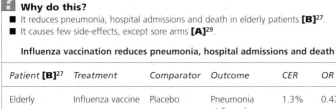

**Why do this?**
- It reduces pneumonia, hospital admissions and death in elderly patients **[B]**[27].
- It causes few side-effects, except sore arms **[A]**[29].

**Influenza vaccination reduces pneumonia, hospital admissions and death**

| Patient **[B]**[27] | Treatment | Comparator | Outcome | CER | OR | NNT |
|---|---|---|---|---|---|---|
| Elderly | Influenza vaccine | Placebo | Pneumonia at ? weeks | 1.3% | 0.47 (0.34 to 0.65) | 150 (120 to 220) |
| | | | Hospitalisation at? weeks | 0.79% | 0.50 (0.35 to 0.72) | 260 (200 to 460) |
| | | | Death at ? weeks | 1.0% | 0.32 (0.24 to 0.44) | 140 (130 to 170) |

**Intramuscular influenza vaccination causes sore arms**

| Patient **[A]**[29] | Treatment | Comparator | Outcome | CER | RRR | NNT |
|---|---|---|---|---|---|---|
| Elderly outpatient | Influenza vaccine im | Placebo im | Sore arm at ? weeks | 4.8% | −330% (−620% to −150%) | −6 (−9 to −5) |

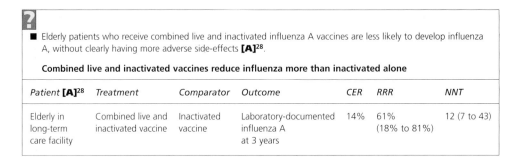

- Elderly patients who receive combined live and inactivated influenza A vaccines are less likely to develop influenza A, without clearly having more adverse side-effects **[A]**[28].

**Combined live and inactivated vaccines reduce influenza more than inactivated alone**

| Patient **[A]**[28] | Treatment | Comparator | Outcome | CER | RRR | NNT |
|---|---|---|---|---|---|---|
| Elderly in long-term care facility | Combined live and inactivated vaccine | Inactivated vaccine | Laboratory-documented influenza A at 3 years | 14% | 61% (18% to 81%) | 12 (7 to 43) |

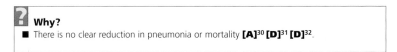

There is no clear benefit from pneumococcal vaccine **[A]**[30].

**Why?**
- There is no clear reduction in pneumonia or mortality **[A]**[30] **[D]**[31] **[D]**[32].

## PROGNOSIS

Death is common **[A]**[7], particularly if your patient is **[B]**[5]:
- admitted to hospital
- elderly
- from a nursing home
- bacteraemic
- requiring intensive care.

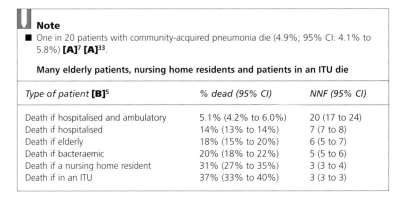

**Note**
- One in 20 patients with community-acquired pneumonia die (4.9%; 95% CI: 4.1% to 5.8%) **[A]**[7] **[A]**[33].

**Many elderly patients, nursing home residents and patients in an ITU die**

| Type of patient **[B]**[5] | % dead (95% CI) | NNF (95% CI) |
|---|---|---|
| Death if hospitalised and ambulatory | 5.1% (4.2% to 6.0%) | 20 (17 to 24) |
| Death if hospitalised | 14% (13% to 14%) | 7 (7 to 8) |
| Death if elderly | 18% (15% to 20%) | 6 (5 to 7) |
| Death if bacteraemic | 20% (18% to 22%) | 5 (5 to 6) |
| Death if a nursing home resident | 31% (27% to 35%) | 3 (3 to 4) |
| Death if in an ITU | 37% (33% to 40%) | 3 (3 to 3) |

Determine your patient's risk of dying in the next month **[A]**[7] using the scoring system shown in Box 2. Sum the components.

## Box 2  Scoring system for predicting the risk of dying in the next month

| Prognostic feature [A][7] | Score |
|---|---|
| Age | (years) for men |
| | (years) – 10 for women |
| Nursing home resident | +10 |
| Coexisting disease | |
| ■ neoplastic disease | +30 |
| ■ liver disease | +20 |
| ■ congestive heart failure | +10 |
| ■ cerebrovascular disease | +10 |
| ■ renal disease | +10 |
| Physical examination findings | |
| ■ altered mental status | +20 |
| ■ respiratory rate 30/min or more | +20 |
| ■ systolic blood pressure < 90 mmHg | +20 |
| ■ temperature ≤ 35°C, or ≥ 40°C | +15 |
| ■ pulse ≥ 125 beats/min | +10 |
| Laboratory and radiographic findings | |
| ■ arterial pH < 7.35 | +30 |
| ■ urea ≥ 11 mmol/l | +20 |
| ■ sodium <130 mmol/l | +20 |
| ■ glucose ≥ 14 mmol/l | +10 |
| ■ haematocrit < 30% | +10 |
| ■ $PO_2$ < 8.0 pKa | +10 |
| ■ pleural effusion | +10 |

| Score [A][7] | Class | Risk of dying |
|---|---|---|
| >130 | V | high |
| 91–130 | IV | moderate |
| 71–90 | III | low |
| < 70 | II | low |
| Aged < 50 years and none of the conditions or physical findings listed | I | low |

## Why?

### A clinical prediction rule can help predict mortality at 30 days

| Score [A][7] | LR (95% CI) | % dead at 30 days (95% CI) | NNF (95% CI) | % admitted to ITU at 30 days (95% CI) | NNF (95% CI) |
|---|---|---|---|---|---|
| > 130 | 7.1 (5.7 to 8.9) | 27% (21% to 33%) | 4 (3 to 5) | 17% (12% to 22%) | 6 (4 to 8) |
| 91–130 | 2.0 (1.5 to 2.5) | 9.3% (6.7% to 12%) | 11 (8 to 15) | 11% (8.5% to 14%) | 9 (7 to 12) |
| 71–90 | 0.18 (0.058 to 0.55) | 0.92% (0.0% to 2.0%) | 110 (51 to inf) | 5.9% (3.0% to 8.8%) | 17 (11 to 33) |
| < 70 | 0.12 (0.040 to 0.37) | 0.63% (0.0% to 1.3%) | 160 (75 to inf) | 4.3% (1.7% to 6.9%) | 23 (15 to 59) |
| Aged < 50 years and none of the conditions or physical findings listed | 0.025 (0.0035 to 0.18) | 0.13% (0.0% to 0.38%) | 770 (260 to inf) | 4.3% (1.4% to 7.3%) | 23 (14 to 72) |

*Note*
- Elderly patients who survive an episode of community-acquired pneumonia remain at increased risk of dying, particularly from pneumonia [A][34].

**Why?**
An episode of pneumonia in the elderly increases the risk of dying, particularly from pneumonia

| Patient | Prognostic factor [A][34] | Outcome | Control rate | RR (95% CI) | NNF+ (95% CI) |
|---|---|---|---|---|---|
| Elderly | Survived community-acquired pneumonia *independent* | Death at 9 years | 48% | 1.5 (1.2 to 1.9) | 5 (3 to 13) |
| | Survived community-acquired pneumonia *independent* | Pneumonia-related death at 9 years | −7.9% | 2.1 (1.3 to 3.4) | 12 (5 to 42) |

**Guideline writer**: Christopher Ball
**CAT writers**: Christopher Ball, Clare Wotton, Robert Phillips

## REFERENCES

| No. | Level | Citation |
|---|---|---|
| 1 | 1a | Heckerling PS, Tape TG, Wigton RS et al. Clinical prediction rule for pulmonary infiltrates. Ann Intern Med 1990; 113: 664–70 |
| 2 | 4 | Research Committee of the British Thoracic Society and Public Health Laboratory Service. Community-acquired pneumonia in adults in British hospitals in 1982–1983: a survey of aetiology, mortality, prognostic factors and outcome. Q J Med 1987; 239: 195–220 |
| 3 | 4 | Farr BM, Kaiser DL, Harrison BD et al. Prediction of microbial aetiology at admission to hospital for pneumonia from the presenting clinical features. Thorax 1989; 44: 1031–5 |
| 4 | 4 | Sopena N, Sabria-Leal M, Pedro-Botet ML et al. Comparative study of the clinical presentation of Legionella pneumonia and other community-acquired pneumonias. Chest 1998; 113: 1195–200 |
| 5 | 2a | Fine MJ, Smith MA, Carson CA et al. Prognosis and outcomes of patients with community-acquired pneumonia: a meta-analysis. JAMA 1995; 274: 134–41 |
| 6 | 1a | Metlay JP, Kapoor WN, Fine MJ et al. Does this patient have community-acquired pneumonia? Diagnosing pneumonia by history and physical examination. JAMA 1997; 278: 1440–5 |
| 7 | 1a | Fine MJ, Auble TE, Yealy DM et al. A prediction rule to identify low-risk patients with community-acquired pneumonia. N Engl Med 1997; 336: 243–50 |
| 8 | 2a | Metlay JP, Kapoor WN, Fine MJ et al. Does this patient have community-acquired pneumonia? Diagnosing pneumonia by history and physical examination. JAMA 1997; 278: 1440–5 |

| No. | Level | Citation |
|-----|-------|----------|
| 9 | 2a | History and physical examination for dyspnea: a review. ACP J Club 1993 Nov–Dec; 119:90. Summary of Mulrow CD et al. Discriminating causes of dyspnea through clinical examination. J Gen Intern Med 1993; 8: 383–92 |
| 10 | 4 | Thrush DN et al. Does significant arterial hypoxemia alter vital signs? J Clin Anesthesia 1997; 9: 355–7 |
| 11 | 4 | Sanyal S, Smith PR, Saha AC et al. Initial microbiologic studies did not affect outcome in adults hospitalized with community-acquired pneumonia. Am J Respir Crit Care Med 1999; 160: 346–8 |
| 12 | 2a – | Reed WW, Byrd GS, Gates RJ et al. Sputum Gram's stain in community-acquired pneumococcal pneumonia: a meta-analysis. West J Med 1996; 165: 197–204 |
| 13 | 4 | Woodhead MA, Arrowsmith J, Chamberlain-Webber R et al. The value of routine microbial investigation in community-acquired pneumonia. Respir Med 1991; 85: 313–17 |
| 14 | 4 | Ruf B, Schurmann D, Horbach I et al. Prevalence and diagnosis of Legionella pneumonia: a 3-year prospective study with emphasis on application of urinary antigen detection. Ann Intern Med 1990; 162: 1341–8 |
| 15 | 4 | MacFarlane JT, Miller AC, Smith WHR et al. Comparative radiographic features of community-acquired legionnaires' disease, pneumococcal pneumonia, mycoplasma pneumonia, and psittacosis. Thorax 1984; 39: 28–33 |
| 16 | 1b | Albaum MN, Hill LC, Murphy M et al. Interobserver reliability of the chest radiograph in community-acquired pneumonia. Chest 1996; 110: 343–50 |
| 17 | 1b | Cantral DE, Tape TG, Reed EC et al. Quantitative culture of bronchoalveolar lavage fluid for the diagnosis of bacterial pneumonia. Am J Med 1993; 95: 601–7 |
| 18 | 1b | Chan R, Hemeryck L, O'Regan M et al. Oral versus intravenous antibiotics for community acquired lower respiratory tract infection in a general hospital: open, randomised controlled trial. BMJ 1995; 310: 1360–2 |
| 19 | 2b | Gleason PP, Meehan TP, Fine JM et al. Associations between initial antimicrobial therapy and medical outcomes for hospitalized elderly patients with pneumonia. Arch Intern Med 1999; 159: 2562–72 |
| 20 | 1b | File TM, Segreti J, Dunbar L et al. Multicenter, randomized study comparing efficacy and safety of intravenous and/or oral levofloxacin versus ceftriaxone and/or cefuroxime axetil in treatment of adults with community-acquired pneumonia. Antimicrob Agents Chemother 1997; 41: 1965–72 |
| 21 | 1b | Aubier M, Verster R, Regamey C et al. Once-daily sparfloxacin versus high-dosage amoxicillin in the treatment of community-acquired, suspected pneumococcal pneumonia in adults. Clin Infect Dis 1998; 26: 1312–20 |
| 22 | 4 | Ewig S, Ruiz M, Torres A et al. Pneumonia acquired in the community through drug-resistant Streptococcus pneumoniae. Am J Respir Crit Care Med 1999; 159: 1835–42 |
| 23 | 1b | Sacks PV, Kanarck D. Treatment of acute pleuritic pain: comparison of indomethicin and a placebo. Am Rev Resp Dis 1973; 108: 666–9 |
| 24 | 2a | Heffner JE et al. Pleural fluid chemical analysis in parapneumonic effusion: a meta-analysis. Am J Respir Crit Care Med 1995; 151: 1700–8 |
| 25 | 1b | Davies RJ et al. Randomised controlled trial of intrapleural streptokinase in community acquired pleural infection. Thorax 1997; 52: 416–21 |

| No. | Level | Citation |
|-----|-------|----------|
| 26 | 1b – | Bouros D et al. Intrapleural streptokinase versus urokinase in the treatment of complicated parapneumonic effusions: a prospective double-blind study. Am J Respir Crit Care Med 1997; 155: 291–5 |
| 27 | 2b | Gross PA, Hermogenes AW, Sacks HS et al. The efficacy of influenza vaccine in elderly persons: a meta-analysis and review of the literature. Ann Intern Med 1995; 123: 518–27 |
| 28 | 1b | Treanor JJ, Mattison HR, Dumyati G et al. Protective efficacy of combined live intranasal and inactivated influenza A virus vaccines in the elderly. Ann Intern Med 1992; 117: 625–33 |
| 29 | 1b | Margolis KL, Nichol KL, Poland GA et al. Frequency of adverse reactions to influenza vaccine in the elderly: a randomized, placebo-controlled trial. JAMA 1990; 264: 1139–41 |
| 30 | 1b | Fine MJ, Smith MA, Carson CA et al. Efficacy of pneumococcal vaccination in adults: a meta-analysis of randomized controlled trials. Arch Intern Med 1994; 154: 2666–77 |
| 31 | 1b – | Ortqvist A, Hedlund J, Burman L-A et al. Randomised trial of 23-valent pneumococcal capsular polysaccharide vaccine in prevention of pneumonia in middle-aged and elderly people. Lancet 1998; 351: 399–403 |
| 32 | 1b – | Koivula I, Sten M, Leinonen M et al. Clinical efficacy of pneumococcal vaccine in the elderly: a randomized, single-blind population-based trial. Am J Med 1997; 103: 281–90 |
| 33 | 1b | Research Committee of the British Thoracic Society and Public Health Laboratory Service. Community-acquired pneumonia in adults in British hospitals in 1982–1983: a survey of aetiology, mortality, prognostic factors and outcome. Q J Med 1987; 239: 195–220 |
| 34 | 1b | Koivula I, Sten M, Makela PH. Prognosis after community-acquired pneumonia in the elderly: a population-based 12-year follow-up study. Arch Intern Med 1999; 159: 1550–5 |

## PREVALENCE

A pulmonary embolism typically presents with breathlessneis, pleuritic pain or chest X-ray changes **[A]**[1].
PE is uncommon in the community **[A]**[2], but a quarter of patients referred to hospital with a suspected PE **[A]**[1] **[A]**[3] **[A]**[4], and a fifth of patients with pleuritic chest pain, have one **[A]**[5]

 **Note**

■ 17% to 32% of patients attending emergency departments with a suspected PE have one **[A]**[1] **[A]**[3] **[A]**[4].

■ 21% of patients with pleuritic chest pain have a PE (95% CI: 15% to 27%) **[A]**[5]:
  − 9.0% of patients < 40 years old
  − 28% of patients > 40 years old.

## CLINICAL FEATURES

Use the following clinical prediction rule to rank patients for their risk of having a PE **[A]**[6]. Remember a PE cannot be safely diagnosed or excluded on history and physical examination alone; imaging studies are necessary **[A]**[3].

1. Ask about risk factors for venous thromboembolism:

   ● recent immobilisation
     − paralysis of a leg
     − surgery or a fracture of the leg with immobilisation within the last 12 weeks
     − recently bedridden > 3 days within the last 4 weeks
   ● previous venous thromboembolism (objective diagnosis)
   ● a strong family history of DVT or PE
     − ≥ 2 family members with objectively proven events
     − a first-degree relative with hereditary thrombophilia
   ● active cancer (ongoing treatment, diagnosed within the last 6 months or having palliative care)
   ● post-partum.

2. Score your patients for the following respiratory points:

   ● dyspnoea or worsening of chronic dyspnoea
   ● pleuritic chest pain
   ● chest pain (non-retrosternal and non-pleuritic)
   ● arterial oxygen saturation < 92% while breathing room air that corrects with 40% $O_2$
   ● haemoptysis
   ● pleural rub.

3. Think about alternative diagnoses (see Differential diagnoses below).

4. Decide if your patient's symptoms are atypical, typical or severe for PE (Table 1).

| Table 1 Classifying symptoms for PE | |
|---|---|
| Severity | Symptoms |
| Atypical | Respiratory or cardiac symptoms not meeting criteria for 'typical' |
| Typical | ≥ 2 respiratory points and any of the following:<br>● heart rate > 90 beats/min<br>● leg symptoms<br>● low-grade fever<br>● results of chest X-ray compatible with PE |
| Severe | Either typical symptoms and all of the following:<br>  ● syncope<br>  ● blood pressure <90 mmHg with heart rate > 100 beats/min<br>  ● receiving ventilation or needs oxygen flow > 40%<br><br>Or typical symptoms and:<br>● new-onset right heart failure (elevated JVP and new S1, Q3, and T3 or RBBB)<br><br>Or all of:<br>● syncope<br>● blood pressure < 90 mmHg with heart rate >100 beats/min<br>● receiving ventilation or needing oxygen flow >40%<br>● new-onset right heart failure (elevated JVP and new S1, Q3, and T3 or RBBB) |

4. Decide on your patient's risk for a PE (Table 2).

| Table 2 Classifying risk for PE | | | |
|---|---|---|---|
| Symptoms for PE | Low risk | Medium risk | High risk |
| Atypical | An alternative diagnosis or no risk factors | No alternative diagnosis and risk factors | |
| Typical | An alternative diagnosis and no risk factors | Any other combination | |
| Severe | | An alternative diagnosis | No alternative diagnosis |

**Why do this?**

When combined with ventilation-perfusion scanning and ultrasound scanning (see below):
- few cases of PE are missed (0.6%: 95% CI: 0.1% to 1.1%) **[A]**[6]
- it helps clinicians agree about the risk of a PE. $K_{interobserver}$ for prediction rule = 0.85 **[A]**[6].

**A clinical prediction rule can help diagnose PE**

| Patient **[A]**[6] | Target disorder (reference standard) | Diagnostic test | LR+ (95% CI) | Post-test probability |
|---|---|---|---|---|
| Suspected PE (pre-test probability 17%) | PE (angiography, ultrasound, V/Q scan, follow-up) | 'High risk' (Table 2) | 9.2 (6.5 to 13) | 66% |
| | | 'Moderate risk' | 1.9 (1.6 to 2.2) | 28% |
| | | 'Low risk' | 0.17 (0.12 to 0.25) | 3% |

In addition, ask about features that might affect your management:

- oral contraceptive pill use **[B]**[7]

**Why?**

- It increases the risk of developing venous thromboembolism.
- Third-generation oral contraceptives are slightly more dangerous than second-generation **[B]**[8] **[B]**[9].
- There is no clear evidence to suggest that women on HRT are at increased risk of venous thromboembolism **[A]**[7].

**Oral contraceptive pill increases the risk of VTE very slightly**

| Patient | Prognostic factor | Outcome | Control rate | OR (95% CI) | NNF+ (95% CI) |
|---|---|---|---|---|---|
| Healthy | Oral contraceptive pill *independent* | VTE | 0.003% | 2.4 (1.6 to 3.5) | 6000 (3400 to 14000) |

**Third-generation contraceptives increase the risk of VTE slightly more than second-generation**

| Outcome **[B]**[8] **[B]**[9] | Risk factor | PEER | OR (95% CI) | NNH (95% CI) |
|---|---|---|---|---|
| VTE | Desogestrel or gestodene compared to levonogestrel *independent* | 0.012% | 2.2 (1.0 to 4.7) | 7000 (2300 to infinity) |

- smoking **[A]**[2]
- hypertension **[A]**[2]
- obesity (BMI > 29) **[A]**[2].

■ These all increase the risk of having a PE **[A]**[2].

**Obesity, heavy smoking and hypertension increase the risk of having a PE**

| Patient | Prognostic factor | Outcome | Control rate | RR (95% CI) | NNF+ (95% CI) |
|---------|-------------------|---------|--------------|-------------|---------------|
| Healthy | BMI > 29.0 *independent* | PE at 16 years | 0.22% | 3.0 (2.0 to 4.7) | 150 (100 to 270) |
| | 25 to 34 cigarettes/day *independent* | PE at 16 years | 0.26% | 1.8 (1.2 to 2.9) | 210 (130 to 320) |
| | ≥ 35 cigarettes/day *independent* | PE at 16 years | 0.26% | 2.1 (1.2 to 3.6) | 180 (110 to 320) |
| | Hypertension *independent* | PE at 16 years | 0.23% | 1.5 (1.2 to 2.0) | 290 (220 to 370) |

## DIFFERENTIAL DIAGNOSIS

### Dyspnoea

Think about other causes of breathlessness. Common causes include **[B]**[10]:

● asthma
● heart failure
● COPD
● arrhythmia
● infection
● interstitial lung disease
● anaemia.

**?** **Why?**
**PE is a rare cause of dyspnoea**

| Causes of dyspnoea **[B]**[10] | % |
|-------------------------------|-----|
| Asthma | 33% |
| Heart failure | 31% |
| COPD | 9% |
| Arrhythmia | 7% |
| Infection | 5% |
| Interstitial lung disease | 4% |
| Anaemia | 2% |
| PE | < 2% |

## Pleuritic Pain

Think about other causes of pleuritic chest pain **[A]**[5] **[B]**[11].
Common causes include:

- viral or idiopathic
- pneumonia
- chest wall trauma
- cancer.

**? Why?**

**Common causes of pleuritic pain are viral or idiopathic and PE**

| Causes of pleuritic pain **[A]**[5] | % (95% CI) |
|---|---|
| Viral or idiopathic | 46% (39% to 54%) |
| PE | 21% (15% to 27%) |
| Pneumonia | 8% (4% to 12%) |
| Other (chest wall trauma, cancer, SLE, TB) | 25% (18% to 31%) |

**Common causes of severe pleuritic pain are pneumonia and PE**

| Severe pleuritic pain **[B]**[11] | % (95% CI) |
|---|---|
| Broncho- or lobar pneumonia | 65 (52 to 78) |
| PE | 29 (17 to 42) |
| Chest injury | 6 (0 to 12) |

## INVESTIGATIONS

- Arterial blood gas **[A]**[12].

**! Note**

■ Arterial blood gases are unhelpful in diagnosing or excluding PE **[A]**[12], but can help rule out other conditions **[A]**[1] **[A]**[3].

**Arterial blood gases are unhelpful in diagnosing or excluding PE**

| Patient **[A]**[12] | Target disorder (reference standard) | Diagnostic test | LR+ (95% CI) | Post-test probability | LRS– (95% CI) | Post-test probability |
|---|---|---|---|---|---|---|
| Suspected PE (pre-test probability 36%) | PE (angiography) | $Po_2 \geq 80$ mmHg (10.2 kPa) | 1.1 (0.98 to 1.1) | 37% | 0.82 (0.61 to 1.1) | 32% |
| | | $Pco_2 \geq 35$ mmHg (4.5 kPa) | 1.0 (0.89 to 1.2) | 37% | 0.97 (0.83 to 1.1) | 35% |

- Chest X-ray **[A]**[1]. Look for any abnormality, particularly:
  - atelectasis or pulmonary parenchymal abnormality
  - pleural effusion
  - pleural-based opacity
  - decreased pulmonary vasculature
  - pulmonary oedema.

**? Why?**

An abnormal chest X-ray makes pulmonary embolism slightly more likely

| Patient **[A]**[1] | Target disorder (reference standard) | Diagnostic test | LR+ (95% CI) | Post-test probability | LR– (95% CI) | Post-test probability |
|---|---|---|---|---|---|---|
| Suspected PE (pre-test probability 21%) | PE (angiography, follow-up) | Abnormal chest X-ray | 1.3 (1.1 to 1.4) | 37% | 0.48 (0.31 to 0.75) | 18% |
| | | Atelectasis or parenchymal abnormality | 1.4 (1.2 to 1.7) | 40% | 0.62 (0.47 to 0.83) | 23% |
| | | Pleural effusion | 1.5 (1.2 to 2.0) | 42% | 0.76 (0.62 to 0.92) | 26% |
| | | Pleural-based opacity | 1.6 (1.2 to 2.3) | 44% | 0.83 (0.71 to 0.96) | 28% |
| | | Decreased pulmonary vasculature | 1.8 (1.1 to 2.9) | 45% | 0.89 (0.81 to 0.99) | 30% |
| | | Pulmonary oedema | 0.34 (0.14 to 0.86) | 14% | 1.1 (1.1 to 1.2) | 34% |

- ECG **[A]**[6]. Look for:
  - new S1, Q3, and T3 (S wave in lead I, Q wave in lead III, T wave inversion in lead III)
  - new right bundle-branch block.

These three tests are not individually very helpful in diagnosing PE, but should be done to rule out other diseases **[A]**[1] **[A]**[3].

- Blood count **[A]**[5].

| Patient [A][5] | Target disorder (reference standard) | Diagnostic test | LR+ (95% CI) | Post-test probability | LR− (95% CI) | Post-test probability |
|---|---|---|---|---|---|---|

**Why?**
A raised white cell count makes a PE slightly more likely

| Patient [A][5] | Target disorder (reference standard) | Diagnostic test | LR+ (95% CI) | Post-test probability | LR− (95% CI) | Post-test probability |
|---|---|---|---|---|---|---|
| Suspected PE (pre-test probability 21%) | PE (V/Q scan, angiography, autopsy) | White cell count >10 ×10$^9$/l | 1.7 (1.2 to 2.6) | 31% | 0.68 (0.47 to 0.98) | 15% |

- D-dimer [A][13] in clinically low-risk cases [A][4]. Use a whole-blood agglutination test [A][4] [A][13].

**Why?**
■ A negative D-dimer, can rule out PE in low-risk cases – post-test probability 0.7%.

**A negative D-dimer can rule out PE in low-risk cases**

| Patient [A][4] | Target disorder (reference standard) | Diagnostic test | LR+ (95% CI) | Post-test probability | LR− (95% CI) | Post-test probability |
|---|---|---|---|---|---|---|
| Suspected PE (pre-test probability 17%) | PE (V/Q scan, venogram, ultrasound, follow-up) | D-dimer positive (Simpli-red whole blood agglutination) | 2.7 (2.4 to 3.0) | 35% | 0.22 (0.16 to 0.31) | 4% |

- Baseline clotting [D].
- Factor Leiden/V and other thrombophilia studies if indicated; consider a haematology referral if positive [D].
- Perform a ventilation-perfusion scan [A][3].

**Why?**
A V/Q scan can help diagnose or exclude a PE

| Patient [A][3] | Target disorder (reference standard) | Diagnostic test | LR (95% CI) | Post-test probability |
|---|---|---|---|---|
| Suspected PE (pre-test probability 27%) | PE (angiogram or follow-up) | High probability V/Q scan | 13 (8.1 to 19) | 82% |
| | | Intermediate probability V/Q scan | 1.1 (0.91 to 1.3) | 29% |
| | | Low probability V/Q scan | 0.38 (0.29 to 0.52) | 12% |
| | | Normal/near normal scan V/Q scan | 0.11 (0.045 to 0.26) | 4% |

**Note**
- Around 60% of all scans are low or intermediate probability **[A]**[3].
- Pre-existing heart/lung disease does not affect the accuracy of the scan, but more patients have non-diagnostic scans **[A]**[14].

Patients with low or intermediate probability scans need further testing **[C]**[15], so base further investigations on the plan given in Table 3.

**Table 3 Basics for further investigations for PE**

| V/Q scan result | PE probability | Next test | if required | If required |
|---|---|---|---|---|
| Normal | Low, moderate or high | Ultrasound<br>● positive: PE<br>● negative: no PE | | |
| Non-high | Low or moderate | Serial ultrasound (day 1, 3, 7, 14)<br>● positive: PE<br>● negative: no PE | | |
| Non-high | High | Ultrasound<br>● positive: PE<br>● negative: venography | Venography<br>● positive: PE<br>● negative: pulmonary angiography | Angiography<br>● positive: PE<br>● negative: no PE |
| High | Low | Ultrasound<br>● positive: PE<br>● negative: venography | Venography<br>● positive: PE<br>● negative: pulmonary angiography | Angiography<br>● positive: PE<br>● negative: no PE |
| High | Moderate or high | PE | | |

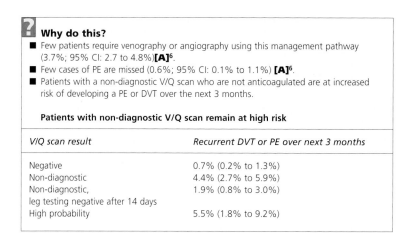
**Why do this?**
- Few patients require venography or angiography using this management pathway (3.7%; 95% CI: 2.7 to 4.8%)**[A]**[6].
- Few cases of PE are missed (0.6%; 95% CI: 0.1% to 1.1%) **[A]**[6].
- Patients with a non-diagnostic V/Q scan who are not anticoagulated are at increased risk of developing a PE or DVT over the next 3 months.

**Patients with non-diagnostic V/Q scan remain at high risk**

| V/Q scan result | Recurrent DVT or PE over next 3 months |
|---|---|
| Negative | 0.7% (0.2% to 1.3%) |
| Non-diagnostic | 4.4% (2.7% to 5.9%) |
| Non-diagnostic, leg testing negative after 14 days | 1.9% (0.8% to 3.0%) |
| High probability | 5.5% (1.8% to 9.2%) |

- Bilateral compression ultrasound **[A]**[16] of the common femoral, popliteal and distal popliteal veins: the test is positive if any vein is not fully compressible.

**Why?**
**Compression ultrasound can help diagnose PE but not rule it out**

| Patient **[A]**[16] | Target disorder (reference standard) | Diagnostic test | LR+ (95% CI) | Post-test probability | LR– (95% CI) | Post-test probability |
|---|---|---|---|---|---|---|
| Suspected PE (pre-test probability 17%) | PE (V/Q scan, angiography) | Positive ultrasound scan | 10 (4.2 to 25) | 90% | 0.73 (0.66 to 0.81) | 13% |

- Venography **[A]**.

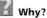
**Why?**
- It is the current reference standard for DVT, but it is not perfect.
  - Some DVT are missed: 2% of patients with a negative venogram develop DVT **[C]**[17].
  - It may not be technically possible (5%) **[C]**[18].
  - Pain is a common side-effect (20%). Serious side-effects are rare **[C]**[18].
  - It may cause DVT **[C]**[18].

- Pulmonary angiography **[A]**.

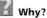
**Why?**
- Pulmonary angiography is the reference standard for pulmonary embolism, however, around 3% of tests are non-diagnostic **[C]**[19].
- Minor complications (urticaria, pruritus, mild renal dysfunction) occur in 5% **[C]**[19].
- 1% of patients have major complications (respiratory distress requiring CPR or intubation; renal failure requiring dialysis; haematoma requiring transfusion of 2+ units) or die **[C]**[19]

**Pulmonary angiography can diagnose and exclude PE**

| Patient **[C]**[19] | Target disorder (reference standard) | Diagnostic test | LR+ (95% CI) | Post-test probability | LR– (95% CI) | Post-test probability |
|---|---|---|---|---|---|---|
| Suspected PE (pre-test probability) 21%) | PE (follow-up or autopsy) | Pulmonary angiography | 170 (64 to 450) | 99% | 0.0026 (0.00037 to 0.019) | 0.15% |

| ? | Pulmonary angiography can have serious complications | |
|---|---|---|
| Complication | % | |
| Non-diagnostic scan | 3.2% (2.1% to 4.2%) | |
| Death | 0.45% (0.06% to 0.84%) | |
| Major complications | 0.81% (0.28% to 1.3%) | |
| Minor complications | 5.4% (4.1% to 6.7%) | |

Other tests that may be helpful include:

- capnography [A][20]; measure the waveform area (area under curve produced by one expiration)

**? Why?**
**A low capnogram waveform area makes a PE much more likely**

| Patient [A][20] | Target disorder (reference standard) | Diagnostic test | LR (95% CI) | Post-test probability |
|---|---|---|---|---|
| Suspected PE (pre-test probability 14%) | PE (V/Q scan, angiography or follow-up) | Capnogram waveform area <25 mmHg.s | 13 (4.2 to 38) | 67% |
| | | 25–50 mmHg.s | 1.2 (0.81 to 1.9) | 16% |
| | | >50 mmHg.s | 0.0 (0.0 to 0.29) | 0% |

- impedance plethysmography

**? Why?**
- It can help diagnose PE but not rule it out [B][21].
- It is a cost-effective method [B][21].

**Impedance plethysmography can help diagnose PE but not rule it out**

| Patient [A][5] | Target disorder (reference standard) | Diagnostic test | LR+ (95% CI) | Post-test probability | LR– (95 % CI) | Post-test probability |
|---|---|---|---|---|---|---|
| Suspected PE (pre-test probability 21%) | PE (V/Q scan, angiography or autopsy) | Abnormal impedance plethysmography | 13 (3.7 to 44) | 77% | 0.74 (0.60 to 0.91) | 16% |

- helical CT [B][22]

| Why? | | | | | | | |
|------|---|---|---|---|---|---|---|
| **A positive helical CT scan makes a PE much more likely** | | | | | | | |
| Patient **[B]**[22] | Target disorder (reference standard) | Diagnostic test | LR+ (95% CI) | Post-test probability | LR– (95% CI) | Post-test probability |
| Suspected PE (pre-test probability 46%) | PE (angiography) | Helical CT | 19 (2.7 to 130) | 93% | 0.23 (0.10 to 0.55) | 15% |

- MRI **[B]**[23].

| Why? | | | | | | | |
|------|---|---|---|---|---|---|---|
| **A positive MRI scan makes a PE much more likely** | | | | | | | |
| Patient **[B]**[22] | Target disorder (reference standard) | Diagnostic test | LR+ (95% CI) | Post-test probability (%) | LR– (95% CI) | Post-test probability (%) |
| Suspected PE (pre-test probability 46%) | PE (angiography) | MRI | 22 (3.2 to 150) | 89% | 0.0 (0.0 to 0.32) | 0.0% |

## THERAPY

- Give oxygen if the patient is hypoxic **[A]**.
- Give analgesia for pleuritic pain, e.g. a NSAID.

| Why do this? | | | | | | |
|------|---|---|---|---|---|---|
| ■ Indometacin reduces severe pleuritic chest pain compared with placebo **[A]**[11]. | | | | | | |
| ■ Indometacin increases FVC and FEV$_1$ and reduces the respiratory rate **[A]**[11]. | | | | | | |
| **Indometacin gives effective pain-relief for severe pleuritic chest pain** | | | | | | |
| Patient **[A]**[11] | Treatment | Comparator | Outcome | CER | RRR | NNT |
| Severe pleuritic chest pain | Indometacin | Placebo | Pain-relief good or excellent at 2 h | 34% | 140% (39% to 320%) | 2 (1 to 4) |

- Give anticoagulation **[A]**[24] (see chapter on **Anticoagulation**).

**Why do this?**
■ It reduces death and recurrent PE **[A]**[24].

Anticoagulation reduces recurrent and fatal PE

| Patient **[A]**[24] | Treatment | Comparator | Outcome | CER | RRR | NNT |
|---|---|---|---|---|---|---|
| Severe pleuritic chest pain | Warfarin | Placebo | Death from PE at 12 months | 26% | 100% | 4 (2 to 15) |
| | | | Recurrent PE at 12 months | 32% | 100% | 3 (2 to 9) |

Use a low-molecular-weight heparin **[D]**[25]**[D]**[26] and warfarin **[A]**[24].

**Why do this?**
■ LMWH is probably as effective and safe as heparin **[D]**[25] **[D]**[26], and no monitoring is needed.

Give warfarin:

- for 6 months for first PE with transient risk factors **[A]**[27]
- indefinitely for:
  - idiopathic cases **[A]**[28]
  - recurrent VTE **[A]**[29].

**Why do this?**
■ 6 months of oral anticoagulant therapy for a first episode of a DVT or PE leads to fewer recurrences of VTE than 6 weeks of therapy without clearly increasing bleeding or mortality **[A]**[27].
■ Indefinite oral anticoagulant therapy for a first idiopathic episode of a DVT or PE leads to fewer recurrences of VTE than 3 months of therapy without clearly increasing bleeding or mortality **[A]**[28].
■ Indefinite oral anticoagulant therapy for a second episode of a DVT or PE leads to fewer recurrent VTE than 6 months of therapy, without clearly increasing bleeding or mortality **[A]**[29].

Indefinite anticoagulation reduces recurrent VTE for idiopathic and recurrent episodes

| Patient | Treatment | Comparator | Outcome | CER | RRR | NNT |
|---|---|---|---|---|---|---|
| First PE or DVT **[A]**[27] | Anticoagulation for 6 months | Anticoagulation for 6 weeks | Recurrent VTE at 2 years | 18% | 48% (26% to 63%) | 12 (8 to 24) |
| First idiopathic PE or DVT **[A]**[28] | Indefinite anticoagulation | Anticoagulation for 3 months | Recurrent VTE at 10 months | 21% | 94% (55% to 99% | 5 (4 to 10) |
| Second PE or DVT **[A]**[29] | Indefinite anticoagulation | Anticoagulation for 6 months | Recurrent VTE at 4 years | 21% | 88% (60% to 96%) | 6 (4 to 10) |

Consider the following in life-threatening cases **[D]**:
- thrombolysis **[D]**[30–33]

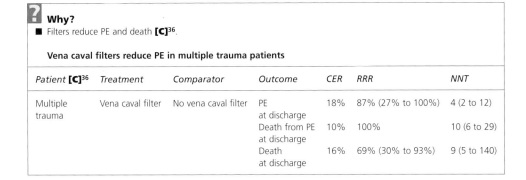

**Why?**
- It improves lung perfusion and ventricular wall movement, but there is no clear effect on mortality or recurrent PE **[D]**[30–33].
- The risk of bleeding is increased **[A]**[34].
- No thrombolytic has been shown to be better than another **[D]**[35].

**Thrombolysis increases the risk of bleeding**

| Patient **[A]**[34] | Treatment | Comparator | Outcome | CER | RRR | NNH |
|---|---|---|---|---|---|---|
| PE | Urokinase | Heparin | Bleeding at 14 days | 45% | −68% (−160% to −8%) | 5 (3 to 28) |
| | | | Severe bleeding at 14 days | 26% | −90% (−270% to −1%) | 8 (4 to 240) |

- embolectomy **[D]**.

## PREVENTION

### Surgery
See chapter on **Deep vein thrombosis** for more details.

### Trauma
Consider vena caval filters in trauma patients with multiple injuries **[C]**[36].

**Why?**
- Filters reduce PE and death **[C]**[36].

**Vena caval filters reduce PE in multiple trauma patients**

| Patient **[C]**[36] | Treatment | Comparator | Outcome | CER | RRR | NNT |
|---|---|---|---|---|---|---|
| Multiple trauma | Vena caval filter | No vena caval filter | PE at discharge | 18% | 87% (27% to 100%) | 4 (2 to 12) |
| | | | Death from PE at discharge | 10% | 100% | 10 (6 to 29) |
| | | | Death at discharge | 16% | 69% (30% to 93%) | 9 (5 to 140) |

**Note**
- In uncomplicated DVT, vena caval filters produce no benefit **[A]**[37].

## PROGNOSIS

Recurrent PE is not common following treatment, **[A]**[38] but mortality is high **[A]**[38] **[A]**[39].

A poor prognosis is associated with:

- cancer **[A]**[38]
- chronic lung disease **[A]**[38]
- left heart failure **[A]**[38]
- immobility **[A]**[39]
- surgery within the last 3 months **[A]**[39]
- a history of thrombophlebitis **[A]**[39].

**Why?**
Cancer, heart failure and chronic lung disease increase the risk of dying following a PE

| Patient | Prognostic factor | Outcome | Control rate | RR (95% CI) | NNF (95% CI) |
|---|---|---|---|---|---|
| PE | Cancer **[A]**[38] *independent* | Death at 1 year | 18% | 4.4 (2.1 to 9.5) | 2 (1 to 5) |
| | Left heart failure **[A]**[38] *independent* | Death at 1 year | 18% | 2.6 (1.2 to 5.7) | 3 (1 to 27) |
| | Chronic lung disease **[A]**[38] *independent* | Death at 1 year | 19% | 3.2 (1.3 to 7.4) | 2 (1 to 17) |
| | Immobilisation **[A]**[39] *not independent* | Death at 1 year | 15% | 1.76 (1.43 to 2.15) | 9 (6 to 16) |
| | Surgery within 3 months **[A]**[39] *not independent* | Death at 1 year | 15% | 1.69 (1.38 to 2.07) | 10 (6 to 18) |
| | History of thrombophlebitis **[A]**[39] *not independent* | Death at 1 year | 15% | 1.34 (1.03 to 1.81) | 20 (8 to 220) |

**Guideline writer**: Chris Ball
**CAT writer**: Chris Ball

**REFERENCES**

| No. | Level | Citation |
|---|---|---|
| 1 | 1b | Stein PD et al. Clinical, laboratory, rentgenographic and electrocardiographic findings in patients with acute pulmonary embolism and no pre-existing cardiac or pulmonary disease. Chest 1991; 100: 598–603 |
| 2 | 1b | Goldhaber SZ et al. A prospective study of risk factors for pulmonary embolism in women. JAMA 1997; 277: 642–5 |
| 3 | 1b | PIOPED Investigators. Value of the ventilation-perfusion scan in acute pulmonary embolism: results of the prospective investigation of pulmonary embolism diagnosis. JAMA 1990; 263: 2753–9 |

| No. | Level | Citation |
| --- | --- | --- |
| 4 | 1b | Ginsberg JS, Wells PS, Kearon C et al. Sensitivity and specificity of a rapid whole-blood assay d-dimer in the diagnosis of pulmonary embolism. Ann Intern Med 1998; 129: 1006–11 |
| 5 | 1b | Hull RD et al. Pulmonary embolism in outpatients with pleuritic chest pain. Arch Intern Med 1988; 148: 838–44 |
| 6 | 1a | Wells PS et al. Use of a clinical model for safe management of patients with suspected pulmonary embolism. Ann Intern Med 1998; 129: 997–1005 |
| 7 | 2a | Doukatis JD et al. A re-evaulation of the risk of venous thromboembolism with the use of oral contraceptives or hormone replacement therapy. Arch Intern Med 1997; 157: 1522–30 |
| 8 | 3b | Vanderbroucke JP et al. Increased risk of venous thromboembolism in oral-contraceptive users who are carriers of factor V Leiden mutation. Lancet 1994; 344: 1453–7 |
| 9 | 3b | Nonfatal venous thromboembolism was associated with oral contraceptives that contain desogestrel and gestodene. ACP J Club 1996 May–June; 124: 79. Evidence-Based Med 1996 May–June; 1: 126. Summary of: Jick H et al. Risk of idiopathic cardiovascular death and nonfatal venous thromboembolism in women using oral contraceptives with differing progestogen components. Lancet 1995; 346: 1589–93 |
| 10 | 2a | History and physical examination for dyspnea: a review. ACP J Club 1993 Nov–Dec; 119: 90. Summary of: Mulrow CD et al. Discriminating causes of dyspnea through clinical examination. J Gen Intern Med. 1993; 8: 383–92 |
| 11 | 2b | Sacks PV, Kanarck D. Treatment of acute pleuritic pain: comparison of indomethacin and a placebo. Am Rev Resp Dis 1973; 108: 666–9 |
| 12 | 1b | Stein PD et al. Arterial blood gas analysis in the assessment of suspected acute pulmonary embolism. |
| 13 | 1a | Becher DM et al. D-dimer testing and acute venous thromboembolism: a shortcut to accurate diagnosis? Arch Intern Med 1996; 156: 939–46 |
| 14 | 1b | Stein PD et al. Diagnostic utility of ventilation-perfusion lung scans in acute pulmonary embolism is not diminished by pre-existing cardiac or pulmonary disease. Chest 1991; 100: 604–6 |
| 15 | 4 | Hull RD et al. Non-invasive stategy for treatment of patients with suspected pulmonary embolism. Arch Intern Med 1994; 154: 289–97 |
| 16 | 1b | Compression ultrasonography had limited value for detecting pulmonary embolism. Evidence-Based Med 1997; 2: 187. Summary of: Turkstra F et al. Diagnostic utility of ultrasonography of leg veins in patients suspected of having pulmonary embolism. Ann Intern Med 1997; 126: 775–81 |
| 17 | 4 | Hull RD et al. Clinical validity of a negative venogram in patients with clinically suspected venous thrombosis. Circulation 1981; 64: 622–4 |
| 18 | 4 | Lensing AW et al. Lower extremity venography with iohexol; results and complications. Radiology 1990; 177: 503–5 |
| 19 | 4 | Stein PD et al. Complications and validity of pulmonary angiography in acute pulmonary embolism. Circulation 1992; 85: 462–8 |
| 20 | 1b | Kline JA, Arunachlam M. Preliminary study of the capnogram waveform area to screen for pulmonary embolism. Ann Emerg Med 1998; 32: 289–96 |
| 21 | 2b | Hull RD et al. Cost-effectiveness of pulmonary embolism diagnosis. Arch Intern Med 1996; 156: 68–72 |

| No. | Level | Citation |
|-----|-------|----------|
| 22 | 2b | Remy-Jordan M et al. Central pulmonary thromboembolism diagnosis with spiral volumetric CT with single breath holding technique: comparison with pulmonary angiogram. Radiology 1992; 185: 381–7 |
| 23 | 2b | Meaney JF et al. Diagnosis of pulmonary embolism with MRI angiography. N Engl J Med 1997; 336: 1422–7 |
| 24 | 1b | Barritt DW, Jordan SC. Anticoagulant drugs in the treatment of pulmonary embolism: a controlled trial. Lancet 1960; i: 1309–12 |
| 25 | 1b– | Columbus Investigators. Low-molecular-weight heparin in the treatment of patients with venous thromboembolism. N Engl J Med 1997; 337: 657–62 |
| 26 | 1b– | Simoneau S et al. A comparison of low-molecular-weight heparin and unfractionated heparin for acute pulmonary embolism. N Engl J Med 1997; 337: 663–9 |
| 27 | 1b | Fewer venous thromboembolism recurrences occurred with 6 months than with 6 weeks of anticoagulant therapy. ACP J Club 1996 Jan–Feb; 124: 9. Evidence-Based Med 1996 Jan Feb; 1:42. Summary of: Schulman S, Rhedin AS, Lindmarker P et al. and the Duration of Anticoagulation Trial Study Group. A comparison of six weeks with six months of oral anticoagulant therapy after a first episode of venous thromboembolism. N Engl J Med 1995; 332:1661–5 |
| 28 | 1b | Kearon C, Gent M, Hirsch J et al. A comparison of three months of anticoagulation with extended anticoagulation for a first episode of idiopathic venous thromboembolism. N Engl J Med 1999; 340: 901–7 |
| 29 | 1b | Schulman S et al. The duration of oral anticoagulation after a second episode of venous thromboembolism. N Engl J Med 1997; 336: 393–8 |
| 30 | 1b– | Ly B et al. A controlled clinical trial of streptokinase and heparin in the treatment of pulmonary embolism. Acta Med Scand 1978; 203: 465–70 |
| 31 | 1b– | Goldhaber SZ et al. Reduced bolus alteplase vs conventional alteplase infusion for pulmonary embolism thrombolysis: an international multicentre randomised trial. The Bolus Alteplase Pulmonary Embolism Group. Chest 1994; 106: 718–24 |
| 32 | 1b– | Goldhaber SZ et al. Alteplase versus heparin in acute pulmonary embolism: a randomised trial assessing right ventricular function and pulmonary perfusion. Lancet 1993; 341: 507–16 |
| 33 | 1b– | Levine M et al. tPA for the treatment of acute pulmonary embolism: a collaborative study by PIOPED investigators. Chest 1990; 97: 528–33 |
| 34 | 1b | Sherry S et al. Urokinase-pulmonary embolism trial. Circulation 1973; 17(suppl 2) |
| 35 | 1b– | Goldhaber SZ et al. Recombinant tissue-type plasminogen activator versus a novel dosing regimen of urokinase in acute pulmonary embolism: a randomised controlled multicenter trial. J Am Coll Cardiol 1992; 20: 24–30 |
| 36 | 4 | Rodriguez JL et al. Early placement of prophylactic vena caval filters in injured patients at high risk for PE. J Trauma 1996; 40: 797–804 |
| 37 | 1b | Decousus H, Leizorovicz A, Parent F et al. A clinical trial of vena caval filters in the prevention of pulmonary embolism in patients with proximal deep-vein thrombosis. N Engl J Med 1998; 338: 409–415 |
| 38 | 1b | Carson JL et al. The clinical course of pulmonary embolism. N Engl J Med 1992; 326: 1240–5 |
| 39 | 1b | Quinn DL et al. A prospective investigation of pulmonary embolism in women and men. JAMA 1992; 268: 1989–96 |

## PREVALENCE

Acute renal failure is defined as:

- oliguria: urine output < 400 ml/day
- rapid (hours to weeks) decline in glomerular filtration rate manifest by increasing serum urea and creatinine.

Acute renal failure is relatively common in inpatients, especially if they have pre-existing renal insufficiency [C][1].

> **Note**
> - 5% of medical and surgical inpatients develop acute renal failure [C][1]:
> - 3% with admission creatinine < 106 µmol/l.
> - 14% with admission creatinine > 106 µmol/l.

## CAUSES

### Pre-renal causes [C][1-5]:

- cardiogenic shock e.g. hypotension from MI, heart failure
- hypovolaemia, e.g. dehydration, haemorrhage, surgery
- sepsis
- liver failure.

### Renal causes [C][1-5]:

- acute tubular necrosis due to ischaemia (i.e. any pre-renal cause if sufficiently severe or prolonged)
- acute tubular necrosis due to drugs or toxins (e.g. aminoglycosides, contrast media)
- acute interstitial nephritis
- vasculitis, atheroemboli, glomerulonephritis, myeloma, systemic sclerosis and malignant hypertension.

### Post-renal causes [C][1-5]:

- obstruction (stones, prostate, tumour).

*Note*
Any of the above may coincide with pre-existing chronic renal insufficiency: called acute-on-chronic renal failure.

### Note

- Causes are commonly multifactorial (63%: 95% CI 55% to 71%) and often iatrogenic in origin (55%) **[C]**[1].

**Acute tubular necrosis and prerenal failure are the commonest causes of acute renal failure**

| Causes of acute renal failure | % (95% CI) |
|---|---|
| Acute tubular necrosis | 45% (41% to 49%) |
| Pre-renal | 21% (18% to 24%) |
| Acute onset chronic renal failure | 13% (10% to 15%) |
| Obstruction (stones, prostate, tumour) | 10% (7.9% to 12%) |
| Acute tubulointerstitial nephritis | 2.0% (1.0% to 3.0%) |
| Secondary glomerulonephritis | 1.6% (0.7% to 2.5%) |
| Primary glomerulonephritis | 1.5% (0.6% to 2.3%) |
| Vasculitis | 1.5% (0.6% to 2.3%) |
| Vascular (atheroembolic or thrombosis) | 1.1% (0.3% to 1.8%) |
| Other or unknown | 3.5% (2.2% to 4.8%) |

**Decreased renal perfusion, surgery and drugs are the commonest causes of in-hospital acute renal failure**

| Causes of in-hospital acute renal failure **[C]**[1] | % (95% CI) |
|---|---|
| Decreased renal perfusion | 42% (33% to 50%) |
| Major surgery | 18% (11% to 24%) |
| Contrast media administration | 12% (6.7% to 18%) |
| Aminoglycoside administration | 7.0% (2.6% to 11%) |
| Hepatorenal syndrome | 3.9% (0.5% to 7.2%) |
| Multifactorial | 3.1% (0.1% to 6.1%) |
| Obstruction | 2.3% (0.0% to 4.9%) |
| Vasculitis | 1.6% (0.0% to 3.7%) |
| Other or unknown | 11% (5.5% to 16%) |

**Hypotension, dehydration and sepsis are the commonest causes of hospital-acquired acute tubular necrosis**

| Causes of acute tubular necrosis **[C]**[2] | % (95% CI) |
|---|---|
| Hypotension | 63% (55% to 71%) |
| Multifactorial | 62% (54% to 70%) |
| Dehydration | 29% (22% to 37%) |
| Sepsis | 26% (19% to 33%) |
| Pigmenturia | 19% (12% to 25%) |
| Aminoglycoside use | 10% (5% to 16%) |
| Radiocontrast | 10% (5% to 16%) |
| Liver disease | 2.1% (0.0% to 4.4%) |

## CLINICAL FEATURES

Ask about:

- previous systemic disease – diabetes, vascular disease
- known renal disease, previous renal function tests
- recent systemic disturbances – MI, GI bleeding, major surgery
- medication – ACE inhibitors, aminoglycosides, radiocontrast, other antibiotics.

Look for evidence of [D]:

- volume contraction
- volume overload
- outflow obstruction
- infection
- joint or skin problems.

## INVESTIGATIONS

- Blood count [D].
- Urea, electrolytes, creatinine, glucose [A]:
  - urea (in mmol/l): creatinine (in μmol/l) ratio [C][6]

| **Why?** |
|---|
| **A urea:creatinine ratio > 0.1 makes pre-renal failure more likely** |

| Patient | Target disorder (reference standard) | Diagnostic test | LR + (95% CI) | Post-test probability | LR– (95% CI) | Post-test probability |
|---|---|---|---|---|---|---|
| Suspected pre-renal failure (pre-test probability 20%) | Pre-renal failure (clinical records) | Urea:creatinine ratio > 0.1 | 3.4 (1.5 to 8.0) | 46% | 0.53 (0.38 to 0.74) | 12% |

- estimate the creatinine clearance [D].

$$Cl_{Cr} \text{ (ml/min)} = \frac{(140 - \text{age}) \times \text{weight (kg)}}{Cr_s \text{ (μmol/l)}} \times (1.2 \text{ for men})$$

  - $Cl_{Cr}$ creatinine clearance; $Cr_s$ serum creatinine.
  - Normal creatinine clearance is around 100 ml/min.
  - This formula is derived for use in steady state (not the case in ARF), but can provide an idea of the severity of the problem (e.g. for drug dose adjustments).
  - If the creatinine is rising, true clearance will be lower (often much lower) than that calculated.
  - If oligoanuric, best estimate of true creatinine clearance is less than 10 ml/min – adjust drugs accordingly.

Consider:

- arterial blood gas, pH [D]
- chest X-ray [D]
- ECG [D].

If no clear cause, also consider [D]:

- calcium
- creatinine kinase
- blood cultures
- autoantibodies (ANA, anti-dsDNA, ANCA, anti-GBM), complement levels, cryoglobulins, immunoglobulins, ESR
- serum and urine electrophoresis – myeloma, lymphoma, amyloid.

Insert a urethral catheter [A] to exclude lower urinary tract obstruction. Record the urine output [D]. Take a urine sample.

- Perform a urine dipstick, and look for:
  - protein
  - leucocytes [B][7]
  - haemoglobin [B][7].

---

**？ Why?**

Urine dipstick for leucocytes can help rule in the presence of leucocytes in the urine

| Patient [B][7] | Target disorder (reference standard) | Diagnostic test | LR (95% CI) | Post-test probability |
|---|---|---|---|---|
| Inpatients or outpatients providing MSU (pre-test probability 24%) | Leucocytes in urine (> 5 leucocytes per high-power view on urine microscopy) | Urine dipstick leucocytes: | | |
| | | large | 14 (8.8 to 22) | 81% |
| | | moderate | 9.0 (6.5 to 12) | 74% |
| | | small | 2.6 (2.1 to 3.1) | 45% |
| | | trace | 0.91 (0.75 to 1.1) | 22% |
| | | negative | 0.20 (0.16 to 0.25) | 6% |
| | | Totally clear dipstick | 0.053 (0.024 to 0.11) | 1% |

Urine dipstick for occult blood can help rule in the presence of blood in the urine

| Patient [B][7] | Target disorder (reference standard) | Diagnostic test | LR (95% CI) | Post-test probability |
|---|---|---|---|---|
| Inpatients or outpatients (pre-test probability 11%) providing MSU | Blood in urine (> 5 erythrocytes per high-power power view on urine microscopy) | Urine dipstick blood: | | |
| | | large | 34 (22 to 54) | 81% |
| | | moderate | 9.0 (6.2 to 13) | 53% |
| | | small | 2.1 (1.6 to 2.9) | 21% |
| | | trace | 0.89 (0.65 to 1.2) | 10% |
| | | negative | 0.18 (0.13 to 0.25) | 2% |
| | | Totally clear dipstick | 0.13 (0.057 to 0.28) | 1% |

**Absence of blood or protein on urine dipstick makes glomerular disease less likely**

| Patient **[B]**[8] | Target disorder (reference standard) | Diagnostic test | LR + (95% CI) | Post-test probability | LR- (95% CI) | Post-test probability |
|---|---|---|---|---|---|---|
| Undergoing renal biopsy (pre-test probability 3%) | Glomerular disease (renal biopsy) | Blood on dipstick | 2.7 (1.6 to 4.5) | 8% | 0.16 (0.067 to 0.38) | 0.5% |
| | | Protein ≥2+ on dipstick | 1.9 (1.2 to 2.9) | 6% | 0.34 (0.17 to 0.66) | 1% |

If differential diagnosis is between pre-renal and acute tubular necrosis, consider urine biochemistry:

**Note**

These indices only valid predictors if:
- no previous diuretics
- previously normal renal function.

- urine sodium **[C]**[4] **[C]**[5] **[C]**[9]
- urine chloride **[C]**[4]
- urine creatinine **[C]**[4] **[C]**[5] **[C]**[9]
- urine osmolality **[C]**[5] **[C]**[9].

**Why?**

**A low urine sodium makes pre-renal failure more likely**

| Patient **[C]**[9] | Target disorder (reference standard) | Diagnostic test | LR (95% CI) | Post-test probability |
|---|---|---|---|---|
| Acute renal failure (pre-test probability 24%) | Pre-renal failure (response to pre-renal therapy) | Urine sodium: < 10 mmol/l | 3.5 (1.6 to 7.4) | 53% |
| | | 10–20 mmol/l | 1.4 (0.56 to 3.6) | 21% |
| | | > 20 mmol/l | 0.41 (0.20 to 0.82) | 12% |

**A low urine chloride makes pre-renal failure more likely**

| Patient **[C]**[4] | Target disorder (reference standard) | Diagnostic test | LR (95% CI) | Post-test probability |
|---|---|---|---|---|
| Acute renal failure (pre-test probability 31%) | Pre-renal failure (response to pre-renal therapy) | Urine chloride: < 10 mmol/l | Infinity (6.9 to infinity) | 100% |
| | | 10–20 mmol/l | 3.6 (1.3 to 9.7) | 62% |
| | | >20 mmol/l | 0.21 (0.088 to 0.52) | 9% |

Use to calculate:

- the fractional excretion of sodium [C]⁴[C]⁵[C]⁹:

$$\frac{[\text{urine Na} \times \text{plasma creatinine}]}{[\text{plasma Na} \times \text{urine creatinine}]} \times 100$$

- the fractional excretion of chloride [C]⁴:

$$\frac{[\text{urine Cl} \times \text{plasma creatinine}]}{[\text{plasma Cl} \times \text{urine creatinine}]} \times 100$$

**? Why?**

**A low fractional excretion of sodium or chloride makes pre-renal failure more likely**

| Patient [C]⁴ | Target disorder (reference standard) | Diagnostic test | LR + (95% CI) | Post-test probability | LR− (95% CI) | Post-test probability |
|---|---|---|---|---|---|---|
| Acute renal failure (pre-test probability 31%) | Pre-renal failure (possible cause and response to pre-renal therapy) | Fractional excretion of sodium ≤ 1% | 10 (3.9 to 26) | 82% | 0.16 (0.055 to 0.45) | 7% |
| | | Fractional excretion of chloride ≤ 1% | 22 (5.8 to 87) | 91% | 0.050 (0.0073 to 0.34) | 2% |

**A high urine osmolality makes pre-renal failure more likely**

| Patient [C]⁹ | Target disorder (reference standard) | Diagnostic test | LR + (95% CI) | Post-test probability | LR− (95% CI) | Post-test probability |
|---|---|---|---|---|---|---|
| Acute renal failure (pre-test probability 24%) | Pre-renal failure (response to pre-renal therapy) | Urine osmolality > 500 mOsmol/kg | 7.9 (1.6 to 38) | 71% | 0.79 (0.62 to 1.0) | 20% |

Send for urine microscopy.
Look out for comments on:

- red blood cell shape [B]⁸
- lymphocytes [B]⁸
- eosinophils [C]¹⁰ [C]¹¹
- casts [B]⁸.

**Why?**
**Absence of dysmorphic red blood cells or the presence of haem-granular casts makes glomerular disease less likely**

| Patient [B][8] | Target disorder (reference standard) | Diagnostic test | LR + (95% CI) | Post-test probability | LR– (95% CI) | Post-test probability |
|---|---|---|---|---|---|---|
| Undergoing renal biopsy (pre-test probability 3%) | Glomerular disease (renal biopsy) | Dysmorphic red blood cells on microscopy | 4.7 (2.3 to 9.6) | 13% | 0.080 (0.026 to 0.24) | 0.2% |
| | | Haem-granular casts on microscopy | 0.66 (0.48 to 0.92) | 2% | 2.3 (1.1 to 5.1) | 6.6% |
| | | Any glomerular abnormality on microscopy | 4.9 (2.2 to 11) | 13% | 0.23 (0.13 to 0.42) | 0.7% |

**Absence of lymphyoctes, eosinophils or haem-granular casts on microscopy make interstitial disease less likely**

| Patient [B][8] | Target disorder (reference standard) | Diagnostic test | LR + (95% CI) | Post-test probability | LR– (95% CI) | Post-test probability |
|---|---|---|---|---|---|---|
| Undergoing renal biopsy (pre-test probability 2%) [B][8] | Interstitial disease (renal biopsy) | Lymphocytes ≥ 10 per 10 high-power fields on microscopy | 3.0 (1.8 to 4.9) | 6% | 0.28 (0.13 to 0.63) | 0.6% |
| | | Haem-granular casts on microscopy | 1.7 (1.2 to 2.2) | 3% | 0.27 (0.089 to 0.79) | 0.5% |
| | | Granular casts ≥ 5 per 10 high-power fields on microscopy | 2.1 (1.2 to 3.6) | 4% | 0.58 (0.35 to 0.96) | 1.2% |
| Under investigation for renal disease (pre-test probability 4.4%) [C][10][C][11] | Interstitial disease (renal biopsy or clinical features) | >1% eosinophils using Hansel's stain on microscopy | 9.1 (4.2 to 20) | 29% | 0.40 (0.16 to 0.99) | 2% |

Exclude obstruction (unless it is clinically obvious) [A]:

● CT or ultrasound scan [A][12]
  Look for hydronephrosis (collecting system dilatation): most patients
  with hydronephrosis have obstruction.

**Why?**
**Ultrasound and CT can help rule out hydronephrosis**

| Patient [A][12] | Target disorder (reference standard) | Diagnostic test | LR + (95% CI) | Post-test probability | LR– (95% CI) | Post-test probability |
|---|---|---|---|---|---|---|
| Acute renal failure (pre-test probability: 14%) | Hydronephrosis (excretory urography) | CT | 11 (5.9 to 19) | 64% | 0.0 (0.0 to 0.17) | 0% |
| | | Ultrasound scan | 6.2 (4.1 to 9.2) | 64% | 0.0 (0.0 to 0.13) | 0% |

**Note**
- 9% of CTs and ultrasound scans are non-diagnostic [A][12].

Obtain a nephrology opinion [D].
Consider performing a renal biopsy if [C][13]:

- clinical signs suggestive of primary renal disease, vascular lesions or systemic disease
- no obvious cause for acute renal failure
- suspected acute interstitial nephritis or drug-induced vasculitis
- oligoanuria thought due to acute tubular necrosis persists beyond 3 weeks without perpetuating factors.

**Why?**
- In selected patients, biopsy findings alter management in 70% of cases (95% CI: 55% to 87%) [C][14].
- Complications are uncommon, but may be severe [B][15].

**Bleeding and unsuitable samples are the commonest complications**

| Complications [B][15] | % (95% CI) |
|---|---|
| Clinically important bleeding | 4.1% (0.9% to 7.4%) |
| Unsuitable sample | 1.4% (0.0% to 3.3%) |
| Nephrectomy for prolonged bleeding (> 30 days) | 0.7% (0.0% to 2.0%) |

## THERAPY

Treat underlying causes [D]:

- resuscitate the patient [A] using crystalloids [A][16]
- relieve any outflow obstruction [A].

**Why do this?**
■ Colloids are not clearly better than crystalloids for resuscitating patients, and may well be harmful **[A]**[16].

Monitor the patient **[D]**, but even if critically ill, avoid immediate routine right heart catheterisation **[B]**[17].

**Why?**
■ Critically ill patients who have right heart catheterisation (Swan-Ganz catheter) as part of initial management strategy are more likely to die **[B]**[17].
■ Costs of care, intensity of care and length of stay in ITU are higher in patients managed by right heart catheterisation **[B]**[17].

**Right heart catheterisation is associated with increased mortality**

| Patient **[B]**[17] | Prognostic factor | Outcome | Control rate | OR (95% CI) | NNF+(95% CI) |
|---|---|---|---|---|---|
| Critically ill | Right heart catheterisation *independent* | Death at 6 months | 46% | 1.21 (1.09 to 1.25) | 21 (18 to 47) |

Provide supportive care.

● Monitor fluid status carefully (e.g. clinical assessment, weight, fluid charts, invasive monitoring) and restrict water and sodium as necessary **[D]**.
● Review medication:
  – avoid potential nephrotoxins (e.g. NSAIDs, aminoglycosides) **[D]**.
  – adjust doses of other medications to account for renal insufficiency **[D]**.
● Regular electrolyes, urea, creatinine: watch for hyperkalaemia **[D]**.

Ask for a nephrology opinion **[D]**.

The following improve urine output without clearly reducing dialysis or death:

● diuretics
  – high-dose loop diuretics, e.g furosemide **[A]**[18]
      i loading dose 120–240 mg furosemide, followed by an infusion of 20 mg/h **[A]**[18]
      ii if unable to give as infusion, give 120 mg over 1 h every 6 h
      iii reduce dose if creatinine falling
      iv titrate dose to urine output

**Why do this?**

■ High-dose loop diuretics increase urine flow in patients treated with dopamine and mannitol, but seizures are more common **[A]**[18].

■ The time to dialysis is longer (~ 3 days), but the duration of dialysis is similar (~ 13 days) **[A]**[18]. However there is no clear effect on mortality or renal recovery **[D]**[19] **[D]**[20] **[D]**[21].

**High-dose loop diuretics increase urine flow, but cause more seizures**

| Patient **[A]**[18] | Treatment | Comparator | Outcome | CER | RRR | NNT |
|---|---|---|---|---|---|---|
| Acute renal failure due to renal causes | High-dose loop diuretics | Placebo | Increase in urine flow at 21 days | 23% | 120% (11% to 340%) | 4 (2 to 12) |
| | | | Seizure at 21 days | 3.3% | −480% (−4200% to 21%) | −6 (−23 to −4) |

● mannitol – single dose of 100 ml of 20% solution, in patients where the underlying problem is uncorrected hypovolaemia **[C]**[22]

**Why do this?**

■ 54% of patients with oliguric acute renal failure due to surgical or obstetrical problems increase their urine output when given mannitol (mean of 80 ml/h).

■ Mannitol 100 ml of 20% solution every 6 h led to hyperosmolality in 16% and pulmonary oedema in 1% of patients **[A]**[18].

● inotropic agents **[C]**[24]
  ● noradrenaline **[C]**[23] – started if systolic blood pressure < 90 mmHg; 0.5 µg/kg per minute with increments of 0.3 0.6 µg/kg per minute to maintain systolic blood pressure > 120/80
● dopamine **[B]**[24] – low dose: 1–3 µg/kg per minute.

**Why do this?**

■ Noradrenaline infusion increases urine output, decreases creatinine levels and increases creatinine clearance in around 80% of patients with septic shock **[C]**[23].

■ Dopamine acutely increases urine output and creatinine clearance in patients with oliguria or established acute renal failure **[B]**[24].

■ Noradrenaline stabilises more patients in hyperdynamic septic shock than dopamine **[A]**[25].

■ The effect on development of acute renal failure, requirement for dialysis, or death is unclear **[A]**[25] **[B]**[24] **[C]**[23].

**Noradrenaline stabilises septic shock better than dopamine**

| Patient **[A]**[20] | Treatment | Comparator | Outcome | CER | RRR | NNT |
|---|---|---|---|---|---|---|
| Hyperdynamic septic shock | Noradrenaline | Dopamine | Haemodynamic stabilisation for at least 6 h | 31% | 200% (43% to 530%) | 2 (1 to 3) |

Dialyse patients who fail to respond **[A]** as advised by a specialist **[D]**.

**Note**
■ Patients require dialysis for an average of 13 days **[A]**[18].
■ An intensive dialysis regimen is not clearly better than a normal regimen in patients with acute renal failure maintaining predialysis urea < 21 mmol/L, creatinine < 440 µmol/L **[D]**[26].

There is no clear benefit from using:

● anaritide
● essential amino acids.

**Why?**
■ Anaritide has little effect on creatinine levels, does not reduce the need for dialysis nor clearly reduce mortality in patients with acute tubular necrosis **[A]**[27].
■ Essential amino acids have no clear effect on mortality in severely ill patients with acute renal failure **[A]**[28].

## PREVENTION

### Contrast medium nephrotoxicity

Use low-osmolality contrast media **[A]**[29], particularly for high-risk patients:

● with pre-existing renal impairment **[A]**[29]
● with diabetes **[B]**[30]
● undergoing angiography **[B]**[30].

**Why do this?**
■ Around 3% of patients develop nephrotoxicity following contrast media studies **[B]**[30].
■ Low-osmolality contrast media cause less nephrotoxicity than high-osmolality contrast media in high-risk patients.

**Low-osmolality contrast media cause less acute renal dysfunction than high-osmolality media**

| Patient [A][29] | Treatment | Comparator | Outcome | CER | OR | NNT |
|---|---|---|---|---|---|---|
| Undergoing contrast study | Low-osmolality contrast media | High-osmolality contrast media | Increase in Cr levels of > 44 µmol/l at ?2 days | 3% | 0.61 (0.48 to 0.77) | 90 (68 to 150) |
| Undergoing contrast study | Low-osmolality contrast media | High-osmolality contrast media | Increase in Cr levels of > 90 µmol/l at ?2 days | 3% | 0.44 (0.26 to 0.73) | 120 (95 to 260) |
| Pre-existing renal impairment undergoing contrast study | Low-osmolality contrast media | High-osmolality contrast media | Increase in Cr levels of > 44 µmol/l at ?2 days | 1.5% | 0.50 (0.36 to 0.70) | 70 (55 to 120) |

**Why do this?**

Angiography, pre-existing renal failure or insulin-dependent diabetes increases the risk of nephrotoxicity

| Patient [B][30] | Prognostic factor | Outcome | Control rate | RR (95% CI) | NNF+ (95% CI) |
|---|---|---|---|---|---|
| Elderly | Angiocardiography *independent* | Nephrotoxicity at 48 h | 3% | 3.44 (1.25 to 6.79) | 14 (6 to 140) |
| | Pre-existing renal insufficiency *independent* | Nephrotoxicity at 48 h | 3% | 3.06 (1.29 to 5.41) | 17 (8 to 120) |
| | Insulin-dependent diabetes mellitus *independent* | Nephrotoxicity at 48 h | 3% | 3.06 (1.19 to 7.80) | 17 (5 to 180) |

Avoid:

- furosemide [A][31]
- mannitol [D][32]

**Why do this?**

■ Furosemide increases the risk of developing acute renal dysfunction in patients with chronic renal insufficiency.
■ Mannitol has no clear effect on preventing acute renal dysfunction.

**Using furosemide increases the risk of acute renal dysfunction following contrast media studies**

| Patient [A][31] | Treatment | Comparator | Outcome | CER | RRR | NNH |
|---|---|---|---|---|---|---|
| Chronic renal insufficiency, undergoing contrast study | Furosemide and 0.45% saline infusion | 0.45% saline infusion | Acute renal dysfunction at 48 h | 11% | −270% (−1100% to −16%) | 3 (2 to 14) |

## Antibiotics: aminoglycosides

**Avoid aminoglycosides** in patients with renal dysfunction (creatinine clearance >60 ml/min or rising creatinine) or with shock, unless there is no good alternative [D].

In patients with either of these problems reconsider choice of antibiotics before subsequent doses [D].

Estimate the patient's renal function when contemplating aminoglycoside treatment:

- calculate the patient's creatinine clearance

$$\text{CrCl (ml/min)} = \frac{(140 - \text{age}) \times \text{weight}}{\text{Cr } (\mu\text{mol/l})} (\times 1.2 \text{ if male})$$

- if the patient is obese, use an estimate of the patient's ideal body weight to calculate creatinine clearance:
  - ideal body weight (kg) for males = 52 kg + 0.72 kg for every cm above 154 cm in height

– ideal body weight (kg) for females = 49 kg + 0.64 kg for every cm above 154 cm in height.

**In patients with creatinine clearance > 60 ml/min,** give aminoglycosides once a day (most commonly 4.5 mg/kg of dose-determining weight (see below)).

**Why do this?**
■ Fewer patients develop nephrotoxicity. There is no clear effect on ototoxicity.
■ More patients are cured.

**Once-daily dosing of aminoglycosides leads to more cures and less nephrotoxicity**

| Patient [A][33] | Treatment | Comparator | Outcome | CER (%) | RRR | NNT |
|---|---|---|---|---|---|---|
| Infection without neutropenia | Once-daily aminoglycoside | Multiple doses per day | Cure at 10 days | 82% | 1.47 (1.13 to 1.94) | 20 (13 to 58) |
| | | | Nephrotoxicity at 10 days | | 0.60 (0.40 to 0.86) | 21 (14 to 62) |

**In obese patients,** use a dose-determining weight calculated as follows:

dose determining weight = ideal body weight + 0.4 (actual body weight – ideal body weight).

**In patients with renal insufficiency** (when there is no good alternative to an aminoglycoside):

● adjust the dose or the dose interval according to the level of dysfunction and according to the clinical circumstances
● aim for trough levels less than 2 µg/ml
● obtain a trough level prior to the second dose
● continue to follow aminoglycoside levels and the serum creatinine.

In all patients, monitor gentamicin levels during therapy, and adjust dose intervals:

● measure a trough level prior to the third dose; if not less than 2 µg/l, increase the dose interval or reduce the dose.

Monitor creatinine levels during therapy (every 2–3 days minimum, more frequently if pre-existing renal dysfunction, shock or critically ill) **[D]**.

Aminoglycoside toxicity can manifest days after the last dose **[D]**.

**Critically ill**
Avoid using:

● albumin **[D]**.

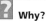 **Why?**
- Albumin infusions for maintenance of colloid osmotic pressure do not clearly preserve renal function, or prevent death in critically ill patients **[D]**[34].
- It increases mortality in critically-ill patients with hypovolaernia, burns or hypoalbuminaemia **[A]**[35].

**Albumin increases mortality in critically-ill patients**

| Patient | Treatment | Comparator | Outcome | CER | OR (95% CI) | NNT (95% CI) |
|---|---|---|---|---|---|---|
| Critically ill **[A]**[35] | Albumin | Saline | Death at discharge | 8.1 | 1.95 (1.37 to 2.78). | 15 (9 to 37) |

## PROGNOSIS

Many patients require dialysis **[C]**[2], but few require it long-term **[C]**[1]**[C]**[2].

 **Note**
- 36% require dialysis (95% CI: 33% to 40%) **[C]**[2].
- 3%, require long-term dialysis (95% CI: 0.0% to 5.8%) **[C]**[1] **[C]**[2].

Mortality is high, particularly if patients require dialysis **[A]**[36].

**Note**
- 45% of patients with acute renal failure die (95% CI: 41% to 49%) **[A]**[36].
- 66% of patients requiring dialysis die (95% CI: 60% to 72%) **[A]**[36].

Patients are more likely to die if they:
- have acute stroke or seizure **[B]**[37]
- have acute myocardial infarction **[B]**[37]
- have oliguria **[B]**[37]**[B]**[38]
- are male **[B]**[37]
- are on mechanical ventilation **[B]**[37]
- have sepsis **[B]**[38].

 **Why?**
**Recent strokes, seizures, heart attacks or the presence of oliguria increases the risk of dying**

| Patient | Prognostic factor | Outcome | Control rate | OR (95% CI) | NNF+(95% CI) |
|---|---|---|---|---|---|
| Acute renal failure | Acute stroke or seizure *independent* | Death at 60 days | 45% | 7.35 (1.92 to 28.1) | 2 (2 to 6) |
| | Acute MI *independent* | Death at 60 days | 45% | 5.90 (2.43 to 14.4) | 3 (2 to 5) |
| | Oliguria *independent* | Death at 60 days | 45% | 4.39 (2.09 to 9.24) | 3 (2 to 6) |
| | Male *independent* | Death at 60 days | 45% | 3.70 (1.75 to 7.82) | 3 (2 to 7) |
| | Mechanical ventilation *independent* | Death at 60 days | 45% | 2.95 (1.53 to 5.68) | 4 (3 to 9) |

Patients on dialysis are more likely to die if they [B][39]:
● have CNS depression after the first week
● required inotropic drug support after the first week
● are elderly.

**Guideline writers**: Catherine Clase, Christopher Ball
**CAT writers**: Catherine Clase, Christopher Ball

## REFERENCES

| No. | Level | Citation |
| --- | --- | --- |
| 1 | 4 | Hou SH et al. Hospital acquired renal insufficiency: a prospective study. Am J Med 1983: 74: 243–8 |
| 2 | 4 | Liano F et al. Epidemiology of acute renal failure: a prospective, multicenter, community-based study. Kidney Int 1996; 50: 811–18 |
| 3 | 4 | Rasmussen HH Ibels LS. Acute renal failure: multivariate analysis of causes and risk factors. Am J Med 1982: 73; 211–18 |
| 4 | 4 | Anderson RJ et al. Urinary chloride concentration in acute renal failure. Mineral Electrolyte Metab 1984: 10; 92–7 |
| 5 | 4 | Miller TR et al. Urinary diagnostic indices in acute renal failure. Ann Intern Med 1978; 89: 47–50 |
| 6 | 4 | Morgan DB et al. Plasma creatinine and urea:creatinine ratio in patients with raised plasma urea. BMJ 1977; 2: 929–32 |
| 7 | 2b | Bonnardeaux A et al. A study on the reliability of dipstick urinalysis. Clin Nephrol 1994; 41: 167–72 |
| 8 | 2b | Marcussen N et al. Analysis of cytodiagnostic urinalysis findings in 77 patients with concurrent renal biopsies. Am J Kidney Dis 1992; 20: 618–28 |
| 9 | 4 | Espinel CH, Gregory AW. Differential diagnosis of acute renal failure. Clin Nephrol 1980; 13: 73–7 |
| 10 | 4 | Corwin HL et al. The detection and interpretation of urinary eosinophils. Arch Pathol Lab Med 1989; 113: 1256–8 |
| 11 | 4 | Nolan CR et al. Eosinophiluria – a new method of detection and definition of the clinical spectrum. N Engl J Med 1986; 315: 1516–19 |
| 12 | 1b | Webb JAW et al. Can ultrasound and computed tomography replace high-dose excretory urography in patients with impaired renal function? Q J Med 1984; 211: 411–25 |
| 13 | 4 | Sraer JD et al. Renal biopsy in acute renal failure. Kidney Int 1975; 8: 60–1A |
| 14 | 4 | Richards NT et al. Knowledge of renal histology alters patient management in over 40% of cases. Nephrol Dial Transplant 1994; 9: 1255–9 |
| 15 | 2b | Sraer JD et al. Renal biopsy in acute renal failure. Kidney Int 1975; 8: 60–1A |
| 16 | 1a – | Schierhout G, Roberts I. Fluid resuscitation with colloid or crystalloid solutions in critically ill patients: a systematic review of randomized trials. BMJ 1998; 316: 961–4 |

| No. | Level | Citation |
|-----|-------|----------|
| 17 | 3b | Connors AF et al. The effectiveness of right heart catheterization in the initial care of critically ill patients. JAMA 1996; 276: 889–97 |
| 18 | 1b | Shilliday IR et al. Loop diuretics in the management of acute renal failure; a prospective, double-blind, placebo-controlled, randomized study. Nephrol Dial Transplant 1997; 12: 2592–6 |
| 19 | lb – | Shilliday IR et al. Loop diuretics in the management of acute renal failure; a prospective, double-blind, placebo-controlled, randomized study. Nephrol Dial Transplant 1997; 12: 2592–2596 |
| 20 | 1b – | Cantarovich F et al. Frusemide in high doses in the treatment of acute renal failure. Postgrad Med J 1971; 47 (suppl): 13–17 |
| 21 | 1b – | Kleinknecht D et al. Furosemide in acute oliguric renal failure: a controlled trial. Nephron 1976; 17: 51–8 |
| 22 | 4 | Luke RG et al. Factors determining response to mannitol in acute renal failure. Am J Med Sci 1970; 259: 168–74. |
| 23 | 4 | Martin C et al. Renal effects of norepinephrine used to treat septic shock patients. Crit Care Med 1990; 18: 282–5 |
| 24 | 2b | Denton MD et al. 'Renal-dose' dopamine for the treatment of acute renal failure: scientific rationale, experimental studies and clinical trials. Kidney Int 1996; 49: 4–14 |
| 25 | 1b | Martin C, Papazian L, Perrin G et al. Norepinephrine or dopamine for the treatment of hyperdynamic septic shock? Chest 1993; 103: 1826–31 |
| 26 | 2b – | Gillum DM et al. The role of intensive dialysis in acute renal failure. Clin Nephrol 1986; 25: 249–55 |
| 27 | 1b | Allgren RL et al. Anaritide in acute tubular necrosis. N Engl J Med 1997; 336: 828–34 |
| 28 | 1b | Naylor CD et al. Does treatment with essential amino acids and hypertonic glucose improve survival in acute renal failure: a meta-analysis. Ren Fail 1987–1988; 10: 141–52 |
| 29 | 1b | Nephrotoxicity of high- and low-osmolality contrast media: a meta-analysis. ACP J Club 1993 Nov–Dec; 119: 74. Barrett BJ, Carlisle EJ. Meta-analysis of the relative nephrotoxicity of high- and low-osmolality iodinated contrast media. Radiology 1993; 188: 171–8 |
| 30 | 2b | Risk for contrast media-induced nephrotoxicity was low for both high and low-contrast media. ACP J Club 1992 July–Aug; 117:29. Revised November 1997. Moore RD, Steinberg EP, Powe NR et al. Nephrotoxicity of high-osmolality versus low-osmolality contrast media: randomized clinical trial. Radiology 1992; 182: 649–55 |
| 31 | 1b | Solomon R, Werner C, Mann D et al. Effects of saline, mannitol, and furosemide on acute decreases in renal function induced by radiocontrast agents. N Engl J Med 1994; 331: 1416–20 |
| 32 | 1b – | Solomon R, Werner C, Mann D, et al. Effects of saline, mannitol, and furosemide on acute decreases in renal function induced by radiocontrast agents. New England Journal of Medicine 1994; 331: 1416–1420 |
| 33 | 1a | Ferriois-Lissost R, Alos-Aliminana M. Effectiveness and safety of once-daily aminoglycosides: a meta-analysis. Am J Health Syst Pharm 1996; 53: 1141–50 |
| 34 | 1b – | Grundmann R, Heistermann S. Postoperative albumin infusion therapy based on colloid osmotic pressure. A prospectively randomized trial. Arch Surg 1985; 120: 911–15 |

| No. | Level | Citation |
| --- | --- | --- |
| 35 | 1a | The Albumin Reviewers (Alderson P, Bunn F, Lefebvre C (et al.) Human albumin administration in critically ill patients (Cochrane Review). In: The Cochrane Library, Issue 3, 1998. Oxford: Update Software |
| 36 | 1b | Liano F et al. Epidemiology of acute renal failure: a prospective, multicenter, community-based study. Kidney Int 1996; 50: 811–18 |
| 37 | 2b | Chertow GM et al. Predictors of mortality and the provision of dialysis in patients with acute tubular necrosis. J Am Soc Nephrol 1998; 9: 692–8 |
| 38 | 2b | Cantarovitch F et al. A simple prognostic index for patients with acute renal failure requiring dialysis. Ren Fail 1996; 18: 585–9 |
| 39 | 2b | Lien J, Chan V. Risk factors influencing survival in acute renal failure treated by hemodialysis. Arch Intern Med 1985; 145: 2067–9 |

## PREVALENCE

Many patients are regular attenders: **[B]** – contact their regular physician and ask how they are normally treated **[D]**.

 **Note**
- 30% of patients with sickle cell disease are admitted to hospital each year **[C]**[1] but a third of all the crises happen in 5% of patients **[B]**[2].
- Genotype is important: patients with SS anaemia and S-$\beta^0$ thalassaemia are more likely to have crises than others **[C]**[1].

Most patients requiring admission present with painful vaso-occlusive crises (Table 1) **[C]**[1].

The presentation varies with the age of the patient **[C]**[1].

| Table 1 Presentation on admission | |
|---|---|
| Type of presentation **[C]**[1] | % of admission diagnoses |
| Vaso-occlusive | 91% (87% to 96%) |
| ■ painful | 88% (83% to 93%) |
| ■ stroke | 1.9% (0.0% to 4.0%) |
| (in children) | |
| ■ renal papillary necrosis | 1.9% (0.0% to 4.0%) |
| Syndromes | 16% (9.9% to 21%) |
| ■ girdle | 8.1% (3.9% to 12%) |
| (from adolescence) | |
| ■ acute chest syndrome | 6.2% (2.5% to 9.9%) |
| ■ hepatic | 0.6% (0.0% to 1.8%) |
| ■ splenic | 0.6% (0.0% to 1.8%) |
| Infective | 7% |

## CLINICAL FEATURES

Think about:
- painful crises
- acute chest syndrome
- infective episodes
- neurological or surgical problems.

Ask about:
if a painful crisis
- where they have pain **[C]**[3]

> **Note**
> ■ Most patients have two or three sites of pain: the commonest sites are the lumbar spine and femur **[C]**[3].

- potential triggers such as cold weather, stress, exertion, alcohol, pregnancy **[C]**[3]

> **Why?**
> ■ There are several potential triggers for sickle cell crisis.
>
> | Sickle cell crisis triggers **[C]**[3] | % of cases |
> | --- | --- |
> | Cold | 35% |
> | Emotional stress | 10% |
> | Physical exertion | 7% |
> | Pregnancy | 5% |
> | Alcohol | 4% |

or if acute chest syndrome **[C]**
- chest pain, fever, dyspnoea and coughing.

> **Why?**
> ■ Patients may present with features of acute chest syndrome.
>
> | Acute chest syndrome **[C]**[4] | % of patients with finding |
> | --- | --- |
> | *Symptoms* | |
> | ■ chest pain | 84% |
> | ■ severe chest pain | 44% |
> | ■ fever | 64% |
> | ■ cough | 63% |
> | ■ short of breath | 47% |
> | ■ productive cough | 44% |
> | | |
> | *Signs* | |
> | ■ chills | 39% |
> | ■ temperature > 39°C | 15% |
> | ■ crackles | 54% |
> | ■ normal chest examination | 28% |
> | ■ decreased percussion | 40% |

Remember to ask about:
- fever and rigors **[C]**

> **Why?**
> ■ Fever is common (42% of patients with a crisis **[C]**[3]), but few have an infection (1.8% of patients with acute chest syndrome have bacteraemia **[C]**[4]).

- abdominal pain [C].
- priapism [C][32].

Look for:
- chest signs [C]
- focal neurological signs [C]
- an acute abdomen [C].

Ask for a surgical opinion if there are signs of an acute abdomen – it may not be due to the crisis!

**Why?**
- Gallstones are common in patients with sickle cell disease [C][5].
- Investigations (including liver function tests and abdominal ultrasound) are not very helpful at distinguishing a vaso-occlusive crisis from an acute abdomen [C][5].

## INVESTIGATIONS

Be guided by the presenting syndrome.
- Blood count [D], reticulocyte count [D].
- Urea and electrolytes, creatinine [D].
- CRP [D].
- Blood cultures [D].
- Pulse oximetry – but beware [C][6].

**Why?**
**Pulse oximetry is unhelpful in excluding hypoxia**

| Patient[C][6] | Target disorder (reference standard) | Diagnostic test | LR+ (95% CI) | Post-test probability | LR– (95% CI) | Post-test probability |
|---|---|---|---|---|---|---|
| Healthy children with sickle cell disease (pre-test probability 37%) | Hypoxia ($SaO_2$ <93% on capillary blood gas) | Pulse oximetry: $SaO_2$ <93% | Infinity (1.3 to infinity) | 100% | 0.71 (0.45 to 1.1) | 29% |

In acute chest syndromes:
- arterial blood gas [D]
- chest X-ray [D].
In the acute abdomen and neurological problems, other imaging may be required.

## THERAPY

Give symptomatic relief and specific therapies where indicated.
- Give oxygen if hypoxic [C][7].

**Note**
- Patients with painful crises who are not hypoxic do not clearly require oxygen **[C]**[7].

In all cases:
- consider broad-spectrum antibiotics **[D]**
- ensure an adequate fluid intake **[D]**
- seek expert advice **[D]**.

For painful crises and acute chest syndromes:
- give analgesia **[A]**.
Give morphine or diamorphine iv or im regularly **[A]** or via patient-controlled analgesia **[D]**[8].

**Why do this?**
- PCA is safe and well-tolerated in patients with sickle cell crises **[D]**[8].

Avoid regular administration of pethidine (meperidine).

**Why do this?**
- Patients with sickle cell disease who have levels of norpethidine >1.0 μg/l (a toxic metabolite of pethidine) are at increased risk of fittingx **[C]**[9].

**Pethidine and sickle cell disease**

| Outcome **[C]**[9] | Risk factor | PEER | OR (95% CI) | NNH (95% CI) |
|---|---|---|---|---|
| Fit | Norpethidine >1.0 μg/l _not independent_ | ? | Infinity (5.5 to inf) | 1 (1 to 200) |

Give regular NSAIDs.**[A]**[10]

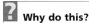
**Why do this?**
- Patients on regular ketorolac and meperidine (pethidine) prn have less pain and stay less time in hospital (around 3 days shorter) **[A]**[10].

Try TENS if the pain is bad **[D]**[11].

**Why do this?**
- Sickle cell patients with crises find TENS a helpful procedure, although the effect on pain relief after 4 h is unclear **[D]**[11].

In patients with acute chest syndrome:
- use incentive spirometry **[A]**[12] – 10 maximal inspirations every 2 h from 8 a.m. to 10 p.m., and at night if awake until chest pain settled.

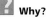
**Why do this?**
- Patients with acute chest pain have fewer pulmonary complications if they breathe deeply every 2 h when awake **[A]**[12].

| Patient | Treatment | Comparator | Outcome | CER | RRR | NNT |
|---|---|---|---|---|---|---|
| Sickle cell disease and acute chest or back pain | Incentive spirometry | No spirometry | Pulmonary complications (atelectasis or infiltrates) at 3 days | 42% | 87% (30% to 100%) | 3 (2 to 8) |

Consider exchange blood transfusions if any of the following are present:
- lung involvement **[C]**[13]
- sequestration syndromes **[D]**
- neurological involvement (stroke, TIA, fits) **[D]**.

**Why do this?**
- Children with sickle cell disease and lung infection, infarction or acute chest syndrome improve clinically following blood transfusion (NNT = 1 at 48 h) **[C]**[13].

**Blood transfusions in sickle cell crises**

| Patient | Treatment | Comparator | Outcome | CER | RRR | NNT |
|---|---|---|---|---|---|---|
| Sickle cell disease and lung infection, infarction or acute chest syndrome | Blood transfusion | No blood transfusion | No clinical improvement at 48 h | 75% | 100% | 1 (1 to 3) |

There is no clear benefit from:
- steroids **[D]**[14]
- cognitive coping therapy **[D]**[15]
- anti-sickling agents, e.g. cetiedil **[D]**[16].

**Why?**
- Methylprednisolone has not been shown to be helpful in children with painful crises from sickle cell disease **[D]**[14].
- Patients with sickle cell disease who have cognitive coping training use more coping strategies and have slightly fewer negative thoughts after 1 month. Other effects are unclear **[D]**[15].
- Cetiedil makes investigators feel better about their patients (NNT = 2), but patients have the same amount of pain and it does not significantly shorten the number of days in hospital **[D]**[16].

## PREVENTION

- Educate your patients about sickle cell crises **[B]**[17].

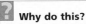
**Why do this?**
- Increased education and information reduce emergency department visits and inpatient days **[B]**[17].

- Give hydroxyurea in severe cases **[A]**[18] – (initial dose 15 mg/kg per day, increase by 5 mg/kg per day every 12 weeks to maximum of 35 mg/kg per day, unless marrow depression noted (neutropenia $< 2.0 \times 10^9/l$, reticulocytes or platelets $<80 \times 10^9 l$; Hb $< 4.5 g/dl$). If this occurs, stop therapy until recovery. Resume at 2.5 mg/kg per day lower).

**Why do this?**
- Patients with more than three crises a year who take hydroxyurea have fewer episodes of acute chest syndrome (NNT = 5) and fewer require blood transfusions.
- Painful crises occur less often (mean of two fewer a year) and take longer to occur (mean of 2 months).

**Hydroxyurea in sickle cell disease**

| Patient [A][18] | Treatment | Comparator | Outcome | CER | RRR | NNT |
|---|---|---|---|---|---|---|
| Frequent sickle cell crises | Hydroxyurea | Placebo | Acute chest syndrome at 21 months | 35% | 53% (25% to 81%) | 5 (4 to 12) |
| Frequent sickle cell crises | Hydroxyurea | Placebo | Need for blood transfusion at 21 months | 50% | 36% (14% to 58%) | 6 (3 to 15) |

- Consider Depo-Provera (medroxyprogesterone acetate) contraception in women **[A]**[19].

**Why do this?**
- Women who take Depo-Provera have fewer painful episodes and fewer episodes of bone pain after 14 months **[A]**[19].

**Depo-Provera in sickle cell disease**

| Patient[A][19] | Treatment | Comparator | Outcome | CER | RRR | NNT |
|---|---|---|---|---|---|---|
| Sickle cell disease | Depo-Provera | Placebo | Bone pain at 14 months | 87% | 30% (2% to 58%) | 4 (2 to 53) |
| Sickle cell disease | Depo-Provera | Placebo | Increase in painful crises at 14 months | 57% | 69% (24% to 100%) | 3 (2 to 7) |

Consider:
- folate [B][20]

**Why do this?**
- Folate supplementation reduces dactylitis in children with homozygous sickle cell (SS) disease and > 2 episodes of dactylitis a year [B][20].
- There is no good evidence to support the use of these drugs in adults.

**Folate reduces dactylitis in children with sickle cell disease**

| Patient [B][20] | Treatment | Comparator | Outcome | CER | RRR | NNT |
|---|---|---|---|---|---|---|
| Children with sickle cell disease and dactylitis > 2 episodes/year | Folate | Placebo | Dactylitis at 1 year | 18% | 83% (22% to 100%) | 7 (4 to 25) |

- regular penicillin prophylaxis.

**Why do this?**
- Daily penicillin V reduces *Streptococcus pneumoniae* infections in children aged < 3 years with sickle cell disease. The effect on other infections and mortality is unclear[A][21].
- Penicillin prophylaxis cannot clearly be safely stopped in children with sickle cell disease over 5 years of age [D][22].
- There is no good evidence to support the use of these drugs in adults.

**Penicillin reduces *S. pneumoniae* in children with in sickle cell disease**

| Patient | Treatment | Comparator | Outcome | CER | RRR | NNT |
|---|---|---|---|---|---|---|
| Children aged < 3 years with sickle cell disease [A][21] | Penicillin V | Vitamin C | *Strep. pneumoniae* infection at 15 months | 12% | 85% (31% to 100%) | 9 (6 to 26) |

There is no clear benefit from:
- routine transfusion therapy in adults.[D][23]

**Why?**
- Regular transfusion therapy does not clearly prevent further TIAs or strokes in sickle cell patients who have had one already [D][23], although it may reduce hospital admissions in children with stroke or intractable painful crises [C][24].

## Surgery
Avoid surgery if possible, especially in patients with severe disease [B][25].

**Why do this?**

- Complications are common: 39% of patients have a serious or life-threatening complication – 9% have a vaso-occlusive crisis **[B]**[25].
- The risk is increased in patients aged > 20 years **[B]**[25].
- The risk of a crisis is increased if patients have had five or more previous hospital admissions **[B]**[25] or have neurological disease **[C]**[24].

**Neurological disease and frequent hospital admissions increase the risk of surgical complications**

| Patient | Prognostic factor | Outcome | Control rate | OR (95% CI) | NNF+(95% CI) |
|---|---|---|---|---|---|
| Cholecystectomy **[B]**[25] | Aged > 20 years | Complication by ?30 days | 27% | 2.01 (1.05 to 3.86) | 6 (3 to 100) |
| Cholecystectomy **[B]**[25] | 5+ previous hospital admission | Sickle cell crisis by ?30 days | 24% | 3.02 (1.19 to 7.65) | 4 (2 to 30) |
| Elective surgery **[C]**[26] | Neurological disease | Complication by 30 days | ~30% | 2.76 (1.48 to 5.12) | 4(3 to 11) |

If surgery is required, keep it simple **[B]**[25].

**Why do this?**

- Complications are more likely when incidental procedures are performed **[B]**[25] or surgery is more risky **[C]**[26].

**Incidental or risky surgical procedures increase the risks of complications**

| Patient | Prognostic factor | Outcome | Control rate (%) | OR (95% CI) | NNF+(95% CI) |
|---|---|---|---|---|---|
| Cholecystectomy **[B]**[25] | Incidental procedure | Complication by ?30 days | 30 | 2.0 (1.22 to 3.29) | 6 (4 to 23) |
| Elective surgery **[A]**[27] | Increased surgical risk | Complication by 30 days | ~30 | 1.76 (1.09 to 2.89) | 7 (4 to 52) |

Transfuse patients before surgery (up to Hb ≥ 10 g/dl).

**Why do this?**
**Crises are more common in patients not transfused pre-operatively [B][25]**

| Patient | Prognostic factor | Outcome | Control rate | OR (95% CI) | NNF+ (95% CI) |
|---|---|---|---|---|---|
| Cholecystectomy | Not transfused pre-operatively *independent* | Sickle cell crisis by ?30 days | 33% | 2.79 (1.16 to 6.69) | 4 (2 to 30) |

There is no clear benefit from:
- aggressive transfusion before surgery (to achieve SS ≤ 30%).

**Why?**

■ Patients who are aggressively transfused pre-operatively are not clearly less likely to have serious or life- threatening complications, but are more likely to develop transfusion reactions.

**Aggressive transfusion pre-operatively increases the risk of transfusion reactions**

| Patient | Treatment | Comparator | Outcome | CER | RRR | NNH |
|---------|-----------|------------|---------|-----|-----|-----|
| Awaiting elective surgery[B][25] | Aggressive transfusion (Hb > 100 g/l and SS ≤ 30%) | Standard transfusion (Hb ≥100 g/l) | Transfusion reactions within 30 days | 7.3% | −92% (−100% to −25%) | 15 (9 to 55) |

## PROGNOSIS

Patients with sickle cell disease die younger **[B]**[28].

**Note**

■ Patients with sickle cell disease have a reduction in life-expectancy**[B]**[28].
  – SS: median age of death – male 42, female 48 (USA).
  – SC: median age of death – male 60, female 68 (small numbers, USA).
■ A third die during acute sickle crises **[B]**[28].

The risk of dying is increased if patients have:
● low-level fetal haemoglobin
● acute chest syndrome
● renal failure
● seizures
● white cell count $> 15 \times 10^9$ g/l.

The following complications are common.
● Acute chest syndrome.

**Note**

■ A third of sickle cell patients have an episode of acute chest syndrome over 10 years. Half of them have more than one **[B]**[29].

Patients are at increased risk if they have:
– younger age
– lower HbF
– anaemia
– raised steady-state white cell count.
It can progress to chronic lung disease, which is often fatal.

> **Note**
> - Patients with frequent acute chest syndromes or aseptic necrosis aged > 20 years are at increased risk of developing chronic lung disease **[B]**[30].
> - Patients with sickle cell anaemia who have chronic lung disease are at a greatly increased risk of dying (NNH = 2 at 17 years) **[B]**[30].

- Cerebrovascular accidents – haemorrhagic in adulthood **[C]**.[31]

Further strokes and death are common.

> **Note**
> - 5% of patients have a stroke **[C]**[31].
> - A third die **[C]**[31].
> - Two-thirds have another within the next 9 years **[C]**[31].

Patients with Hb-SS are at increased risk **[C]**[31].

> **Why?**
> Hb-SS increases the risk of stroke

| Outcome **[C]**[31] | Risk factor | PEER | OR (95% CI) | NNH (95% CI) |
|---|---|---|---|---|
| Stroke | Hb-SS *not independent* | 5% | 5.6 (1.3 to 24) | 16 (4 to 790) |

- Priapism.

> **Note**
> - ~ 40% of men with sickle cell anaemia have an episode of priapism in 1 year **[C]**[32].
> - The majority of episodes do not require hospital treatment **[C]**[32].

Give oral stilboestrol 5 mg daily to patients with frequent attacks **[A]**[33].

> **Why do this?**
> - Stilboestrol stops stuttering priapism in patients with sickle cell anaemia who have more than two attacks a week **[A]**[33].
> Stilboestrol stops stuttering priapism

| Patient **[A]**[33] | Treatment | Comparator | Outcome | CER | RRR | NNT |
|---|---|---|---|---|---|---|
| Stuttering priapism with > 2 attacks per week | Stilboestrol | Placebo | Continuing attacks at 2 weeks | 80% | 100% | 1 (1 to 2) |

**Guideline writer**: Christopher Ball
**CAT writers**: Nick Shenker, Christopher Ball

## REFERENCES

| No. | Level | Citation |
| --- | --- | --- |
| 1 | 4 | Brozovic M et al. Acute admissions of patients with sickle cell disease who live in Britain. BMJ 1987; 294: 1206–8 |
| 2 | 2c | Platt OS et al. Pain in sickle cell disease: rates and risk factors. N Engl J Med 1991; 325: 11–16 |
| 3 | 4 | Serjeant GR et al. The painful crisis of homozygous sickle cell disease: clinical features. Br J Haematol 1994; 87: 586–91 |
| 4 | 4 | Vichinsky EP et al. Acute chest syndrome in sickle cell disease: clinical presentation and course. Blood 1997; 89: 1787–92 |
| 5 | 4 | Serafini A et al. Diagnostic studies in patients with sickle cell anaemia with acute abdominal pain. Arch Intern Med 1987; 147: 1061–2 |
| 6 | 4 | Pianosi P et al. Pulse oximetry in sickle cell disease. Arch Dis Child 1993; 68: 735–38 |
| 7 | 4 | Khoury H, Grimsley E. Oxygen inhalation in non-hypoxic sickle cell patients during vaso-occlusive crisis. Blood 1995; 86: 3998 |
| 8 | 1b – | Gonzalez et al. Intermittent injection versus patient-controlled analgesia for sickle-call crisis pain Arch Intern Med 1991; 151: 1373–8 |
| 9 | 4 | Pryle et al. Toxicity of norpethidine in sickle cell crisis. BMJ 1992; 304: 1478 |
| 10 | 1b | Perlin E et al. Enhancement of pain control with ketorolac trimethamine in patients with sickle cell vaso-occlusive crisis: Am J Hematol 1994; 46: 43–7 |
| 11 | 1b – | Wang WC et al. Transcutaneous nerve stimulation treatment of sickle cell pain crises. Acta Haematol 1988; 80: 99–102 |
| 12 | 1b | Bellett PS et al. Incentive spirometry to prevent acute pulmonary complications in sickle cell disease. N Engl J Med 1995; 333: 699–703 |
| 13 | 4 | Mallouh AA, Asha M. Beneficial effect of blood transfusion in children with sickle cell syndrome. Arch J Dis Childhood, 1988; 142: 178 |
| 14 | 1b – | Griffin TC et al. High dose methylprednisolone therapy for pain in children and adolescents with sickle cell disease. N Engl J Med 1994; 330: 733–7 |
| 15 | 1b – | Gil KM et al. Effects of cognitive coping skills training on coping strategies and experimental pain sensation in African-American adults with sickle cell disease. Health Psychol 1996; 15: 3–10 |
| 16 | 1b – | Benjamin LJ et al. A collaborative, double-blind randomised study of cetiedil citrate in sickle-cell crisis. Blood 1986; 67: 1442–7 |
| 17 | 2a | Elander J, Midence K. A review of the evidence about factors affecting quality of pain management in sickle cell disease. Clin J Pain 1996; 12: 180–3 |
| 18 | 1b | Charoche S et al. Effect of hydroxyurea on frequency of painful crises in sickle cell anaemia. N Engl J Med 1995; 332: 1317–22 |
| 19 | 1b | De Ceulaer K et al. Medroxyprogesterone acetate and homozygous sickle cell disease. Lancet 1982; ii: 229–31 |
| 20 | 2b | Rabb LM et al. A trial of folate supplementation in children with homozygous sickle cell disease. Br J Haematol 1983; 54: 589–94 |

| No. | Level | Citation |
|-----|-------|----------|
| 21 | 1b | Gaston MH. Prophylaxis with oral penicillin in children with sickle cell anemia: a randomised trial. N Engl J Med 1986; 314: 1593–9 |
| 22 | 1b − | Falletta JM et al. Discontinuation of penicillin prophylaxis in children with sickle cell anaemia. J Pediatr 1995; 127: 685–90 |
| 23 | 2b − | Russell MO et al. Effect of transfusion therapy on arteriographic abnormalities and on recurrence of stroke in sickle cell disease. Blood 1984; 63: 162–9 |
| 24 | 4 | Styles L et al. Effects of long-term transfusion regimen on sickle-related illnesses. J Pediatr 1994; 125: 909 |
| 25 | 2b | Haberkern CM et al. Cholecystectomy in sickle cell anaemia patients: perioperative outcome of 364 cases from the national pre-operative transfusion study. Blood 1997; 89: 1533–42 |
| 26 | 4 | Vichinsky EP et al. A comparison of conservative and aggressive transfusion regimens in perioperative management of sickle cell disease. N Engl J Med 1995; 333: 206–13 |
| 27 | 1b | Vichinsky EP et al. A comparison of conservative and aggressive transfusion regimens in perioperative management of sickle cell disease: NEJM 1995; 333: 206–13 |
| 28 | 2b | Platt OS et al. Mortality in sickle cell disease: life expectancy and risk factors for early death. N Engl J Med 1994; 330: 1639–44 |
| 29 | 2b | Castro O et al. The acute chest syndrome in sickle cell disease: incidence and risk factors. Blood 1994; 84: 643–9 |
| 30 | 3b | Powars D et al. Sickle cell chronic lung disease: prior morbidity and risk of pulmonary failure. Medicine 1988; 67: 66–75 |
| 31 | 4 | Powars D et al. The natural history of stroke in sickle cell disease. Am J Med 1978; 65: 461–71 |
| 32 | 4 | Fowler JE et al. Priapism associated with the sickle cell hemoglobinopathies: prevalence, natural history and sequelae. J Urol 1991; 145: 65–8 |
| 33 | 1b | Serjeant GR et al. Stilboestrol and stuttering priapism in homozygous sickle cell disease. Lancet 1985; ii: 1274–6 |

## PREVALENCE

Status epilepticus is defined as:

- continuous seizures for >30 min
- two or more seizures without full recovery of consciousness between seizures.

Status epilepticus is uncommon **[C]**[1] **[C]**[2], although patients over 60 years of age presenting with a first fit are often in status epilepticus **[C]**[3].

> **Note**
> ■ Status epilepticus occurs in 3% to 7% of patients with fits **[C]**[1] **[C]**[2].
> ■ 30% of elderly patients with a first seizure present in status **[C]**[3].

## CAUSES

Common causes include:

- discontinued or irregular anticonvulsant use
- alcohol withdrawal
- stroke
- metabolic/anoxic causes.

Rarer causes include:

- infection
- tumour
- trauma
- drug overdoses.

> **Note**
> **Causes of status epilepticus**
>
> | **[B]**[4] **[B]**[5] **[C]**[2] **[C]**[6] | % |
> | --- | --- |
> | Discontinued or irregular anticonvulsant use | 23% to 50% |
> | Alcohol withdrawal | 14% to 28% |
> | Stroke | 23% |
> | Metabolic/anoxic | 12% |
> | Infection | 5% to 6% |
> | Tumour | 4% |
> | Trauma | 4% |
> | Drug overdose | 2% |
> | Unknown | 14% |

## CLINICAL FEATURES

Look for a cause **[D]**[7].
Ask about:

- previous fits
- trauma
- medication
- alcohol and street drugs.

Look for:

- focal neurological signs
- signs of infection
- drug misuse.

Exclude:

- hypoxia
- hypoglycaemia.

Think about status epilepticus in patients in a coma.
Signs can be subtle. Look for twitching of extremities, mouth and eyes,
but these may be absent.

 **Why?**
- Patients in a coma who have rhythmic clonic movements are at increased risk of having status epilepticus **[A]**[8].
- Patients in a coma may display no clinical signs of status epilepticus, but still have it **[A]**[8].
- A fifth of patients with status epilepticus may not be convulsing **[C]**[2].

Watch out for pseudoseizures. These are more likely if **[C]**[9]:

- there is no clear cause for fitting
- the patient has a psychiatric history
- the patient is conscious yet having seizures with bilateral motor activity
- attacks seem atypical
- the patient resists examination
- the patient calls out.

**Why?**

**Unexplained seizures, a psychiatric history or atypical fits increase the chance of a pseudoselzure**

| Patient | Target disorder (reference standard) | Diagnostic test | LR+ (95% CI) | LR– (95% CI) |
|---|---|---|---|---|
| Suspected pseudoseizure **[C]**⁹ | Pseudoseizure (diagnosed by a senior neurologist) | Unexplained illness | >100 (3.0 to infinity) | 0.38 (0.19 to 0.76) |
| | | Psychiatric history | 10 (1.5 to 67) | 0.25 (0.092 to 0.68) |
| | | Conscious yet having seizure with bilateral motor activity | 8.0 (1.2 to 55) | 0.42 (0.21 to 0.84) |
| | | Attacks thought atypical by staff | 6.5 (1.8 to 23) | 0.0 (0.0 to 0.24) |
| | | Resisting examination | 4.5 (1.2 to 17) | 0.36 (0.16 to 0.85) |
| | | Vocalisation | 4.0 (1.0 to 15) | 0.45 (0.22 to 0.94) |

These are less likely if patients have **[C]**⁹:
- extensor plantar during seizures.

**Why?**

| Patient | Target disorder (reference standard) | Diagnostic test | LR+ (95% CI) | LR– (95% CI) |
|---|---|---|---|---|
| Suspected pseudoseizure **[C]**⁹ | Pseudoseizure (diagnosed by a senior neurologist) | Extensor plantar during seizures | 0.36 (0.16 to 0.80) | 4.5 (1.2 to 17) |

- If in doubt, treat the patient for status epilepticus, but watch for medication side-effects.

**Why?**
- Medication-related complications are common **[C]**⁹:
  - respiratory arrest: 61% (95% CI: 32% to 91%)
  - infection: 54% (95% CI: 31% to 92%).
- In one study, 70% of patients with pseudoseizures were still on anticonvulsants after 2 years **[C]**⁹.

## INVESTIGATIONS

- Vital signs [D][10].
- Pulse oximetry.
- ECG monitoring.
- Rapid blood glucose assay (see chapter on **Hypoglycaemia**).
- Urea, electrolytes, calcium.
- Anticonvulsant drug levels.
- Blood count.
- Arterial blood gas.
- Consider requesting an early EEG in unclear cases.

Once stable, consider:

- liver function tests
- toxicology screen
- CT or MRI head
- lumbar puncture
- EEG.

## THERAPY

Check airway, breathing, circulation [A].
- Oxygen [B][4].

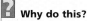

**Why do this?**
- Patients who become hypoxic are at increased risk of dying [B][4].

- Lorazepam [A][11] 0.1 mg/kg iv at 2 mg/min;

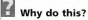

**Why do this?**
- It is faster than diazepam, phenobarbital (10 min faster) or phenytoin (25 min faster) at terminating seizures [A][11].
- It is better than phenytoin at terminating seizures, but is not clearly different from diazepam with or without phenytoin, or phenobarbital [D][12] [D][13].

**Lorazepam stops more seizures than phenytoin**

| Patient | Treatment | Comparator | Outcome | CER | RBI | NNT |
|---------|-----------|------------|---------|-----|-----|-----|
| Status epilepticus [A][11] | Lorazepam | Phenytoin | Termination of seizures at 60 min | 42% | 29% (1% to 64%) | 8 (4 to 160) |

- or diazepam [A][11] 0.15 mg/kg iv at 5 mg/min.
An alternative route is rectally; using larger doses [A][14].

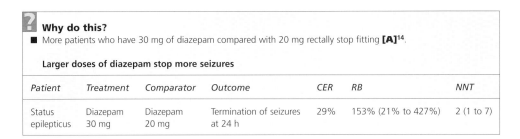

**Why do this?**
- More patients who have 30 mg of diazepam compared with 20 mg rectally stop fitting **[A]**[14].

**Larger doses of diazepam stop more seizures**

| Patient | Treatment | Comparator | Outcome | CER | RB | NNT |
|---------|-----------|------------|---------|-----|-----|-----|
| Status epilepticus | Diazepam 30 mg | Diazepam 20 mg | Termination of seizures at 24 h | 29% | 153% (21% to 427%) | 2 (1 to 7) |

Fits often continue **[B]**[15].

**Note**
- Around a half of patients with generalised status epilepticus stop fitting on first medication; this falls to only a quarter in patients in a coma.

If they do, try:

- phenobarbital **[A]**[16] 15 mg/kg iv at 100 mg/min;

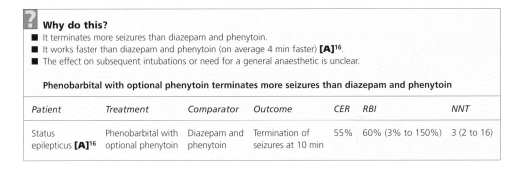

**Why do this?**
- It terminates more seizures than diazepam and phenytoin.
- It works faster than diazepam and phenytoin (on average 4 min faster) **[A]**[16].
- The effect on subsequent intubations or need for a general anaesthetic is unclear.

**Phenobarbital with optional phenytoin terminates more seizures than diazepam and phenytoin**

| Patient | Treatment | Comparator | Outcome | CER | RBI | NNT |
|---------|-----------|------------|---------|-----|-----|-----|
| Status epilepticus **[A]**[16] | Phenobarbital with optional phenytoin | Diazepam and phenytoin | Termination of seizures at 10 min | 55% | 60% (3% to 150%) | 3 (2 to 16) |

then

- phenytoin **[B]**[15] **[B]**[5] 18 mg/kg iv at 50 mg/min.

**Why do this?**
- No studies have shown which medication is best to use next if there is no response to benzodiazepines **[D]**[12] **[D]**[13].

If fits continue (especially if >1 h) **[B]**[4], intubate and anaesthetise with either:

- propofol **[D]**[18]
- midazolam **[D]**[19] **[D]**[20]

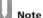
**Note**

■ Propofol is not clearly as good as high-dose barbiturates in terminating seizures or reducing death in patients with refractory status epilepticus **[D]**[18].

Watch for side-effects of medication: they are common, so monitor patients continuously **[A]**[11].

**Note**

■ Hypoventilation occurs in ~10% to 15%, hypotension in ~30% to 60%, cardiac rhythm disturbance in ~5% to 9% **[A]**[11].

On recovery, fully conscious patients not on medication can be rapidly loaded with oral phenytoin (try 18 mg/kg) **[D]**[21].

**Why do this?**

■ Few patients have side-effects (7.8%; 95% CI: 0.46% to 15%) **[D]**[21].
■ Phenytoin capsules or suspension are probably equally effective in loading patients who are conscious following a seizure **[D]**[21].

## PROGNOSIS

Few patients die **[B]**[4].

**Note**

■ 2% die within 1 month **[B]**[4].

Patients are at increased risk of dying if **[B]**[4]:

● seizures continue for >1 h
● they become hypoxic
● they are old.

**Why?**
Seizures lasting over an hour, anoxia and increasing age increase the risk of dying

| Patient | Prognostic factor | Outcome | Control rate | OR (95% CI) | NNF+ (95% CI) |
|---|---|---|---|---|---|
| Status epilepticus **[B]**[4] | Seizure duration >1 h *independent* | Death at 1 month | 2.0% | 9.79 (2.14 to 44.9) | 7 (2 to 46) |
| | Anoxia *independent* | Death at 1 month | 2.0% | 3.66 (1.47 to 9.09) | 20 (7 to 110) |
| | Age (per 10 years) *independent* | Death at 1 month | 2.0% | 1.39 (1.06 to 1.81) | 130 (65 to 860) |

**Guideline writer**: Christopher Ball
**CAT writer**: Christopher Ball

## REFERENCES

| No. | Level | Citation |
|-----|-------|----------|
| 1 | 4 | Oxbury JM, Whitty CW. Causes and consequences of status epilepticus in adults: a study of 86 cases. Brain 1971; 91: 733–44 |
| 2 | 4 | Dunne JW et al. Non-convulsive status epilepticus: a prospective study. Q J Med 1986; 62: 117–27 |
| 3 | 4 | Sung CY, Chu NS. Status epilepticus in the elderly: etiology, seizure type and outcome. Acta Neurol Scand 1989; 80: 51–6 |
| 4 | 2b | Towne AR et al. Determinants of mortality in status epilepticus. Epilepsia 1994; 35: 27–34 |
| 5 | 2b | Shaner DM et al. Treatment of status epilepticus: a prospective comparison of diazepam and phenytoin versus phenobarbital and optional phenytoin. Neurology 1988; 38: 202–7 |
| 6 | 4 | Aminoff MJ, Simon RP. Status epilepticus – causes, clinical features and consequences in 98 patients. Am J Med 1980; 69: 657–66 |
| 7 | 5 | Lowenstein DH, Alldredge BK. Status epilepticus. N Engl J Med 1998; 338: 970–6 (Narrative review) |
| 8 | 2b | Lowenstein DH, Aminoff MJ. Clinical and EEG feature of status epilepticus in comatose patients. Neurology 1992; 42: 100–4 |
| 9 | 4 | Howell SJ et al. Pseudostatus epilepticus. Q J Med 1989; 71: 507–19 |
| 10 | 5 | Working Group on Status Epilepticus. Treatment of convulsive status epilepticus: recommendations of the epilepsy foundation of America's working group on status epilepticus. JAMA 1993; 270: 854–9 |
| 11 | 1b | Trieman DM et al. A comparison of four treatments for generalised convulsive status epilepticus. N Engl J Med 1998; 339: 792–8. |
| 12 | 1 | Trieman DM et al. A comparison of four treatments for generalised convulsive status epilepticus: NEJM 1998; 339: 792–8 |
| 13 | 1b– | Leppik IE et al. A double-blind study of lorazepam and diazepam in status epilepticus. JAMA 1983; 249: 1452–4 |
| 14 | 1b | Remy C et al. Intrarectal diazepam in epileptic adults. Epilepsia 1992; 33: 353–7 |
| 15 | 2b | Trieman DM et al. A comparison of four treatments for generalised convulsive status epilepticus. NEJM 1998; 339: 792–8 |
| 16 | 1b | Shaner DM et al. Treatment of status epilepticus: a prospective comparison of diazepam and phenytoin versus phenobarbital and optional phenytoin. Neurol 1998; 38: 202–7 |
| 17 | 1b– | Shaner DM et al. Treatment of status epilepticus: a prospective comparison of diazepam and phenytoin versus phenobarbital and optional phenytoin. Neurol 1998; 38: 202–7 |
| 18 | 2b– | Stecker MM et al. Treatment of refractory status epilepticus with proprofol: clinical and pharmacokinetic findings. Epilepsia 1998; 39: 18–26 |
| 19 | 5 | Parent JM, Lowenstein DH. Treatment of refractory generalized status epilepticus with continuous infusion of midazolam. Neurology 1994; 44: 1837–40 |
| 20 | 5 | Kumar A, Bleck TP. Intravenous midazolam for the treatment of refractory status epilepticus. Crit Care Med 1992; 20: 483–8 |
| 21 | 1b– | Osborn HH et al. Single-dose oral phenytoin loading. Ann Emerg Med 1987; 16: 407–12 |

## PREVALENCE

Most patients have an ischaemic stroke **[A]**[1]. Most ischaemic strokes involve the anterior circulation **[A]**[1].

> **Note**
> ■ 80% of patients presenting with a stroke have a cerebral infarction (95% CI: 78% to 84%) **[A]** [1].

## CLINICAL FEATURES

Ask about risk factors for stroke:

● hypertension (particularly a diastolic BP ≥ 100 mmHg) **[A]**[2] **[A]**[3] **[B]**[4]

> **?** **Why?**
> **Hypertension increases the risk of a stroke**
>
> | Patient [A][2] | Prognostic factor | Outcome | Control rate | OR (95% CI) | NNF+ (95% CI) |
> |---|---|---|---|---|---|
> | Healthy | Diastolic BP 100–109 mmHg *independent* | Stroke at 10 years | 0.20% | 1.80 (1.60 to 2.00) | 690 (560 to 930) |
> | | Diastolic BP ≥ 110 mmHg *independent* | Stroke at 10 years | | 3.60 (3.00 to 4.00) | 220 (190 to 280) |

● atrial fibrillation **[A]**[5] **[A]**[6]

> **?** **Why?**
> A fifth of patients with atrial fibrillation will have a stroke within 5 years (19%; 95% CI: 19% to 20%) **[A]**[6].
>
> **AF increases the risk of stroke, especially with other risk factors**
>
> | Strokes per year [A][7] | No other risk factors (95% CI) | 1+ other risk factor (95% CI) |
> |---|---|---|
> | Aged < 65 | 1.0% (0.3% to 3.1%) | 4.9% (3.0% to 8.1%) |
> | Aged 65–75 | 4.3% (2.7% to 7.1%) | 5.7% (3.9% to 8.3%) |
> | Aged > 75 | 3.5% (1.6% to 7.7%) | 8.1% (4.7% to 14%) |

● diabetes mellitus **[A]**[3] **[B]**[4] **[B]**[7] **[B]**[8]

| | | | | | |
|---|---|---|---|---|---|
| **Why?** Diabetes increases the risk of a stroke | | | | | |
| Patient | Prognostic factor | Outcome | Control rate | RR (95% CI) | NNF+ (95% CI) |
| Hypertension | Diabetes mellitus **[B]**[8] independent | Stroke at 4.5 years | 5.5% | 1.80 (1.26 to 2.57) | 23 (12 to 70) |

- smoking **[A]**[9]**[B]**[3]

| | | | | | |
|---|---|---|---|---|---|
| **Why?** Smoking increases the risk of having a stroke | | | | | |
| Patient | Prognostic factor | Outcome | Control rate | RR (95% CI) | NNF+ (95% CI) |
| Healthy **[A]**[9] | Smoker: 1–19 cigarettes per day independent Smoker: ≥ 20 cigarettes per day independent | Non-fatal stroke at 9.7 years | 1.4% | 1.86 (1.04 to 3.33) 2.71 (1.84 to 3.98) | 83 (32 to 1800) 42 (24 to 85) |

- high cholesterol **[A]**[10]

| |
|---|
| **Why?** ■ A high cholesterol (> 5.2 mmol/l) increases the risk of dying from a non-haemorrhagic stroke – the higher the cholesterol, the greater the risk **[A]**[10]. |

- history of stroke or TIA **[B]**[4] particularly with other risk factors **[B]**[5] **[B]**[8]

| | | | | | |
|---|---|---|---|---|---|
| **Why?** Hypertension: a previous stroke increases the risk of another | | | | | |
| Patient | Prognostic factor | Outcome | Control rate | RR (95% CI) | NNF+ (95% CI) |
| Hypertension | History of stroke **[B]**[8] independent | Stroke at 4.5 years | 5.5% | 2.13 (1.00 to 4.56) | 16 (5 to infinity) |

- ischaemic heart disease **[B]**[5] **[B]**[11]

| | | | | |
|---|---|---|---|---|
| **Why?** Ischaemic heart disease and aortic atheroma increases the risk of a stroke | | | | |
| Outcome | Risk factor | PEER | OR (95% CI) | NNH (95% CI) |
| Stroke or TIA **[B]**[4] | Coronary heart disease independent | 2% | 2.20 (1.20 to 4.20) | 44 (17 to 260) |
| Ischaemic stroke or TIA **[B]**[12] | Ascending aortic or arch atheroma independent | 2% | 7.10 (2.70 to 18.4) | 8 (3 to 29) |

- infection within the previous week **[B]**[4]

| | | | | |
|---|---|---|---|---|
| **?** **Why?** A recent infection increases the risk of a stroke | | | | |
| *Outcome* | *Risk factor* | *PEER* | *OR (95% CI)* | *NNH (95% CI)* |
| Stroke or TIA **[B]**[4] | Infection within 1 week *independent* | 2% | 4.60 (1.90 to 11.3) | 15 (6 to 58) |

- oral contraceptive pill use **[B]**[13]

| | | | | |
|---|---|---|---|---|
| **?** **Why?** Oral contraceptive pill use, particularly if a smoker, increases the risk of stroke | | | | |
| *Outcome* **[B]**[13] | *Risk factor* | *PEER* | *OR (95% CI)* | *NNH (95% CI)* |
| First-ever stroke | Current user of oral contraceptives *independent* | 0.1% | 2.50 (1.50 to 4.00) | 670 (330 to 2000) |
| | Smokes and current user of oral contraceptives *independent* | | 2.90 (1.50 to 5.70) | 530 (210 to 2000) |
| | Ever used oral contraceptives *independent* | | 1.50 (1.10 to 2.00) | 2000 (1000 to 10 000) |
| | Smokes and former user of oral contraceptives *independent* | | 1.80 (1.10 to 2.80 | 1300 (560 to 10 000) |
| | Oral contraceptives with high progestogen content *independent* | | 6.70 (1.60 to 28.5) | 180 (37 to 1700) |
| | Oral contraceptives with high oestrogen content *independent* | | 5.80 (1.50 to 22.8) | 210 (46 to 2000) |
| | Oral contraceptives with intermediate progestogen content *independent* | | 3.60 (1.60 to 8.20) | 380 (140 to 1700) |
| | Oral contraceptives with intermediate oestrogen content *independent* | | 2.90 (1.70 to 5.00) | 530 (250 to 1400) |

The risk of stroke increases with increasing numbers of risk factors **[B]**[14,15].

| | |
|---|---|
| **?** **Why?** The risk of stroke increases with increasing numbers of risk factors | |
| *Number of prognostic factors* **[B]**[14] **[B]**[15] | *Rate of thromboembolism* |
| ≥ 3 | 19% (12% to 30%) |
| 1 or 2 | 6.0% (4.1% to 8.8%) |
| 0 | 1.0% (0.2% to 4.0%) |

Also ask about:
- a history of depression [A][16].

| | | Why? | | | |
|---|---|---|---|---|---|
| | | Depression increases the risk of a stroke | | | |
| Patient [A][16] | Prognostic factor | Outcome | Control rate | OR (95% CI) | NNF + (95% CI) |
| Well | Depression *independent* | Death from stroke at 29 years | 2.5% | 1.54 (1.06 to 2.22) | 22 (14 to 141) |

A stroke is less likely with:
- hormone replacement therapy [A][17]

| | | Why? | | | |
|---|---|---|---|---|---|
| | | Postmenopausal hormone use reduces the risk of stroke | | | |
| Patient [A][17] | Prognostic factor | Outcome | Control rate | OR (95% CI) | NNF+ (95% CI) |
| Postmenopausal women | Postmenopausal hormone use *independent* | Stroke at 11 years | 13% | 0.69 (0.14 to 1.00) | −27 (−9 to infinity) |

- alcohol consumption [A][18].

| | | Why? | | | |
|---|---|---|---|---|---|
| | | Moderate alcohol consumption reduces ischaemic stroke, but increases subarachnoid haemorrhage | | | |
| Patient | Prognostic factor | Outcome | Control rate | RR (95% CI) | NNF+ (95% CI) |
| Female nurse [A][18] | 1.5–4.9 g alcohol per day *independent* | Ischaemic stroke at 10 years | 0.08% | 0.40 (0.20 to 0.90) | −2100 (−13 000 to −1600) |
| | 5.0–14.9 g alcohol per day *independent* | | | 0.30 (0.10 to 0.70) | −1800 (−4200 to −1400) |
| | 5.0–14.9 g alcohol per day *independent* | Subarachnoid haemorrhage at 10 years | 0.03% | 3.70 (1.00 to 13.8) | 1300 (280 to infinity) |

Look for:
- a carotid bruit [A][19] [A][20], particularly with a history of TIA or diabetes [A][21]

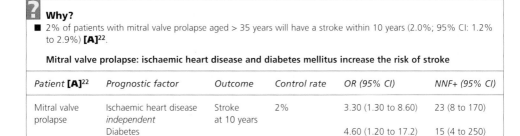

**? Why?**

■ A seventh of patients admitted with acute stroke, TIA or retinal stroke will have severe carotid stenosis 13% (95% CI: 11% to 16%) **[A]**[21].

**A carotid bruit increases the risk of another stroke**

| Patient **[A]**[19] | Prognostic factor | Outcome | Control rate | OR (95% CI) | NNF+ (95% CI) |
|---|---|---|---|---|---|
| Retinal infarct | Carotid bruit *independent* | Stroke at 4 years | 10% | 5.10 (1.30 to 20.0) | 4 (2 to 38) |

**An ipsilateral carotid bruit makes severe carotid stenosis slightly more likely but is not diagnostic**

| Patient **[A]**[20] | Target disorder (reference standard) | Diagnostic test | LR+ (95% CI) | Post-test probability | LR– (95% CI) | Post-test probability |
|---|---|---|---|---|---|---|
| Recent or recurrent TIA or non-disabling stroke (pre-test probability 13%) | >70% carotid stenosis (angiography) | Ipsilateral bruit | 1.6 (1.4 to 1.8) | 19% | 0.61 (0.54 to 0.69) | 8% |

■ mitral valve prolapse **[A]**[22].

**? Why?**

■ 2% of patients with mitral valve prolapse aged > 35 years will have a stroke within 10 years (2.0%; 95% CI: 1.2% to 2.9%) **[A]**[22].

**Mitral valve prolapse: ischaemic heart disease and diabetes mellitus increase the risk of stroke**

| Patient **[A]**[22] | Prognostic factor | Outcome | Control rate | OR (95% CI) | NNF+ (95% CI) |
|---|---|---|---|---|---|
| Mitral valve prolapse | Ischaemic heart disease *independent* | Stroke at 10 years | 2% | 3.30 (1.30 to 8.60) | 23 (8 to 170) |
| | Diabetes *independent* | | | 4.60 (1.20 to 17.2) | 15 (4 to 250) |

Assess your patient's functional status, specifically looking at **[B]**[23]:
- upper limb motor function
- proprioception
- ability to stand and walk

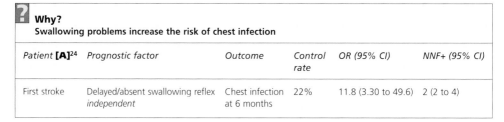

> **? Why?**
>
> **Upper limb motor function, proprioception and standing and walking ability help predict independence**
>
> | Patient [B][23] | Prognostic factor | Outcome | Control rate | Unadjusted RR (95% CI) | NNF+ (95% CI) |
> |---|---|---|---|---|---|
> | Stroke | None to slight upper limb motor function weakness *independent* | Functional independence at 4 months | 30% | 2.33 (1.52 to 3.56) | 2 (1 to 6) |
> | | With none to slight difficulty with proprioception *independent* | | 23% | 2.56 (1.43 to 4.60) | 3 (1 to 10) |
> | | Postural function of walking or standing *independent* | | | 2.69 (1.61 to 4.50) | 2 (1 to 7) |

> **Note**
> - Loss of memory recall, difficulty with problem-solving, lower limb motor function, comprehension, ability to express oneself and normal or abnormal hand on two point discrimination did not usefully predict return to independence **[B][23]**.

- dysphagia **[A][24]**

> **? Why?**
>
> **Swallowing problems increase the risk of chest infection**
>
> | Patient [A][24] | Prognostic factor | Outcome | Control rate | OR (95% CI) | NNF+ (95% CI) |
> |---|---|---|---|---|---|
> | First stroke | Delayed/absent swallowing reflex *independent* | Chest infection at 6 months | 22% | 11.8 (3.30 to 49.6) | 2 (2 to 4) |

- visual neglect **[C][25]**

> **? Why?**
> - It is common – a third of patients with anterior circulation infarction have visual neglect (33%; 95% CI: 25% to 40%) **[C][25]**

- urinary incontinence **[B][26]**

> **? Why?**
>
> **Urinary incontinence is associated with an increased risk of dying**
>
> | Patient | Prognostic factor | Outcome | Control rate | RR (95% CI) | NNF+ (95% CI) |
> |---|---|---|---|---|---|
> | Ischaemic stroke **[B][26]** | Urinary incontinence *independent* | Death at 1 year | ?20% | 7.32 (2.52 to 21.3) | 1 (1 to 3) |

- a reduced level of consciousness [A][27] [B][28].

> **?** **Why?**
>
> **A reduced level of consciousness on admission is associated with an increased risk of dying**

| Patient | Prognostic factor | Outcome | Control rate | RR (95% CI) | NNF+ (95% CI) |
|---|---|---|---|---|---|
| First stroke or TIA [A][27] | Altered consciousness *independent* | Death at discharge | 5.9% | 9.53 (6.16 to 14.7) | 3 (2 to 5) |

Classify your patient's type of stroke (based on maximal deficit) (Table 1) [A][1].

**Table 1  The clinical features of stroke subtypes**

| Stroke subtype | Features |
|---|---|
| Lacunar infarcts (LACI) | Pure motor or sensory stroke, sensorimotor stroke or ataxic hemiparesis |
| Total anterior circulation infarcts (TACI) | A combination of new higher cerebral dysfunction (e.g. dysphasia), homonymous visual field defect, and ipsilateral motor or sensory deficit of at least two areas of face, arm and leg |
| Partial anterior circulation infarcts (PACI) | Only 2 of 3 components of TACI; higher cerebral dysfunction alone or with motor/sensory deficit more restricted than for LACI |
| Posterior circulation infarcts (POCI) | Brainstem or cerebellar dysfunction |

> **?** **Why?**
>
> **Classifying the type of stroke helps determine probability of recovery, recurrent stroke and death**

| Stroke subtype [A][1] | % of patients (95% CI) | Recurrent stroke at 1 year | Death at 1 year | Functionally independent at 1 year |
|---|---|---|---|---|
| LACI | 20% (17% to 23%) | 9% (4% to 14%) | 11% (6% to 16%) | 62% |
| TACI | 14% (11% to 16%) | 6% (2% to 12%) | 60% (50% to 70%) | 4% |
| PACI | 27% (24% to 31%) | 17% (12% to 23%) | 16% (11% to 22%) | 55% |
| POCI | 19% (16% to 22%) | 20% (13% to 27%) | 19% (12% to 25%) | 62% |
| Unclassified | 20% (17% to 23%) | | | |

## INVESTIGATIONS

- Blood count **[D]**.
- Urea and electrolytes, creatinine **[D]**.
- Glucose **[A]**[29] **[A]**[30] **[B]**[28].

| ? Why? An elevated glucose on admission increases the risk of recurrent ischaemic stroke and death | | | | | |
|---|---|---|---|---|---|
| Patient | Prognostic factor | Outcome | Control rate | RR (95% CI) | NNF+ (95% CI) |
| Ischaemic stroke **[A]**[30] | 5.5 mmol/l increase in admission glucose *independent* | Recurrent stroke at 5 years | 22% | 1.40 (1.10 to 1.70) | |
| Ischaemic stroke **[A]**[30] | admission glucose > 7.7 mmol/l *independent* | Death at 5 years | 44% | 1.70 (1.40 to 2.80) | 4 (2 to 7) |

- Serum lipids **[A]**[10].
- ECG **[C]**[31].

| ? Why? ECG abnormalities make a stroke more likely | | | | | |
|---|---|---|---|---|---|
| Patient | Prognostic factor | Outcome | Control rate | RR (95% CI) | NNF+ (95% CI) |
| Hypertension | ECG abnormalities *independent* | Stroke | 5.5% | 1.47 (1.09 to 1.99) | 39 (18 to 200) |

■ Arrhythmias are common in patients with TIAs **[C]**[31].

**Sick sinus syndrome is common with TIA**

| Arrhythmias found with TIA **[C]**[31] | % (95% CI) |
|---|---|
| Episodic sick sinus syndrome | 32% (23% to 41%) |
| Bradyarrhythmia | 18% (11% to 26%) |
| Bradytachyarrhythmia | 14% (7.2% to 21%) |
| Atrial fibrillation or flutter | 5.0% (0.73% to 9.3%) |

- Chest X-ray **[D]**.
- CT or MRI of the head **[B]**[32].

> ? Why?
> ■ Clinical features alone cannot safely diagnose or exclude an ischaemic stroke from a haemorrhagic stroke **[B]**[32].

**Note**

■ Clinicians agree moderately about involvement of middle cerebral artery territory in acute ischaemic stroke **[B]**[33].

Consider:
● echocardiography in young patients **[C]**[34]

**Why?**

■ 40% of patients under 55 with an ischaemic stroke have a patent foramen ovale (95% CI: 28% to 52%) **[C]**[34].

For patients willing to have carotid endarterectomy, consider:
● carotid ultrasound **[A]**[35] **[A]**[36] or magnetic resonance angiography **[A]**[36] followed by angiography if indicated **[A]**.

**Why?**

MR angiography or duplex ultrasonography alone cannot safely diagnose or exclude significant stenosis

| Patient | Target disorder (reference standard) | Diagnostic test | LR+ (95% CI) | Post-test probability | LR– (95% CI) | Post-test probability |
|---|---|---|---|---|---|---|
| Suspected carotid artery disease **[A]**[36] (pre-test probability 33%) | >70% carotid artery stenosis (angiography) | MR angiography | 3.6 (1.8 to 4.5) | 61% | 0.10 (0.04 to 0.24) | 4% |
| | | Duplex ultrasonography | 4.6 (2.4 to 8.8) | 68% | 0.23 (0.09 to) 0.57 | 10% |
| Suspected carotid artery disease **[A]**[35] (pre-test probability ?50%) | >50% carotid artery stenosis | Doppler ultrasonography | 6.0 | 75% | 0.19 | 9% |
| | | Duplex ultrasonography | 5.7 | 86% | 0.18 | 16% |

**THERAPY**

Admit your patient to a stroke unit **[A]**[37] **[A]**[38], if available,

**Why do this?**
- Patients who are admitted to stroke units are less likely to die, require institutional care or become dependent compared with those admitted to a general ward **[A]**[37].
- Patients on stroke units spend less time in hospital (on average 2 days fewer) **[A]**[37].

**Stroke units reduce death, dependency and the need for institutional care**

| Patient [A][37] | Treatment | Comparator | Outcome | CER | OR | NNT |
|---|---|---|---|---|---|---|
| Stroke | Admitted to stroke unit (usually within 7 days of onset) | Admitted to general ward | Death at 6–12 months | 26% | 0.83 (0.71 to 0.97) | 29 (17 to 170) |
| | | | Death or institutional care at 6–12 months | 46% | 0.77 (0.68 to 0.88) | 16 (11 to 32) |
| | | | Death or dependency at 6–12 months | 62% | 0.75 (0.65 to 0.87) | 14 (9 to 30) |

and provide:
- intensive physiotherapy **[A]**[39] and occupational therapy **[A]**[39], **[A]**[40].

 **Why do this?**
- Occupational therapy helps improve functional status (on average, an increase of 4 points on the extended activities of daily living scale) **[A]**[40].
- Intensive physiotherapy and occupational therapy lead to greater improvements in activities of daily living than does conventional care **[A]**[39].

The benefits of thrombolysis are mixed **[A]**[41] – it cannot currently be recommended as routine therapy **[D]**.

Thrombolysis is applicable for patients who understand the risks **[D]** and:
- present within 3–6 h of symptom onset **[D]**[42] with a clear neurological deficit **[D]**
- have a CT scan which excludes a haemorrhagic stroke **[A]**
- have neurological deficit that is neither very mild nor very severe **[D]**
- have no recent trauma or surgery **[D]**, or no active peptic ulcer disease **[D]**.

**Why?**
- Thrombolysis reduces dependency at 3 months **[A]**[41], but not clearly at 1 year **[D]**[43].
- Patients given thrombolysis are more likely to die particularly early and from intracranial haemorrhage **[A]**[41].
- No thrombolytic agent or dose has been shown to be clearly better than another **[D]**[44].
- Neurologists and radiologists only correctly interpret 83% of CT scans (95% CI: 65% to 100%), and emergency physicians only 67% of scans (95% CI: 43% to 91%) for eligibility for thrombolysis **[C]**[45].

**Thrombolysis kills more patients, but reduces dependency in those that survive**

| Patient | Treatment | Comparator | Outcome | CER | OR | NNT |
|---|---|---|---|---|---|---|
| Acute ischaemic stroke **[A]**[41] | Thrombolysis | Placebo | Death at 7–10 days | 10% | 1.85 (1.48 to 2.32) | −14 (−25 to −10) |
| | | | Fatal intracranial haemorrhage at 7–10 days | 1.0% | 4.15 (2.96 to 5.84) | −32 (−51 to −21) |
| | | | Any intracranial haemorrhage | 2.5% | 3.53 (2.79 to 4.45) | −17 (−24 to −13) |
| | | | Death at 1–3 months | 16% | 1.21 (1.13 to 1.52) | −37 (−59 to −16) |
| | | | Death or dependency at 1–3 months | 59% | 0.83 (0.73 to 0.94) | 22 (13 to 67) |

**Alteplase reduces dependency**

| Patient | Treatment | Comparator | Outcome | CER | OR | NNT |
|---|---|---|---|---|---|---|
| Acute ischaemic stroke **[A]**[46] | Alteplase | Placebo | Independence at 3 months | 46% | −8.2% (−15% to −1.3%) | 12 (7 to 75) |

There is no clear benefit from:
- haemodilution **[D]**[47]

 **Why?**
- Patients with acute ischaemic stroke who receive haemodilution compared with no treatment are not clearly less likely to die **[D]**[47].

- prostacyclin **[D]**[48]

**Why?**
- Patients with acute ischaemic stroke who receive prostacyclin compared with placebo are not clearly less likely to die **[D]**[48].

- piracetam **[D]**[49]

**Why?**

■ Patients with acute ischaemic stroke who take piracetam compared with placebo are not clearly less likely to die or be dependent **[D]**[49].

● pentoxifylline, propentofylline, pentifylline **[D]**[50]

 **Why?**

■ Patients with acute ischaemic stroke who receive pentoxifylline, propentofylline or pentifylline compared with placebo are not clearly less likely to die **[D]**[50].

● fibrinogen-depleting agents **[D]**[51]

 **Why?**

■ Fibrinogen-depleting agents have no clear effect on reducing death or disability following an acute ischaemic stroke or an intracranial haemorrhage **[D]**[51].

● corticosteroids **[D]**[52]

 **Why?**

■ Patients with acute ischaemic stroke who receive corticosteroids compared with placebo are not clearly less likely to die **[D]**[52].

● gangliosides **[D]**[52]

 **Why?**

■ Patients with acute ischaemic stroke who receive gangliosides compared with placebo are not clearly less likely to die **[D]**[53].

● theophylline **[D]**[54]

 **Why?**

■ Theophylline has no clear effect on early mortality following an acute ischaemic stroke **[D]**[53].

● glycerol **[D]**[55].

**Why?**

■ Patients with an ischaemic stroke who receive glycerol compared with placebo are less likely to be dead at 2 weeks, but not at 1 year **[D]**[55].

**Glycerol reduces mortality at 2 weeks but not at 1 year**

| Patient | Treatment | Comparator | Outcome | CER | OR | NNT |
|---|---|---|---|---|---|---|
| Stroke **[A]**[55] | Glycerol | Placebo or no treatment | Death at 2 weeks | 27% | 0.58 (0.36 to 0.91) | 11 (7 to 55) |
| | | | Death at one year | 47% | 0.82 (0.54 to 1.23) | 20 (NNT = 7 to infinity, NNH = 19 to infinity) |

## Intracranial haemorrhage

There is no clear benefit from:

● haematoma evacuation **[D]**[56] **[D]**[57].

**Why?**

■ Patients with a supratentorial intracranial haemorrhage who have craniotomy and haematoma evacuation compared with medical therapy are not clearly less likely to die or be dependent **[D]**[56] **[D]**[57].

## PREVENTION

## Acute ischaemic stroke or transient ischaemic attack

Give patients with suspected ischaemic stroke aspirin within 48 h **[A]**[58] or as soon as an intracranial haemorrhage has been excluded **[D]**[59].

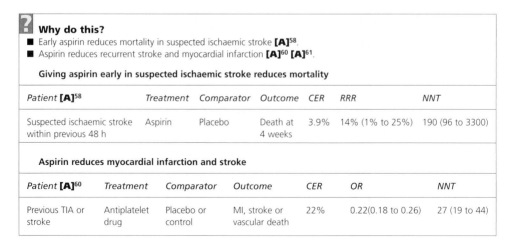

**Why do this?**

■ Early aspirin reduces mortality in suspected ischaemic stroke **[A]**[58].
■ Aspirin reduces recurrent stroke and myocardial infarction **[A]**[60] **[A]**[61].

**Giving aspirin early in suspected ischaemic stroke reduces mortality**

| Patient **[A]**[58] | Treatment | Comparator | Outcome | CER | RRR | NNT |
|---|---|---|---|---|---|---|
| Suspected ischaemic stroke within previous 48 h | Aspirin | Placebo | Death at 4 weeks | 3.9% | 14% (1% to 25%) | 190 (96 to 3300) |

**Aspirin reduces myocardial infarction and stroke**

| Patient **[A]**[60] | Treatment | Comparator | Outcome | CER | OR | NNT |
|---|---|---|---|---|---|---|
| Previous TIA or stroke | Antiplatelet drug | Placebo or control | MI, stroke or vascular death | 22% | 0.22(0.18 to 0.26) | 27 (19 to 44) |

Consider adding dipyridamole [A][62].

**Why do this?**

■ Aspirin and dipyridamole reduces recurrent stroke more effectively than aspirin, but increases the risk of moderate or severe bleeding. There is no clear effect on mortality [A][62].

**Dipyridamole added to aspirin reduces stroke better than aspirin alone, but causes more bleeding**

| Patient [A][62] | Treatment | Comparator | Outcome | CER | RRR | NNT |
|---|---|---|---|---|---|---|
| Recent TIA or ischaemic stroke | Aspirin or dipyridamole | Aspirin | Stroke at 2 years | 13% | 29% (14% to 42%) | 25 (16 to 57) |
| | | | Moderate or severe bleed at 2 years | | −140% (−280% to −48%) | −48 (−99 to −31) |

Alternatives include:
● clopidrogel [A][63]

**Why do this?**

■ Clopidrogel reduces stroke, myocardial infarction and death more effectively than aspirin [A][62].

**Clopidrogel reduces stroke, MI and death better than aspirin**

| Patient [A][63] | Treatment | Comparator | Outcome | CER | RRR | NNT |
|---|---|---|---|---|---|---|
| Recent ischaemic stroke, recent MI or peripheral vascular disease | Clopidrogel | Aspirin | Stroke, MI or death at 2 years | 15% | 7.0% (0.0% to 13%) | 100 (50 to 160 000) |

● ticlopidine [A][64].

**Why do this?**

■ Ticlopidine reduces recurrent stroke, myocardial infarction and vascular death [A][64].
■ It is more effective than aspirin at reducing stroke, though there is no clear difference in mortality [A][65].
■ However, adverse effects severe enough to discontinue therapy are common (particularly neutropenia) [A][64] [A][65].

**Ticlopidine reduces recurrent stroke, MI and vascular death**

| Patient [A][64] | Treatment | Comparator | Outcome | CER | RRR | NNT |
|---|---|---|---|---|---|---|
| Recent thromboembolic stroke [A][64] | Ticlopidine | Placebo | Stroke, MI or vascular death at 3 years | 25% | 2.0% (0.0% to 36%) | 19 (10 to 760) |
| | | | Discontinued therapy due to adverse effects | 2.8% | −320% (−620% to −140%) | −11 (−17 to −8) |
| Recent TIA or minor stroke [A][64] | Ticlopidine | Aspirin | Stroke | 14% | 18% (1% to 32%) | 40 (21 to 560) |
| | | | Adverse effect | 53% | −17% (−10% to −24%) | −11 (−18 to −8) |

Anticoagulate patients with atrial fibrillation [A][66].

 **Why do this?**
■ It reduces recurrent stroke and other vascular events, but major extracranial bleeds are more common [A][66].

**Patients with AF who are anticoagulated have fewer recurrent strokes, but more major extracranial bleeds**

| Patient | Treatment | Comparator | Outcome | CER | OR | NNT |
|---|---|---|---|---|---|---|
| Stroke and AF [A][66] | Anticoagulation | Aspirin | Recurrent stroke at 2 years | 23% | 0.36 (0.22 to 0.58) | 8 (6 to 12) |
| | | | All vascular events at 2 years | 33% | 0.55 (0.37 to 0.82) | 9 (6 to 24) |
| | | | Major extracranial bleed at 2 years | 0.93% | 4.32 (1.55 to 12.10) | −34 (−200 to −11) |

 **Note**
■ Early anticoagulation in all strokes has no effect on death, dependence or recurrent stroke [A][67].
■ Patients are less likely to have deep vein thrombosis or pulmonary embolism, but are more likely to have a major extracranial bleed [A][68].
■ Anticoagulation for presumed non-embolic ischaemic stroke or transient-ischaemic attack has no clear effect on death or recurrent stroke [A][68].

**Early anticoagulation reduces DVT and PE, but causes more extracranial bleeding**

| Patient | Treatment | Comparator | Outcome | CER | OR | NNT |
|---|---|---|---|---|---|---|
| Stroke [A][69] | Anticoagulation within 2 weeks of stroke | No anticoagulation | DVT during treatment period | 44% | 0.21 (0.15 to 0.29) | 3 (3 to 4) |
| | | | Symptomatic PE during treatment period | 0.93% | 0.61 (0.45 to 0.83) | 280 (200 to 640) |
| | | | Major extracranial haemorrhage | 3.6% | 0.76 (0.65 to 0.88) | −120 (−240 to −81) |

There is no clear benefit from:
● immediate anticoagulation [D][70].

 **Why?**
■ Patients with embolic stroke who receive immediate anticoagulation compared with waiting 10 days are not clearly less likely to have recurrent embolism, haemorrhagic infarction or die [D][70].

● indobufen [A][71].

 **Why?**
■ It is not clearly better than warfarin at reducing recurrent strokes, and causes more adverse effects [A][71].

Treat:

● hypertension **[A]**⁷²

 **Why do this?**

■ It reduces recurrent strokes, fatal strokes and major cardiovascular events, though there is no clear reduction in mortality **[A]**⁷².

**Treating hypertension reduces further strokes and major cardiovascular events**

| Patient | Treatment | Comparator | Outcome | CER | RRR | NNT |
|---|---|---|---|---|---|---|
| Previous stroke or TIA **[A]**⁷² | Blood pressure-lowering medication | Placebo | Stroke at ? years | 9.5% | 26% (14% to 37%) | 40 (26 to 84) |
| | | | Fatal stroke at ? years | 3.3% | 28% (5% to 46%) | 110 (58 to 700) |
| | | | Major cardiovascular events at ? years | 11% | 20% (7 to 30%) | 45 (27 to 130) |

● high cholesterol using a statin **[A]**⁷³ **[A]**⁷⁴

 **Why do this?**

■ Statins reduce death and recurrent stroke in patients with ischaemic heart disease, previous stroke and a high cholesterol level **[A]**⁷³ **[A]**⁷⁴.

**Statins reduce death and recurrent stroke in high-risk patients with high cholesterol levels**

| Patient | Treatment | Comparator | Outcome | CER | OR | NNT |
|---|---|---|---|---|---|---|
| Previous stroke and high cholesterol level **[A]**⁷³ | Statin | Placebo | Recurrent stroke at ? years | 2.3% | 0.68 (0.55 to 0.85) | 140 (98 to 300) |
| | | | Death at ? years | 6.2% | 0.79 (0.69 to 0.91) | 81 (55 to 190) |

Encourage patients to stop smoking **[A]**⁷⁵.

**Why do this?**

**Stopping smoking or never smoking reduces the risk of stroke**

| Patient | Prognostic factor | Outcome | Control rate | RR (95% CI) | NNF + (95% CI) |
|---|---|---|---|---|---|
| Healthy **[A]**⁷⁵ | Never smoked *independent* | Stroke at 12 years | 0.38% | 0.39 (0.30 to 0.52) | 430 (380 to 550) |
| | Stopped smoking 2–4 years ago *independent* | | | 0.21 (0.04 to 0.96) | 330 (270 to 6600) |

There is no clear benefit from:
- altering blood pressure early [D][76].

 **Why?**
- Patients with acute ischaemic or haemorrhagic stroke who were given interventions to alter blood pressure compared with placebo are not clearly less likely to die [D][76].

Consider:
- giving an ACE inhibitor to patients with one other cardiovascular risk factor (hypertension, elevated total cholesterol levels, low high-density lipoprotein cholesterol levels, cigarette smoking or documented microalbuminuria) [A][77].

 **Why do this?**
- Patients at high-risk for cardiovascular disease who take ramipril are less likely to die, have a stroke, myocardial infarction or cardiac arrest or develop heart failure [A][77].
- Many patients stop therapy, particularly owing to cough [A][77].

**Ramipril reduces death and cardiovascular complications in patients at high risk for cardiovascular disease**

| Patient | Treatment | Comparator | Outcome | CER | RRR | NNT |
|---|---|---|---|---|---|---|
| Previous stroke, MI or peripheral vascular disease and at least one other cardiovascular risk factor | Ramipril 5 mg bd | Placebo | Death from any cause at 5 years | 12% | 15% (5% to 24%) | 55 (32 to 180) |
| | | | MI at 5 years | 12% | 19% (9% to 2%8) | 44 (28 to 99) |
| | | | Stroke at 5 years | 4.9% | 30 (15% to 43%) | 68 (44 to 150) |
| | | | Heart failure at 5 years | 12% | 22% (12% to 31%) | 39 (26 to 77) |
| | | | Cardiac arrest at 5 years | 1.3% | 36% (4 to 58%) | 220 (120 to 2400) |
| | | | Discontinued therapy permanently at 5 years | 31% | −6% (−13% to −0.086%) | −52 (−3500 to −26) |
| | | | Treatment discontinued due to cough at 5 years | 1.9% | −300% (−410% to −220%) | −18 (−22 to −16) |

Consider performing carotid endarterectomy in patients with:
● carotid stenosis > 50% **[A]**[78] **[A]**[79]

**Why do this?**
■ Though there is a small increased risk of early disabling stroke or death following carotid endarterectomy, in the long term it reduces stroke and death **[A]**[78] **[A]**[79].
■ It is cost-effective in symptomatic patients **[A]**[80].

**Carotid endarterectomy reduces stroke and death in patients with symptomatic carotid stenosis > 70%**

| Patient | Treatment | Comparator | Outcome | CER | OR | NNT |
|---|---|---|---|---|---|---|
| Symptomatic carotid to artery stenosis > 70% | Carotid endarterectomy | Medical therapy | Disabling stroke or death at 1 year | 14% | 0.48 (0.33 to 0.70) | 15 (11 27) |
| Symptomatic carotid artery stenosis 50–69% | | | | 18% | 0.69 (0.51 to 0.94) | 21 (13 to 110) |
| Symptomatic carotid artery stenosis < 50% | | | | 11% | 1.23 (1.0 to 1.51) | −44 (inf to −21) |
| Symptomatic carotid artery stenosis | Carotid endarterectomy | Medical therapy | Disabling stroke or death at 30 days | 1.2% | 2.23 (1.55 to 3.22) | −72 (−160 to −40) |

using patch angioplasty **[A]**[81]

**Why do this?**
■ Patients who have patch angioplasty compared with primary closure are less likely to have a stroke. There is no clear effect on mortality **[A]**[81].
■ Polytetrafluoroethylene patching is not clearly better than vein patching at preventing stroke **[D]**[82].

**Patch angioplasty reduces early stroke**

| Patient **[A]**[81] | Treatment | Comparator | Outcome | CER | OR | NNT |
|---|---|---|---|---|---|---|
| Carotid endarterectomy | Patch | No patch | Stroke at 30 days | 4.2% | 0.38 (0.15 to 0.97) | 39 (28 to 820) |

Give patients low-dose aspirin **[A]**[83].

**Why do this?**
■ It leads to fewer strokes and myocardial infarction than high-dose aspirin **[A]**[83].

**Carotid endarterectomy: low-dose aspirin prevents more strokes and MIs than high-dose aspirin**

| Patient **[A]**[83] | Treatment | Comparator | Outcome | CER | RRR | NNT |
|---|---|---|---|---|---|---|
| Undergoing carotid endarterectomy | Aspirin 81 or 325 mg daily | Aspirin 650 mg or 1300 mg daily | Stroke | 6.7% | 32% (7% to 50%) | 46 (26 to 220) |
| | | | MI | 2.5% | 1.3% (0.35% to 2.3%) | 75 (43 to 290) |

Avoid carotid endarterectomy for patients with:
- a carotid stenosis < 50% **[A]**[78].

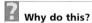 **Why do this?**
- Carotid endarterectomy increases the risk of disabling stroke or death **[A]**[78].

There is no clear benefit from:
- shunting **[D]**[84]

 **Why?**
- Shunting during endarterectomy has no clear effect on subsequent stroke or death **[D]**[83].

- local anaesthetic **[D]**[85].

**Why?**
- Patients who have carotid endarterectomy performed under local anaesthetic compared with general anaesthetic are not clearly more likely to have a stroke or die **[D]**[85].

Surgical complications are more likely with:
- increasing age **[B]**[84]
- female sex **[B]**[87]
- non-elective admission **[B]**[86]

 **Why?**

**Increasing age, female sex or a non-elective admission increase the risk of surgical complications**

| Patient | Prognostic factor | Outcome | Control rate | OR (95% CI) | NNF+ (95% CI) |
|---|---|---|---|---|---|
| Undergoing carotid endarterectomy **[B]**[87] | Female _independent_ | Stroke or death at ?30 days | 8.6% | 1.44 (1.14 to 1.83) | 30 (16 to 92) |
| | Age (>75 versus <74 years) _independent_ | | | 1.36 (1.09 to 1.71) | 36 (19 to 140) |
| Undergoing carotid endarterectomy **[B]**[86] | Non-elective admission _independent_ | Death at discharge | 1.2% | 2.43 | 60 |

- associated stroke risk factors
  - atrial fibrillation [B][84]
  - congestive heart failure [B][86] [B][88]
  - hypertension [B][86]
  - a recent stroke or TIA [B][89] particularly if more severe [B][87]

---

**? Why?**

**Stroke risk factors increase the risk of surgical complications**

| Patient | Prognostic factor | Outcome | Control rate | OR (95% CI) | NNF+ (95% CI) |
|---|---|---|---|---|---|
| Undergoing carotid endarterectomy [B][87] | Hypertension *independent* | Stroke or death at ?30 days | 8.6% | 1.82 (1.37 to 2.41) | 17 (10 to 36) |
| Undergoing carotid endarterectomy [B][90] | History of congestive heart failure *independent* | Stroke or death at 30 days | 8.6% | 2.60 (1.20 to 5.60) | 9 (4 to 65) |
| Carotid endarterectomy [B][86] | Atrial fibrillation *independent* | Death at discharge | 1.2% | 2.02 | 84 |
| Undergoing carotid endarterectomy [B][86] | Monocular versus cerebral TIA *independent* | Stroke or death at ?30 days | 8.6% | 0.49 (0.37 to 0.66) | −24 (−36 to 19) |

**A more severe stroke increases the risk of surgical complications**

| Patient | Prognostic factor | Outcome | Control rate | RR (95% CI) | NNF + (95% CI) |
|---|---|---|---|---|---|
| Undergoing carotid endarterectomy [B][91] | Evolving stroke *independent* | Death, stroke, MI at 30 days | 11% | 7.58 (1.54 to 15.0) | 1 (1 to 17) |
|  | Recent stroke *independent* |  |  | 2.42 (1.10 to 4.84) | 6 (2 to 91) |
|  | Carotid TIA *independent* |  |  | 1.74 (1.06 to 2.79) | 12 (5 to 150) |

---

- associated cardiovascular disease
  - history of angina [B][90] or a recent MI [B][91]
  - peripheral vascular disease [B][89]
  - mitral or aortic valve disease [B][86]

---

**? Why?**

**A recent MI increases the risk of surgical complications**

| Patient | Prognostic factor | Outcome | Control rate | RR (95% CI) | NNF+ (95% CI) |
|---|---|---|---|---|---|
| Undergoing carotid endarterectomy [B][91] | MI within past 6 months *independent* | Death, stroke, MI at 30 days | 11% | 2.87 (1.09 to 6.41) | 5 (2 to 100) |

<table>
<tr><td colspan="6">❓ **Why?**<br>**Angina, peripheral vascular disease and valve disease increase the risk of surgical complications**</td></tr>
</table>

| Patient | Prognostic factor | Outcome | Control rate | OR (95% CI) | NNF+ (95% CI) |
|---|---|---|---|---|---|
| Undergoing carotid endarterectomy **[B]**[90] | History of angina *independent* | Stroke or death at 30 days | 8.6% | 1.90 (1.03 to 3.40) | 15 (6 to 430) |
| Undergoing carotid endarterectomy **[B]**[87] | Peripheral vascular disease *independent* | Stroke or death at ? 30 days | 8.6% | 2.19 (1.40 to 3.60) | 12 (6 to 33) |
| Carotid endarterectomy **[B]**[86] | Mitral valve disorder *independent* | Death at discharge | 1.2% | 1.81 | 110 |
| | Aortic valve disorder *independent* | | | 2.61 | 54 |

- diffuse carotid artery stenosis **[B]**[87]
- no antiplatelet cover during surgery **[B]**[87]

<table>
<tr><td colspan="6">❓ **Why?**<br>**Diffuse carotid artery stenosis or no antiplatelet cover during surgery increases the risk of complications**</td></tr>
</table>

| Patient | Prognostic factor | Outcome | Control rate | OR (95% CI) | NNF+ (95% CI) |
|---|---|---|---|---|---|
| Undergoing carotid endarterectomy **[B]**[89] | Occlusion of contralateral internal carotid artery *independent* | Stroke or death at ? 30 days | 8.6% | 1.91 (1.35 to 2.69) | 15 (9 to 37) |
| | Stenosis of distal ipsilateral internal carotid artery *independent* | | | 1.56 (1.03 to 2.36) | 24 (10 to 430) |
| | Stenosis of ipsilateral external carotid artery *independent* | | | 1.61 (1.05 to 2.47) | 22 (10 to 260) |
| Undergoing carotid endarterectomy **[B]**[89] | No perioperative antiplatelet medication *independent* | Stroke or death at ? 30 days | 8.6% | 2.50 (1.40 to 4.50) | 10 (5 to 33) |

- low annual operating volumes for surgeons and hospitals **[B]**[86] and the surgeon's place of training **[B]**[91].

<table>
<tr><td colspan="2">❓ **Why?**<br>**Surgeons performing few operations in hospitals with few operations are associated with increased mortality**</td></tr>
</table>

| **[B]**[86] | Mortality rate (95% CI) |
|---|---|
| Surgeon performing < 5 operatios per year in a hospital with ≥ 100 procedures a year | 2.0% (1.5% to 2.6%) |
| Surgeon performing ≥ 5 operation per year in a hospital with ≤ 100 procedures a year | 0.94% (0.73% to 1.2%) |

**Why?**

**Surgical training affects operative complication rate**

| Patient | Prognostic factor | Outcome | Control rate (%) | RR (95% CI) | NNF+ (95% CI) |
|---|---|---|---|---|---|
| Undergoing carotid endarterectomy **[B]**[91] | Surgeons not trained in North America or Western Europe working in the USA *independent* | Death, stroke, MI at 30 days | 11% | 1.91 (1.12 to 3.13) | 10 (4 to 76) |

# REHABILITATION

## Spasticity

Consider using:

- baclofen **[A]**[92]

**Why do this?**

■ It helps improve muscle tone in spasticity, but side-effects are common and there is no clear improvement in incapacity **[A]**[92].

**Spasticity: baclofen causes side-effects**

| Patient | Treatment | Comparator | Outcome | CER | RRR | NNT |
|---|---|---|---|---|---|---|
| Stroke with spasticity for at least 3 months **[A]**[92] | Baclofen | Placebo | Side-effects at 6 weeks | 15% | −230% (−930% to −8%) | 3 (2 to 12) |

- botulinum toxin for spastic foot **[A]**[93]

**Why do this?**

■ It helps improve ankle movement and gait for patients with a spastic foot **[A]**[93].

■ Patients with arm spasticity who receive botulinum toxin in addition to spasticity therapy are not clearly more likely to improve than patients who have spasticity therapy alone **[D]**[94].

- acupuncture for patients with severe hemiparesis **[A]**[95].

**Why do this?**

■ Acupuncture helps improve walking, motor function, balance and activities of daily living (on average 2 points) **[A]**[95].

■ Patients given acupuncture are more likely to be discharged home **[A]**[95].

**Patients with severe hemiparesis given acupuncture are more likely to be living at home after a year**

| Patient | Treatment | Comparator | Outcome | CER | RRR | NNT |
|---|---|---|---|---|---|---|
| Severe hemiparesis **[A]**[95] | Acupuncture and rehabilitation | Rehabilitation | Living at home at 1 year | 66% | −36% (−80% to −3%) | 4 (2 to 28) |

## Dysphagia

Consider inserting percutaneous endoscopic gastrostomy tube for patients with persistent dysphagia **[A]**[96], unless they have **[C]**[97]:

- GI abnormalities
- ascites or hepatomegaly
- clotting disorders.

**Why do this?**

■ Patients who receive PEG feeding compared with nasogastric tube feeding are less likely to die, and are more likely to put on weight **[A]**[96].

■ PEG feeding is less likely to fail than nasogastric tube feeding. There is no clear difference in the complication rate **[A]**[98].

**Dysphagia: fewer patients die and more gain weight on PEG feeding than nasogastric tube feeding**

| Patient | Treatment | Comparator | Outcome | CER | RRR | NNT |
|---------|-----------|------------|---------|-----|-----|-----|
| Stroke and persistent dysphagia for ≥ 8 days**[A]**[96] | PEG tube feeding | Nasogastric tube feeding | Death at 6 weeks | 57% | 78% (14% to 94%) | 2 (1 to 7) |
| | | | Weight gain at 1 week | 13% | −64% (−97% to −32%) | 2 (1 to 3) |
| Neurological disease and dysphagia for ≥ 4 weeks **[A]**[98] | PEG tube feeding | Nasogastric tube feeding | Treatment failure | 95% | 100% | 1 (1 to 1) |

There is no clear benefit from:
- aggressive management by a dysphagia therapist **[D]**[99]

**Why?**

■ A therapist-selected diet and supervision is not clearly better than a patient-selected diet combined with swallowing exercises at reducing pneumonia, dehydration or malnutrition.

- electromyographic biofeedback **[D]**[100]**[D]**[101]

**Why?**

■ There is no clear improvement in gait **[D]**[100] or range of motion in the paralysed limb **[D]**[101].

- sensorimotor stimulation **[D]**[102]

**Why?**

■ Patients with arm hemiplegia who receive sensorimotor stimulation compared with sham treatment are not clearly more likely to have less impairment or disability **[D]**[102].

- leg and arm training[D][103]

**Why?**
- Though patients have some improvement in dexterity, there is no clear improvement in activities of daily living or walking **[D]**[103].

- spatiomotor cueing for visual neglect **[D]**[104]

**Why?**
- Patients with partial anterior circulation infarction and visual neglect who receive spatiomotor cueing compared with conventional rehabilitation are not clearly more likely to be discharged home **[D]**[104].

- functional electrostimulation[D][105]

**Why?**
- It may increase muscle strength recovery, but the effect on function is unclear **[D]**[105].

## Discharge

Consider:
- community rehabilitation[D][106]

**Why?**
- Patients achieve similar functional levels when rehabilitated in the community compared with hospital and are not clearly less satisfied with care. There is no clear difference in mortality **[D]**[106].
- Community-based rehabilitation is probably more cost-effective **[C]**[107].

with home physiotherapy **[A]**[108].

**Why do this?**
- It is more effective than day hospital attendance at achieving independent movement and walking, and fewer patients are still being treated at 6 months **[A]**[108].

**Home physiotherapy is more effective than day hospital for post-stroke rehabilitation**

| Patient | Treatment | Comparator | Outcome | CER | RRR (%) | NNT |
|---------|-----------|------------|---------|-----|---------|-----|
| Stroke **[A]**[108] | Home physiotherapy | Day hospital care | Independence in functional movement at 6 months | 31% | −86% (−200% to −16%) | 4 (2 to 12) |
| | | | Independence in functional ambulation at 6 months | 23% | −93% (−240% to −9%) | 5 (3 to 24) |
| | | | Still receiving treatment at 6 months | | 59% (27% to 77%) | 3 (2 to 8) |

There is no clear benefit from:
- managing patients with stroke in the community **[D]**[109]

 **Why?**
- Patients with stroke who received 'hospital-at-home' care compared with hospital admission are not clearly less likely to die or become dependent **[D]**[109].

- family careworkers **[D]**[110].

 **Why?**
- Providing family careworkers does not clearly improve social functioning or general health compared with standard care **[D]**[110].

## PROGNOSIS

### Deterioration
Many patients with stroke will get worse over the next few days **[B]**[111].

**Why?**
**A third of patients with a haemorrhage or non-cardioembolic infarction worsen**

| Type of stroke **[B]**[111] | % with neurological worsening (95% CI) |
|---|---|
| Brain haemorrhage | 38% (33% to 43%) |
| Cardioembolic infarction | 15% (13% to 18%) |
| Non-cardioembolic infarction | 34% (32% to 36%) |

- 41% of patients with acute thromboembolic ischaemic stroke will deteriorate over the first 48 h (95% CI: 31% to 51%) **[A]**[112].
- A quarter of patients with an intracranial haemorrhage deteriorate within 24 h of admission (23%; 95% CI: 15% to 32%) **[A]**[113]

The risk of early deterioration is increased with **[B]**[111]:
- posterior circulation stroke
- reduced level of consciousness
- hypertension.

The risk of early deterioration following an ischaemic stroke is increased with **[A]**[112]:
- high systolic blood pressure at admission
- carotid vascular territory involvement
- elevated initial glycaemia.

The risk of early deterioration following an intracranial haemorrhage is increased with [A]¹¹⁴:
- ventricular extension
- intracerebral haemorrhage volume ≥ 30 ml.

**Why?**
Ventricular extension and a large bleed increase the risk of deterioration within 24 h

| Patient [A]¹¹⁴ | Prognostic factor | Outcome | Control rate | OR (95% CI) | NNF+ (95% CI) |
|---|---|---|---|---|---|
| Intracerebral haemorrhage | Ventricular extension | Deterioration at 24 h | 11% | 4.67 (1.30 to 16.7) | 4 (2 to 36) |
| | Intracerebral haemorrhage volume ≥ 30 ml | | 10% | 6.78 (1.89 to 24.4) | 3 (2 to 14) |

## Functional outcome

Patients with more severe strokes are less likely to be functionally independent [A]¹.

**Note**
Patients with more severe strokes are less likely to be functionally independent

| Stroke subtype [A]¹ | Functionally independent at 1 year |
|---|---|
| LACI | 62% |
| TACI | 4% |
| PACI | 55% |
| POCI | 62% |

Patients are less likely to have a good function outcome with [B]¹¹⁵:
- increasing age
- a severe deficit
- bilateral or right-sided stroke
- incontinence
- dysphagia
- no committed caregiver.

None the less, many patients return to work [B]¹¹⁶.

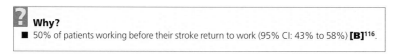

**Why?**
- 50% of patients working before their stroke return to work (95% CI: 43% to 58%) [B]¹¹⁶.

Patients are more likely to return to work if they have **[B]**[116]:
- no apraxia
- normal muscle strength
- a desk job.

 **Why?**
No apraxia, normal muscle strength or a white-collar job increases the probability of returning to work

| Patient **[B]**[116] | Prognostic factor | Outcome | Control rate | OR (95% CI) | NNF+ (95% CI) |
|---|---|---|---|---|---|
| Stroke | No apraxia *independent* | Return to work at ? months | 50% | 5.16 | 3 |
| | Normal muscle strength *independent* | | | 4.2 | 3 |
| | White collar job *independent* | | | 1.4 | 11 |

## Depression
Watch out for depression **[B]**[117]**[B]**[118].

 **Why?**
- It is common – 47% of patients are clinically depressed at 12 months (95% CI: 42% to 53%) **[B]**[117]**[B]**[118].
- Many caregivers also get depressed (40%; 95% CI: 33% to 47%) **[B]**[117].

The risk of depression is increased with increasing age, and reduced with an active rehabilitation programme **[B]**[117].

 **Why?**
Increasing age and no active rehabilitation increase the risk of depression

| Patient **[B]**[117] | Prognostic factor | Outcome | Control rate | OR (95% CI) | NNF+ (95% CI) |
|---|---|---|---|---|---|
| Stroke | Aged >70 years *independent* | Depression at 1 year | 47% | 1.64 (1.02 to 2.62) | 8 (4 to 200) |
| | Active rehabilitation programme *independent* | | 55% | 0.55 (0.34 to 0.88) | −7 (−31 to −4) |

Many patients will develop dementia **[B]**[119].

**Why?**
■ A third of patients will develop dementia within 5 years (32%; 95% CI: 25% to 39%) **[B]**[119].

## Seizures

Watch out for seizures within the first few days **[A]**[120].

**Why?**
■ 2.4% of patients with a first stroke will have a seizure within 48 h (95% CI; 1.5% to 3.2%) **[B]**[121].
■ 6.1% of patients with an ischaemic stroke will have seizures within the first week (95% CI: 4.1% to 8.2%) **[B]**[122].

The risk is increased with:
● a cortical involvement **[B]**[121]
● an acute agitated confusional state **[B]**[121]
● an anterior hemisphere infarct **[B]**[122].

**Why?**
Early seizures are more likely with an acute agitated confusional state or cortical involvement

| Patient | Prognostic factor | Outcome | Control rate | OR (95% CI) | NNF+ (95% CI) |
|---------|-------------------|---------|--------------|-------------|---------------|
| First stroke **[B]**[121] | Cortical involvement *independent* | Seizures at 48 h | 0.25% | 6.01 (2.54 to 14.2) | 81 (31 to 261) |
| | Acute agitated confusional state *independent* | | 2.1% | 4.44 (1.43 to 13.8) | 15 (5 to 113) |
| First ischaemic stroke **[B]**[122] | Anterior hemisphere infarct *independent* | Early seizures at 1 week | 2.0% | 4.00 (1.20 to 13.7) | 18 (5 to 250) |

A few patients will go on to have late seizures **[B]**[120] **[B]**[122].

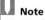

**Note**
■ 8% of patients will have a seizure in the next 2 years (95% CI: 5.8% to 10%) **[B]**[120]**[B]**[122] – half will be recurrent (3.8%; 95% CI: 2.3% to 5.3%) **[B]**[120].

The risk of seizures is increased with:
● a haemorrhagic first stroke **[B]**[120]
● seizure onset within 24 h of stroke **[B]**[120] **[B]**[122]
● recurrent stroke **[B]**[122].

**Why?**
**A haemorrhagic stroke and early seizures increase the risk of having a seizure at 2 years**

| Patient [B][122] | Prognostic factor | Outcome | Control rate | OR (95% CI) | NNF+ (95% CI) |
|---|---|---|---|---|---|
| First stroke | Haemorrhagic first stroke *independent* | Seizure at 2 years | 8% | 10.2 (3.70 to 27.9) | 6 (5 to 8) |
| | Early onset seizure *independent* | Seizure at 2 years | | 7.52 (2.46 to 23.0) | 55 (50 to 81) |

## Dysphagia

Swallowing problems are common [A][24].

**Note**
- Half of patients with a first stroke will have continued swallowing problems, a chest infection or aspiration at 6 months [A][24].
- A fifth will develop a chest infection at 6 months (22%; 95% CI: 15 to 30%) [A][24].

The risk of continued swallowing problems, a chest infection or aspiration is increased with a delayed or absent swallowing reflex on admission [A][24].

**Why?**
**Swallowing problems increase the risk of chest infection**

| Patient [A][24] | Prognostic factor | Outcome | Control rate | OR (95% CI) | NNF+ (95% CI) |
|---|---|---|---|---|---|
| First stroke | Delayed/absent swallowing reflex *independent* | Chest infection at 6 months | 22% | 11.8 (3.30 to 49.6) | 2 (2 to 4) |

Dysphagia, chest infection or aspiration are more likely with [A][24]:
- penetration of food
- delayed oral transit
- increasing age
- male sex.

**Why?**
**Swallowing problems, increasing age and male sex increase the risk of swallowing complications**

| Patient [A][24] | Prognostic factor | Outcome | Control rate | OR (95% CI) | NNF+ (95% CI) |
|---|---|---|---|---|---|
| First stroke | Penetration of food | Swallowing abnormality, chest infection or aspiration at 6 months *independent* | 51% | 14.0 (4.00 to 51.0) | 2 (2 to 3) |
| | Delayed oral transit | | 51% | 14.0 (4.00 to 50.0) | 2 (2 to 3) |
| | Increasing age | | 57% | 5.00 (1.40 to 21.0) | 3 (3 to 13) |
| | Male sex | | 39% | 5.00 (1.50 to 18.0) | 3 (2 to 10) |

### Recurrence

Recurrent strokes are common **[A]**[30]**[B]**[123]**[B]**[124], though the risk is lower for patients with a TIA or minor stroke **[A]**[125]**[A]**[126].

**Note**

■ A fifth of patients with a first stroke will have another within 5 years (20%; 95% CI: 17% to 23%) **[B]**[124].

■ 10% of patients with an ischaemic stroke will have another stroke within 13 months (95% CI: 8.5% to 12%) **[A]**[127]; 22% will have had another stroke at 5 years (95% CI: 18% to 27%) **[A]**[30] **[B]**[123].

■ 12% of patients with a minor stroke will have a major stroke within 10 years (95% CI: 8% to 15%) **[A]**[125]; 27%. of patients will have a recurrent stroke or die within 2 years (95% CI: 20% to 34%) **[A]**[126].

**Stroke subtypes help predict risk of recurrent stroke**

| Stroke subtype **[A]**[1] | Recurrent stroke |
|---|---|
| LACI | 9% (4% to 14%) |
| TACI | 6% (2% to 12%) |
| PACI | 17% (12% to 23%) |
| POCI | 20% (13% to 27%) |

The risk of recurrence is increased following an ischaemic stroke with **[A]**[127]:

● increasing age **[B]**[123]
● a prior stroke **[A]**[127]
● diabetes mellitus **[A]**[127]**[B]**[123] or elevated glucose levels on admission **[A]**[30]
● hypertension at discharge **[A]**[30]
● heavy alcohol use **[A]**[30].

**Why?**
**Ischaemic stroke: diabetes, a previous stroke or hypertension increases the risk of a recurrent stroke**

| Patient | Prognostic factor | Outcome | Control rate | RR (95% CI) | NNF+ (95% CI) |
|---|---|---|---|---|---|
| Ischaemic stroke **[A]**[127] | Diabetes *independent* | Recurrent stroke at 1 year | 10% | 1.66 (1.14 to 2.42) | 15 (7 to 71) |
| | Prior stroke *independent* | | | 1.74 (1.19 to 2.55) | 14 (6 to 53) |
| Ischaemic stroke **[A]**[30] | Heavy alcohol use *independent* | Recurrent stroke at 5 years | 22% | 2.50 (1.40 to 4.40) | 3 (1 to 11) |
| | Hypertension at discharge *independent* | | | 1.60 (1.01 to 2.60) | 8 (3 to 460) |
| | 5.5 mmol/l increase in admission glucose *independent* | | | 1.40 (1.10 to 1.70) | |

| | | | | | |
|---|---|---|---|---|---|
| **?** **Why?** | | | | | |
| **Ischaemic stroke: increasing age increases the risk of having a stroke** | | | | | |
| *Patient* | *Prognostic factor* | *Outcome* | *Control rate* | *RR (95% CI)* | *NNF+ (95% CI)* |
| First ischaemic stroke **[B]**[123] | Age increase of 10 years *independent* | Recurrent stroke at 5 years | 25% | 1.20 (1.10 to 1.36) | |

The risk of a recurrent stroke following a TIA or minor stroke is increased with:

- increasing age **[A]**[126]
- recurrent minor strokes or a lacunar stroke **[A]**[125]
- diabetes mellitus **[A]**[126]
- hypertension **[A]**[125]
- a prior MI **[A]**[125].

| | | | | | |
|---|---|---|---|---|---|
| **?** **Why?** | | | | | |
| **Minor stroke: increasing age and diabetes increase the risk of death or a recurrent stroke** | | | | | |
| *Patient* | *Prognostic factor* | *Outcome* | *Control rate* | *RR (95% CI)* | *NNF+ (95% CI)* |
| TIA or minor stroke **[A]**[126] | Age >65 years | Recurrent stroke or death at 2 years | 27% | 2.55 (1.23 to 5.25) | 1 (1 to 8) |
| | Diabetes mellitus | | | 2.78 (1.47 to 5.27) | 2 (1 to 8) |

| | | | | | |
|---|---|---|---|---|---|
| **Minor stroke: recurrent minor strokes, hypertension or a previous MI increases the risk of a major stroke** | | | | | |
| *Patient* **[A]**[125] | *Prognostic factor* | *Outcome* | *Control rate* | *OR (95% CI)* | *NNF+ (95% CI)* |
| First stroke and minor or no disability | Recurrent minor strokes | Major stroke at 10 years | ?10% | 2.80 (1.30 to 6.20) | 7 (3 to 38) |
| | Lacunar stroke | | 8.2% | 3.10 (1.90 to 4.60) | 7 (5 to 16) |
| | Prior MI | | ?10% | 2.90 (1.30 to 6.80) | 7 (3 to 38) |
| | Hypertension | | 4.7% | 3.00 (1.40 to 6.40) | 12 (5 to 57) |

**Death**

Many patients die **[B]**[123] though the risk is lower with a minor stroke or TIA **[A]**[1][A][125].

> **Note**
> - A third of patients with any stroke are dead within a year (38%; 95% CI: 34% to 42%) **[B]**[26].
> - A tenth of patients admitted to hospital with an ischaemic stroke will die within 30 days (8.9%; 95% CI: 4.3% to 14%) **[A]**[128]. A third are dead within 12 months (28%; 95% CI: 23% to 33%) **[B]**[26], and 44% are dead within 5 years (95% CI: 39% to 50%) **[A]**[30] **[B]**[123].
> - 15% with a first-ever stroke or TIA die in hospital (95% CI: 13% to 17%) **[A]**[129], 30% of patients with a first stroke and minor disability are dead within 10 years (95% CI: 25% to 35%) **[A]**[125] **[A]**[130].
> - Half of patients with an intracranial haemorrhage die in hospital (51%; 95% CI: 43% to 58%) **[A]**[113].
>
> **Stroke subtypes help predict which patients will die**
>
> | Stroke subtype **[A]**[1] | Death at 1 year (%) |
> | --- | --- |
> | LACI | 11% (6% to 16%) |
> | TACI | 60% (50% to 70%) |
> | PACI | 16% (11% to 22%) |
> | POCI | 19% (12% to 25%) |

The risk of dying following a stroke is increased with **[B]**[28]:
- fever on admission
- drowsy or comatose at first examination
- increasing age
- an elevated glucose on admission.

> **Why?**
> **Fever, decreased consciousness, old age and high blood glucose increase the risk of dying**
>
> | Patient | Prognostic factor | Outcome | Control rate | OR (95% CI) | NNF+ (95% CI) |
> | --- | --- | --- | --- | --- | --- |
> | Stroke **[B]**[28] | Fever | Death at 30 days | 15% | 3.40 (1.20 to 9.50) | 4 (2 to 40) |
> | | Drowsy or comatose at first examination | | 15% | 9.70 (3.70 to 27.7) | 2 (1 to 4) |
> | | Age >75 years | | 17% | 3.70 (1.30 to 11.9) | 4 (2 to 24) |
> | | Glycaemia >6.7 mmol/l | | 12% | 3.00 (1.20 to 8.30) | 6 (2 to 48) |

The risk of dying following an ischaemic stroke is increased with:
- increasing age **[A]**[30] **[A]**[123] **[A]**[131]
- a severe **[A]**[30] or worsening stroke **[B]**[132]
- atrial fibrillation **[A]**[131]**[B]**[123]
- ischaemic heart disease (particularly if an early-onset) **[B]**[123] or intermittent claudication **[B]**[26]
- smoking **[A]**[131]
- heart failure **[B]**[28] **[B]**[123]
- an elevated glucose on admission **[A]**[30]
- urinary incontinence **[B]**[26]
- unpartnered marital status **[B]**[26].

**❓ Why?**

### Stroke risk factors and increasing age increase the risk of dying

| Patient | Prognostic factor | Outcome | Control rate | OR (95% CI) | NNF+ (95% CI) |
|---|---|---|---|---|---|
| Ischaemic stroke [A]131 | Smoking *independent* | Death at 30 days | 30% | 1.87 (1.07 to 3.27) | 7 (4 to 70) |
| | Atrial fibrillation *independent* | | 21% | 1.84 (1.04 to 3.27) | 9 (4 to 154) |
| | Increasing age (per 10 years) *independent* | | | 1.66 (1.27 to 2.17) | |
| First ischaemic stroke [B]123 | Ischaemic heart disease by age 50 years *independent* | Death at 5 years | 69% | 3.14 (2.05 to 4.81) | 5 (4 to 8) |
| | Ischaemic heart disease by age 60 years *independent* | | | 2.26 (1.68 to 3.04) | 7 (6 to 10) |
| | Ischaemic heart disease by age 70 years *independent* | | | 1.63 (1.35 to 1.97) | 11 (8 to 17) |

### A severe stroke, heart failure or urinary incontinence increase the risk of dying

| Patient | Prognostic factor | Outcome | Control rate | RR (95% CI) | NNF+ (95% CI) |
|---|---|---|---|---|---|
| Ischaemic stroke [A]30 | Major hemispheric or basilar syndrome *independent* | Death at 5 years | 44% | 2.00 (1.30 to 3.00) | 2 (1 to 8) |
| | Admission glucose > 7.7 mmol/l *independent* | | | 1.70 (1.40 to 2.80) | 4 (2 to 7) |
| | Congestive heart failure *independent* | | | 2.60 (1.70 to 4.10) | 2 (1 to 4) |
| | Lacunar syndrome *independent* | | | 0.56 (0.32 to 0.92) | –4 (–21 to –3) |
| Ischaemic stroke [B]26 | Urinary incontinence *independent* | Death at 1 year | ?20% | 7.32 (2.52 to 21.3) | 1 (1 to 3) |
| | Unpartnered marital status *independent* | | | 2.42 (1.08 to 5.43) | 4 (1 to 62) |

### A worsening stroke increases mortality

| Patient | Outcome | % (95% CI) | NNF (95% CI) |
|---|---|---|---|
| First ischaemic stroke [B]132 | Early neurological improvement at 30 days | 22% (16% to 29%) | 5 (3 to 6) |
| | Mortality in improving patients at 30 days | 2.9% (–2.7% to 8.6%) | 34 (12 to inf) |
| | Mortality in stable patients at 30 days | 17% (8.7% to 25%) | 6 (4 to 11) |
| | Mortality in deteriorating patients at 30 days | 38% (22% to 55%) | 3 (2 to 5) |

The risk of dying following a TIA or minor stroke is increased with [A][135]:

- increasing age [A][125] [A][133]
- diabetes mellitus [A][133]
- atrial fibrillation [A][125]
- ischaemic heart disease [A][125] [A][133] or intermittent claudication [A][133]
- hypercholesterolaemia [A][125]
- minor disability [A][123], including dysarthria [A][125], cranial nerve palsy [A][129] or limb weakness [A][129]
- seizures in hospital or altered consciousness [A][129]
- intraventricular haemorrhage [A][129]
- vomiting [A][129].

**? Why?**

**Minor stroke or TIA: stroke risk factors and increasing age increase the risk of dying**

| Patient [A][125] | Prognostic factor | Outcome | Control rate | OR (95% CI) | NNF+ (95% CI) |
|---|---|---|---|---|---|
| First stroke and minor or no disability | Age ≥65 years *independent* | Death at 10 years | 9.3% | 1.07 (1.05 to 1.09) | 170 (130 to 240) |
| | Minor disability *independent* | | 9.7% | 3.40 (2.20 to 5.20) | 6 (4 to 11) |
| | Prior MI *independent* | | ?10% | 1.80 (1.10 to 3.10) | 15 (6 to 110) |
| | Non-valvular atrial fibrillation *independent* | | ?10% | 2.00 (1.10 to 3.70) | 12 (5 to 110) |
| | Hypercholesterolaemia *independent* | | 14% | 1.80 (1.20 to 2.70) | 11 (6 to 42) |
| TIA [A][133] | Male *independent* | Stroke, MI or vascular death at 2 years | 15% | 1.60 (1.30 to 2.00) | 14 (9 to 27) |
| | Dysarthria *independent* | | | 1.30 (1.10 to 1.60) | 27 (14 to 80) |
| | Diabetes mellitus *independent* | | | 1.90 (1.50 to 2.50) | 10 (6 to 17) |
| | Intermittent claudication *Independent* | | | 1.60 (1.20 to 2.30) | 14 (7 to 40) |

**First stroke or TIA: early seizures, and altered consciousness increase the risk of dying**

| Patient [A][129] | Prognostic factor | Outcome | Control rate | RR (95% CI) | NNF+ (95% CI) |
|---|---|---|---|---|---|
| First stroke or TIA | Early seizures *independent* | Death at discharge | 17% | 6.17 (2.13 to 17.9) | 3 (2 to 8) |
| | Altered consciousness *independent* | | 5.9% | 9.53 (6.16 to 14.7) | 3 (2 to 5) |
| | Intraventricular haemorrhage *independent* | | 14% | 7.55 (3.33 to 17.1) | 2 (2 to 5) |
| | Cranial nerve palsy *independent* | | 16% | 4.68 (2.18 to 10.1) | 3 (2 to 8) |
| | Limb weakness *independent* | | 4.5% | 3.27 (1.67 to 6.45) | 11 (5 to 36) |
| | Vomiting *independent* | | 15% | 1.94 (1.02 to 3.71) | 10 (4 to 400) |

The risk of dying from an intracranial haemorrhage is increased with
[A][113]:

- ventricular extension
- intracerebral haemorrhage volume ≥ 30 ml
- an initial GCS < 12.

**Why?**

Intraventricular haemorrhage: ventricular extension, a large bleed or a GCS < 12 increases the risk of dying

| Patient [A][113] | Prognostic factor | Outcome | Control rate | OR (95% CI) | NNF+ (95% CI) |
|---|---|---|---|---|---|
| Intracranial haemorrhage | Ventricular extension *independent* | Death at discharge | 23% | 6.66 (2.85 to 15.6) | 2 (2 to 4) |
| | Intracerebral haemorrhage volume ≥ 30 ml *independent* | | 26% | 4.23 (1.82 to 9.82) | 3 (2 to 8) |
| | Initial GCS < 12 *independent* | | 31% | 3.23 (1.46 to 7.14) | 4 (2 to 12) |

**Guideline writer**: Christopher Ball
**CAT writers**: Clare Wotton, Nick Shenker, Christopher Ball

## REFERENCES

| No. | Level | Citation |
|---|---|---|
| 1 | 1b | Bamford J, Sandercock P, Dennis M et al. Classification and natural history of clinically identifiable subtypes of cerebral infarction. Lancet 1991; 337: 1521–6 |
| 2 | 1b | MacMahon S, Peto R, Cutler J et al. Blood pressure, stroke, and coronary heart disease. Part 1: Prolonged differences in blood pressure: prospective observational studies corrected for the regression dilution bias. Lancet 1990; 335: 765–74 |
| 3 | 1b | Rastenyte D, Tuomilehto J, Domarkiene S, et al. Risk factors for death from stroke in middle-aged Lithuanian men: Results from a 20-year prospective study. Stroke 1996; 27: 672–676 |
| 4 | 3b | Grau AJ, Buggle F, Heindl S et al. Recent infection as a risk factor for cerebrovascular ischemia. Stroke 1995; 26: 373–9 |
| 5 | 1b | Wolf PA, Abbott RD, Kannel WB. Atrial fibrillation as an independent risk factor for stroke: the Framingham Study. Stroke 1991; 22: 983–8 |
| 6 | 1b | Wolf PA, Mitchell JB, Baker CS et al. Impact of atrial fibrillation on mortality, stroke, and medical costs. Arch Intern Med 1998; 158: 229–34 |
| 7 | 1a | Atrial Fibrillation Investigators et al. Risk factors for stroke and efficacy of antithrombotic therapy in atrial fibrillation: analysis of pooled data from five randomised controlled trials. Arch Intern Med 1994; 154(13): 1449–57 |
| 8 | 2b | Davis BR, Vogt T, Frost PH et al. Risk factors for stroke and type of stroke in persons with isolated systolic hypertension. Stroke 1998; 29: 1333–40 |
| 9 | 1b | Robbins AS, Manson JE, Lee I-M et al. Cigarette smoking and stroke in a cohort of US male physicians. Ann Intern Med 1994; 120: 458–62 |

| No. | Level | Citation |
|-----|-------|----------|
| 10 | 1b | Iso H, Jacobs DR, Wentworth D et al. Serum cholesterol levels and six-year mortality from stroke in 350 977 men screened for the multiple risk factor intervention trial. N Engl J Med 1989; 320: 904–10 |
| 11 | 2b | European Atrial Fibrillation Trial Study Group. Optimal oral anticoagulation therapy in patients with non-rheumatic atrial fibrillation and recent cerebral ischemia. N Engl J Med 1995; 333: 5–10 |
| 12 | 3b | Jones EF, Kalman JM, Calafiore P et al. Proximal aortic atheroma: an independent risk factor for cerebral ischaemia. Stroke 1995; 26: 218–24 |
| 13 | 3b | Hannaford PC, Croft PR, Kay CR et al. Oral contraceptives and stroke: evidence from the Royal College of General Practitioners' Oral Contraception Study. Stroke 1994; 25: 935–42 |
| 14 | 1b | Stroke Prevention in Atrial Fibrillation Investigators. Predictors of thrombembolism in atrial fibrillation: clinical features of patients at risk. Ann Intern Med 1992; 116: 1–5 |
| 15 | 2b | Stroke Prevention in Atrial Fibrillation Investigators. Predictors of thromboembolism in atrial fibrillation: echocardiographic features of patients at risk. Ann Intern Med 1992; 116: 6–12 |
| 16 | 1b | Everson SA, Roberts RE, Goldberg DE et al. Depressive symptoms and increased risk of stroke mortality over a 29-year period. Arch Intern Med 1998; 158: 1133–8 |
| 17 | 1b | Finucane FF, Madans JH, Bush TL et al. Decreased risk of stroke among postmenopausal hormone users: results from a national cohort. Arch Intern Med 1993; 153: 73–9 |
| 18 | 1b | Stampfer MJ, Colditz GA, Willett WC et al. A prospective study of moderate alcohol consumption and the risk of coronary disease and stroke in women. N Eng J Med 1988; 319: 267–73 |
| 19 | 1b | Hankey GJ, Slattery JM, Warlow CP. Prognosis and prognostic factors of retinal infarction: a prospective cohort study. B J Med 1991; 302: 499–504 |
| 20 | 1b | Sauve JS, Thorpe KE, Sackett DL et al. Can bruits distinguish high-grade from moderate symptomatic carotid stenosis? Ann Intern Med 1994; 120: 633–7 |
| 21 | 1b | Mead GE, Wardlaw JM, Lewis SC et al. Can simple clinical features be used to identify patients with severe carotid stenosis on Doppler ultrasound? J Neurol Neurosurg Psychiatry 1999; 66: 16–19 |
| 22 | 2b | Orencia AJ, Petty GW, Khandheria BK et al. Risk of stroke with mitral valve prolapse in population-based cohort study. Stroke 1995; 26: 7–13 |
| 23 | 2b | Prescott RJ, Garraway WM, Akhtar AJ. Predicting functional outcome following acute stroke using a standard clinical examination. Stroke 1982; 13: 641–7 |
| 24 | 1b | Mann G, Hankey GJ, Cameron D. Swallowing function after stroke: prognosis and prognostic factors at 6 months. Stroke 1999; 30: 744–8 |
| 25 | 4 | Kalra L, Perez I, Gupta S et al. The influence of visual neglect on stroke rehabilitation. Stroke 1997; 28: 1386–91 |
| 26 | 2b | Anderson CS, Jamrozik KD, Broadhurst RJ et al. Predicting survival for 1 year among different subtypes of stroke: results from the Perth Community Stroke Study. Stroke 1994; 25: 1935–44 |
| 27 | 1b | Arboix A, Comes E, Massons J et al. Relevance of early seizures for in-hospital mortality in acute cerebrovascular disease. Neurology 1996; 47: 1429–35 |
| 28 | 2b | Azzimondi G, Bassein L, Nonino F et al. Fever in acute stroke worsens prognosis: a prospective study. Stroke 1995; 26: 2040–3 |

| No. | Level | Citation |
|-----|-------|----------|
| 29 | 1b | Davalos A, Cendra E, Teruel J et al. Deteriorating ischemic stroke: risk factors and prognosis. Neurology 1990; 40: 1865–9 |
| 30 | 1b | Sacco RL, Shi T, Zamanillo MC et al. Predictors of mortality and recurrence after hospitalized cerebral infarction in an urban community: The Northern Manhattan Stroke Study. Neurology 1994; 44: 626–34 |
| 31 | 4 | Koudstaal PJ, van Gijn J, Klootwijk AP et al. Holter monitoring in patients with transient and focal ischaemic attacks of the brain. Stroke 1986; 17: 192–5 |
| 32 | 2a | Panzer RJ, Feibel JH, Barker WH et al. Predicting the likelihood of hemorrhage in patients with stroke. Arch Intern Med 1985; 145: 1800–3 |
| 33 | 2b | Marks MP, Holmgren EB, Fox AJ et al. Evaluation of early computed tomography findings in acute ischemic stroke. Stroke 1999; 30: 389–92 |
| 34 | 4 | Lechat P, Mas JL, Lascault G et al. Prevalence of patent foramen ovale in patients with stroke. N Engl J Med 1988; 318: 1148–52 |
| 35 | 1a | Blakeley DD, Oddone EZ, Hasselblad V et al. Noninvasive carotid artery testing: a meta-analytic review. Ann Intern Med 1995; 122: 360–7 |
| 36 | 1b | Mittl RL, Broderick M, Carpenter JP et al. Blinded-reader comparison of magnetic resonance angiography and duplex ultrasonography for carotid artery bifurcation stenosis. Stroke 1994; 25: 4–10 |
| 37 | 1a | Stroke Unit Trialists' Collaboration. Organised inpatient (stroke unit) care for stroke (Cochrane Review). In: The Cochrane Library, Issue 2, 1999. Oxford: Update Software |
| 38 | 1b | Indredavik B, Bakke F, Slordahl SA, et al. Stroke unit treatment: 10-year follow-up. Stroke 1999; 30: 1524–7 |
| 39 | 1a | Kwakkel G, Wagenaar RC, Koelman TW et al. Effects of intensity of rehabilitation after stroke: a research synthesis. Stroke 1997; 28: 1550–6 |
| 40 | 1b | Walker MF, Gladman JRF, Lincoln NB et al. Occupational therapy for stroke patients not admitted to hospital: a randomised controlled trial. Lancet 1999; 354: 278–80 |
| 41 | 1a | Wardlaw JM, Yamaguchi T, del Zappo G. Thrombolysis for acute ischaemic stroke (Cochrane Review). In: The Cochrane Library, Issue 2, 1999. Oxford: Update Software |
| 42 | 1a – | Wardlaw JM, Yamaguchi T, del Zappo G: Thrombolysis for acute ischaemic stroke. The Cochrane Library, Issue 2, Oxford: Update Software 1999. |
| 43 | 1b – | Kwiatkowski TG, Libman RB, Frankel M et al. Effects of tissue plasminogen activator for acute ischemic stroke at one year. N Engl J Med 1999; 340: 1781–7 |
| 44 | 1a – | Liu M, Wardlaw J. Thrombolysis (different doses, routes of administration and agents) for acute ischaemic stroke (Cochrane Review). In: The Cochrane Library, Issue 2, 1999. Oxford: Update Software |
| 45 | 4 | Schriger DL, Kalafut M, Starkman S et al. Cranial computed tomography interpretation in acute stroke: physician accuracy in determining eligibility for thrombolytic therapy. JAMA 1998; 279: 1293–7 |
| 46 | 1b | Hacke W, Kaste M, Fieschi C et al. Randomised double-blind placebo-controlled trial of thrombolytic therapy with intravenous alteplase in acute ischaemic stroke (ECASS II). Lancet 1998; 352: 1245–51 |
| 47 | 1a – | Asplund K, Israelsson K, Schampi I. Haemodilution for acute ischaemic stroke (Cochrane Review). In: The Cochrane Library, Issue 2, 1999. Oxford: Update Software |

| No. | Level | Citation |
|-----|-------|----------|
| 48 | 1a – | Bath P, Bath F. Prostacyclin and analogues for acute ischaemic stroke (Cochrane Review). In: The Cochrane Library, Issue 2, 1999. Oxford: Update Software |
| 49 | 1a – | Ricci S, Celani MG, Cantisani AT et al. Piracetam for acute ischaemic stroke (Cochrane Review). In: The Cochrane Library, Issue 2, 1999. Oxford: Update Software |
| 50 | 1a – | Bath PMW, Bath FJ, Asplund K. Pentoxifylline, propentofylline and pentifylline for acute ischaemic stroke (Cochrane Review). In: The Cochrane Library, Issue 2, 1999. Oxford: Update Software |
| 51 | 1a – | Liu M, Counsell C, Wardlaw J. Fibrinogen depleting agents for acute ischaemic stroke (Cochrane Review). In: The Cochrane Library, Issue 2, 1999. Oxford: Update Software |
| 52 | 1a – | Qizilbash N, Lewington SL, Lopez-Arrieta JM. Corticosteroids for acute ischaemic stroke (Cochrane Review). In: The Cochrane Library, Issue 2, 1999. Oxford: Update Software |
| 53 | 1a – | Candelise L, Ciccone A. Gangliosides for acute ischaemic stroke (Cochrane Review). In: The Cochrane Library, Issue 2, 1999. Oxford: Update Software |
| 54 | 1a – | Mohiuddin AA, Bath FJ, Bath PMW. Theophylline, aminophylline, caffeine and analogues for acute ischaemic stroke. (Cochrane Review). In: The Cochrane Library, Issue 2, 1999. Oxford: Update Software |
| 55 | 1a – | A Rogvi-Hansen B, Boysen G. Glycerol for acute ischaemic stroke. (Cochrane Review). In: The Cochrane Library, Issue 2, 1999. Oxford: Update Software |
| 56 | 1b – | Morgenstern LB, Frankowski RF, Shedden P et al. Surgical treatment for intracerebral hemorrhage (STICH): a single-centre, randomized clinical trial. Neurology 1998; 51: 1359–63 |
| 57 | 1a – | Prasad K, and Shrivastava A: The Cochrane Library, Issue 2, Oxford: Update Software. Surgery for primary supratentorial intracerebral haemorrhage (Cochrane Review) 1999; 2: |
| 58 | 1b | CAST (Chinese Acute Stroke Trial) Collaborative Group. CAST: randomised placebo-controlled trial of early aspirin use in 20 000 patients with acute ischaemic stroke. Lancet 1997; 349: 1641–9 |
| 59 | 1b – | International Stroke Trial Collaborative Group. The International Stroke Trial (IST): a randomised trial of aspirin, subcutaneous heparin, both, or neither among 19 435 patients with acute ischaemic stroke. Lancet 1997; 349: 1569–81 |
| 60 | 1b | Antiplatelet Trialists' Collaboration. Collaborative overview of randomised trials of antiplatelet therapy I: prevention of death, MI and stroke by prolonged antiplatelet therapy in various categories of patients. BMJ 1994; 308: 81–106 |
| 61 | 1a | Johnson ES, Lanes SF, Wentworth CE et al. A metaregression analysis of the dose response effect of aspirin on stroke. Arch Intern Med 1999; 159: 1248–53 |
| 62 | 1b | Diener H, Cunha L, Forbes C et al. European Stroke Prevention Study 2. Dipyridamole and acetylsalicylic acid in the secondary prevention of stroke. J Neurol Sci 1996; 143: 1–13 |
| 63 | 1b | CAPRIE Steering Committee. A randomised, blinded, trial of clopidogrel versus aspirin in patients at risk of ischaemic events (CAPRIE). Lancet 1996; 348: 1329–39 |
| 64 | 1b | Gent M, Blakely JA, Easton JD et al. The Canadian American ticlopidine study (CATS) in thromboembolic stroke. Lancet 1989; i: 1215–20 |
| 65 | 1b | Hass WK, Easton JD, Adams HP et al. A randomized trial comparing ticlopidine hydrochloride with aspirin for the prevention of stroke in high-risk patients. N Engl J Med 1989; 321: 501–7 |

| No. | Level | Citation |
|-----|-------|----------|
| 66 | 1a | Koudstaal P. Secondary prevention following stroke or transient ischemic attack in patients with nonrheumatic atrial fibrillation: anticoagulant therapy versus control (Cochrane Review). In: The Cochrane Library, Issue 4, 1998. Oxford: Update Software |
| 67 | 1a | Gubitz G, Counsell C, Sandercock P et al. Anticoagulants for acute ischaemic stroke (Cochrane Review). In: The Cochrane Library Issue 1, 1999. Oxford: Update Software |
| 68 | 1a | Liu M, Counsell C, Sandercock P. Anticoagulants for acute ischaemic stroke (Cochrane Review). In: The Cochrane Library, Issue 2, 1999. Oxford: Update Software |
| 69 | 1a | Gubitz G, Counsell C, Sandercock P et al. Anticoagulants for acute ischaemic stroke (Cochrane Review). In: The Cochrane Library, Issue 1, 1999. Oxford: Update Software |
| 70 | 1b – | Cerebral Embolism Study Group. Immediate anticoagulation of embolic stroke: a randomized trial. Stroke 1983; 14: 668–76 |
| 71 | 1b | Morocutti C, Amabile G, Fattapposta F et al. Indobufen versus warfarin in the secondary prevention of major vascular events in nonrheumatic atrial fibrillation. Stroke 1997; 28: 1015–21 |
| 72 | 1a | The INDANA Project Collaborators. Effect of antihypertensive treatment in patients having already suffered from stroke: gathering the evidence. Stroke 1997; 28: 2557–62 |
| 73 | 1a | Hebert PR, Gaziano JM, Chan KS et al. Cholesterol lowering with statin drugs, risk of stroke, and total mortality. JAMA 1997; 278: 313–21 |
| 74 | 1a | Crouse III JR, Byington RP, Hoen HM et al. Reductase inhibitor monotherapy and stroke prevention. Arch Intern Med 1997; 157: 1305–10 |
| 75 | 1b | Kawachi I, Colditz GA, Stampfer MJ et al. Smoking cessation and decreased risk of stroke in women. JAMA 1993; 269: 232–6 |
| 76 | 1a – | Blood Pressure in Acute Stroke Collaboration (BASC). Interventions for deliberately altering blood pressure in acute stroke (Cochrane Review). The Cochrane Library, Issue 2, 1999. Oxford: Update Software |
| 77 | 1b | The Heart Outcomes Prevention Evaluation Study Investigators. Effects of an angiotension-converting-enzyme inhibitor, ramipril on death from cardiovascular causes, myocardial infarction, and stroke in high-risk patients. N Engl J Med 2000; 342: 145–53 |
| 78 | 1a | Cina CS, Clase CM, Haynes RB. Carotid endarterectomy for symptomatic carotid stenosis (Cochrane Review). In: The Cochrane Library, Issue 3, 1999. Oxford: Update Software |
| 79 | 1b | Barnett HJM, Taylor DW, Eliasziw M et al. Benefit of carotid endarterectomy in patients with symptomatic moderate or severe stenosis. N Engl J Med 1998; 339: 1415–25 |
| 80 | 1a | Holloway RG, Benesch CG, Rahilly CR. A systematic review of cost-effectiveness research of stroke evaluation and treatment. Stroke 1999; 30: 1340–9 |
| 81 | 1a | Counsell C, Salinas C, Warlow C, et al. Patch angioplasty versus primary closure for carotid endarterectomy (Cochrane Review). In: The Cochrane Library, Issue 2, 1999. Oxford: Update Software |
| 82 | 1a – | Counsell C, Warlow C, Naylor R. Patches of different types for carotid patch angioplasty (Cochrane Review). In: The Cochrane Library, Issue 2, 1999. Oxford: Update Software |
| 83 | 1b | Taylor DW, Barnett HJM, Haynes RB et al. Low-dose and high-dose acetylsalicylic acid for patients undergoing carotid endarterectomy: a randomised controlled trial. Lancet 1999; 353: 2179–84 |

| No. | Level | Citation |
|-----|-------|----------|
| 84 | 1a – | Counsell C, Salinas R, Naylor R et al. Routine or selective carotid artery shunting for carotid endarterectomy (and different methods of monitoring in selective shunting) (Cochrane Review). In: The Cochrane Library, Issue 2, 1999. Oxford: Update Software |
| 85 | 2a – | Tangkanakul C, Counsell C, Warlow C. Local versus general anaesthesia for carotid endarterectomy (Cochrane Review). In: The Cochrane Library, Issue 2, 1999. Oxford: Update Software |
| 86 | 2b | Hannan EL, Popp AJ, Tranmer B et al. Relationship between provider volume and mortality for carotid endarterectomy in New York State. Stroke 1998; 29: 2292–7 |
| 87 | 2a | Rothwell PM, Slattery J, Warlow CP. Clinical and angiographic predictors of stroke and death from carotid endarterectomy: systematic review. BMJ 1997; 315: 1571–1577 |
| 88 | 2b | Wong JH, Findlay M, Suarez-Almazor ME. Regional performance of carotid endarterectomy: appropriateness, outcomes, and risk factors for complications. Stroke 1997; 28: 891–8 |
| 89 | 2b | Brook RH, Park RE, Chassin MR et al. Carotid endarterectomy for elderly patients: predicting complications. Ann Intern Med 1990; 113: 747–53 |
| 90 | 2b | Wong JH, Findlay M, Suarez-Almazor ME. Regional performance of carotid endarterectomy: appropriateness, outcomes, and risk factors for complications. Stroke 1997; 28: 891–8 |
| 91 | 2b | Brook RH, Park RE, Chassin MR et al. Carotid endarterectomy for elderly patients: predicting complications. Ann Intern Med 1990; 113: 747–53 |
| 92 | 1b | Medaer R, Hellebuyk H, Van Den Brande E et al. Treatment of spasticity due to stroke: a double-blind, cross-over trial comparing baclofen with placebo. Acta Ther 1991; 17: 323–31 |
| 93 | 1b | Burbaud P, Wiart L, Dubos JL et al. A randomised, double blind, placebo controlled trial of botulinum toxin in the treatment of spastic foot in hemiparetic patients. J Neurol Neurosurg Psychiatry 1996; 61: 265–9 |
| 94 | 1b – | Simpson DM, Alexander DN, O'Brien CF et al. Botulinium toxin type A in the treatment of upper extremity spasticity: a randomized, double-blind, placebo-controlled trial. Neurology 1996; 46: 1306–10 |
| 95 | 1b | Johansson K, Lindgren I, Widner H et al. Can sensory stimulation improve the functional outcome in stroke patients? Neurology 1993; 43: 2189–92 |
| 96 | 1b | Norton B, Homer-Ward M, Donnelly MT et al. A randomised prospective comparison of percutaneous endoscopic gastrostomy and nasogastric tube feeding after acute dysphagic stroke. BMJ 1996; 312: 13–16 |
| 97 | 2b | Park RH, Allison MC, Lang J et al. Randomised comparison of percutaneous endoscopic gastrostomy and nasogastric tube feeding in patients with persisting neurological dysphagia. BMJ 1992; 304: 1406–9 |
| 98 | 1b | Park RH, Allison MC, Lang J et al. Randomised comparison of percutaneous endoscopic gastrostomy and nasogastric tube feeding in patients with persisting neurological dysphagia: British Medical Journal 1992; 304: 1406–1409 |
| 99 | 1b – | DePippo KL, Holas MA, Reding MJ et al. Dysphagia therapy following stroke: a controlled trial. Neurology 1994; 44: 1655–60 |
| 100 | 1a – | Moreland JD, Thomson MA, Fuoco AR. Electromyographic biofeedback to improve lower extremity function after stroke: a meta-analysis. Arch Phys Med Rehabil 1998; 79: 134–40 |
| 101 | 1b – | Glanz M, Klawansky S, Stason W et al. Biofeedback therapy in poststroke rehabilitation: a meta-analysis of the randomized controlled trials. Arch Phys Med Rehabil 1995; 76: 508–15 |

| No. | Level | Citation |
|---|---|---|
| 102 | 1b − | Feys HM, De Weerdt WJ, Selz BE et al. Effect of a therapeutic intervention for the hemiplegic upper limb in the acute phase after stroke: a single-blind, randomized, controlled multicenter trial. Stroke 1998; 29: 785–92 |
| 103 | 1b − | Kwakkel G, Wagenaar RC, Twisk JWR et al. Intensity of leg and arm training after primary middle-cereberal-artery stroke: a randomised trial. Lancet 1999; 354: 191–6 |
| 104 | 1b − | Kalra L, Perez I, Gupta S et al. The influence of visual neglect on stroke rehabilitation. Stroke 1997; 28: 1386–1391 |
| 105 | 1a − | Glanz M, Klawansky S, Stason W et al. Functional electrostimulation in poststroke rehabilitation: a meta-analysis of the randomized controlled trials. Arch Phys Med Rehabil 1996; 77: 549–53 |
| 106 | 1b − | Rudd AG, Wolfe CDA, Tiling K et al. Randomised controlled trial to evaluate early discharge scheme for patients with stroke. BMJ 1997; 315: 1039–44 |
| 107 | 4 | Beech R, Rudd AG, Tilling K et al. Economic consequences of early inpatient discharge to community-based rehabilitation for stroke in an inner-London teaching hospital. Stroke 1999; 30: 729–35 |
| 108 | 1b | Young JB, Forster A. The Bradford community stroke trial: results at six months. BMJ 1992; 304: 1085–9 |
| 109 | 1a − | Langhorne P, Dennis MS, Kalra L et al. Services for helping acute stroke patients avoid hospital admission (Cochrane Review). In: The Cochrane Library, Issue 4, 1999. Oxford: Update Software |
| 110 | 1b − | Dennis M, O'Rourke S, Slattery J et al. Evaluation of a stroke family care worker: results of a randomised controlled trial. BMJ 1997; 314: 1071–7 |
| 111 | 2b | Yamamoto H, Bogousslavsky J, van Melle G. Different predictors of neurological worsening in different causes of stroke. Arch Neurol 1998; 55: 481–3 |
| 112 | 1b | Davalos A, Cendra E, Teruel J et al. Deteriorating ischemic stroke: risk factors and prognosis. Neurology 1990; 40: 1865–9 |
| 113 | 1b | Qureshi AI, Safdar K, Weil J et al. Predictors of early deterioration and mortality in black Americans with spontaneous intracerrebral hemorrhage. Stroke 1995; 26: 1764–7 |
| 114 | 1b | Qureshi AI, Safdar K, Weil J et al. Predictors of early deterioration and mortality in black Americans with spontaneous intracerrebral hemorrhage. Stroke 1995; 26: 1764–7 |
| 115 | 2b | Ween JE, Alexander MP, D'Esposito M et al. Factors predictive of stroke outcome in a rehabilitation setting. Neurology 1996; 47: 388–92 |
| 116 | 2b | Saeki S, Ogata H, Okubo T et al. Return to work after stroke: a follow-up study. Stroke 1995; 26: 399–401 |
| 117 | 2b | Kotila M, Numminen H, Waltimo O et al. Depression after stroke: results of the FINNSTROKE study. Stroke 1998; 29: 368–72 |
| 118 | 2b | Kauhanen M, Korpelainen JT, Hiltunen P et al. Poststroke depression correlates with cognitive impairment and neurological deficits. Stroke 1999; 30: 1875–80 |
| 119 | 2c | Bornstein NM, Gur AY, Treves TA et al. Do silent brain infarctions predict the development of dementia after first ischaemic stroke? Stroke 1996; 27: 904–5 |
| 120 | 1b | Burn J, Dennis M, Bamford J et al. Epileptic seizures after a first stroke: the Oxfordshire community stroke project. BJM 1997; 315: 1582–7 |

| No. | Level | Citation |
|-----|-------|----------|
| 121 | 2b | Arboix A, Garcia-Eroles L, Massons JB et al. Predictive factors of early seizures after acute cerebrovascular diseases. Stroke 1997; 28: 1590–4 |
| 122 | 2b | So EL, Annegers JF, Hauser WA et al. Population-based study of seizure disorders after cerebral infarction. Neurology 1996; 46: 350–5 |
| 123 | 2b | Petty GW, Brown RD, Whisnant JP et al. Survival and recurrence after first cerebral infarction: a population-based study in Rochester, Minnesota, 1975 through 1989. Neurology 1998; 50: 208–16 |
| 124 | 2c | Burn J, Dennis M, Bamford J et al. Long-term risk of recurrent stroke after a first-ever stroke: the Oxfordshire community stroke project. Stroke 1994; 25: 333–7 |
| 125 | 1b | Prencipe M, Culasso F, Rasura M et al. Long-term prognosis after a minor stroke: 10-year mortality and major stroke recurrence rates in a hospital-based cohort. Stroke 1998; 29: 126–32 |
| 126 | 1b | Kernan WN, Horwitz RI, Brass LM et al. A prognostic system for transient ischemia or minor stroke. Ann Intern Med 1991; 114: 552–7 |
| 127 | 1b | Hier DB, Foulkes MA, Swiontoniowski M et al. Stroke recurrence within 2 years after ischemic infarction. Stroke 1991; 22: 155–61 |
| 128 | 1b | Matchar DB, Divine GW, Heyman A et al. The influence of hyperglycemia on outcome of cerebral infarction. Ann Intern Med 1992; 117: 449–56 |
| 129 | 1b | Arboix A, Comes E, Massons J et al. Relevance of early seizures for in-hospital mortality in acute cerebrovascular disease. Neurology 1996; 47: 1429–35 |
| 130 | 1b | Dippel DWJ, Koudstaal PJ. We need stronger predictors of major vascular events in patients with a recent transient ischaemic attack or nondisabling stroke. Stroke 1997; 28: 774–6 |
| 131 | 1b | Lin H-J, Wolf PA, Kelly-Hayes M et al. Stroke severity in atrial fibrillation: The Framingham Study. Stroke 1996; 27: 1760–4 |
| 132 | 2b | Toni D, Fiorelli M, Bastianello S et al. Acute ischaemic strokes improving during the first 48 hours of onset: predictability, outcome, and possible mechanism. Stroke 1997; 28: 10–14 |

## CAUSES

Syncope is a transient loss of consciousness. Common causes of syncope include [B]1-3:

- cardiovascular
  - arrhythmias (tachycardias and bradycardias)
  - aortic stenosis
  - myocardial infarction
  - aortic dissection
  - pulmonary embolism
- neurological
  - seizure
  - transient ischaemic attack
  - subclavian steal
  - carotid sinus hypersensitivity
- non-cardiovascular
  - vasovagal
  - orthostatic hypotension
  - drugs
  - situational syncope (micturition, defecation, post-prandial)
  - psychogenic
  - hypoglycaemia.

**Note**
Common causes include vasovagal syncope and arrhythmias

| Cause | Medical referral [B]1 | Emergency department [B]2 | Elderly in a long-term care facility [B]3 | Young [C]4 |
|---|---|---|---|---|
| *Cardiovascular* | 25% | | | 3% |
| ■ arrhythmia | | 4% | 7% | |
| – ventricular tachycardia | 11% | | | |
| – sick sinus syndrome | 3% | | | |
| – bradycardia, 2nd-or 3rd-degree heart block | 3% | | | |
| – supraventricular tachycardia | 2% | | | |
| ■ aortic stenosis | 2% | | 5% | |
| *Neurological* | | | | |
| ■ seizure disorder | 2% | 9% | 3% | |
| ■ TIAs | 2% | | | |
| *Non-cardiovascular* | 29% | | | |
| ■ vasovagal syncope | 8% | 37% | | 12% |
| ■ situational syncope | 7% | | | 3% |
| – micturition | | 2% | | |
| – defecation | | | 5% | |
| – post-prandial | | | 8% | |
| ■ orthostatic hypotension | 10% | 8% | 6% | 2% |
| ■ drug-induced syncope | 2% | | 11% | 0% |
| ■ volume depletion | | | 4% | |
| ■ hypoglycaemic | | 2% | | |
| ■ psychiatric | 0.7% | 0.6% | | 39% |
| *unknown* | 41% | 38% | 26% | 33% |

## CLINICAL FEATURES

Perform a careful history and physical examination **[C]**[5].

**Why?**
- 45% of patients with syncope can have a diagnosis made on the basis of history and physical examination alone (95% CI: 40% to 49%)**[C]**[5].

Ask about:
- the syncopal episode and situation **[D]**, particularly
- any nausea or vomiting before collapse **[A]**[6]

**Why?**
**Lack of nausea and vomiting increases the risk of an arrhythmia**

| Patient **[A]**[5] | Prognostic factor | Outcome | Control rate | RR (95% CI) | NNF+(95% CI) |
|---|---|---|---|---|---|
| Unexplained syncope | Absence of nausea or vomiting before syncope *independent* | Syncope due to cardiac arrhythmia at 1 year | 20% | 7.1 (1.6 to 33.3) | 2 (1 to 12) |

- whether the syncopal episode occurred on exertion **[B]**[7]

**Why?**
**Exertional syncope makes aortic stenosis much more likely**

| Patient **[B]**[7] | Target disorder (reference standard) | Diagnostic test | LR+ (95% CI) | Post-test probability | LR– (95% CI) | Post-test probability |
|---|---|---|---|---|---|---|
| Elderly patient with syncope (pre-test probability 5%) | Aortic stenosis (imaging studies) | Effort syncope | Infinity (1.3 to infinity) | 100% | 0.76 (0.67 to 0.86) | 4% |

- any tongue biting, post-collapse disorientation or 'blueness' if collapse observed **[C]**[8]

**Why?**
Tongue biting and disorientation make collapse likely to be seizures

| Patient [C][8] | Target disorder (reference standard) | Diagnostic test | LR+ (95% CI) | Post-test probability | LR– (95% CI) | Post-test probability |
|---|---|---|---|---|---|---|
| Patients with recurrent collapse ?seizure (pre-test probability 9%) | Seizure (composite reference standard) | Tongue biting | 7.3 (2.3 to 23) | 42% | 0.62 (0.48 to 0.81) | 6% |
| | | Witnessed disorientation after the event | 5.03 (2.7 to 9.2) | 33% | 0.18 (0.08 to 0.37) | 1.7% |
| | | Witnessed 'blueness' during event | 16 (2.1 to 110) | 61% | 0.72 (0.59 to 0.88) | 6.6% |

- when the patient last ate [A][9]

**Why?**
- Post-prandial hypotension occurs in a third of elderly patients – around 1% become symptomatic from this [A][9].

- any cardiovascular disease, particularly
  - known arrhythmias [A][10]

**Why?**
- Ventricular arrhythmias increase the risk of dying.
- Three-quarters of patients with sick sinus syndrome are symptomatic – commonly with syncope (45%), palpitations (30%) or light-headedness (27%) [C][11].
- Symptoms of dizziness and fainting do not help predict arrhythmias [A][12].

  - heart failure [A][13]
  - ischaemic heart disease [A][13]
  - aortic stenosis [D]

**Why?**
Heart failure and ischaemic heart disease increase the risk of dying

| Patient [A][13] | Prognostic factor | Outcome | Control rate | OR (95% CI) | NNF+(95% CI) |
|---|---|---|---|---|---|
| Unexplained syncope | Congestive heart failure *independent* | Death at 2 years | 16% | 4 (1.9 to 8.1) | 4 (2 to 10) |
| Unexplained syncope | Mild heart disease *independent* | Death at 1 year | 9% | 77 (1.6 to 36.4) | 2 (1 to 19) |
| | Severe heart disease *independent* | Death at 1 year | | 13.5 (2.6 to 70.5) | 1 (1 to 7) |

- chest pain **[D]**

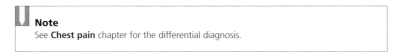

**Note**

See **Chest pain** chapter for the differential diagnosis.

- previous episodes of syncope **[A]**[5] or seizures **[D]**

**Why?**

**Frequently recurrent syncope increases the risk of recurrence**

| Patient **[A]**[5] | Prognostic factor | Outcome | Control rate | OR (95% CI) | NNF+ (95% CI) |
|---|---|---|---|---|---|
| Syncope | 4 or more episodes of syncope in last year *independent* | Recurrent syncope at 1 year | 34% | 3.8 (2.1 to 7.0) | 1 (1 to 3) |

- previous psychiatric problems **[C]**[14]

**Why?**

- Psychiatric problems account for some unexplained cases: 24% of patients have evidence of major depression or panic disorder (95% CI: 14% to 33%) **[C]**[14].

**Two or more psychiatric diagnoses increase the risk of recurrent syncope**

| Patient **[A]**[5] | Prognostic factor | Outcome | Control rate | OR (95% CI) | NNF+(95% CI) |
|---|---|---|---|---|---|
| Syncope | 2 or more psychiatric diagnoses *independent* | Recurrent syncope at 1 year | 34% | 2.3 (1.0 to 1.6) | 2 (5 to infinity) |

- current medication use **[B]**[3] **[B]**[15]

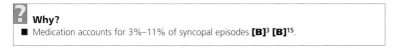

**Why?**

- Medication accounts for 3%–11% of syncopal episodes **[B]**[3] **[B]**[15].

- family history of unexplained syncope or sudden death **[C]**[16].

**Why?**
- Long QT syndrome is a rare, inherited but treatable cause of syncope and sudden death.
- 80% of patients experience syncope, 45% have a family history of sudden death at <50 years [C][16].

Look for:

- cardiovascular causes:
  - an irregular [B][17] or slow-rising pulse [B][3]
  - apical-carotid delay [B][3]

**Why?**

**An irregular pulse makes an arrhythmia more likely**

| Patient[B][17] | Target disorder (reference standard) | Diagnostic test | LR+ (95% CI) | Post-test probability | LR– (95% CI) | Post-test probability |
|---|---|---|---|---|---|---|
| Undergoing Holter monitoring (pre-test probability 53%) | Arrhythmia (Holter monitoring) | Irregular pulse | 8.9 (1.2 to 69) | 91% | 0.97 (0.94 to 0.99) | 52% |

- No other clinical features usefully diagnose or exclude arrhythmias.

**A slow-rising carotid pulse and apical-carotid delay help diagnose aortic stenosis**

| Patient [B][3] | Target disorder (reference standard) | Diagnostic test | LR+ (95% CI) | Post-test probability | LR– (95% CI) | Post-test probability |
|---|---|---|---|---|---|---|
| Elderly patient with syncope (pre-test probability 5%) | Aortic stenosis (imaging studies) | Slow rise of carotid pulse | 130 (33 to 560) | 87% | 0.62 (0.51 to 0.75) | 3% |
| | | Apical-carotid delay | Infinity (2.4 to infinity) | 100% | 0.05 (0.01 to 0.31) | 0.3% |

- heart murmurs, particularly aortic stenosis [B][3]:
  - listen for a reduced or absent second heart sound, or a fourth heart sound
  - listen for a murmur loudest in late systole and radiating to the right carotid

**Why?**

**Heart sounds and a murmur loudest in late systole help diagnose aortic stenosis**

| Patient [B][3] | Target disorder (reference standard) | Diagnostic test | LR+ (95% CI) | Post-test probability | LR−(95% CI) | Post-test probability |
|---|---|---|---|---|---|---|
| Elderly patient with syncope (pre-test probability 5%) | Aortic stenosis (imaging studies) | Reduced or absent 2nd heart sound | 50 (24 to 100) | 72% | 0.45 (0.34 to 0.58) | 2% |
| | | 4th heart sound | 2.5 (2.1 to 3.0) | 12% | 0.26 (0.14 to 0.49) | 1% |
| | | Any murmur | 2.4 (2.2 to 2.7) | 11% | 0.0 (0.0 to 0.13) | 0% |
| | | Murmur loudest in late systole | 100 (25 to 410) | 84% | 0.31 (0.22 to 0.44) | 2% |
| | | Radiation to right carotid | 1.4 (1.3 to 1.5) | 7% | 0.10 (0.13 to 0.40) | 0.5% |

- injuries
- neurological causes
  - decreased level of consciousness [D] and any focal neurological signs [D]

- other causes
  - perform carotid sinus massage to look for carotid sinus hypersensitivity [D] – it is safe [B][18]

**Why?**

■ Few patients have a TIA or minor stroke following carotid sinus massage, and most neurological deficits recover (0.44%; 95% CI: 0.11% to 0.76%) [B][18].

- orthostatic hypotension [B][2] [B][3] [B][15].

## INVESTIGATIONS

- Blood count [D].
- Urea and electrolytes, creatinine [D].
- Glucose [D].
- Cardiac enzymes [B] (see **Myocardial Infaction** chapter for more details).
- Creatinine kinase [A][19]

| **❓ Why?**<br>**A raised CK makes a seizure much more likely** | | | | | | |
|---|---|---|---|---|---|---|
| Patient **[A]**[19] | Target disorder (reference standard) | Diagnostic test | LR+ (95% CI) | Post-test probability | LR− (95% CI) | Post-test probability |
| Transient loss of consciousness (pre-test probability 44%) | Tonic-clonic seizure (chart review) | CK ≥ 188 units/litre | 23 (3.2 to 170) | 95% | 0.58 (0.45 to 0.76) | 31% |

- 12-lead ECG. Look for:
  - ischaemic changes **[A]**[20]
  - evidence of arrhythmias **[A]**.

| **❓ Why?**<br>■ An ECG helps diagnose a cause in 11% of cases (95% CI: 7% to 15%) **[B]**[15]. | | | | | | |
|---|---|---|---|---|---|---|
| **No ischaemic changes on the first ECG make acute cardiac ischaemia less likely** | | | | | | |
| Patient **[A]**[21] | Target disorder (reference standard) | Diagnostic test | LR+ (95% CI) | Post-test probability | LR− (95% CI) | Post-test probability |
| Transient loss of consciousness (pre-test probability 7%) | Cardiac ischaemia (serial ECG, cardiac enzymes and records) | Ischaemic abnormalities on ECG | 2.1 (1.8 to 2.4) | 14% | 0.0 (0.0 to 0.29) | 0% |

| **An abnormal ECG increases the risk of an arrhythmia** | | | | | |
|---|---|---|---|---|---|
| Patient **[A]**[5] | Prognostic factor | Outcome | Control rate | RR (95% CI) | NNF+ (95% CI) |
| Unexplained syncope | Abnormalities on ECG *independent* | Syncope due to cardiac arrhythmia at 1 year | 20% | 23.5 (7.0 to 78.7) | 2 (1 to 2) |

Consider the following if seizures are suspected:

- EEG **[C]**[22]
- hyperventilation test (at least two symptoms associated with episode reproduced) **[C]**[22].

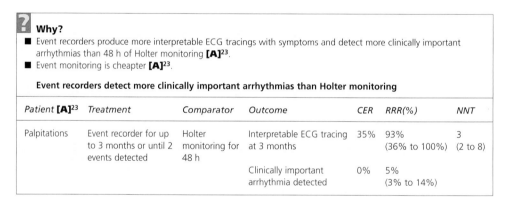

**Why?**
Epileptiform features on an EEG makes a seizure more likely, and a positive hyperventilation test less likely

| Patient [C][22] | Target disorder (reference standard) | Diagnostic test | LR+ (95% CI) | Post-test probability | LR– (95% CI) | Post-test probability |
|---|---|---|---|---|---|---|
| Unexplained transient loss of consciousness (pre-test probability 38%) | Seizure (clinical features) | Epileptiform EEG | 7.4 (2.7 to 21) | 82% | 0.63 (0.50 to 0.81) | 28% |
| | | Hyperventilation test | 0.29 (0.13 to 0.62) | 15% | 1.9 (1.4 to 2.8) | 54% |

If there is no clear cause, consider:

- event recorders [A][23]

**Why?**
- Event recorders produce more interpretable ECG tracings with symptoms and detect more clinically important arrhythmias than 48 h of Holter monitoring [A][23].
- Event monitoring is cheaper [A][23].

**Event recorders detect more clinically important arrhythmias than Holter monitoring**

| Patient [A][23] | Treatment | Comparator | Outcome | CER | RRR(%) | NNT |
|---|---|---|---|---|---|---|
| Palpitations | Event recorder for up to 3 months or until 2 events detected | Holter monitoring for 48 h | Interpretable ECG tracing at 3 months | 35% | 93% (36% to 100%) | 3 (2 to 8) |
| | | | Clinically important arrhythmia detected | 0% | 5% (3% to 14%) | |

or Holter monitoring [B][15] worn for at least 24 h [C][24].

**Why?**
- Holter monitoring over 72 h detects twice as many arrhythmias as monitoring for 24 h [C][24].
- It can help diagnose a cause in 27% of cases (95% CI: 21% to 33%) [B][14].

| Day [C][24] | Major arrhythmia detected (95% CI) |
|---|---|
| 1 | 15% (8.3% to 23%) |
| 2 | 11% (5.1% to 20%) |
| 3 | 4.2% (0.8% to 12%) |

**Note**

- Symptoms of dizziness and fainting are common in patients with syncope, but few are associated with arrhythmias (1.0%; 95% CI: 0.49% to 1.5%) **[C]**[25].

**Dizziness and fainting make a major arrhythmia less likely**

| Patient **[C]**[25] | Target disorder (reference standard) | Diagnostic test | LR+ (95% CI) | Post-test probability | LR– (95% CI) | Post-test probability |
|---|---|---|---|---|---|---|
| Unexplained syncope (pre-test probability 9%) | Major arrhythmia (24 h ECG) | Dizziness and fainting | 0.25 (0.12 to 0.56) | 2% | 1.2 (1.1 to 1.2) | 10% |

There is no clear benefit from:

- tilt table testing **[B]**[26]

**Why?**

- Patients with a history of syncope have a positive test more often than healthy controls **[A]**[26].
- Those with a positive test are not clearly different in terms of prognosis **[C]**[27].
- Treatment regimens for recurrent syncope have only been tested on patients with positive tilt tests **[A]**[29] **[A]**[30] **[A]**[31].

- electrophysiological studies **[B]**[32]

**Why?**

- Electrophysiological studies detect abnormal rhythms in many patients with unexplained syncope **[C]**[33] **[C]**[34], but few are true arrhythmias (24%; 95% CI: 4% to 43%) and electrophysiological studies induce many unrelated ones (14%; 95% CI: 0% to 30%) **[B]**[35].
- Abnormal studies do not clearly predict further syncopal episodes or mortality **[C]**[33].
- 20% of patients require DC cardioversion out of induced arrhythmias **[B]**[36].

- signal-averaged ECG **[A]**[37].

**Why?**

- It does not usefully predict inducible ventricular tachycardia on electrophysiological study **[A]**[37].

**THERAPY**

- Treat individual diagnoses appropriately **[D]**.
- Insert a pacemaker in patients with severe recurrent vasovagal syncope **[A]**[29].

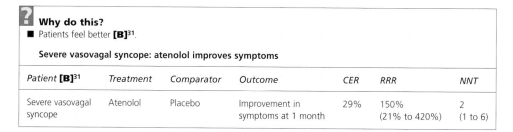

**? Why do this?**
■ It reduces recurrent episodes **[A]**[29].

**Severe vasovagal syncope: a permanent pacemaker reduces recurrent episodes**

| Patient **[A]**[29] | Treatment | Comparator | Outcome | CER | RRR | NNT |
|---|---|---|---|---|---|---|
| Recurrent vasovagal syncope (at least 6 episodes) | Permanent pacemaker | No pacemaker | Recurrent syncope at 12 months | 70% | 68% (33% to 85%) | 2 (1 to 4) |

Alternatives include:
● atenolol **[B]**[31]

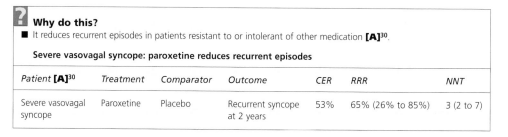

**? Why do this?**
■ Patients feel better **[B]**[31].

**Severe vasovagal syncope: atenolol improves symptoms**

| Patient **[B]**[31] | Treatment | Comparator | Outcome | CER | RRR | NNT |
|---|---|---|---|---|---|---|
| Severe vasovagal syncope | Atenolol | Placebo | Improvement in symptoms at 1 month | 29% | 150% (21% to 420%) | 2 (1 to 6) |

● paroxetine **[A]**[30].

**? Why do this?**
■ It reduces recurrent episodes in patients resistant to or intolerant of other medication **[A]**[30].

**Severe vasovagal syncope: paroxetine reduces recurrent episodes**

| Patient **[A]**[30] | Treatment | Comparator | Outcome | CER | RRR | NNT |
|---|---|---|---|---|---|---|
| Severe vasovagal syncope | Paroxetine | Placebo | Recurrent syncope at 2 years | 53% | 65% (26% to 85%) | 3 (2 to 7) |

## PROGNOSIS

Recurrent episodes are common **[A]**[38] and can be distressing **[C]**[39].

**Note**
■ A third of patients who attend hospital with syncope have another episode, many within 1 year (34%; 95% CI: 29% to 38%) **[A]**[38].
■ Patients typically have more than one recurrence – in one study a mean of seven over 2.5 years **[A]**[38].
■ However, no one specific cause of syncope favours recurrence, and recurrent syncope is not clearly associated with death or major morbidity **[A]**[38] **[A]**[40].
■ Recurrent syncope is associated with raised levels of psychosocial and physical distress **[C]**[39].

Recurrent syncope is more likely if [A][5]:

- patient aged 45 or less
- four or more episodes of syncope in the last year
- two or more psychiatric diagnoses.

---

**? Why?**

Recurrent syncope, psychiatric problems and a young age increase the risk of recurrence

| Patient [A][5] | Prognostic factor | Outcome | Control rate | OR (95% CI) | NNF+ (95% CI) |
|---|---|---|---|---|---|
| Syncope | Aged 45 or less *independent* | Recurrent syncope at 1 year | 34% | 1.9 (1.1 to 3.4) | 3 (1 to 29) |
| | 4 or more episodes of syncope in the last year *independent* | Recurrent syncope at 1 year | 34% | 3.8 (2.1 to 7.0) | 1 (1 to 3) |
| | 2 or more psychiatric diagnoses *independent* | Recurrent syncope at 1 year | 34% | 2.3 (1.0 to 1.6) | 2 (5 to inf) |

---

Use the following clinical prediction rule to rank patients for risk of cardiac arrhythmia or death (Table 1) [A][10]:

- aged > 45 years
- history of congestive heart failure
- history of ventricular arrhythmias
- abnormal ECG
  - atrial fibrillation or flutter, or multifocal atrial tachycardia
  - junctional or paced rhythm
  - frequent or repetitive PVC (including ventricular tachycardia)
  - PR interval < 0.10 mm
  - Mobitz I with other abnormalities, Mobitz II or complete heart block
  - conduction disorder: left axis deviation, bundle-branch block, intraventricular delay
  - ventricular hypertrophy
  - old myocardial infarction.

**Table 1 Risk of arrhythmia or death**

| Risk factors [A][10] | Risk of arrhythmia within a year | Risk of dying within a year |
|---|---|---|
| 3+ | High | High |
| 2 | Medium | Medium |
| 1 | Low | Low |
| 0 | Low | Low |

**Note**

**Four factors can help predict arrhythmia and death**

| Risk factors [A][10] | Arrhythmia within a year | NNF (95% CI) | Death at 1 year (95% CI) | NNF (95% CI) |
|---|---|---|---|---|
| 3+ | 45% (29% to 62%) | 2 (2 to 4) | 27% (12% to 43%) | 4 (2 to 8) |
| 2 | 18% (12% to 25%) | 5 (4 to 8) | 16% (10% to 22%) | 6 (4 to 10) |
| 1 | 6% (2% to 11%) | 15 (9 to 64) | 8% (3% to 14%) | 12 (7 to 32) |
| 0 | 3% (0% to 7%) | 30 (14 to infinity) | 1% (0% to 3%) | 91 (31 to infinity) |

Cardiac arrhythmias are a common cause of unexplained syncope and are more likely with [A][5]:

- no history of nausea or vomiting prior to syncope
- an abnormal ECG.

**Note**

■ A fifth of patients with unexplained syncope will go on to be diagnosed with a cardiac arrhythmia (20%; 95% CI: 15 to 25%) [A][5] [A][10].

**Lack of nausea and vomiting and an abnormal ECG increase the risk of an arrhythmia**

| Patient [A][5] | Prognostic factor | Outcome | Control rate | RR (95% CI) | NNF+ (95% CI) |
|---|---|---|---|---|---|
| Unexplained syncope | Absence of nausea or vomiting before syncope *independent* | Syncope due to cardiac arrhythmia at 1 year | 20% | 7.1 (1.6 to 33.3) | 2 (1 to 12) |
| | Abnormalities on ECG *independent* | Syncope due to cardiac arrhythmia at 1 year | 20% | 23.5 (7.0 to 78.7) | 2 (1 to 2) |

Death is relatively common in the next year [A][5] [A][10][A][15], particularly suddenly [A][9].

**Note**

■ Around 1 in 10 patients presenting to the emergency department with syncope unexplained on history and examination are dead within 1 year (9% to 14%) [A][5] [A][9] [A][14]; 1 in 13 die suddenly (7%; 95% CI: 4% to 10%) [A][9].

Death is more likely with:

- age > 45 years [A][10]
- heart disease [A][5]

| **Why?** Heart disease increases the risk of dying | | | | | |
|---|---|---|---|---|---|
| *Patient* **[A]**[5] | *Prognostic factor* | *Outcome* | *Control rate* | *RR (95% CI)* | *NNF+ (95% CI)* |
| Unexplained syncope | Mild heart disease *independent* | Death at 1 year | 9% | 7.7 (1.6 to 36.4) | 2 (1 to 19) |
| | Severe heart disease *independent* | | | 13.5 (2.6 to 70.5) | 1 (1 to 7) |

- congestive heart failure **[A]**[13] or left ventricular ejection fraction <30% **[A]**[41]
- a history of cardiac arrhythmias **[A]**[10]
- serum creatinine > 177 μmol/l **[A]**[11]
- an abnormal ECG **[A]**[10], particularly
  - frequent (> 10/h) or repetitive (≥2 consecutive) premature ventricular contractions **[A]**[12]
  - sinus pause > 2 s **[A]**[13].

| **Why?** Heart and renal failure and certain arrhythmias increase the risk of dying | | | | | |
|---|---|---|---|---|---|
| *Patient* **[A]**[13] | *Prognostic factor* | *Outcome* | *Control rate* | *OR (95% CI)* | *NNF+(95% CI)* |
| Unexplained syncope | Congestive heart failure *independent* | Death at 2 years | 16% | 4 (1.9 to 8.1) | 4 (2 to 10) |
| | Creatinine > 2.0 mg/dl *independent* | Death at 2 years | 16% | 7.9 (3.3 to 18.9) | 2 (2 to 4) |
| | Frequent or repetitive PVCs *independent* | Death at 2 years | 16% | 3.7 (1.8 to 7.5) | 4 (2 to 11) |
| | Sinus pause > 2 s *independent* | Death at 2 years | 16% | 3.3 (1.1 to 9.6) | 4 (2 to 77) |

| **Frequent or repetitive premature ventricular contractions increase the risk of sudden death** | | | | | |
|---|---|---|---|---|---|
| *Patient* **[A]**[13] | *Prognostic factor* | *Outcome* | *Control rate* | *OR (95% CI)* | *NNF+(95% CI)* |
| Unexplained syncope | Frequent or repetitive PVCs *independent* | Sudden death at 2 years | 7% | 14.9 (4 to 55.7) | 2 (1 to 6) |

If no cardiovascular or neurological cause is found following investigation, recurrences are rare **[A]**[40].

| **Note** |
|---|
| ■ 3.3% of patients with isolated syncope in the community (no cardiovascular or neurological cause if found) have a recurrent episode over 26 years (95% CI: 2.8% to 3.8%) **[A]**[40]. |

**Guideline writer**: Christopher Ball
**CAT writers**: Christopher Ball, Robert Phillips, Clare Wotton

## REFERENCES

| No. | Level | Citation |
| --- | --- | --- |
| 1 | 2b | Kapoor WN. Evaluation of patients with syncope. Medicine 1990; 69: 160–175 |
| 2 | 2b | Martin GJ et al. Prospective evaluation of syncope. Ann Emerg Med 1984; 13: 499–504 |
| 3 | 3b | Lipsitz LA et al. Syncope in institutionalised elderly: the impact of multiple pathological conditions and situational stress. J Chronic Dis 1986; 39: 619–30 |
| 4 | 4 | Koenig D et al. Syncope in young adults: evidence for a combined medical and psychiatric approach. J Intern Med 1992; 232: 169–76 |
| 5 | 4 | Oh JH, Hanusa BH, Kapoor WN. Do symptoms predict cardiac arrhythmias and mortality in patients with syncope? Arch Intern Med 1999; 159: 375–80 |
| 6 | 1a | Oh JH, Hanusa BH, Kapoor WN. Do symptoms predict cardiac arrhythmias and mortality in patients with syncope? Arch of Intern Med 1999; 159: 375–80 |
| 7 | 2a | Etchells E et al. Does this patient have an abnormal systolic murmur? JAMA 1997; 277: 564–71 |
| 8 | 4 | Hoefnagales WA et al. Transient loss of consciousness: the value of history for distinguishing seizure from syncope. J Neurol 1991; 238: 39–43 |
| 9 | 1b | Vaitkevicius PV et al. Frequency and importance of post-prandial blood pressure reduction in elderly nursing-home patients. Ann Intern Med 1991; 115: 865–70 |
| 10 | 1a | Martin TP et al. Risk stratification of patients with syncope. Ann Emerg Med 1997; 29: 459–66 |
| 11 | 4 | Rubenstein JJ et al. Clinical spectrum of the sick sinus syndrome. Circulation 72; 46: 5–11 |
| 12 | 1b | Clark PI et al. Arrhythmias detected by ambulatory monitoring: lack of correlation with symptoms of dizziness and syncope. Chest 1980; 77: 722–4 |
| 13 | 1b | Kapoor WN et al. Prolonged ECG monitoring in patients with syncope: importance of frequency or repetition of ventricular ectopy. Am J Med 1987; 82: 20–8 |
| 14 | 4 | Linzer M et al. Psychiatric syncope: a new look at an old disease. Psychosomatics 1990; 31: 181–8 |
| 15 | 2c | Kapoor WN, Karpf M, Wieand S et al. Prospective evaluation and follow-up of patients with syncope. N Engl J Med 1983; 309: 197–204 |
| 16 | 4 | Moss AJ et al. The long QT syndrome prospective longitudinal study of 328 families. Circulation 1991; 84: 1136–44 |
| 17 | 2b | Zeldis SM et al. Cardiovascular complaints: correlation with 24 hour electrocardiographic monitoring. Chest 1980; 78: 456–62 |
| 18 | 2b | Munro NC et al. Incidence of complications after carotid sinus massage in older patients with syncope. J Am Geriatr Soc 1994; 42: 1248–51 |
| 19 | 1b | Libman MD et al. Seizure versus syncope: measuring serum creatinine kinase in the emergency department. J Gen Intern Med 1991; 6: 408–12 |

| No. | Level | Citation |
| --- | --- | --- |
| 20 | 1b | Georgeson S et al. Acute cardiac ischemia in patients with syncope: importance of initial electrocardiogram. J Gen Intern Med 1992; 7: 379–86 |
| 21 | 1b | Georgeson S et al. Acute cardiac ischemia in patients with syncope: importance of initial electrocardiogram. J Gen Intern Med 1992; 7: 379–86 |
| 22 | 4 | Hoefnagles WA et al. Syncope or seizure? The diagnostic value of the EEG and hyperventilation test in transient loss of consciousness. J Neurol Neurosurg Psychiatry 1991; 54: 953–6 |
| 23 | 1b | Event recorders provided better data and were more cost-effective than 48-hour Holter monitoring in detecting arrhythmias. Evidence-Based Med 1996 July-Aug; 1: 159. Summary of: Kinlay S et al. Cardiac event recorders yield more diagnoses and are more cost-effective than 48-hour Holter monitoring in patients with palpitations. A controlled clinical trial. Ann Intern Med 1996; 124: 16–20 |
| 24 | 4 | Bach E et al. The duration of Holter monitoring in patients with syncope: is 24 hours long enough? Arch Intern Med 1990; 150: 1073–8 |
| 25 | 4 | Gibson TC, Heitzman MR. Diagnostic efficacy of 24 hour electrocardiographic monitoring for syncope. Am J Cardiol 1984; 53: 1013–17 |
| 26 | 2a | Kapoor WN et al. Upright tilt testing in evaluating syncope: a comprehensive literature review. Am J Med 1994; 97: 78–88 |
| 27 | 1b | Oribe E, Caro S, Perera R et al. Syncope: the diagnostic value of head-up tilt testing. PACE 1997; 20(1): 874–79 |
| 28 | 4 | Grimm W, Degenhardt M, Hoffman J et al. Syncope recurrence can better be predicted by history than by head-up tilt testing in untreated patients with neurally-mediated syncope. Eur Heart J 1997; 18: 1465–69 |
| 29 | 1b | Connolly SJ, Sheldon R, Roberts RS et al. The North American Vasovagal Pacemaker Study (VPS): a randomized trial of permanent cardiac pacing for the prevention of vasovagal syncope. J Am Coll Cardiol 1999; 33: 16–20 |
| 30 | 1b | Di Girolamo E et al. Effects of paroxetine hydrochloride, a selective serotonin reuptake inhibitor on refractory vasovagal syncope: a randomized, double-blind, placebo-controlled study. J Am Coll Cardiol 1999; 33: 1227–30 |
| 31 | 2b | Mahonda N et al. Randomised double-blind, placebo controlled study of oral atenolol in patients with unexplained syncope and +ve upright tilt-table test results. Am Heart J 1995; 130: 1250–3 |
| 32 | 2b | Fujimara O et al. The diagnostic sensitivity of electrophysiologic testing in patients with syncope caused by transient bradycardia. N Engl J Med 1989; 321: 1703–7 |
| 33 | 4 | Doherty JU et al. Electophysiologic evaluation and follow-up characteristics of patients with recurrent unexplained syncope or presyncope. Am J Cardiol 1985; 55: 703–8 |
| 34 | 4 | Denes P, Ezri MD. The role of electrophysiologic studies in the management of patients with unexplained syncope. Pacing Clin Electrophysiol 1985; 8: 424–35 |
| 35 | 2b | Fujimara O et al. The diagnostic sensitivity of electrophysiologic testing in patients with syncope caused by transient bradycardia. N Engl J Med 1989; 321: 1703–7 |

| No. | Level | Citation |
| --- | --- | --- |
| 36 | 2c | Horowitz LN et al. Risks and complications of clinical cardiac electrophysiologic studies: a prospective analysis of 1000 consecutive patients. J Am Coll Cardiol 1987; 9: 1261–8 |
| 37 | 1b | Steinberg JS et al. Use of the signal-averaged ECG for predicting inducible ventricular tachycardia in patients with unexplained syncope: relation to clinical variables in a multivariate analysis. J Am Coll Cardiol 1994; 23: 99–106 |
| 38 | 1b | Kapoor WN et al. Diagnostic and prognostic implications of recurrences in patients with syncope. Am J Med 1987; 83: 700–8 |
| 39 | 4 | Linzer M et al. Impairment of physical and psychosocial function in recurrent syncope. Clin Epidemiol 1991; 44: 1037–43 |
| 40 | 1b | Savage DD et al. Epidemiological features of isolated syncope: the Framingham Study. Stroke 1985; 16: 626–9 |
| 41 | 1b | Middlekauf HR et al. Prognosis after syncope: impact of LVF. Am Heart J 93; 125: 121–5 |

Think about cardiac arrhythmias in patients with:
- palpitations
- dyspnoea **[B]**[1]

**Why?**
- 7% of patients attending hospital with dyspnoea have an arrhythmia **[B]**[1].

- chest pain
- dizziness or syncope
- cardiac arrest.

Ask about:
- any nausea or vomiting before collapse **[A]**[2]

**Why?**
**Lack of nausea and vomiting increases the risk of an arrhythmia**

| Patient **[A]**[2] | Prognostic factor | Outcome | Control rate | RR (95% CI) | NNF+ (95% CI) |
|---|---|---|---|---|---|
| Unexplained syncope | Absence of nausea or vomiting before syncope *independent* | Syncope due to cardiac arrhythmia at 1 year | 20% | 7.1 (1.6 to 33.3) | 2 (1 to 12) |

- any cardiovascular disease, particularly
  - known arrhythmias **[A]**[3]

**Why?**
- Ventricular arrhythmia increases the risk of dying.
- Three-quarters of patients with sick sinus syndrome are symptomatic – commonly with syncope (45%), palpitations (30%) or light-headedness (27%) **[C]**[4].
- Symptoms of dizziness and fainting do not help predict arrhythmias **[A]**[5].

  - ischaemic heart disease **[D]**.

Look for:
- an irregular pulse **[B]**[6]

**Why?**
**An irregular pulse makes an arrhythmia more likely**

| Patient **[B]**[6] | Target disorder (reference standard) | Diagnostic test | LR+ (95% CI) | Post-test probability | LR– (95% CI) | Post-test probability |
|---|---|---|---|---|---|---|
| Undergoing Holter monitoring (pre-test probability 53%) | Arrhythmia (Holter monitoring) | Irregular pulse | 8.9 (1.2 to 69) | 91% | 0.97 (0.94 to 0.99) | 52% |

- cannon waves in the jugular vein [C][7]

**Why?**
No cannon waves makes a ventricular tachycardia less likely

| Patient [C][7] | Target disorder (reference standard) | Diagnostic test | LR+ (95% CI) | Post-test probability | LR– (95% CI) | Post-test probability |
|---|---|---|---|---|---|---|
| Tachycardia (pre-test probability ? 50%) | Ventricular tachycardia (induced rhythm) | Slow independent jugular venous pulse (cannon waves) | 3.8 (1.8 to 8.2) | 79% | 0.067 (0.0097 to 0.46) | 6% |
| | | Variable amplitude of first heart sound | Infinity (4.0 to infinity) | 10% | 0.45 (0.28 to 0.73) | 31% |

- variable amplitude of the first heart sound [C][7].

**Why?**
A variable first heart sound makes a ventricular tachycardia more likely

| Patient [C][7] | Target disorder (reference standard) | Diagnostic test | LR+ (95% CI) | Post-test probability | LR– (95% CI) | Post-test probability |
|---|---|---|---|---|---|---|
| Tachycardia (pre-test probability ? 50%) | Ventricular tachycardia (induced rhythm) | Variable amplitude of first heart sound | Infinity (4.0 to infinity) | 100% | 0.45 (0.28 to 0.73) | 31% |

- Perform carotid sinus massage [D] – it is safe if there is no bruit [B][8].

**Why?**
- Few patients have a transient ischaemic attack or minor stroke following carotid sinus massage, and most neurological deficits recover (0.44%; 95% CI: 0.11% to 0.76%) [B][8].

## INVESTIGATIONS

- Urea, electrolytes, creatinine.
- Calcium, magnesium [D].
- Cardiac enzymes [D].
- Thyroid function tests.
- 12-lead ECG [A].

Consider further testing if the diagnosis is uncertain and your patient is stable.

- Event recorders [A][9]

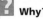 

**Why?**
- Event recorders produce more interpretable ECG tracings with symptoms and detect more clinically important arrhythmias than 48 h of Holter monitoring **[A]**[9].
- Event monitoring is cheaper **[A]**[9].

**Event recorders detect more clinically important arrhythmias than Holter monitoring**

| Patient [A][9] | Treatment | Comparator | Outcome | CER | RRR | NNT |
|---|---|---|---|---|---|---|
| Palpitations | Event recorder for up to 3 months or until two events detected | Holter monitoring for 48 h | Interpretable ECG tracing at 3 months | 35% | 93% (36% to 100%) | 3 (2 to 8) |
| | | | Clinically important arrhythmia detected | 0% | | 5 (3 to 14) |

or Holter monitoring **[B]**[10] worn for as long as possible **[C]**[11].

**Why?**
- Holter monitoring over 72 h detects twice as many arrhythmias as does monitoring for 24 h **[C]**[11].
- It can help diagnose a cause in 27% of cases (95% CI: 21% to 33%) **[B]**[10].

**Holter monitoring detects more arrhythmias the longer it is worn**

| Day [C][11] | Major arrhythmia detected (95% CI) |
|---|---|
| 1 | 15% (8.3% to 23%) |
| 2 | 11% (5.1% to 20%) |
| 3 | 4.2% (0.8% to 12%) |

**Note**
- Symptoms of dizziness and fainting are common in patients with syncope, but few are associated with arrhythmias (1.0%; 95% CI: 0.49% to 1.5%) **[C]**[12].

**Dizziness and fainting make a major arrhythmia less likely**

| Patient [C][12] | Target disorder (reference standard) | Diagnostic test | LR+ (95% CI) | Post-test probability | LR– (95% CI) | Post-test probability |
|---|---|---|---|---|---|---|
| Unexplained syncope (pre-test probability 9%) | Major arrhythmia (24 h ECG) | Dizziness and fainting | 0.25 (0.12 to 0.56) | 2% | 1.2 (1.1 to 1.2) | 10% |

## THERAPY

If uncertain about the source of the arrhythmia:
try carotid sinus massage or ask the patient to perform a Valsalva
manoeuvre [D].

> **? Why do this?**
> ■ Neither technique is clearly better at causing reversion to sinus rhythm [D][13].

Give
● adenosine [A][14] 3 mg, 6 mg, 9 mg, or 12 mg [A][14], unless the patient is
on dipyridamole [A][15].

> **? Why do this?**
> ■ It terminates 90% of episodes of paroxysmal SVT, but 20% report moderate or severe adverse reactions – these commonly include facial flushing, chest discomfort and dyspnoea [A][14].
> ■ It is as effective as verapamil for cardioversion of SVT [A][14].
> ■ It has no effect on ventricular arrhythmias, but may help reveal atrial flutter or fibrillation [D].
> ■ Dipyridamole potentiates the effect of adenosine [A][15].
>
> **Larger doses of adenosine terminate more arrhythmias**
>
> | Patient [A][14] | Treatment | Comparator | Outcome | CER | RRR | NNT |
> |---|---|---|---|---|---|---|
> | Paroxysmal SVT | Adenosine 3 mg | Placebo | Cardioversion at 8 min | 7.8% | 350% (88% to 990%) | 4 (3 to 6) |
> | | Adenosine 6 mg | Placebo | Cardioversion at 8 min | 9.3% | 560% (210% to 1300%) | 2 (2 to 2) |
> | | Adenosine 9 mg | Placebo | Cardioversion at 8 min | 13% | 540% (230% to 1100%) | 1 (1 to 2) |
> | | Adenosine 12 mg | Placebo | Cardioversion at 8 min | 14% | 550% (250% to 1100%) | 1 (1 to 1) |

If a central line is *in situ*, use it [A][16].

> **? Why do this?**
> ■ More arrhythmias are terminated at low doses [A][16].
> **SVT: 3 mg adenosine via a central line is more likely to terminate the arrhythmia than via a peripheral line**
>
> | Patient | Treatment | Comparator | Outcome | CER | RRR | NNT |
> |---|---|---|---|---|---|---|
> | SVT [A][16] | 3 mg adenosine via central vein | 3 mg adenosine via peripheral vein | Arrhythmia terminated at 10 min | 37% | 110% (26% to 250%) | 3 (2 to 6) |

## Acute-onset atrial flutter
● Control the ventricular rate [A] using:
 – digoxin [D].
 Alternatives include:
 – calcium-channel blockers: verapamil [A][16] [A][17] or diltiazem [A][18]
 – beta-blockers: esmolol [A][19] or sotalol [A][20].

**Why?**
- Verapamil slows the ventricular rate (on average by 40 beats/min) **[A]**[18] **[A]**[20], and helps cardioversion **[A]**[18].
- Diltiazem slows the ventricular rate (on average by 20 beats/min) **[A]**[19].
- Esmolol **[A]**[20] or sotalol **[A]**[21] slows the ventricular rate, but neither has any clear effect on cardioversion.

**Atrial flutter: verapamil helps conversion to sinus rhythm**

| Patient | Treatment | Comparator | Outcome | CER | RRR | NNT |
|---|---|---|---|---|---|---|
| Atrial flutter **[A]**[18] | Verapamil | Placebo | Sinus rhythm | 0% | 100% | 3 (1 to 25) |

- Consider cardioversion to sinus rhythm **[A]** if your patient fails to revert spontaneously **[D]**.

 **Note**
- Half of patients with acute AF revert spontaneously within 18 h **[B]**[22].

Options include:

- DC cardioversion **[A]** particularly if your patient is haemodynamically unstable.

  Cardioversion is more likely to be successful if **[A]**[23]:
  - the onset of this episode of arrhythmia is recent
  - your patient is young.

 **Why do this?**
- Cardioversion with atrial flutter is more successful than atrial fibrillation – 96% revert (95% CI: 91% to 100%), and patients are more likely to remain in sinus rhythm long-term **[A]**[23].

- Anticoagulate the patient before and after cardioversion **[C]**[24].

 **Why do this?**
- Anticoagulation preceding and up to a month after cardioversion reduces thromboembolism **[C]**[24].

**Anticoagulation reduces thromboembolism following cardioversion**

| Patient | Treatment | Comparator | Outcome | CER | RRR | NNT |
|---|---|---|---|---|---|---|
| Undergoing DC cardioversion for AF or flutter **[C]**[24] | Anticoagulation | No anticoagulation | Thromboembolism at 6 weeks | 2.2% | 100% | 45 (25 to 220) |

Consider:

- giving an infusion of ibutilide before cardioversion **[A]**[25].

**Why do this?**

■ It increases the chance that patients will remain in sinus rhythm **[A]**[25].

**Pre-treatment with ibutilide helps maintain sinus rhythm following DC cardioversion**

| Patient **[A]**[24] | Treatment | Comparator | Outcome | CER | RRR | NNT |
|---|---|---|---|---|---|---|
| Acute AF or flutter | Ibutilide before cardioversion | Placebo before cardioversion | Sinus rhythm at 12 months | 72% | −39% (−65% to −17%) | 4 (2 to 6) |

There is no clear benefit from:
● transoesophageal echocardiography **[B]**[26]

**Why?**

■ Using transoesophageal echocardiography to predict which patients require anticoagulation **[B]**[26], or when cardioversion should occur **[D]**[27], has no clear effect on subsequent embolic events.

An alternative is pharmacological cardioversion, using any of:

**Note**

■ No one method of pharmacological cardioversion is definitively better than another – studies are small and have short follow-up, so some of the differences noted below may be due to chance. In addition, adverse effects from cardioversion and effects on mortality are unclear.

● flecainide **[A]**[27]

**Why do this?**

■ Flecainide is more effective at cardioversion than verapamil **[A]**[28].
■ Watch for severe hypotension **[A]**[29].

**Flecainide is more effective at cardioversion than procainamide, digoxin or verapamil**

| Patient | Treatment | Comparator | Outcome | CER | RRR | NNT |
|---|---|---|---|---|---|---|
| Paroxysmal atrial flutter **[A]**[28] | Flecainide | Verapamil | Sinus rhythm at 1 h | 5.0% | 1300% (100% to 9600%) | 2 (1 to 2) |
| Recent-onset AF **[A]**[29] | Flecainide | Digoxin | Severe hypotension at 6 h | 5.9% | −270% (−100% to −9%) | −6 (−37 to −3) |

● ibutilide **[A]**[30]

**Why do this?**
- Ibutilide is more effective at cardioversion than procainamide **[A]**[31], sotalol **[A]**[32] or placebo **[A]**[30].
- However, it increases the risk of ventricular tachycardias **[A]**[30], but still causes fewer overall adverse effects than procainamide **[A]**[31].

**Ibutilide is effective at cardioversion but causes ventricular tachycardia**

| Patient | Treatment | Comparator | Outcome | CER | RRR | NNT |
|---|---|---|---|---|---|---|
| Recent-onset AF or flutter **[A]**[30] | Ibutilide | Placebo | Sinus rhythm at 1.5 h | 2.5% | 1800% (380% to 7400%) | 2 (2 to 3) |
| | | | Polymorphic VT at 24 h | 0.0% | | −11 (−21 to −7) |
| Recent-onset AF or flutter **[A]**[31] | Ibutilide | Procainamide | Sinus rhythm at 24 h | 18% | 220% (79% to 470%) | 3 (2 to 4) |
| | | | Adverse effects | 47% | 39% (1% to 63%) | 5 (3 to 76) |
| Recent-onset AF or flutter **[A]**[32] | Ibutilide | Sotalol | Sinus rhythm at 1 h | 11% | 65% (33% to 82%) | 5 (3 to 9) |

- amiodarone **[A]**[32].

**Why do this?**
- Amiodarone is more effective at cardioversion than digoxin **[A]**[33].

**Amiodarone is more effective at cardioversion than digoxin or verapamil**

| Patient | Treatment | Comparator | Outcome | CER | RRR | NNT |
|---|---|---|---|---|---|---|
| Acute atrial flutter **[A]**[33] | Amiodarone | Digoxin | Sinus rhythm at 24 h | 71% | −50% (−72% to −1%) | 5 (2 to 170) |

## Supraventricular tachycardia
Try carotid sinus massage or ask the patient to perform a Valsalva manoeuvre **[D]**.

**Why do this?**
- Neither technique is clearly better at causing reversion to sinus rhythm **[D]**[34].

Give:
- adenosine **[A]**[14] 3 mg, 6 mg, 9 mg, 12 mg **[A]**[14]; unless the patient is on dipyridamole **[A]**[15].

**Why do this?**

- It terminates 90% of episodes of paroxysmal SVT, but 20% report moderate or severe adverse reactions – commonly facial flushing, chest discomfort and dyspnoea **[A]**[14].
- It is as effective as verapamil for cardioversion **[A]**[14].
- Dipyridamole potentiates the effect of adenosine **[A]**[15].

**Larger doses of adenosine terminate more arrhythmias**

| Patient [A][14] | Treatment | Comparator | Outcome | CER | RRR | NNT |
|---|---|---|---|---|---|---|
| Paroxysmal SVT | Adenosine 3 mg | Placebo | Cardioversion at 8 min | 7.8% | 350% (88% to 990%) | 4 (3 to 6) |
| | Adenosine 6 mg | Placebo | Cardioversion at 8 min | 9.3% | 560% (210% to 1300%) | 2 (2 to 2) |
| | Adenosine 9 mg | Placebo | Cardioversion at 8 min | 13% | 540% (230% to 1100%) | 1 (1 to 2) |
| | Adenosine 12 mg | Placebo | Cardioversion at 8 min | 14% | 550% (250% to 1100%) | 1 (1 to 1) |

If a central line is *in situ*, use it **[A]**[16].

**Why do this?**

- More arrhythmias are terminated at low doses **[A]**[16].

**SVT: 3 mg adenosine via a central line is more likely to terminate the arrhythmia than via a peripheral line**

| Patient | Treatment | Comparator | Outcome | CER | RRR | NNT |
|---|---|---|---|---|---|---|
| SVT [A][16] | 3 mg adenosine via central vein | 3 mg adenosine via peripheral vein | Arrhythmia terminated at 10 min | 37% | 110% (26% to 250%) | 3 (2 to 6) |

If this fails, consider one of:

- DC cardioversion **[A]**
- calcium-channel blockers: diltiazem, at least 0.15 mg/kg **[A]**[35]

**Why do this?**

- Doses of 0.15 mg/kg of verapamil are more effective than placebo at cardioversion **[A]**[35]

**SVT: diltiazem is more effective at cardioversion than placebo**

| Patient | Treatment | Comparator | Outcome | CER | RRR | NNT |
|---|---|---|---|---|---|---|
| Paroxysmal SVT [A][35] | Diltiazem 0.15 mg/kg | Placebo | Sinus rhythm at 17 min | 25% | −240% (−590% to −64%) | 2 (1 to 3) |

- beta-blockers: esmolol **[D]**[36], nadolol **[A]**[37]

**Why do this?**
- Esmolol is probably as effective as propranolol at cardioversion **[D]**[36].
- Nadolol is more effective than placebo at slowing the ventricular rate and achieving cardioversion **[A]**[37].

**SVT: nadolol helps slow the ventricular rate and cardioversion**

| Patient | Treatment | Comparator | Outcome | CER | RRR | NNT |
|---------|-----------|------------|---------|-----|-----|-----|
| Paroxysmal SVT **[A]**[37] | Nadolol | Placebo | Ventricular rate < 100, or sinus rhythm at ? minutes | 20% | −59% (−88% to −29%) | 2 (1 to 3) |

- sotalol 1.5 mg/kg over 10 min **[B]**[37]

**Why do this?**
- It helps reversion to sinus rhythm **[B]**[38].

**SVT: sotalol helps reversion to sinus rhythm**

| Patient **[B]**[38] | Treatment | Comparator | Outcome | CER | RRR | NNT |
|---------|-----------|------------|---------|-----|-----|-----|
| Paroxysmal SVT or AF | Sotalol | Placebo | Reversion to sinus rhythm at 30 min | 15% | −460% (−1500% to −92%) | 1 (1 to 2) |

- propafenone **[B]**[39].

**Why do this?**
- It terminates most episodes of SVT (84%; 95% CI: 78% to 90%) **[B]**[39].

## Wolf-Parkinson-White syndrome

Terminate the rhythm using:

- adenosine **[D]**
- amiodarone **[D]**
- flecainide **[D]**
- procainamide **[D]**
- esmolol **[D]**
- diltiazem 0.25 mg/kg **[A]**[40].

**Why do this?**
- Diltiazem helps terminate SVT due to re-entrant pathways **[A]**[40].

**Wolf-Parkinson-White syndrome: diltiazem is more effective than placebo at cardioversion**

| Patient | Treatment | Comparator | Outcome | CER | RRR | NNT |
|---------|-----------|------------|---------|-----|-----|-----|
| SVT due to re-entrant pathway **[A]**[40] | Diltiazem **[A]**[40] | Placebo | Termination of arrhythmia at 15 min | 19% | 350% (100% to 890%) | 2 (1 to 2) |

Avoid using digoxin or verapamil – they may exacerbate the problem **[D]**.

## Ventricular tachycardias

- Cardiovert patients who are haemodynamically compromised **[A]**.
- Give iv amiodarone (initial rapid infusion, 150 mg over 10 min; loading infusion, 1 mg/min for 6 h; maintenance infusion, 0.52 mg/min for the remainder of 48 h) **[A]**[41].

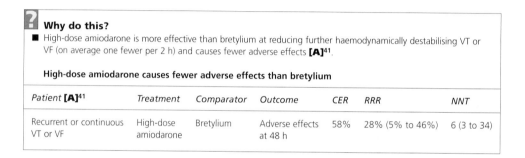

### Why do this?
- High-dose amiodarone is more effective than bretylium at reducing further haemodynamically destabilising VT or VF (on average one fewer per 2 h) and causes fewer adverse effects **[A]**[41].

**High-dose amiodarone causes fewer adverse effects than bretylium**

| Patient **[A]**[41] | Treatment | Comparator | Outcome | CER | RRR | NNT |
|---|---|---|---|---|---|---|
| Recurrent or continuous VT or VF | High-dose amiodarone | Bretylium | Adverse effects at 48 h | 58% | 28% (5% to 46%) | 6 (3 to 34) |

Alternatives include:

- sotalol (100 mg iv over 5 min) **[A]**[41].
- procainamide (a bolus of 10 mg/kg at a rate of 100 mg/min) **[A]**[42].

### Why do this?
- Sotalol **[A]**[42] or procainamide **[A]**[43] is more effective than lidocaine at terminating VT.

**Sotalol or procainamide stops VT better than lidocaine**

| Patient | Treatment | Comparator | Outcome | CER | RRR | NNT |
|---|---|---|---|---|---|---|
| VT | Sotalol **[A]**[42] | Lidocaine | Termination of arrhythmia at 15 min | 18% | −51% (−80% to −22%) | 2 (1 to 5) |
| Monomorphic VT | Procainamide **[A]**[43] | Lidocaine | Termination of arrhythmia at 15 min | 21% | −57% (−88% to −29%) | 2 (1 to 3) |

*Note*
- Do not treat patients with a recent myocardial infarction who have frequent premature ventricular contractions with class Ic antiarrhythmics **[A]**[44] **[A]**[45].

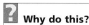**Why?**
■ Patients who receive flecainide or encainide are at increased risk of dying **[A]**[44] **[A]**[45].

**Flecainide or encainide kills patients with a recent MI and frequent PVCs**

| Patient | Treatment | Comparator | Outcome | CER | RRR | NNH |
|---|---|---|---|---|---|---|
| Recent MI and frequent PVCs | Flecainide or encainide **[A]**[44] **[A]**[45] | Placebo | Death or cardiac arrest | 3.5% | −140% (−270% to −53%) | 21 (14 to 40) |

## PREVENTION

### Paroxysmal atrial flutter
Consider long-term antiarrhythmic therapy in symptomatic cases **[D]**.
Start medication in hospital **[A]**[45].

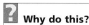**Why do this?**
■ Although few patients have serious complications, it is more cost-effective to start antiarrhythmics in hospital than in clinic **[A]**[46].

Consider using one of:

● flecainide – at least 50 mg twice daily **[A]**[47] **[A]**[48]

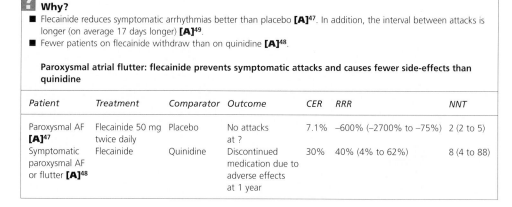**Why?**
■ Flecainide reduces symptomatic arrhythmias better than placebo **[A]**[47]. In addition, the interval between attacks is longer (on average 17 days longer) **[A]**[49].
■ Fewer patients on flecainide withdraw than on quinidine **[A]**[48].

**Paroxysmal atrial flutter: flecainide prevents symptomatic attacks and causes fewer side-effects than quinidine**

| Patient | Treatment | Comparator | Outcome | CER | RRR | NNT |
|---|---|---|---|---|---|---|
| Paroxysmal AF **[A]**[47] | Flecainide 50 mg twice daily | Placebo | No attacks at ? | 7.1% | −600% (−2700% to −75%) | 2 (2 to 5) |
| Symptomatic paroxysmal AF or flutter **[A]**[48] | Flecainide | Quinidine | Discontinued medication due to adverse effects at 1 year | 30% | 40% (4% to 62%) | 8 (4 to 88) |

● sotalol – at least 120 mg twice daily **[A]**[50].

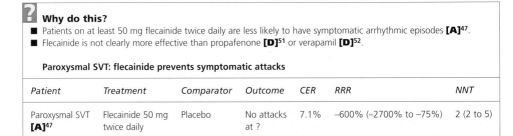

**? Why?**

■ Sotalol reduces recurrent symptomatic episodes compared with placebo, but only at doses of at least 120 mg twice daily **[A]**[50].

**Paroxysmal atrial flutter: sotalol reduces recurrent symptomatic episodes**

| Patient | Treatment | Comparator | Outcome | CER | RRR | NNT |
|---|---|---|---|---|---|---|
| Symptomatic AF or flutter **[A]**[50] | Sotalol 120 mg twice daily | Placebo | Recurrent symptomatic episodes at 1 year | 70% | 27% (3% to 45%) | 5 (3 to 43) |

### Paroxysmal SVT

Consider anti-arrhythmic medication for patients with recurrent symptomatic arrhythmias **[D]**. Start medication in hospital **[A]**[46].

**? Why do this?**

■ Although few patients have serious complications, it is more cost-effective to start antiarrhythmics in hospital than in clinic **[A]**[46].

Consider using one of:

● flecainide 50 mg twice daily **[A]**[47]

**? Why do this?**

■ Patients on at least 50 mg flecainide twice daily are less likely to have symptomatic arrhythmic episodes **[A]**[47].
■ Flecainide is not clearly more effective than propafenone **[D]**[51] or verapamil **[D]**[52].

**Paroxysmal SVT: flecainide prevents symptomatic attacks**

| Patient | Treatment | Comparator | Outcome | CER | RRR | NNT |
|---|---|---|---|---|---|---|
| Paroxysmal SVT **[A]**[47] | Flecainide 50 mg twice daily | Placebo | No attacks at ? | 7.1% | −600% (−2700% to −75%) | 2 (2 to 5) |

● sotalol 80 mg or 160 mg po twice daily **[A]**[52]

**? Why do this?**

■ It reduces recurrent episodes of SVT **[A]**[53].

**Paroxysmal SVT: sotalol reduces recurrent episodes**

| Patient **[A]**[53] | Treatment | Comparator | Outcome | CER | RRR | NNT |
|---|---|---|---|---|---|---|
| Paroxysmal SVT or AF | Sotalol | Placebo | Recurrent episode at 1–4 weeks | 89% | 38% (22% to 51%) | 3 (2 to 5) |

● propafenone 600 mg **[B]**[54].

**Why do this?**

■ It reduces symptomatic arrhythmias, without clearly causing intolerable side-effects, unlike 900 mg propafenone daily **[B]**[54].

**Paroxysmal SVT: propafenone reduces symptomatic arrhythmias**

| Patient **[B]**[54] | Treatment | Comparator | Outcome | CER | RRR | NNT |
|---|---|---|---|---|---|---|
| Paroxysmal SVT or AF | Propafenone 600 mg | Placebo | Symptomatic arrhythmia at 3 months | 71% | 49% (29% to 64%) | 3 (2 to 5) |
| | Propafenone 900 mg | Placebo | Symptomatic arrhythmia at 3 months | 63% | 89% (72% to 96%) | 2 (1 to 2) |
| | | | Intolerable adverse events at 3 months | 1.7% | −1600% (−12000% to −130%) | −4 (−7 to −3) |

## Ventricular arrhythmias

Consider:

● amiodarone **[A]**[55]

**Why do this?**

■ Fewer patients die **[A]**[55].

**Amiodarone reduces the risk of dying suddenly**

| Patient **[A]**[55] | Treatment | Comparator | Outcome | CER | OR | NNT |
|---|---|---|---|---|---|---|
| At risk of sudden death | Amiodarone | Placebo, sotalol, propranolol | Death at ? 1 year | 26% | 0.81 (0.69 to 0.94) | 26 (16 to 86) |
| | | | Sudden death at ? 1 year | 13% | 0.70 (0.58 to 0.85) | 28 (20 to 57) |

● inserting an implantable defibrillator **[A]**[56–58] with endocardial leads **[B]**[59].

**Why do this?**

■ It reduces mortality better than antiarrhythmic drug therapy **[A]**[56–58].
■ Defibrillators with endocardial leads prevent death more effectively than ones with epicardial leads, but are harder to insert **[B]**[59].
■ However, implantable defibrillators are not clearly more effective than amiodarone and are less cost-effective **[A]**[60].

**Implantable defibrillators reduce mortality compared with conventional therapy**

| Patient | Treatment | Comparator | Outcome | CER | RRR | NNT |
|---|---|---|---|---|---|---|
| Near-fatal ventricular arrhythmia **[A]**[56] | Implantable defibrillator | Amiodarone or sotalol | Death at 18 months | 24% | 34% (15% to 49%) | 12 (8 to 30) |
| Previous VT/VF arrest following MI **[A]**[58] | Implantable defibrillator | Conventional therapy | Death at 2 years | 36% | 61% (8% to 86%) | 5 (2 to 150) |
| Recent MI and asymptomatic episode of VT **[A]**[57] | Implantable defibrillator | Conventional therapy | Death at 5 years | 39% | 59% (31% to 76%) | 4 (3 to 9) |
| Cardiac arrest or VF **[B]**[59] | Defibrillator with endocardial leads | Defibrillator with epicardial leads | Death at 3 years | 11% | 72% (53% to 83%) | 13 (9 to 20) |
| | | | Successful implantation at ? weeks | 99.7% | −13% (−16% to −10%) | −8 (−10 to −6) |

> **Note**
> ■ Half of patients will receive a shock in the next 2 years (46%; 95% CI: 35% to 56%). This is more likely **[B]**[61]:
>   – in women
>   – with a low ejection fraction
>   – with antiarrhythmic therapy other than amiodarone.

Consider adding one of the following:

- amiodarone **[B]**[61]
- metoprolol **[A]**[62]
- sotalol **[A]**[63].

>  **Why do this?**
> ■ Patients on amiodarone have fewer shocks than patients on other antiarrhythmics **[B]**[61].
> ■ Patients on sotalol have fewer shocks than on placebo, but there is no clear effect on mortality **[A]**[63].
> ■ Metoprolol is more effective than sotalol at preventing shocks, but there is no clear effect on mortality **[A]**[62].
>
> **Metoprolol is more effective than sotalol at reducing shocks from implanted defibrillators**
>
> | Patient | Treatment | Comparator | Outcome | CER | RRR | NNT |
> |---|---|---|---|---|---|---|
> | Implantable defibrillator for VT **[A]**[63] | Sotalol | Placebo | Defibrillator shock at 12 months | 48% | 38% (17% to 54%) | 5 (3 to 13) |
> | Implantable defibrillator for VT **[A]**[62] | Sotalol | Metoprolol | Defibrillator shock at ? months | 20% | −140% (−410% to −15%) | −4 (−14 to −2) |

There is no clear benefit from:
- propafenone **[D]**[64]

> 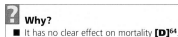 **Why?**
> ■ It has no clear effect on mortality **[D]**[64].

- allocating therapy using electrophysiological testing **[D]**[65]

> **Why?**
> ■ Allocated antiarrhythmic medication on the basis of electrophysiological testing compared with Holter monitoring is not clearly less likely to have recurrent arrhythmias and is worse at predicting long-term efficacy **[A]**[66].

- surgery (subendocardial resection and left ventricular endoaneurysmorrhaphy) **[C]**[67].

**Note**
- A quarter of patients who receive surgery are dead within 3 years (28%; 95% CI: 10% to 46%) **[C]**[67].

## PROGNOSIS

### Atrial flutter
Recurrent episodes are common in patients with paroxysmal atrial flutter **[B]**[68] **[B]**[69].
Patients who are cardioverted are more likely to remain in sinus rhythm if they have **[A]**[23]:

- non-rheumatic mitral valve disease
- low NYHA functional class.

**Note**
- Only a third of patients are still in sinus rhythm at 2 years (36%; 95% CI: 30% to 42%) **[A]**[23].
- Fewer patients in atrial flutter than in atrial fibrillation relapse following cardioversion. **[A]**[23]

### SVT
Recurrent episodes are common in patients with paroxysmal SVT. **[B]**[69] **[B]**[52] **[B]**[53]

**Note**
- Around 70% of patients on no medication will have a recurrent episode within 3 months **[B]**[53].

### Ventricular arrhythmias
Recurrent episodes are common **[B]**[71].
Many patients die, particularly suddenly **[B]**[72–75].

**Note**
- Roughly half of patients with ventricular tachycardias will have another episode within 12 months **[B]**[70].
- A quarter to a third are dead within 1 year – many suddenly **[B]**[72–75].

**Guideline writer**: Christopher Ball
**CAT writers**: Christopher Ball, Nick Shenker, Clare Wotton

# REFERENCES

| No. | Level | Citation |
|---|---|---|
| 1 | 2a | History and physical examination for dyspnea: a review. ACP J Club 1993 Nov Dec; 119:90. Summary of: Mulrow CD et al. Discriminating causes of dyspnea through clinical examination. J Gen Intern Med 1993; 8: 383–92 |
| 2 | 1a | Oh JH, Hanusa BH, Kapoor WN. Do symptoms predict cardiac arrhythmias and mortality in patients with syncope? Arch Intern Med 1999; 159: 375–380 |
| 3 | 1a | Martin TP et al. Risk stratification of patients with syncope. Ann Emerg Med 1997; 29: 459–66 |
| 4 | 4 | Rubenstein JJ et al. Clinical spectrum of the sick sinus syndrome. Circulation 72; 46: 5–11 |
| 5 | 1b | Clark PI et al. Arrhythmias detected by ambulatory monitoring: lack of correlation with symptoms of dizziness and syncope. Chest 1980; 77: 722–4 |
| 6 | 2b | Zeldis SM et al. Cardiovascular complaints: correlation with 24 hour electrocardiographic monitoring. Chest 1980; 78: 456–62 |
| 7 | 4 | Garratt CJ, Griffiths MJ, Young G et al. Value of physical signs in the diagnosis of ventricular tachycardia. Circulation 1994; 90: 3103–7 |
| 8 | 2b | Munro NC et al. Incidence of complications after carotid sinus massage in older patients with syncope. J Am Geriatr Soc 1994; 42: 1248–51 |
| 9 | 1b | Event recorders provided better data and were more cost-effective than 48-hour Holter monitoring in detecting arrhythmias. Evidence-Based Med 1996 July to Aug; 1: 159. Summary of: Kinlay S et al. Cardiac event recorders yield more diagnoses and are more cost-effective than 48-hour Holter monitoring in patients with palpitations: a controlled clinical trial. Ann Intern Med 1996; 1: 124: 16–20 |
| 10 | 2c | Kapoor WN, Karpf M, Wieand S et al. Prospective evaluation and follow-up of patients with syncope. N Engl J Med 1983; 309: 197–204 |
| 11 | 4 | Bach E et al. The duration of Holter monitoring in patients with syncope: is 24 hours long enough? Arch Intern Med 1990; 150: 1073–8 |
| 12 | 4 | Gibson TC, Heitzman MR. Diagnostic efficacy of 24 hour electrocardiographic monitoring for syncope. Am J Cardiol 1984; 53: 1013–17 |
| 13 | 2b– | Lim SH, Anantharaman V, Teo WS et al. Comparison of treatment of supraventricular tachycardia by Valsalva maneuver and carotid sinus massage. Ann Emerg Med 1998; 31: 30–35 |
| 14 | 1b | DiMarco JP, Miles W, Akhtar M et al. Adenosine for paroxysmal supraventricular tachycardia: dose ranging and comparison with verapamil. Assessment in placebo-controlled, multicenter trials. Ann Intern Med 1990; 113: 104–10 |
| 15 | 1b | Conradson TB, Dixon CM, Clarke B et al. Cardiovascular effects of infused adenosine in man, potentiation by dipyridamote. Acta Physiological Scandinavia 1987; 129: 387–91 |
| 16 | 1b | McIntosh-Yellin NL, Drew BJ, Scheinmann MM. Efficacy of central intravenous bolus administration of adenosine for termination of supraventricular tachycardia. J Am Coll Cardiol 1993; 22: 741–5 |
| 17 | 1b | Platia EV et al. Esmolol versus verapamil in the acute treatment of atrial fibrillation or atrial flutter. Am J Cardiol 1989; 63: 925–9 |

| No. | Level | Citation |
|-----|-------|----------|
| 18 | 1b | Tommaso C et al. Atrial fibrillation and flutter: immediate control and conversion with intravenously administered verapamil. Arch Intern Med 1983; 143: 877–81 |
| 19 | 1b | Salerno DM et al. Efficacy and safety of intravenous diltiazem for treatment of atrial fibrillation and flutter. Am J Cardiol 1989; 63: 1046–51 |
| 20 | 1b | Platia EV et al. Esmolol versus verapamil in the acute treatment of atrial fibrillation or atrial flutter. Am J Cardiol 1989; 63: 925–9 |
| 21 | 1b | Sung RJ et al. Intravenous sotalol for the termination of supraventricular tachycardia and atrial fibrillation and flutter: a multicenter randomized, double-blind, placebo-controlled trial. Am Heart J 1995; 129: 739–48 |
| 22 | 2b | Falk RH et al. Digoxin for converting recent-onset atrial fibrillation to sinus rhythm. Ann Intern Med 1987; 106: 503 |
| 23 | 1b | Van Gelder IC et al. Prediction of uneventful cardioversion and maintenance of sinus rhythm from direct-current electrical cardioversion of chronic atrial fibrillation and flutter. Am J Cardiol 1991; 68: 41–6 |
| 24 | 4 | Zeiler Arnold A et al. Role of prophylactic anticoagulation for direct current cardioversion in patients with atrial fibrillation or atrial flutter. J Am Coll Cardiol 1992; 19: 851–5 |
| 25 | 1b | Oral H, Souza JJ, Michaud GF et al. Facilitating transthoracic cardioversion of atrial fibrillation with ibutilide pretreatment. N Engl J Med 1999; 340: 1849–54 |
| 26 | 2a | Moreyra E, Finkelhor RS, Cebul RD. Limitations of transesophageal echocardiography in the risk assessment of patients before nonanticoagulated cardioversion from atrial fibrillation and flutter: an analysis of pooled trials. Am Heart J 1995; 129: 71–5 |
| 27 | 1b– | Klein AL et al. Cardioversion guided by transoesophageal echocardiography: the ACUTE pilot study. Ann Intern Med 1997; 126: 200–9 |
| 28 | 1b | Suttorp MJ et al. Intravenous flecainide versus verapamil for acute conversion of paroxsymal atrial fibrillation or flutter to sinus rhythm. Am J Cardiol 1989; 63: 693–6 |
| 29 | 1b | Donovan KD et al. Efficacy of flecainide for the reversion of acute onset atrial fibrillation. Am J Cardiol 1992; 70: 50A–55A |
| 30 | 1b | Stambler BS et al. Efficacy and safety of repeated intravenous doses of ibutilide for rapid conversion of atrial flutter or fibrillation. Circulation 1996; 94: 1613–21 |
| 31 | 1b | Volgman AS et al. Conversion efficacy and safety of intravenous ibutilide compared with intravenous procainamide in patients with atrial flutter or fibrillation. J Am Coll Cardiol 1998; 31: 1414–19 |
| 32 | 1b | Vos MA et al. Superiority of ibutilide (a new class III agent) over DL-sotalol in converting atrial flutter and atrial fibrillation. Heart 1998; 79: 568–75 |
| 33 | 1b | Hou ZY. Acute treatment of recent-onset atrial fibrillation and flutter with a tailored dosing regimen of intravenous amiodarone: a randomised digoxin-controlled study. Eur Heart J 1995; 16: 521–8 |
| 34 | 2b– | Lim SH, Anantharaman V, Teo WS et al. Comparison of treatment of supraventricular tachycardia by Valsalva maneuver and carotid sinus massage. Ann Emerg Med 1998; 31: 30–5 |
| 35 | 1b | Dougherty AH, Jackman WM, Naccarelli GV et al. Acute conversion of paroxysmal supraventricular tachycardia with intravenous diltiazem. Am J Cardiol 1992; 70: 587–92 |

| No. | Level | Citation |
|-----|-------|----------|
| 36 | 1b– | The Esmolol Multicenter Study Research Group. Efficacy and safety of esmolol vs propranolol in the treatment of supraventricular tachyarrhythmias: a multicenter double-blind clinical trial. Am Heart J 1985; 110: 913–22 |
| 37 | 1b | Olukotun AY, Klein GJ. Efficacy and safety of intravenous nadolol for supraventricular tachycardia. Am J Cardiol 1987; 60: 59–62 |
| 38 | 2b | Jordaens L, Gorgels A, Stroobandt R et al. Efficacy and safety of intravenous sotalol for termination of paroxysmal supraventricular tachycardia. Am J Cardiol 1991; 68: 35–40 |
| 39 | 2a | Reimold SC, Maisel WH, Antman EM. Propafenone for the treatment of supraventricular tachycardia and atrial fibrillation: a meta-analysis. Am J Cardiol 1998; 82: 66–71 |
| 40 | 1b | Huycke EC, Sung RJ, Dias VC et al. Intravenous diltiazem for termination of reenterant supraventricular tachycardia: a placebo-controlled randomised double-blind multicenter study. Am Coll Cardiol 1989; 13: 538–44 |
| 41 | 1b | Kowey PR, Levine JH, Herre JM et al. Randomized, double-blind comparison of intravenous amiodarone and bretylium in the treatment of patients with recurrent, hemodynamically destabilizing ventricular tachycardia or fibrillation. Circulation 1995; 92: 3255–63 |
| 42 | 1b | Ho DSW, Zecchin RP, Richards DAB et al. Double-blind trial of lignocaine versus sotalol for acute termination of spontaneous sustained ventricular tachycardia. Lancet 1994; 344: 18–23 |
| 43 | 1b | Gorgels APM, van den Dool A, Hofs A et al. Comparison of procainamide and lidocaine in terminating sustained monomorphic ventricular tachycardia. Am J Cardiol 1996; 78: 43–6 |
| 44 | 1b | Echt DS et al. Mortality and morbidity of patients receiving encainide, flecainide, or placebo: the Cardiac Arrhythmia Suppression Trial. N Engl J Med 1991; 324: 781–8 |
| 45 | 1b | CAST investigators: Special report. Preliminary report: effect of encainide and flecainide on mortality in a randomized trial of arrhythmia suppression after myocardial infarction. NEJM 1989: 321: 406–12 |
| 46 | 1b | Simons GR, Eisenstein EL, Shaw LJ et al. Cost effectiveness of inpatient initiation of antiarrhythmic therapy for supraventricular tachycardias. Am J Cardiol 1997; 80: 1551–7 |
| 47 | 1b | Pritchett ELC, Datorre SD, Platt ML et al. Flecainide acetate treatment of paroxysmal supraventricular tachycardia and paroxysmal atrial fibrillation: dose-response studies. J Am Coll Cardiol 1991; 17: 297–303 |
| 48 | 1b | Naccarelli GV et al. Prospective comparison of flecainide and quinidine for the treatment of paroxysmal atrial fibrillation/flutter. Am J Cardiol 1996; 77: 53A–59A |
| 49 | 1b | Anderson JL et al. Prevention of symptomatic recurrences of paroxysmal atrial fibrillation in patients initially tolerating antiarrhythmic therapy: a multicenter, double-blind cross-over study of flecainide and placebo with transtelephonic monitoring. Circulation 1989; 80: 1557–1570 |
| 50 | 1b | Benditt DG, Williams JH, Jin J et al. Maintenance of sinus rhythm with oral d,l-sotalol therapy in patients with symptomatic atrial fibrillation and/or atrial flutter. Am J Cardiol 1999; 84: 270–7 |
| 51 | 1b | Chimenti M et al. Safety of flecainide versus propfanone for the long-term management of symptomatic paroxysmal supraventricular tachyarrhythmias; report from the Flecainide and Propafenone Italian Study (FAPIS) group. Eur Heart J 1995; 16: 1943–51 |
| 52 | 1b– | Dorian P, Naccarelli GV, Coumel P et al. A randomized comparison of flecainide versus verapamil in paroxysmal supraventricular tachycardia. Am J Cardiol 1996; 77: 89–95 |

| No. | Level | Citation |
|-----|-------|----------|
| 53 | 1b | Wanless RS et al. Multicenter comparative study of the efficacy and safety of sotalol in the prophylactic treatment of patients with paroxysmal supraventricular tachyarrhythmias. Am Heart J 1997; 133: 441–6 |
| 54 | 2b | UK Propafenone PSVT Study Group. A randomized placebo-controlled trial of propafenone in the prophylaxis of paroxysmal supraventricular tachycardia and paroxysmal atrial fibrillation. Circulation 1995; 92: 2550–7 |
| 55 | 1a | Sim I, McDonald KM, Lavori PW et al. Quantitative overview of randomised trials of amiodarone to prevent sudden cardiac death. Circulation 1997; 96: 2823–9 |
| 56 | 1b | The Antiarrhythmics Versus Implantable Defibrillators (AVID) Investigators. A comparison of antiarrhythmic-drug therapy with implantable defibrillators in patients resuscitated from near-fatal ventricular arrhythmias. N Engl J Med 1997; 337: 1576–83 |
| 57 | 1b | Moss AJ, Hall WJ, Cannom DS et al. Improved survival with an implanted defibrillator in patients with coronary disease at high risk for ventricular arrhythmia. N Engl J Med 1996; 335: 1933–40 |
| 58 | 1b | Wever EF, Hauer RN, van Capelle F et al. Randomized study of implantable defibrillator as first-choice therapy versus conventional strategy in postinfarct sudden death survivors. Circulation 1995; 91: 2195–203 |
| 59 | 2b | The PCD Investigator Group. Clinical outcome of patients with malignant ventricular tachyarrhythmias and a multiprogrammable implantable cardioverter-defibrillator implanted with or without thoracotomy: an international multicenter study. J Am Coll Cardiol 1994; 23: 1521–30 |
| 60 | 1b | Owens DK, Sanders GD, Harris RA et al. Cost-effectiveness of implantable cardioverter defibrillators relative to amiodarone for prevention of sudden cardiac death. Ann Intern Med 1997; 126: 1–12 |
| 61 | 2b | Dolack GL. Clinical predictors of implantable cardioverter-defibrillator shocks (results of the CASCADE trial). Am J Cardiol 1994; 73: 237–41 |
| 62 | 1b | Seidl K, Hauer B, Schwick NG et al. Comparison of metoprolol and sotalol in preventing ventricular tachyarrhythmias after the implantation of a cardioverter/defibrillator. Am J Cardiol 1998; 82: 744–8 |
| 63 | 1b | Pacifico A, Hohnloser SH, Williams JH et al. Prevention of implantable-defibrillator shocks by treatment with sotalol. N Eng J Med 1999; 340(24): 1855–62 |
| 64 | 1b | Siebels J, Kuck K-H and the CASH Investigators. Implantable cardioverter defibrillator compared with antiarrhythmic drug treatment in cardiac arrest survivors (the Cardiac Arrest Study Hamburg). Am Heart J 1994; 127: 1139–44 |
| 65 | 1b | Steinbeck G, Anderson D, Bach P et al. A comparison of electrophysiologically guided antiarrhythmic drug therapy with beta-blocker therapy in patients with symptomatic, sustained ventricular tachyarrhythmias. N Engl J Med 1992; 327: 987–92 |
| 66 | 1b | Mason JW et al. Comparison of electrophysiologic testing with Holter monitoring to predict antiarrhythmic-drug efficacy for ventricular tachyarrhythmias. N Engl J Med 1993; 329: 445–51 |
| 67 | 4 | Rastegar H, Link MS, Foote CB, et al. Perioperative and long-term results with mapping-guided subendocardial resection and left ventricular endoaneurysmorrhaphy. Circulation 1996; 94: 1041–1048 |
| 68 | 2b | Naccarelli GV et al. Prospective comparison of flecainide and quinidine for the treatment of paroxysmal atrial fibrillation/flutter. Am J Cardiol 1996; 77: 53A–59A |

| No. | Level | Citation |
|-----|-------|----------|
| 69 | 2b | Benditt DG, Williams JH, Jin J et al. Maintenance of sinus rhythm with oral d, l-sotalol therapy in patients with symptomatic atrial fibrillation and/or atrial flutter. Am J Cardiol 1999; 84: 270–7 |
| 70 | 2b | Chimenti M et al. Safety of flecainide versus propafenone for the long-term management of symptomatic paroxysmal supraventricular tachyarrhythmias; report from the Flecainide and Propafenone Italian Study (FAPIS) group. Eur Heart J 1995; 16: 1943–51 |
| 71 | 2b | Pacifico A, Hohnloser SH, Williams JH et al. Prevention of implantable-defibrillator shocks by treatment with sotalol. N Engl J Med 1999; 340: 1855–62 |
| 72 | 2a | Sim I, McDonald KM, Lavori PW et al. Quantitative overview of randomised trials of amiodarone to prevent sudden cardiac death. Circulation 1997; 96: 2823–29 |
| 73 | 2b | The Antiarrhythmics Versus Implantable Defibrillators (AVID) Investigators. A comparison of antiarrhythmic-drug therapy with implantable defibrillators in patients resuscitated from near-fatal ventricular arrhythmias. N Eng J Med 1997; 337: 1576–83 |
| 74 | 2b | Moss AJ, Hall WJ, Cannom DS, et al. Improved survival with an implanted defibrillator in patients with coronary disease at high risk for ventricular arrhythmia. The New England Journal of Medicine 1996; 335: 1933–1940 |
| 75 | 2b | Wever EF, Hauer RN, van Capelle F et al. Randomized study of implantable defibrillator as first-choice therapy versus conventional strategy in postinfarct sudden death survivors. Circulation 1995; 91: 2195–203 |

What are we to do when the irresistible force of the need to offer clinical advice meets with the immovable object of flawed evidence? All we can do is our best: give the advice, but alert the advisees to the flaws in the evidence on which it is based.

The ancestor of these levels was created by Suzanne Fletcher and Dave Sackett twenty years ago when they were working for the Canadian Task Force on the Periodic Health Examination[i]. They generated 'levels of evidence' for ranking the validity of evidence about the value of preventive manoeuvres, and then tied them as 'grades of recommendations' to the advice given in the report.

The levels have evolved over the ensuing years, most notably as the basis for recommendations about the use of anti-thrombotic agents [ii], have grown increasingly sophisticated [iii], and have even started to appear in a new generation of evidence-based textbooks that announce, in bold marginal icons, the grade of each recommendation that appears in the texts in bold icons [iv].

However, their orientation remained therapeutic/preventive, and when a group of members of the Centre embarked on creating EBOC, the need for levels and grades for diagnosis, prognosis, and harm became overwhelming and the current version of their efforts appears here. They are the work of Chris Ball, Dave Sackett, Bob Phillips, Brian Haynes, and Sharon Straus, with lots of encouragement and advice from their colleagues.

Periodic updates will appear at http://cebm.jr2.ox.ac.uk/docs/levels.html#levels, and readers are invited to suggest ways that they might be improved or further developed.

A final, cautionary note: these levels and grades speak only to the validity of evidence about prevention, diagnosis, prognosis, therapy, and harm. Other strategies, described elsewhere in the Centre's pages, must be applied to the evidence in order to generate clinically useful measures of its potential clinical implications and to incorporate vital patient-values into the ultimate decisions.

---

[i] Canadian Task Force on the Periodic Health Examination: The periodic health examination. CMAJ 1979;121:1193-1254.

[ii] Sackett DL. Rules of evidence and clinical recommendations on use of antithrombotic agents. Chest 1986; 89 (2 suppl.):2S-3S.

[iii] Cook DJ, Guyatt GH, Laupacis A, Sackett DL, Goldberg RJ. Clinical recommendations using levels of evidence for antithrombotic agents. Chest 1995; 108(4 Suppl):227S-230S

[iv] Yusuf S, Cairns JA, Camm AJ, Fallen EL, Gersh BJ. Evidence-Based Cardiology. London: BMJ Publishing Group; 1998

| Grade of recommendation | Level of evidence | Therapy/Prevention, Aetiology/Harm | Prognosis | Diagnosis | Economic analysis |
|---|---|---|---|---|---|
| [A] | 1a | SR (with *homogeneity**) of RCTs | SR (with *homogeneity**) of inception cohort studies; or a CPG validated on a test set | SR (with *homogeneity**) of Level 1 diagnostic studies; or a CPG validated on a test set | SR (with *homogeneity**) of Level 1 economic studies |
| | 1b | Individual RCT (with narrow *confidence interval*†) | Individual inception cohort study with ≥ 80% follow-up | Independent blind comparison of patients from an *appropriate spectrum*** of patients, all of whom have undergone both the diagnostic test and the reference standard | Analysis comparing all (critically validated) alternative outcomes against appropriate cost measurement, and including a sensitivity analysis incorporating clinically sensible variations in important variables |
| | 1c | *All or none*§ | All or none case-series | Absolute *SpPins* and *SnNouts*†† | Clearly *as good or better*‡‡ but cheaper. Clearly as bad or worse but more expensive. Clearly better or worse at the same cost |
| [B] | 2a | SR (with *homogeneity**) of cohort studies | SR (with *homogeneity**) of either retrospective cohort studies or untreated control groups in RCTs | SR (with *homogeneity**) of Level ≥2 diagnostic studies | SR (with *homogeneity**) of Level ≥2 economic studies |
| | 2b | Individual cohort study (including low quality RCT; e.g. <80% follow-up) | Retrospective cohort study or follow-up of untreated control patients in an RCT; or CPG not validated in a test set | Any of: <br>• independent blind or objective comparison <br>• study performed in a set of non-consecutive patients, or confined to a narrow spectrum of study individuals (or both) all of whom have undergone both the diagnostic test and the reference standard <br>• a diagnostic CPG not validated in a test set | Analysis comparing a limited number of alternative outcomes against appropriate cost measurement, and including a sensitivity analysis incorporating clinically sensible variations in important variables |
| | 2c | 'Outcomes' research | 'Outcomes' research | | |
| [B] | 3a | SR (with *homogeneity**) of case-control studies | | | |
| | 3b | Individual case-control study | | Independent blind or objective comparison of an *appropriate spectrum***, but the reference standard was not applied to all study patients | Analysis without accurate cost measurement, but including a sensitivity analysis incorporating clinically sensible variations in important variables |

| | | quality cohort and case-control studies§§ | quality prognostic cohort studies*** | |
|---|---|---|---|---|
| | | | | • reference standard was unobjective, unblinded or not independent<br>• positive and negative tests were verified using separate reference standards<br>• study was performed in an *inappropriate spectrum** of patients | Analysis with no sensitivity analysis |
| [D] | 5 | Expert opinion without explicit critical appraisal, or based on physiology, bench research or 'first principles' | Expert opinion without explicit critical appraisal, or based on physiology, bench research or 'first principles' | Expert opinion without explicit critical appraisal, or based on economic theory |

SR, systematic review; RCT, randomised controlled trial; CPG, clinical practice guide.

1. These levels were generated in a series of iterations among members of the NHS R&D Centre for Evidence-Based Medicine (Christopher Ball, Dave Sackett, Robert Phillips, Brian Haynes, and Sharon Straus).

2. Recommendations based on this approach apply to 'average' patients and may need to be modified in light of an individual patient's unique biology (risk, responsiveness, etc.) and preferences about the care they receive.

3. Users can add a minus-sign (–) to denote the level that fails to provide a conclusive answer because of:
   - **either** a single result with a wide confidence interval (e.g. such that an ARR in an RCT is not statistically significant but whose confidence intervals fail to exclude clinically important benefit or harm)
   - **or** a systematic review with troublesome (and statistically significant) heterogeneity
   - such evidence is inconclusive, and therefore can only generate Grade D recommendations.

**Notes**

\* By homogeneity we mean a systematic review that is free of worrisome variations (heterogeneity) in the directions and degrees of results between individual studies. Not all systematic reviews with statistically significant heterogeneity need be worrisome, and not all worrisome heterogeneity need be statistically significant. As noted above, studies displaying worrisome heterogeneity should be tagged with a minus sign (–) at the end of their designated level

\** An appropriate spectrum is a cohort of patients who would normally be tested for the target disorder. An inappropriate spectrum compares patients already known to have the target disorder with patients diagnosed with another condition

‡ See note #3 above for advice on how to understand, rate and use trials or other studies with wide confidence intervals

§ Met when *all* patients died before the Rx became available, but some now survive on it; or when some patients died before the Rx became available, but *none* now die on it

†† An 'Absolute SpPin' is a diagnostic finding whose Specificity is so high that a Positive result rules-in the diagnosis. An 'Absolute SnNout' is a diagnostic finding whose Sensitivity is so high that a Negative result rules-out the diagnosis

‡‡ Good, better, bad and worse refer to the comparisons between treatments in terms of their clinical risks and benefits

§§ By poor quality *cohort* study we mean one that failed to clearly define comparison groups and/or failed to measure exposures and outcomes in the same (preferably blinded), objective way in both exposed and non-exposed individuals and/or failed to identify or appropriately control known confounders and/or failed to carry out a sufficiently long and complete follow-up of patients. By poor quality *case-control* study we mean one that failed to clearly define comparison groups and/or failed to measure exposures and outcomes in the same (preferably blinded), objective way in both cases and controls and/or failed to identify or appropriately control known confounders

\*** By poor quality prognostic cohort study we mean one in which sampling was biased in favour of patients who already had the target outcome, or the measurement of outcomes was accomplished in <80% of study patients, or outcomes were determined in an unblinded, non-objective way, or there was no correction for confounding factors.

If you want to find out more about practising and teaching EBM, we'd encourage you to grab the nearest copy of *Evidence-based Medicine*[v]. Written by David Sackett and some of the other top EBM exponents, it provides a fun, rapid and easy introduction to some of these ideas. The book has an associated website at http://www.library.utoronto.ca/medicine/ebm/, which provides more in-depth information. The Centre for Evidence-based Medicine's website at http://cebm.jr2.ox.ac.uk also provides teaching materials and information on courses.

---

[v] Sackett DL, Straus SE, Richardson WS et al. Evidence-based Medicine: how to practice and teach EBM. 2nd edn. Edinburgh: Churchill Livingstone; 2000

(Adapted with permission from David Sackett et al, Evidence-based Medicine: how to practice and teach EBM. 2nd edn. Edinburgh: Churchill Livingstone; 2000)

**Absolute risk reduction (ARR)**. See **treatment effects**

**'All-or-none'**. Where **all** patients die/ fail without the intervention, and some survive/ succeed with it (e.g. antibiotics for menigococcal meninigitis); or where many patients die/ fail without the intervention and **none** die/ fail with it.

**Case-control study**. A study which involves identifying patients who have the outcome of interest (cases) and control patients without the same outcome, and looking back to see if they had the exposure of interest.

**Case series**. A report on a series of patients with an outcome of interest. No control group is involved.

**Clinical practice guideline**. A systematically developed statement designed to assist clinician and patient decisions about appropriate health care for specific clinical circumstances

**Cohort study**. Involves identification of two groups (cohorts) of patients, one which did receive the exposure of interest, and one which did not, and following these cohorts forward for the outcome of interest.

**Confidence interval (CI)**. The range within which we would expect the true value of a statistical measure to lie. The CI is usually accompanied by a percentage value which shows the level of confidence that the true value lies within this range. For example, for an NNT of 10 with a 95% CI of 5 to 15, we would have a 95% confidence that the true NNT value was between 5 and 15.

**Control event rate (CER)**. See **treatment effects**.

**Decision analysis (or clinical decision analysis)**. The application of explicit, quantitative methods that quantify prognoses, treatment effects and patient values in order to analyze a decision under conditions of uncertainity.

**Event rate**. The proportion of patients in a group in whom the event is observed. Thus, if out of 100 patients the event is observed in 27, the event rate is 0.27. Control event rate (CER) and experimental event rate (EER) are used to refer to this in control and experimental groups of patients, respectively. The patient expected event rate (PEER) refers to the rate of events we'd expect in a patient who received no treatment or conventional treatment. See **treatment effects.**

**Evidence-based health care**. Extends the application of the principles of evidence-based medicine (see below) to all professions associated with health care, including purchasing and management.

**Evidence-based medicine**. The conscientious, explicit and judicious use of current best evidence in making decisions about the care of individual patients. The practice of evidence-based medicine means integrating individual clinical expertise and our patients' own values and expectations with the best available external clinical evidence from systematic research. (See also Sackett DS, et al. EBM : What it is and what it isn't. BMJ 1996; 312: 71–2.)

**Experimental event rate (EER)**. See **treatment effects**.

**Incidence**. The proportion of new cases of the target disorder in the population at risk during a specified time interval.

**Inception cohort**. A group of patients who are assembled near the onset of a target disorder.

**Intention-to-treat analysis**. A method of analysis for randomized trials in which all patients randomly assigned to one of the treatments are analyzed together, regardless of whether or not they completed or received that treatment.

**Likelihood ratios (LR)**. The likelihood that a given test result would be expected in a patient with the target disorder compared with the likelihood that the same result would be expected in a patient without the target disorder.
- **Positive likelihood ratio (LR +)**. A measure of how much a positive test pushes you towards making the diagnosis. The greater the positive LR, the better the test is at diagnosing the target disorder. Likelihood ratios of 10 or more indicate a very useful test—when applied to pre-test probabilities of 33% or more, such tests will generate post-test probabilities of 83% or more.
- **Negative likelihood ratio (LR +)**. A measure of how much a negative test pushes you away from making the diagnosis. The lower the negative LR, the better the test is at excluding the target disorder. Likelihood ratios of 0.1 or less indicate a very useful test— when applied to pre-test probabilities of 33% or less, such tests will generate post-test probabilities of 5% or less.

---

**Calculation of sensitivity/specificity/LR**

|  | Disease positive | Disease negative |
|---|---|---|
| Test positive | a | b |
| Test negative | c | d |

- Sensitivity = $\dfrac{a}{(a + c)}$

- Specificity = $\dfrac{d}{(b + d)}$

- $LR+ = \dfrac{\text{sensitivity}}{(1 - \text{specificity})} = \dfrac{a}{(a + c)} \div \dfrac{b}{(b + d)}$

- $LR- = \dfrac{(1 - \text{specificity})}{\text{sensitivity}} = \dfrac{c}{(a + c)} \div \dfrac{d}{(b + d)}$

- Pre-test probability = $\dfrac{(a + c)}{(a + b + c + d)}$

---

**Number needed to follow (NNF)**. The number of patients that need to be followed to see one bad outcome: the lower the NNF, the more common the outcome. NNF = 1/(event rate).

**Number extra needed to follow (NNF+)**. The number of patients with a certain risk factor (compared to without that risk factor) that need to be followed to see one extra bad outcome: the lower the NNF+, the worse the risk factor.

---

**Calculation of number extra needed to follow**

- **using odds ratios**

$$NNF+ = \frac{PEER\ (OR - 1) + 1}{PEER\ (OR - 1) \times (1 - PEER)}$$

- **using relative risk**

$$NNF+ = \frac{1}{PEER\ (1 - RR)}$$

---

**Number needed to harm (NNH)**. The number of patients that need to be treated to cause one bad outcome: the lower the NNH, the more harmful the treatment. See **treatment effects.**

**Number needed to treat (NNT)**. The number of patients that need to be treated to prevent one bad outcome: the lower the NNT, the better the treatment. See **treatment effects.**

**Odds ratios (OR)**. The ratio of the odds of having the target disorder in the experimental group relative to the odds in favour of having the target disorder in the control group (in cohort or systematic reviews), or the odds in favour of being exposed in subjects with the target disorder divided by the odds in favour of being exposed in the control subjects (without the target disorder).

---

**Calculation or OR/RR for trimethoprin-sulfamethoxazole prophylaxis in cirrhosis**

|  | Adverse outcome occurs (infectious complication) | Adverse outcome does not occur (no infectious complication) | Totals |
|---|---|---|---|
| Exposed to treatment (experimental) | a = 1 | b = 29 | a + b = 30 |
| Not exposed to treatment (control) | c = 9 | d = 21 | c + d = 30 |
| Total | a + b = 10 | b + d =50 | a + b + c + d =60 |

- CER = c/(c + d) = 30%
- EER = a/(a + b) = 3.3%
- Control event odds = c/d = 0.43
- Experimental event odds = a/b = 0.034
- Relative risk = EER/CER = 0.11
- Relative odds = odds ratio = (a/b)/(c/d) = ad/bc = 0.08

'Outcomes' study. The observation of a defined population at a single point in time or time interval. Exposure and outcome are determined simultaneously.

Patient expected event rate. See treatment effects.

Overview. See systematic review.

Post-test probability. The proportion of patients with a particular test result who have the target disorder. Patients with suspected pulmonary embolism with a high probability ventilation-perfusion scan have a post-test probability of 82%, i.e. most but not all have a PE. Alternatively, consider any patient with a high probability v/q scan as having a 82% chance of having a PE.

Pre-test probability (prevalence). The proportion of people with the target disorder in the population at risk at a specific time (point prevalence) or time interval (period prevalence). For example, for patients referred to hospital with suspected pulmonary embolism, the pre-test probability is 30%; that is, only a third actually have a PE confirmed on subsequent investigations. Alternatively, consider any patient with a suspected PE as having a 30% chance of actually having one.

Randomised controlled trial (RCT). A group of patients is randomised into an experimental group (which receives the intervention under study) and a control group (which receives standard therapy or placebo). These groups are followed up for the variables/ outcomes of interest.

Relative risk (RR). The incidence (or risk) of an adverse outcome in patients with a prognostic factor relative to the risk in patients without that factor (equivalent to risk ratio)

Relative risk reduction. See treatment effects.

Risk ratio (RR). The ratio of risk in the treated group (EER) to the risk in the control group (CER)—used in randomized trials and cohort studies (equivalent to relative risk). RR = EER/CER.

Systematic review (SR). A summary of the medical literature that uses explicit methods to perform a thorough literature search and critical appraisal of individual studies and that uses appropriate statistical techniques to combine these valid studies.

Treatment effects. The evidence-based medicine journals (*Evidence-based Medicine* and *ACP Journal Club*) have achieved consensus on some terms they use to describe both the good and bad effects of therapy. We will bring them to life with a synthesis of three randomized trials in diabetes which individually showed that several years of intensive insulin therapy reduced the proportion of patients with worsening retinopathy to 13% from 38%, raised the proportion of patients with satisfactory haemoglobin A1c levels to 60% from 30%, and increased the proportion of patients with at least one episode of symptomatic hypoglycaemia to 47% to 23%. Note that in each case the first number constitutes the 'experimental event rate' (EER) and the second number the 'control event rate' (CER). We will use the following terms and calculation to describe these effects of treatment:

*When the experimental treatment reduces the probability of a bad outcome (worsening diabetic retinopathy)*

- **RRR (relative risk reduction)**. Calculated as $|EER - CER|/CER$, and accompanied by a 95% confidence interval (CI). In the case of worsening diabetic retinopathy, $|EER - CER|/CER = |13\% - 38\%|/ 38\% = 66\%$.

- **ARR (absolute risk reduction)**. The absolute arithmetic difference in rates of bad outcomes between experimental and control participants in a trial, calculated as $|EER - CER|$, and accompanied by a 95% CI. In this case, $|EER - CER| = |13\% - 38\%| = 25\%$.

- **NNT (number needed to treat)**. The number of patients who need to be treated to achieve one additional favorable outcome, calculated as $1/ARR$ and accompanied by a 95% CI. In this case, $1/ARR = 1/25\% = 4$.

| Calculations for the occurrence of diabetic retinopathy in IDDMs | | | | |
|---|---|---|---|---|
| Occurrence of diabetic retinopathy at 5 years among insulin-dependent diabetics in the DCCT trial | | Relative risk reduction (RRR) | Absolute risk reduction (ARR) | Number needed to treat (NNT) |
| Usual insulin regimen (CER) | Intensive insulin regimen (EER) | $\dfrac{|EER - CER|}{CER}$ | $|EER - CER|$ | $1/ARR$ |
| 13% | 38% | $\dfrac{|13\% - 38\%|}{38\%}$ | $\begin{array}{c}|13\% - 28\%| \\ = 25\%\end{array}$ | 1/25% = 4 pts for 6 years with |

*When the experimental treatment increases the probability of a good outcome (satisfactory haemoglobin A1c levels)*

- **RBI (relative benefit increase)**. The proportional increase in rates of good outcomes between experimental and control patients in a trial, calculated as $|EER - CER|/CER$, and accompanied by a 95% confidence interval (CI). In the case of satisfactory haemoglobin A1c levels, $|EER - CER|/CER = |60\% - 30\%|/30\% = 100\%$.

- **ABI (absolute benefit increase)**. The absolute arithmetic difference in rates of good outcomes between experimental and control patients in a trial, calculated as $|EER - CER|$, and accompanied by a 95% CI. In this case, $|EER - CER| = |60\% - 30\%| = 30\%$.

- **NNT (number needed to treat)**. The number of patients who need to be treated to achieve one additional good outcome, calculated as 1/ARR and accompanied by a 95% CI. In this case, 1/ARR = 1/30% = 3.

*When the experimental treatment increases the probability of a bad outcome (episodes of hypoglycaemia)*

- **RRI (relative risk increase)**. The proportional increase in rates of bad outcomes between experimental and control patients in a trial, calculated as $|EER - CER|/CER$, and accompanied by a 95% confidence interval (CI). In the case of hypoglycaemic episodes, $|EER - CER|/CER = |57\% - 23\%|/57\% = 60\%$. (RRI is also used in assessing the impact of 'risk factors' for disease).

- **ARI (absolute risk increase)**. The absolute arithmetic difference in rates of bad outcomes between experimental and control patients in a trial, calculated as $|EER - CER|$, and accompanied by a 95% CI. In this case, $|EER - CER| = |57\% - 23\%| = 34\%$. (ARI is also used in assessing the impact of 'risk factors' for disease.)

- **NNH (number needed to harm)**. The number of patients who, if they received the experimental treatment, would lead to one additional patient being harmed, compared with patients who received the control treatment, calculated as 1/ARR, and accompanied by a 95% CI. In this case, 1/ARR = 1/34% = 3.

| | |
|---|---|
| ABI | absolute benefit increase |
| ACE inhibitors | angiotension converting enzyme inhibitors |
| AF | atrial fibrillation |
| ANA | anti-nuclear antibodies |
| ANCA | anti-neutrophilic cytoplasmic antibodies |
| anti-dsDNA | anti-double-stranded DNA antibodies |
| anti-GBM | anti-glomerular basement membrane antibodies |
| ARF | acute renal failure |
| ARI | absolute risk increase |
| ARR | absolute risk reduction |
| AST | aspartate transaminase |
| BMI | body mass index |
| CDAI | Crohn's disease activity index |
| CEA | carcioembryonic antigen |
| CER | control event rate |
| CI | confidence interval |
| CNS | central nervous system |
| CK | creatine kinase |
| Cl | chloride |
| CO | carbon monoxide |
| COPD | chronic obstructive pulmonary disease |
| CPR | cardiopulmonary resuscitation |
| CRP | C-reactive protein |
| CT | computer tomography |
| CVP | central venous pressure |
| DKA | diabetic ketoacidosis |
| DVT | deep vein thrombosis |
| ECG | electrocardiogram |
| ED | emergency department |
| EER | experimental event rate |
| ESR | erythrocyte sedimentation rate |
| $FEV_1$ | forced expiratory volume at one second |
| G | gauge |
| GCS | Glasgow Coma Scale |
| GI | gastrointestinal |
| h | hours |
| HbCO | carboxyhaemoglobin |

| | |
|---|---|
| $HbO_2$ | oxyhaemoglobin |
| $HCO_3$ | bicarbonate |
| IBD | inflammatory bowel disease |
| im | intramuscular |
| INR | international normalised ratio |
| ITU | intensive therapy unit |
| iv | intravenous |
| JVP | jugular venous pressure |
| K | potassium |
| LDH | lactate dehydrogenase |
| LR | likelihood ratio |
| min | minutes |
| MCV | mean cell volume |
| MI | myocardial infarction |
| MRI | magnetic resonance imaging |
| Na | sodium |
| NNF | number needed to follow |
| NNF+ | number extra needed to follow |
| NNH | number needed to harm |
| NNT | number needed to treat |
| NSAIDs | non-steroidal anti-inflammatory drugs |
| NYHA | New York Heart Association |
| OR | odds ratio |
| PCA | patient controlled analgesia |
| PE | pulmonary embolism |
| PEG | percutaneous endoscopic gastrostomy |
| RBI | relative benefit increase |
| RCT | randomised controlled trial |
| RR | relative risk or risk ratio |
| RRI | relative risk increase |
| RRR | relative risk reduction |
| sc | subcutaneously |
| SLE | systemic lupus erythematosis |
| SR | systematic review |
| SVT | supraventricular tachycardia |
| TB | tuberculosis |
| TIA | transient ischaemic attack |
| VF | ventricular fibrillation |
| VT | ventricular tachycardia |

# Index

# X